T0075317

KAPLAN & SADOCK'S POCKET HANDBOOK OF PSYCHIATRIC DRUG TREATMENT

EIGHTH EDITION

KAPLAN & SADOCK'S POCKET HANDBOOK OF PSYCHIATRIC DRUG TREATMENT

EIGHTH EDITION

SAMOON AHMAD, M.D.

Clinical Professor
Department of Psychiatry
NYU Grossman School of Medicine
New York, New York

Wolters Kluwer

Philadelphia • Baltimore • New York • London
Buenos Aires • Hong Kong • Sydney • Tokyo

Acquisitions Editor: Chris Teja
Development Editor: Ariel S. Winter
Editorial Coordinator: Sean Hanrahan
Editorial Assistant: Kristen Kardoly
Marketing Manager: Kirsten Watrud
Production Project Manager: Kirstin Johnson
Manager, Graphic Arts & Design: Stephen Druding
Manufacturing Coordinator: Beth Welsh/Lisa Bowling
Prepress Vendor: Aptara, Inc.

8th edition

Library of Congress Cataloging-in-Publication Data available upon request.

978-1-9751-6899-5

QUADM0423

Dedicated to
my parents Naseem and Riffat,
my wife Kim, and son Daniel

S.A.

Preface

I was in my residency when the first edition of *Pocket Handbook of Psychiatric Drug Treatment* was published. As a resident learning the complexities of psychopharmacology, it seemed like an overwhelming task, but this book was a blessing. It provided succinct and concise information that was practical and allowed me to make clinical pharmacologic decisions without delving into excessive details.

Upon completion of my residency, I was fortunate to work with my mentor Dr. Benjamin Sadock who inspired me to take an active role in contributing to various textbooks, including previous volumes of this work. Dr. Virginia Sadock, also a co-author in this series, has also been a mentor, friend, and a teacher who has been a constant source of encouragement. In addition, the late Dr. Norman Sussman, who was a co-author on the book and an amazing teacher, helped me learn to simplify the complexities of pharmacology and present it in a simple-to-read format. Over the years, I served as a contributing and consulting editor and am very fortunate to take on the challenge of being the sole author of the eighth edition of this book.

Goals of This Book

The current edition has been updated with new drugs as well as information about drug selection and use that reflects both research data and clinical experience. Since the last edition, numerous drugs have been given additional indications and this book has been revised to reflect those changes and to describe some of the common off-label uses for medications. As it is a common practice to use medications beyond FDA-approved indications, clinicians should be well-versed in the potential benefits of these off-label uses, as well as their associated risks. This information is presented in a simple and concise manner. The book format also provides charts on dosage and side effects in an easy-to-read format for the busy clinician.

Organization of This Book

I have attempted to keep the format similar to previous editions but made changes in the organization of information that the clinician would find easily accessible and practical. Moreover, the chapters have been reorganized so that they follow the same template whenever possible. As in the previous editions, the drugs are presented based on their pharmacologic category and mechanism of action rather than their indications wherever possible. The eighth edition also has some new additions in the form of visual aids and icons that will be helpful to find information readily.

New Additions to This Book

The eighth edition also contains some new chapters that may come as a surprise that I will briefly discuss.

Icons and Other Visual Aids

For added convenience, each chapter is color-coded and has a thumb tab to help clinicians quickly flip between chapters. Additionally, the adverse effects, drug–drug interactions, and cytochrome P450 interactions for each drug are more prominently labeled. In chapters that focus on just one drug, these icons appear at the very beginning of the chapter. In chapters that focus on multiple drugs, a chart will be included at the very start of the chapter with this information. The icons will then be included in the subsection within the chapter that focuses on the drug. My hope is that these icons will act as quick refreshers for clinicians requiring a mere glance.

Application of Schedule I Drugs

There is no doubt that the field of psychiatry is rapidly changing, and this may be a consequence of the limitations of achieving long-lasting or partial-to-poor therapeutic response with conventional treatments for numerous conditions. Consequently, in recent times, there has been a growing interest in treatments considered outside the domain of conventional psychopharmacology including psychedelics, cannabis, and other drugs. This edition for the first time has dedicated chapters to many of these substances that were once considered purely drugs of abuse. I have attempted to provide the reader with a simple guide to understanding how these drugs can be used in a clinical setting. In some cases, use of these drugs continues to be prohibited outside of research settings, but their application seems to be on the horizon.

Metabolic Disorders and Obesity

The interrelationship between psychiatric and metabolic disorders is well established. On the one hand, metabolic disorders are common comorbidities among psychiatric patients. On the other, use of psychotropic medications, particularly atypical antipsychotics, may contribute or lead to weight gain, as well as an increased risk of metabolic disorders. This edition has a dedicated chapter to understanding this complex relationship and provides guidance for screening, investigations, treatment strategies, and suggestions for managing these comorbidities. Clinicians are becoming more familiar with the use of drugs for obesity and the chapter on weight-loss drugs has been updated to reflect use of both FDA-approved as well as off-label medicines with associated risks.

Pharmacogenomics and Neuromodulation

Personalized medicine has been on the forefront of cutting-edge research for years, so a new chapter on pharmacogenomic testing has been added. For the first time, readers will also find a chapter on nondrug treatment approaches that focuses on neuromodulation and brain stimulation.

Purpose of This Series

As with previous editions of the *Pocket Handbook of Psychiatric Drug Treatment*, the purpose of this book is to be a quick and easy-to-navigate reference point for clinicians and to provide them with a concise description of the many drugs used in psychiatry. My hope is that the efforts to create a more uniform template for each chapter and to expand the number of treatments covered within this volume better serve this purpose and ultimately the clinician.

Acknowledgments

This book owes its very existence to my mentor and colleague Benjamin J. Sadock, M.D., Menas S. Gregory Professor of Psychiatry, NYU Grossman School of Medicine, who was the original author to take on this effort seven editions ago. His wisdom, guidance, graciousness, and friendship helped me become a better clinician, thinker, and writer—which in turn landed me this opportunity to step into his shoes as this edition's author. Ben and his wife Virginia—also a prior co-author—are my absolute role models and lifelong friends. I am profoundly honored and appreciative of the time we have spent together over the years.

Maryanne Badaracco, M.D., Director and Chief of Psychiatry, Bellevue Hospital, has been deeply supportive of my pursuit of academic excellence during my 30-year career at Bellevue. I additionally extend my gratitude to Charles Marmar, M.D., Peter H. Schub Professor and Chair of the Department of Psychiatry, NYU Grossman School of Medicine, for his leadership and encouragement.

Jay Fox, my research and editorial assistant, earns new stripes with all of our undertakings. I am extremely fortunate to have him as a wingman. Thank you, Jay.

Thanks to my publisher Wolters Kluwer for advancing highly relevant and important topics, and for their consistent support. Collaboration is at the foundation of any success, and for that, I owe special thanks to Chris Teja, Acquisitions Editor, for his measured tone and approach and for ensuring a seamless process.

Above all, my heartfelt thanks goes to my family. We have all pitched in to get through so much over the past few years. Without your trust in me, and your love, none of this would be possible.

Samoon Ahmad, M.D.
Clinical Professor, Department of Psychiatry
NYU Grossman School of Medicine
New York, New York

Contents

Table A
Index to Book by Generic Name of Drug

(continued)

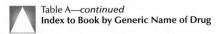

Table A—*continued*
Index to Book by Generic Name of Drug

(continued)

Table A—*continued*
Index to Book by Generic Name of Drug

(continued)

Table A—*continued*
Index to Book by Generic Name of Drug

(continued)

Table A—*continued*
Index to Book by Generic Name of Drug

(continued)

Table A—*continued*
Index to Book by Generic Name of Drug

(continued)

Table A—*continued*
Index to Book by Generic Name of Drug

(continued)

Table A—*continued*
Index to Book by Generic Name of Drug

(continued)

Table A—*continued*
Index to Book by Generic Name of Drug

General Principles of Psychopharmacology

1

Introduction

Historically, psychopharmacology is considered purely in the biologic realm. Treatment of psychiatric disorders requires more than one approach and eliminating the concept of how to implement psychopharmacology in conjunction with other modalities would be a disservice to our patients. I propose that the concept of psychodynamic psychopharmacology can overcome this barrier and even help our patients understand the complexity of psychopharmacologic principles.

This concept has become more relevant since numerous medicines in our armamentarium are U.S. Food and Drug Administration (FDA) approved for more than one disorder and are often used off-label for a host of other conditions. Explaining these complex scientific matters, including FDA-approved versus off-label use, requires a skillful psychodynamic approach, especially with patients who are weary of long-term side effects, dependence, and withdrawal symptoms, and may be particularly apprehensive about the use of these medicines beyond their approved indications.

Considering the above facts, it is evident that every clinician should know the basic principles of psychopharmacology, including pharmacodynamics and pharmacokinetics, and be able to explain these complicated facts to the patient in simple terms. As psychopharmacology has progressed, so has our understanding of the complexity of receptor profiles and drug interactions. This is especially important today as it is becoming more acceptable to use drugs that were once considered a taboo and purely recreational with no approved medical indications. The most notable example is cannabis, whether it contains the intoxicant delta-9 tetrahydrocannabinol (THC) or solely the nonintoxicating cannabidiol (CBD). However, stigmas are dissipating with respect to many drugs that were once considered to be not only illicit but extremely dangerous. The use of lysergic acid diethylamide (LSD), psilocybin, 3,4-methylenedioxymethamphetamine (MDMA), ketamine, and host of others are being researched for various medical and psychiatric conditions. Many patients are already using them on their own for treatment of chronic pain, sleep disorders, and many other conditions. CBD products are openly available on the market.

While taboos about the use of these drugs may be fading, they do still pose dangers when used without supervision and many of them can interact with various psychotropic drugs and cause adverse events without proper dose adjustments. This is especially relevant with CBD, which may impact the liver's cytochrome P450 (CYP) enzyme system and require close monitoring of liver function. Understanding these important new developments and being able to translate this information to our patients is not only medically necessary but vital to their well-being.

This chapter will address these basic principles of psychopharmacology as well as encompass some of the newer concepts like pharmacogenetic testing and its relevance to clinical practice. It also includes section on drug approval and regulatory process, as well as use in special populations.

Historically, psychiatric drugs have been categorized into four main classes.

1. Antipsychotic drugs or neuroleptics used to treat psychosis
2. Antidepressant drugs used to treat depression
3. Antimanic drugs or mood stabilizers used to treat bipolar disorder
4. Antianxiety drugs or anxiolytics used to treat anxious states (which are also effective as hypnotics in high dosages)

This categoric classification is problematic for the following reasons.

Today, most psychiatric drugs have numerous indications and are used to treat a variety of disorders. Furthermore, many nonpsychiatric drugs are now used to treat a host of psychiatric conditions. For example, propranolol is often used to treat social anxiety disorder, while prazosin has been shown to be effective in treating nightmares in post-traumatic stress disorder (PTSD). Listed below are some other reasons that further complicate this classification method.

1. Drugs introduced as treatments for schizophrenia, agents such as the second-generation antipsychotics (SGAs), are also indicated for the management of bipolar and depressive disorders.
2. Drugs from all four categories are used to treat symptoms and disorders such as insomnia, eating disorders, behavioral disturbances associated with dementia, and impulse-control disorders.
3. Drugs such as clonidine (Catapres), propranolol (Inderal), verapamil (Isoptin), modafinil (Provigil), and gabapentin (Neurontin) can effectively treat a variety of psychiatric disorders and do not fit easily into the traditional classification of drugs.
4. Some descriptive psychopharmacologic terms are arbitrary and overlap in meaning. For example, anxiolytics decrease anxiety, sedatives produce a calming or relaxing effect, and hypnotics produce sleep. However, most anxiolytics function as sedatives and at high doses can be used as hypnotics, and all hypnotics at low doses can be used for daytime sedation.

Classification

In recent times, the definition of psychotropic drugs has evolved and instead of describing them by their clinical indication, the better approach has been to classify them based on mechanism of action. This is a fundamental shift in psychiatric thinking. It is also preferable to think of drugs in terms of their pharmacologic actions rather than their therapeutic indications, as these often change and overlap. However, despite these concerns, most clinicians tend to adhere to the older classification. Therefore, this book uses the classification in which each drug is discussed according to its pharmacologic category. Each drug is described in terms of its pharmacologic actions, including pharmacodynamics and pharmacokinetics. Indications, contraindications, drug–drug interactions, and adverse side effects are also discussed.

Table A (see p. xii) lists each psychotherapeutic drug according to its generic name, trade name, and chapter title and number in which it is discussed.

Pharmacologic Actions

The main determinants of the clinical effects of a drug on an individual are determined by its pharmacokinetic and pharmacodynamic properties. In simple terms, pharmacokinetics describes *what the body does to the drug,* and pharmacodynamics describes *what the drug does to the body.* Pharmacokinetic data trace the *absorption, distribution, metabolism,* and *excretion* of the drug in the body. Pharmacodynamic data measure the *effects* of the drug on cells in the brain and other tissues of the body.

Pharmacokinetics

Absorption. Drugs reach the brain through the bloodstream. Orally administered drugs dissolve in the fluid of the gastrointestinal (GI) tract—depending on their lipid solubility and the GI tract's local pH, motility, and surface area—and are then absorbed into the blood.

Stomach acidity may be reduced by proton pump inhibitors, such as omeprazole (Prilosec), esomeprazole (Nexium), and lansoprazole (Prevacid); by histamine H_2 receptor blockers, such as cimetidine (Tagamet), famotidine (Pepcid), nizatidine (Axid), and ranitidine (Zantac); or by antacids. Gastric and intestinal motility may be either slowed by anticholinergic drugs or increased by dopamine receptor antagonists (DRAs), such as metoclopramide (Reglan). Food can also increase or decrease the rate and degree of drug absorption.

As a rule, parenteral administration can achieve therapeutic plasma concentrations more rapidly than can oral administration. However, some drugs are deliberately emulsified in an insoluble carrier matrix for intramuscular (IM) administration, which results in the drug's gradual release over several weeks. These formulations are called *depot* preparations. Intravenous (IV) administration is the quickest route for achieving therapeutic blood concentrations, but it also carries the highest risk of sudden and life-threatening adverse effects.

Distribution and Bioavailability. Drugs that circulate bound to plasma proteins are called *protein bound,* and those that circulate unbound are called *free.* Only the free fraction can pass through the blood–brain barrier.

The *distribution* of a drug to the brain is governed by the brain's regional blood flow, the blood–brain barrier, and the drug's affinity with its receptors in the brain. High cerebral blood flow, high lipid solubility, and high receptor affinity promote the therapeutic actions of the drug.

A drug's *volume of distribution* is a measure of the apparent space in the body available to contain the drug, which can vary with age, sex, adipose tissue content, and disease state. A drug that is very lipid soluble, such as diazepam (Valium), and thus is extensively distributed in adipose tissue, may have a short duration of clinical activity despite a very long elimination half-life.

Bioavailability refers to the fraction of the total amount of administered drug that can subsequently be recovered from the bloodstream. Bioavailability is an important variable because the FDA regulations specify that the bioavailability of a generic formulation can differ from that of the brand-name formulation by no more than 30%.

Metabolism and Excretion

Metabolic Routes.   The four major metabolic routes for drugs are *oxidation, reduction, hydrolysis,* and *conjugation.* Metabolism usually yields inactive metabolites that are readily excreted. However, metabolism also transforms many inactive prodrugs into therapeutically active metabolites.

The liver is the principal site of *metabolism,* and bile, feces, and urine are the major routes of *excretion.* Psychotherapeutic drugs can also be excreted in sweat, saliva, tears, and breast milk.

Quantification of Metabolism and Excretion.   Four important parameters regarding metabolism and excretion are time of *peak plasma concentration, half-life, first-pass effect,* and *clearance.*

The time between the administration of a drug and the appearance of *peak plasma concentrations* varies according to the route of administration and rate of absorption.

A drug's *half-life* is the amount of time it takes for metabolism and excretion to reduce a particular plasma concentration by half. This is not the same as duration of action. The clinical effects of a drug may persist long after a drug has been cleared from the body. A drug administered steadily at time intervals shorter than its half-life will reach 97% of its steady-state plasma concentration after five half-lives.

The *first-pass effect* refers to the initial metabolism of orally administered drugs within the portal circulation of the liver and is described as the fraction of absorbed drug reaching the systemic circulation unmetabolized.

Clearance is a measure of the amount of the drug excreted from the body in a specific period of time.

Pharmacogenomic Testing.   Pharmacogenomics can lead to a better understanding of how our genes influence the response to pharmacologic treatments. Such individualized approach can lower the patient's risk of side effects and consequently lead to better compliance and improved odds of treatment response.

Several companies now offer pharmacogenetic testing, though psychiatrists have not yet incorporated this into regular practice. This is due to a knowledge gap among clinicians, absence of recommendation by the FDA, and lack of endorsement by many expert panels. In addition, many insurance companies which were initially hesitant to cover the cost of testing are now willing to entertain reimbursement. It is imperative that clinicians begin to understand the pharmacogenomic principles and their clinical applications and to incorporate their use in their clinical practice when necessary.

There are numerous sets of genes responsible and in theory, pharmacodynamic gene testing of the serotonin transporter (SLC6A4) may help predict response and adverse effects of selective serotonin reuptake inhibitor (SSRI) and serotonin–norepinephrine reuptake inhibitor (SNRI) antidepressants. Mutation affecting another serotonin receptor, 2C ($5\text{-}HT_{2C}$), may predict weight gain with atypical antipsychotics. The pharmacokinetic genes (discussed below) affecting specific CYP450 enzymes (CYP1A2, CYP2B6, CYP2C9, CYP2C19, CYP2D6, CYP3A4/5) may predict rate of metabolism of medications and predict dose adjustment. Despite the limitations and clinical utility of pharmacogenomic testing, psychiatrists should familiarize themselves with genetic terminology, genes, and alleles affecting various psychotropic medications as well as understand metabolizing factors that may impact the use of psychotropic medicines and inform the patients about potential issues and individualizing treatment choices. For more details on this subject, see *Chapter 43: Pharmacogenomic Testing.*

Drug Selection. Although all FDA-approved psychotropics are similar in overall effectiveness for their indicated disorder, they differ considerably in their pharmacology and in their efficacy and adverse effects on individual patients. The ability of a drug to prove effective, thus, is only partially predictable and is dependent on often poorly understood patient variables. Nevertheless, it is possible that some drugs have a niche in which they can be uniquely helpful for a subgroup of patients without demonstrating any overall superiority in efficacy. No drug is universally effective, and no evidence indicates the unambiguous superiority of any single agent as a treatment for any major psychiatric disorders. The only exception, clozapine (Clozaril), has been approved by the FDA as a treatment for cases of treatment-refractory schizophrenia.

Cytochrome P450 Enzymes. The CYP enzyme system is responsible for the inactivation of most psychotherapeutic drugs. It is so named because the heme-containing enzymes strongly absorb light at a wavelength of 450 nm. Although present throughout the body, these enzymes act primarily in the endoplasmic reticulum of the hepatocytes and the cells of the intestine. Therefore, cellular pathophysiology, such as that caused by viral hepatitis or cirrhosis, may affect the efficiency of drug metabolism by the CYP enzymes.

The human CYP enzymes comprise several distinct families and subfamilies. In the CYP nomenclature, the family is denoted by a numeral, the subfamily by a capital letter, and the individual member of the subfamily by a second numeral (c.g., 2D6). Persons with genetic polymorphisms in the CYP genes that encode inefficient versions of CYP enzymes are considered *poor metabolizers.*

There are two mechanistic processes involving the CYP system: induction and inhibition (Table 1-1).

TABLE 1-1: Comparison of Metabolic Inhibition and Metabolic Induction		
	Inhibition	Induction
Mechanism	Direct chemical effect on existing enzyme	Increased synthesis of metabolizing enzyme
Immediate exposure needed	Yes	No
Prior exposure needed	No	Yes
Rate of onset	Rapid	Slow
Rate of offset	Rapid	Slow
In vitro study	Straightforward (cell homogenates)	Difficult (requires intact cells in culture)

Induction.   Expression of the CYP genes may be induced by alcohol, certain drugs (barbiturates, anticonvulsants), or smoking. For example, an inducer of CYP3A4, such as cimetidine, may increase the metabolism and decrease the plasma concentrations of a substrate of 3A4, such as alprazolam (Xanax).

Inhibition.   Certain drugs are not substrates for a particular enzyme but may nonetheless indirectly inhibit the enzyme and slow its metabolism of other drug substrates. For example, concurrent administration of a CYP2D6 inhibitor, such as fluoxetine (Prozac), may inhibit the metabolism and thus raise the plasma concentrations of CYP2D6 substrates, including amitriptyline (Elavil). If one CYP enzyme is inhibited, then its substrate accumulates until it is metabolized by an alternate CYP enzyme. Table 1-2 lists representative psychotropic drug substrates of human CYPs along with representative inhibitors. The Indiana University School of Medicine has produced a far more exhaustive table that includes a commonly prescribed and used drugs that interact with CYP substrates (see website https://drug-interactions.medicine.iu.edu/MainTable.aspx).

TABLE 1-2: Representative Psychotropic Drug Substrates of Human Cytochrome P450s Along with Representative Inhibitors

CYP3A	CYP2D6	CYP2C19
Substrates	Substrates	Substrates
Triazolam (Halcion)	Desipramine (Norpramin)	Diazepam[a]
Alprazolam (Xanax)	Nortriptyline (Aventyl)	Amitriptyline[a]
Midazolam (Versed)	Paroxetine (Paxil)	Citalopram[a]
Quetiapine (Seroquel)	Venlafaxine (Effexor)	Inhibitors
Nefazodone (Serzone)	Tramadol (Ultram)	Fluvoxamine
Buspirone (BuSpar)	Fluoxetine[a] (Prozac)	Omeprazole (Prilosec)
Trazodone (Desyrel)	Citalopram[a]	
Ramelteon (Rozerem)	Inhibitors	
Zolpidem[a] (Ambien)	Quinidine (Cardioquin)	
Amitriptyline[a] (Endep)	Fluoxetine	
Imipramine[a] (Tofranil)	Paroxetine	
Haloperidol[a] (Haldol)	Bupropion (Wellbutrin, Zyban)	
Citalopram[a] (Celexa)	Terbinafine (Lamisil)	
Clozapine[a] (Clozaril)	Diphenhydramine (Benadryl)	
Diazepam[a] (Valium)		
Inhibitors		
Ritonavir (Norvir)		
Ketoconazole (Nizoral)		
Itraconazole (Sporanox)		
Nefazodone		
Fluvoxamine (Luvox)		
Erythromycin (E-Mycin)		
Clarithromycin (Biaxin)		

[a]Partial substrate.

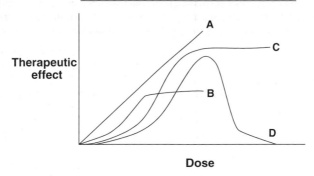

Examples of Dose–Response Curves

FIGURE 1-1 The dosage–response curves plot the therapeutic effect as a function of increasing dose, often calculated as the log of the dose. Drug A has a linear dosage response, drugs B and C have sigmoidal curves, and drug D has a curvilinear dosage–response curve. Although smaller doses of drug B are more potent than are equal doses of drug C, drug C has a higher maximum efficacy than does drug B. Drug D has a therapeutic window such that both low and high doses are less effective than midrange doses.

Pharmacodynamics

The major pharmacodynamic considerations include *molecular site of action*; the *dose–response curve*; the therapeutic index; and the development of tolerance, dependence, and withdrawal symptoms.

Molecular Site of Action. Psychotropic drugs may act at any of several molecular sites in brain cells. Some activate (agonists) or inactivate (antagonists) receptors for a specific neurotransmitter. Other drugs, particularly antidepressant drugs, bind to and block transporters that normally take up serotonin or norepinephrine from the synaptic cleft into the presynaptic nerve ending (reuptake inhibitors).

Some drugs block the passage of cations or anions through ion channels embedded in cellular membranes (channel inhibitors or blockers). Other drugs bind to and inhibit catabolic enzymes that normally inactivate neurotransmitters, thereby prolonging the life span of the active neurotransmitters (e.g., monoamine oxidase inhibitors [MAOIs]). Finally, several drugs have numerous molecular sites of action, although the sites that are therapeutically relevant may remain unknown.

Dose–Response Curves. The dosage–response curve plots the clinical response to the drug as a function of drug concentration (Fig. 1-1). *Potency* refers to comparisons of the dosages of different drugs required to achieve a certain effect. For example, haloperidol (Haldol) is more potent than chlorpromazine (Thorazine) because about 2 mg of haloperidol is required to achieve the same therapeutic effect as 100 mg of chlorpromazine. However, haloperidol and chlorpromazine are equal in their *clinical efficacy*—that is, the maximum achievable clinical response.

Therapeutic Index.   The *therapeutic index* is a relative measure of a drug's toxicity or safety. It is defined as the ratio of the median toxic dosage (TD_{50})—the dosage at which 50% of persons experience toxic effects—to the median effective dosage (ED_{50})—the dosage at which 50% of persons experience therapeutic effects. For example, haloperidol has a high therapeutic index, as evidenced by the wide range of dosages in which it is prescribed without monitoring of plasma concentrations. Conversely, lithium (Eskalith, Lithobid, and Lithonate) has a low therapeutic index, thereby requiring the close monitoring of plasma concentrations to avoid toxicity.

Persons exhibit both interindividual and intraindividual variation in their responses to a specific drug. An individual may be hyporeactive, normally reactive, or hyperreactive to a particular drug. For example, whereas some persons require 50 mg a day of sertraline (Zoloft), other persons require 200 mg a day for control of their symptoms. An unpredictable, non–dosage-related drug response is called *idiosyncratic*. For example, diazepam administered as a sedative paradoxically causes agitation in some persons.

Tolerance, Dependence, and Withdrawal Symptoms.   A person who becomes less responsive to a particular drug over time is said to develop *tolerance* to the effects of the drug. The development of tolerance can be associated with the appearance of physical *dependence,* which is the necessity to continue administering the drug to prevent the appearance of *withdrawal symptoms* (also called discontinuation syndrome).

Drug Interactions

Drug interactions may be either pharmacokinetic or pharmacodynamic, and they vary greatly in their potential to cause serious problems. Pharmacokinetic drug interactions concern the effects of drugs on their respective plasma concentrations, and pharmacodynamic drug interactions concern the effects of drugs on their respective receptor activities.

Pharmacodynamic drug–drug interactions causing additive biochemical changes may trigger toxic adverse effects. For example, MAOIs when co-administered with either tricyclic antidepressants or SSRIs, may precipitate a serotonin syndrome in which serotonin is metabolized slowly and thus accumulates in excessive concentrations. The interaction of disulfiram (Antabuse) and alcohol is another example of toxicity caused by pharmacodynamic drug interactions.

Some clinically important drug interactions are well studied and well proven; other interactions are well documented but have only modest effects; and still, other interactions are true but unproven, although reasonably plausible. Clinicians must remember that (1) animal pharmacokinetic data are not always readily generalizable to humans; (2) in vitro data do not necessarily replicate the results obtained under in vivo conditions; (3) single-case reports can contain misleading information; and (4) studies of acute conditions should not be uncritically regarded as relevant to chronic, steady-state conditions.

An additional consideration is one of phantom drug interactions. The person may be taking only drug A and then later receive both drug A and drug B. The clinician may then notice some effect and attribute it to the induction of metabolism. In fact, what may have occurred is that the person was more compliant at one point in the observation period than in another or there may have been some other effect of which the clinician was unaware. The clinical literature may contain reports of phantom drug interactions that are rare or nonexistent.

Informed clinicians need to keep these considerations in mind and to focus on the clinically important interactions, not on the ones that may be mild, unproven, or entirely phantom. At the same time, clinicians should maintain an open and receptive attitude toward the possibility of pharmacokinetic and pharmacodynamic drug interactions.

Drug Selection

There is no psychotropic drug that is effective in all patients with a given diagnosis. The ability of a drug to prove effective is only partially predictable and depends on the properties of the drug and the biology of the patient. Decisions about drug selection and use are made on a case-by-case basis, relying on the individual judgment of the physician. There are three factors in drug selection: (1) the drug, (2) the patient, and (3) the expertise and judgment of the prescribing physician. Each of these components affects the probability of a successful outcome.

An often-overlooked consideration in drug selection involves possible long-term consequences of being on a particular drug. For example, when starting antidepressant treatment in a young woman, thought needs to be given to which drug would be less problematic should she become pregnant and need to remain on medication. Paroxetine (Paxil), as an example, carries a higher risk of birth defects and would not be the best choice of medication in this instance. Another reason that paroxetine would not be the most appropriate agent for this patient group is its more severe withdrawal syndrome, which would make it more difficult for a woman who wants to discontinue medication in order to become pregnant. Similarly, drugs such as ziprasidone (Geodon) or escitalopram (Lexapro) that can prolong the QT interval may be reasonable choices for a healthy adult with no congenital long QT interval, but may be problematic if that patient needs to be treated for a medical problem with other medications that prolong the QT interval. Thinking long term is important because many psychiatric disorders are chronic and involve treatment over extended periods.

Therapeutic Indications

A therapeutic indication is a psychiatric diagnosis, as defined in the 11th revision of the *International Statistical Classification of Diseases and Related Health Problems* (ICD-11) or the fifth edition text revision of the *Diagnostic and Statistical Manual of Mental Disorders* (DSM-5-TR), for which a specific drug ameliorates signs or symptoms. Drugs are approved on the basis of carefully designed large-scale clinical trials that prove the drug is safe and that clinical improvement is attributable to the drug and not to the placebo. The FDA then grants a manufacturer the official right to advertise the drug as safe and effective for that therapeutic indication.

Clinicians must distinguish between official and unofficial therapeutic indications. This is necessary because many drugs are in fact safe and effective for treating not only those indications proven in FDA-scale trials but also for a much broader range of indications described in smaller trials.

Drug Approval Process in the United States

Under the Federal Food, Drug, and Cosmetic (FD&C) Act, initially passed in 1938 and subsequently heavily amended, the FDA has the authority to (1) control the initial availability of a drug by approving only those new drugs that demonstrate both safety and effectiveness and (2) ensure that the drug's proposed labeling is truthful and contains all pertinent information for the safe and effective use of that drug. An additional concentration of government regulation is directed by the Drug Enforcement Administration (DEA), which classifies drugs according to their abuse potential (Table 1-3). Clinicians are advised to exercise increased

TABLE 1-3: Characteristics of Drugs at Each DEA Level		
Schedule (Control Level)	Characteristics of Drug at Each Schedule	Examples of Drugs at Each Schedule
I	High abuse potential No accepted use in medical treatment in the United States at the present time; therefore, not for prescription use Can be used for research	LSD, heroin, marijuana, peyote, PCP, mescaline, psilocybin, nicocodeine, nicomorphine
II	High abuse potential Severe physical dependence liability Severe psychological dependence liability No refills; no telephone prescriptions	Amphetamine, opium, morphine, codeine, hydromorphone, phenmetrazine, amobarbital, secobarbital, pentobarbital, ketamine, methylphenidate
III	Abuse potential lower than levels I and II Moderate or low physical dependence liability High psychological liability Prescriptions must be rewritten after 6 months or five refills	Glutethimide, methyprylon, nalorphine, sulfonmethane, benzphetamine, phendimetrazine, chlorphentermine, compounds containing codeine, morphine, opium, hydrocodone, dihydrocodeine, diethylpropion, dronabinol
IV	Low abuse potential Limited physical dependence liability Limited psychological dependence liability Prescriptions must be rewritten after 6 months or five refills	Phenobarbital, benzodiazepines,[a] chloral hydrate, ethchlorvynol, ethinamate, meprobamate, paraldehyde
V	Lowest abuse potential of all controlled substances	Narcotic preparations containing limited amounts of nonnarcotic active medicinal ingredients

[a]In New York State, benzodiazepines are treated as schedule II substances, which require a triplicate prescription for a maximum of 3 months' supply.
DEA, Drug Enforcement Administration; LSD, lysergic acid diethylamide; PCP, phencyclidine.

TABLE 1-4: Phases of Drug Development
Nonclinical (Preclinical) Studies. Nonclinical studies that are sufficient to establish a tolerable dose and to identify the target organs of toxicity for a new drug must be conducted before first use of a new chemical entity in humans. A standard battery of animal studies and in vitro studies is required.
Phase I. Phase I studies represent the initial introduction of the new drug into humans. These studies, usually conducted in healthy volunteers, typically in closely monitored (often inpatient) settings, serve to characterize the absorption, distribution, metabolism, and excretion of the compound; to identify overt toxicities associated with drug administration; and to establish a tolerable dose for use in further studies.
Phase II. Phase II includes the initial controlled clinical efficacy studies. These studies typically include carefully selected patients with the disease or condition under study and are usually well controlled, closely monitored, and optimized for the collection of efficacy data. In phase II, exploratory work is undertaken to help determine the optimal doses of the drug.
Phase III. After preliminary evidence suggesting the effectiveness of the drug has been established in phase II trials, additional information about effectiveness and safety is needed to evaluate the overall risk–benefit relationship of the drug and to provide an adequate basis for product labeling. Phase III studies, expanded controlled and uncontrolled trials, provide this information.
Phase IV. After the drug has been approved, subsequent postmarketing activities may be conducted in phase IV. Studies to elucidate new indications or adverse effects and risks occur in this phase.

caution when prescribing controlled substances, especially drugs categorized as Schedule I or Schedule II.

In general, the FDA not only ensures that a new medication is safe and effective but also that a new medication compares favorably with existing agents used for the same indications. The new agent is usually not approvable unless it is at least equivalent in safety and efficacy to existing agents, if not superior. Table 1-4 summarizes the phases of research that lead to approval of a new drug.

Off-Label Uses

After a drug has been approved for commercial use, the clinician may, as part of the practice of medicine, lawfully prescribe a different dosage for a person or otherwise vary the conditions of use from what is approved in the package labeling without notifying the FDA or obtaining its approval. In other words, the FD&C Act does not limit the manner in which a clinician may use an approved drug.

However, although clinicians may treat persons with an approved drug for unapproved purposes—that is, for indications not included on the drug's official labeling—without violating the FD&C Act, this practice exposes the clinician to increased risk for medical malpractice liability. This is a significant concern because the failure to follow the FDA-approved label may create an inference that the clinician is varying from the prevailing standard of care. Clinicians may, however, prescribe medication for any reason they believe to be medically indicated for the welfare of the person. This clarification is important in view of the increasing regulation of clinicians by federal, state, and local governmental agencies. Appropriate documentation detailing the reason, risks, benefits, and patient consent is recommended.

Off-label drug use for treatment of mental disorders most frequently occurs when a patient has repeatedly failed to experience an adequate response to, or could not tolerate, standard therapies. A good example of recent off-label drug use involves utilization of drugs that are believed to act on the glutamate system. A growing body of evidence suggests that glutamate (glutamic acid), the most abundant excitatory neurotransmitter in the brain, is involved in the pathophysiology of several disorders. The most notable example of glutamate-modulating drug therapy is the use of ketamine infusions and an esketamine (Spravato) nasal spray to treat treatment-refractory depression. At this time, only the latter is indicated for use in treating treatment-resistant depression. Other glutamatergic drugs being used outside of their FDA-approved indication include riluzole (Rilutek) in cases of severe obsessive–compulsive disorder (OCD), topiramate (Topamax) for weight loss, pregabalin (Lyrica) for anxiety, and memantine (Namenda) for depression. With the exception of esketamine, the degree to which any of these drugs benefit a large number of patients in need of an unconventional pharmacologic intervention remains to be determined. With all of these drugs, symptom severity and a history of failure of conventional pharmacotherapy typically determine whether it is decided to use these agents.

When using a drug for an unapproved indication or in a dose outside the usual range, the clinician should document the reason for these treatment decisions in the person's chart. If a clinician is in doubt about a treatment plan, they should consult a colleague or suggest that the person under treatment obtain a second opinion.

Precautions and Adverse Effects

Overall, psychotropic drugs are remarkably safe, especially during short-term use. Only a few drugs—such as lithium, clozapine (Clozaril), valproic acid (Depakene), and carbamazepine (Tegretol)—require close laboratory monitoring. In addition, the FDA has established guidelines for use of second-generation antipsychotic agents. In addition to weight, waist circumference, and blood pressure monitoring, it also requires blood tests to monitor changes in blood glucose and lipid levels at regular intervals. Appropriate documentation of monitoring, testing, and interventions are recommended.

Precautions

Before use of a drug, it is important to be prepared to safely manage any expected adverse effects. Clinicians should be fully aware of any warnings and precautions in the product literature and should anticipate how to respond at least to the more common adverse effects listed.

Adverse Effects

Adverse effects are an unavoidable risk of medication treatment. Although it is impossible to have an encyclopedic knowledge of all possible adverse drug effects, prescribing clinicians should be familiar with the more common adverse effects as well as those with serious medical consequences. Even though the FDA requires that product information contain the results of clinical trials, many of the listed adverse effects are not actually causally associated with use of the drug, and it is common for adverse effects to be missed during clinical trials. It is thus important for clinicians to follow reports of treatment-associated adverse

TABLE 1-5: Potential Adverse Effects Caused by Blockade of Muscarinic Acetylcholine Receptors
Blurred vision
Constipation
Decreased salivation
Decreased sweating
Delayed or retrograde ejaculation
Delirium
Exacerbation of asthma (through decreased bronchial secretions)
Hyperthermia (through decreased sweating)
Memory problems
Narrow-angle glaucoma
Photophobia
Sinus tachycardia
Urinary retention

events during the postmarketing period. No single text or document, including the product information, contains a complete list of possible treatment emergent events.

It is always best to anticipate expected adverse effects, as well as rare but potentially problematic adverse effects, and to consider whether those effects will be unacceptable to the patient. For example, sexual dysfunction, weight gain, daytime sedation, sweating, nausea, and constipation may predictably cause some patients to discontinue treatment. It is thus important to discuss potential adverse effects with the patient and to determine if a problem with compliance is likely to arise. Persons generally have decreased trouble with adverse effects if they have been warned to expect them.

Drug adverse effects can largely be explained by their interactions with several neurotransmitter systems, both in the brain and in the peripheral nervous system. Older psychotherapeutic drugs, for example, commonly cause anticholinergic effects (Table 1-5) or bind to dopaminergic, histaminergic, and adrenergic receptors, resulting in the adverse effects listed in Table 1-6.

Newer agents tend to have either more specific neurotransmitter activity or combinations of effects that make them better tolerated than older agents. Nevertheless, some of the adverse effects of the newer agents remain problematic (Table 1-7), and in some cases—such as nausea, weight gain, and sexual dysfunction, all the result of serotonergic activity—these effects are more common than with the older drugs. It is usually not possible to predict which persons will not tolerate a serotonergic agent.

Treatment of Common Adverse Effects.   Psychotherapeutic drugs may cause a wide range of adverse effects. The management of a particular adverse effect is similar, regardless of which psychotherapeutic drug the person is taking. If

TABLE 1-6: Potential Adverse Effects of Psychotherapeutic Drugs and Associated Neurotransmitter Systems	
Antidopaminergic	Antihistaminergic
Endocrine dysfunction	Hypotension
Hyperprolactinemia	Sedation
Menstrual dysfunction	Weight gain
Sexual dysfunction	Multiple neurotransmitter systems
Movement disorders	Agranulocytosis (and other blood dyscrasias)
Akathisia	Allergic reactions
Dystonia	Anorexia
Parkinsonism	Cardiac conduction abnormalities
Tardive dyskinesia	Nausea and vomiting
Antiadrenergic (primarily α)	Seizures
Dizziness	
Postural hypotension	
Reflex tachycardia	

possible, another drug with similar benefits but fewer adverse effects should be used instead. In each drug section in this text, common adverse effects and their treatments are described in detail.

Sexual Dysfunction. Some degree of sexual dysfunction may occur with the use of many psychotropic drugs. This is by far the most common adverse effect associated with the use of SSRIs. About 50% to 80% of persons taking an SSRI report some sexual dysfunction, such as decreased libido, impaired ejaculation and erection, or inhibition of female orgasm.

As a rule, the best approach to pharmacologic management of sexual dysfunction involves either switching from the SSRI to mirtazapine (Remeron) or bupropion (Wellbutrin), as these drugs are unlikely to cause sexual dysfunction. If the use of an SSRI is deemed unavoidable, adding a prosexual agent such as bupropion may be enough to reverse the sexual inhibition caused by SSRIs. The best-tolerated and most potent prosexual drugs currently available are the phosphodiesterases (PDEs), such as sildenafil (Viagra), vardenafil (Levitra), and tadalafil (Cialis).

Anxiety, Akathisia, Agitation, and Insomnia. Many persons initiating treatment with serotonergic antidepressants (e.g., fluoxetine) experience an increase in psychomotor activation in the first 2 to 3 weeks of use. The agitating effects of SSRIs modestly increase the risk of acting out suicidal impulses in persons at risk for suicide. During the initial period of SSRI treatment, persons at risk for self-injury should maintain close contact with the clinician or should be hospitalized, depending on the clinician's assessment of the risk for suicide.

The insomnia and anxiety associated with use of serotonergic drugs can be counteracted by administration of a benzodiazepine or trazodone (Desyrel) for the first several weeks. If the agitation is extreme or persists beyond the initial 3-week period, another type of antidepressant drug, such as mirtazapine or a tricyclic agent, should be considered. Both typical and atypical antipsychotic medications are associated with movement disorders.

TABLE 1-7: Common Adverse Effects Associated with Newer Psychotropic Drugs

Movement disorders

First-generation antipsychotics (the DRAs) are the most common cause of medication-induced movement disorders. The introduction of SDAs has greatly reduced the incidence of these adverse effects, but varying degrees of dose-related parkinsonism, akathisia, and dystonia still occur. Risperidone (Risperdal) most closely resembles the older agents in terms of these adverse effects. Olanzapine (Zyprexa) also causes more EPS than clinical trials suggested. There have been rare reports of SSRI-induced movement disorders, ranging from akathisia to tardive dyskinesia.

Sexual dysfunction

The use of psychiatric drugs may be associated with sexual dysfunction—decreased libido, impaired ejaculation and erection, and inhibition of female orgasm. In clinical trials with the SSRIs, the extent of sexual adverse effects was grossly underestimated because data were based on spontaneous reports by patients. The rate of sexual dysfunction in the original fluoxetine (Prozac) product information, for example, was <5%. In subsequent studies in which information about sexual adverse effects was elicited by specific questions, the rate of SSRI-associated sexual dysfunction was found to be between 35% and 75%. In clinical practice, patients are not likely to report sexual dysfunction spontaneously to the physician, so it is important to ask about this adverse effect. In addition, some forms of sexual dysfunction may be related to the primary psychiatric disorder. Nevertheless, if sexual dysfunction emerges after pharmacotherapy has begun and the primary response to treatment has been positive, it may be worthwhile to attempt to treat the symptoms. Long lists of possible antidotes to these adverse effects have evolved, but few interventions are consistently effective, and few have more than anecdotal evidence to support their use. The clinician and patient should consider the possibility of sexual adverse effects with a patient when selecting a drug and switching treatment to another drug that is less or not at all associated with sexual dysfunction if this adverse effect is not acceptable to the patient.

Weight gain

Weight gain accompanies the use of many psychotropic drugs as a result of retained fluid, increased caloric intake, decreased exercise, or altered metabolism. Weight gain may also occur as a symptom of disorder, as in bulimia or atypical depression, or as a sign of recovery from an episode of illness. Treatment-emergent increase in body weight is a common reason for noncompliance with a drug regimen. No specific mechanisms have been identified as causing weight gain, and it appears that the histamine and serotonin systems mediate changes in weight associated with many drugs used to treat depression and psychosis. Metformin (Glucophage) has been reported to facilitate weight loss among patients whose weight gain is attributed to use of serotonin–dopamine reuptake inhibitors and valproic acid (Depakene). Valproate and olanzapine have been linked to the development of insulin resistance, which could induce appetite increase, with subsequent weight increase.

Weight gain is a noteworthy adverse effect of clozapine (Clozaril) and olanzapine. Genetic factors that regulate body weight, as well as the related problem of diabetes mellitus, seem to involve the 5-HT_{2C} receptor. There is a genetic polymorphism of the promoter region of this receptor, with significantly less weight gain in patients with the variant allele than in those without this allele. Drugs with a strong 5-HT_{2C} affinity would be expected to have a greater effect on body weight of patients with a polymorphism of the 5-HT_{2C} receptor promoter region.

Weight loss

Initial weight loss is associated with SSRI treatment but is usually transient, with most weight being regained within the first few months. Bupropion (Wellbutrin) has been shown to cause modest weight loss that is sustained. When combined with diet and lifestyle changes, bupropion can facilitate more significant weight loss. Topiramate (Topamax) and zonisamide (Zonegran), marketed as treatments for epilepsy, produce sometimes substantial, sustained loss of weight.

Glucose changes

Increased risk of glucose abnormalities, including diabetes mellitus, is associated with weight increase during psychotropic drug therapy. Data are not conclusive, but olanzapine is associated with more frequent reports than other SDAs of abnormalities in fasting glucose levels, as well as in reported cases of hyperosmolar diabetes and ketoacidosis.

(continued)

TABLE 1-7: Common Adverse Effects Associated with Newer Psychotropic Drugs *(continued)*

Hyponatremia

    Hyponatremia is associated with oxcarbazepine (Trileptal) and SSRI treatment, especially in elderly patients. Confusion, agitation, and lethargy are common symptoms.

Cognitive

    Cognitive impairment means a disturbance in the capacity to think. Some agents, such as the benzodiazepine agonists, are recognized as causes of cognitive impairment. However, other widely used psychotropics, such as the SSRIs, lamotrigine (Lamictal), gabapentin (Neurontin), lithium (Eskalith), TCAs, and bupropion, are also associated with varying degrees of memory impairment and word-finding difficulties. In contrast to the benzodiazepine-induced anterograde amnesia, these agents cause a more subtle type of absentmindedness. Drugs with anticholinergic properties are likely to worsen memory performance.

Sweating

    Severe perspiration unrelated to ambient temperature is associated with TCAs, SSRIs, and venlafaxine (Effexor). This adverse effect is often socially disabling. Attempts can be made to treat this adverse effect with α-agents, such as terazosin (Hytrin) and oxybutynin (Ditropan).

Cardiovascular

    Newer agents are less prone to having direct cardiac effects. Many older agents, such as TCAs and phenothiazines, affected blood pressure and cardiac conduction. The drug thioridazine (Mellaril), which has been in use for decades, has been shown to prolong the QTc interval in a dose-related manner and may increase the risk of sudden death by delaying ventricular repolarization and causing torsades de pointes. Newer drugs are now routinely scrutinized for evidence of cardiac effects. A promising treatment for psychosis, sertindole (Serlect), was not marketed because the FDA would have required a black box warning. Slight QTc effects noted with ziprasidone (Geodon) delayed the marketing of that drug. High-normal and high-dose olanzapine may cause prolongation of the PR interval and atrioventricular conduction delay.

    The management of specific adverse effects for individual drugs is covered in their respective chapters.

Rash

    Any medication is a potential source of a drug rash. Some psychotropics, such as carbamazepine (Tegretol) and lamotrigine, have been linked to an increased risk of serious exfoliative dermatitis, so patients should be informed about the seriousness of widespread lesions that occur above the neck and involve the mucous membranes. If such symptoms manifest, a patient should be instructed at the time the medication is prescribed to go immediately to an emergency department and not to first attempt to contact the prescribing psychiatrist.

BP, blood pressure; DRA, dopamine receptor antagonist; EPS, extrapyramidal side effects; FDA, Food and Drug Administration; 5-HT$_{2C}$, serotonin type 2C; QTc, quick test corrected for heart rate; SDA, serotonin–dopamine antagonist; SSRI, selective serotonin reuptake inhibitor; TCA, tricyclic antidepressant.

Gastrointestinal Upset and Diarrhea.   Most of the body's serotonin is synthesized in the GI tract, and serotonergic drugs, particularly sertraline (Zoloft), venlafaxine (Effexor), and fluvoxamine (Luvox), may therefore produce mildly to moderately severe stomach pain, nausea, and diarrhea, usually only for the first few weeks of therapy. Sertraline is most likely to cause loose stools, and fluvoxamine is most likely to cause nausea.

    These symptoms may be minimized by initiating treatment with a very small dosage and administering the drug after eating. Dietary alteration, such as the BRAT diet (*b*ananas, *r*ice, *a*pples, and *t*oast), may reduce loose stools. These symptoms usually abate over time, but some patients never accommodate and must switch to another drug.

Gastrointestinal Bleeding. Drugs that inhibit the serotonin reuptake transporter, most notably the SSRIs and SNRIs, are associated with increased tendency toward bleeding. Most commonly, this involves GI bleeding. Patients who are taking anticoagulant drugs or who use aspirin or nonsteroidal anti-inflammatory drugs are most at risk and should be monitored for this adverse effect, and those agents should be used only if needed.

Headache. A small fraction of persons initiating therapy with any psychotherapeutic drug may experience mildly to moderately severe headache. These headaches often respond to over-the-counter analgesics, but it may be necessary for some persons to switch to another medication.

Anorexia. SSRIs may produce a short-term suppression of appetite. The same is true of bupropion. In patients who are already dangerously underweight, these agents should be used with caution and treatment closely monitored. Fluoxetine (60 mg per day) in the context of a comprehensive program of behavioral management is an approved treatment for bulimia and is also useful for treatment of anorexia nervosa. Unless a comprehensive therapeutic program is available, SSRIs should be used cautiously by persons with eating disorders.

Weight Gain. Most commonly used drugs cause weight gain. The mechanisms can be as diverse as fluid retention, stimulation of appetite, or alteration in metabolism. Olanzapine (Zyprexa), clozapine (Clozaril), quetiapine (Geodon), and mirtazapine are associated with early, frequent, and sometimes extreme or persistent increases in body weight. SSRIs may be associated with more gradual or late-emergent weight gain that may be resistant to weight loss through diet and exercise. In these instances, some form of diet and exercise regimen should be attempted to salvage an otherwise effective treatment regimen. No drug has yet been shown to suppress the appetite safely in all persons though FDA has approved such drugs but should be used with caution, especially in patients with existing psychiatric disorders. These include bupropion–naltrexone (Contrave), phentermine–topiramate (Qsymia), liraglutide (Saxenda), and orlistat (Xenical). The most effective appetite suppressants, the amphetamines, are not used generally because of concerns about abuse. The off-label use of topiramate monotherapy in dosages of 25 to 200 mg daily, or zonisamide (Zonegran), 50 to 150 mg daily, may help to reverse drug-induced weight gain that results from increased caloric intake. Of note, cognitive problems should be monitored in case of topiramate usage with weekly dosage increment of no more than 25 mg.

Edema can be treated by elevating the affected body parts or by administering a diuretic. If the person adds a diuretic to a regimen of lithium or cardiac medications, the clinician must monitor blood concentrations, blood chemistries, and vital signs.

Orlistat (Xenical) does not suppress appetite; instead, it blocks absorption of fat from the intestine. Therefore, it reduces caloric intake from fatty foods but not from carbohydrates or proteins. Because orlistat causes retention of dietary fats in the intestines, it frequently causes excessive flatulence.

Somnolence. Many psychotropic drugs cause sedation. Some persons may self-medicate this adverse effect with caffeine, but this practice may worsen orthostatic hypotension.

It is important for the clinician to alert the patient to the possibility of sedation and to document that the person was advised not to drive or operate dangerous equipment if sedated by medications. Fortunately, some of the newer generations of antidepressant and antipsychotic drugs are much less likely to cause sedation than were their predecessors, and the newer drugs should be substituted for the sedating medications when possible. Modafinil (Provigil) can be added to counteract residual sedative effects of psychotropic drugs.

Dry Mouth.   Dry mouth is caused by the blockade of muscarinic acetylcholine receptors. When persons attempt to relieve the dry mouth by constantly sucking on sugar-containing hard candies, they increase their risk for dental cavities. They can avoid the problem by chewing sugarless gum or sucking on sugarless hard candies.

Some clinicians recommend the use of a 1% solution of pilocarpine (Salagen), a cholinergic agonist, as a mouthwash three times daily. Other clinicians suggest bethanechol tablets, another cholinergic agonist, 10 to 30 mg once or twice daily. It is best to start with 10 mg once a day and to increase the dose slowly. Adverse effects of cholinomimetic drugs, such as bethanechol, include tremor, diarrhea, abdominal cramps, and excessive eye watering.

Blurred Vision.   The blockade of muscarinic acetylcholine receptors causes mydriasis (pupillary dilation) and cycloplegia (ciliary muscle paresis), resulting in blurred vision. The symptom can be relieved by cholinomimetic eye drops. A 1% solution of pilocarpine can be prescribed as one drop, four times daily. Alternatively, bethanechol can be used as it is used for dry mouth. Topiramate, an anticonvulsant often used to treat drug-induced weight gain, can cause glaucoma and subsequent blindness. Patients should be informed to immediately report any change in vision when using topiramate.

Urinary Retention.   The anticholinergic activity of many psychotherapeutic drugs can lead to urinary hesitation, dribbling, urinary retention, and increased urinary tract infections. Elderly persons with prostatic enlargement are at increased risk for these adverse effects. Ten to 30 mg of bethanechol three to four times daily is usually effective in the treatment of the urologic adverse effects.

Constipation.   The anticholinergic activity of psychotherapeutic drugs can cause constipation. This is particularly concerning with clozapine which can cause paralytic ileus, a life-threatening condition and has specific guidelines for bowel monitoring and prophylactic use of stool softeners. The first line of treatment for psychotropic-induced constipation involves the prescribing of bulk laxatives, such as Citrucel, FiberCon, Konsyl, or Metamucil. If this treatment fails, cathartic laxatives, such as Milk of Magnesia, or other laxative preparations can be tried. Prolonged use of cathartic laxatives can result in a loss of their effectiveness. Bethanechol, 10 to 30 mg three to four times daily, can also be used.

Orthostatic Hypotension.   Orthostatic hypotension is caused by the blockade of α_1-adrenergic receptors. Elderly people are at particular risk for development of orthostatic hypotension. The risk of hip fractures from falls is significantly elevated in persons who are taking psychotherapeutic drugs.

Most simply, the person can be instructed to get up slowly and to sit down immediately if dizziness is experienced. Treatments for orthostatic hypotension include avoidance of caffeine, intake of at least 2 L of fluid per day, addition of salt to food (unless prescribed by a physician), reassessment of the dosages of any antihypertensive medications, and wearing support hose. Fludrocortisone (Florinef) is rarely needed.

Overdose.   An extreme adverse effect of drug treatment is an attempt by a person to commit suicide by overdosing on a psychotherapeutic drug. Clinicians should be aware of the risk and attempt to prescribe the safest possible drugs.

It is good clinical practice to write nonrefillable prescriptions for small quantities of drugs when suicide is a consideration. In extreme cases, an attempt should be made to verify that persons are taking the medication and not hoarding the pills for a later overdosage attempt. Persons may attempt suicide just as they are beginning to get better. Clinicians, therefore, should continue to be careful about prescribing large quantities of medication until the person has almost completely recovered, and such patients should be seen at least weekly.

Another consideration for clinicians is the possibility of an accidental overdose, particularly by children in the household. Persons should be advised to keep psychotherapeutic medications in a safe place.

Discontinuation (Withdrawal) Syndromes.   The transient emergence of mild symptoms upon discontinuation or reduction of dosage is associated with a number of drugs, including paroxetine (Paxil), venlafaxine (Effexor), duloxetine (Cymbalta), sertraline (Zoloft), fluvoxamine (Luvox), and the tricyclic and tetracyclic drugs. More severe discontinuation symptoms are associated with lithium (rebound mania), DRAs (tardive dyskinesias), and benzodiazepines (anxiety and insomnia).

Signs and symptoms of the discontinuation syndrome after SSRI use consist of agitation, nausea, disequilibrium, and dysphoria. The syndrome is more likely to occur if the plasma half-life of the agent is brief, if the drug is taken for at least 2 months, or if higher dosages are used and if the drug is stopped abruptly. The symptoms are time limited and can be minimized by a gradual reduction of the dosage.

Dosage and Clinical Guidelines

Diagnosis and the Identification of Target Symptoms

Treatment with psychotherapeutic drugs begins with formation of a therapeutic bond between the doctor and the person seeking treatment. The initial interview is devoted to defining the clinical problem as comprehensively as possible, with special attention paid to the identification of specific target symptoms whose improvement will indicate that the drug therapy is effective.

Medication History.   Past and present medication history discusses the use of all prescription, nonprescription, herbal, and illicit drugs ever taken, including caffeine, ethanol, cannabis, and nicotine; the sequence in which the drugs were used; the dosages used; the therapeutic effects; the adverse effects; details of any overdosages; and the reasons for discontinuing any drug.

Persons and their families are often ignorant about what drugs have been used before, in what dosages, and for how long. This ignorance may reflect the tendency of clinicians not to explain drug trials before writing prescriptions. Clinicians should provide written records of drug trials for each person to present to future caregivers.

A caveat to obtaining a history of drug response from persons is that because of their mental disorders, they may inaccurately report the effects of a previous drug trial. If possible, therefore, the persons' medical records should be obtained to confirm their reports.

Explaining Rationale, Risks, Benefits, and Treatment Alternatives

The use of psychotropic drugs should not be oversimplified into a one diagnosis–one pill approach. Many variables impinge on a person's psychological response to drug treatment. Some persons may view a drug as a panacea, and other persons may view a drug as an assault. Compliance with the dosing regimen is improved by providing a person with ample opportunities to ask questions at the time of prescribing, distributing written material that reinforces proper use of the medication, streamlining the medication regimen to the extent possible, and ensuring that office visits begin at the scheduled appointment time.

Choice of Drug

Previous Drug History.   A specific drug should be selected according to the patient's history of drug response (compliance, therapeutic response, and adverse effects), the person's family history of drug response, and the profile of adverse effects expected for that particular person. If a drug has previously been effective in treating a person or a family member, the same drug should be used again unless there is some specific reason not to use the drug.

Adverse Effect Profile.   Psychotropic drugs of a single class are equally efficacious but do differ in their adverse effect profile. A drug should be selected that is least likely to exacerbate any pre-existing disorders, whether medical or psychiatric, and that has probable adverse effects that are acceptable to the patient. Nevertheless, idiosyncratic reactions may occur.

Assessment of Outcome

Clinical improvements that occur during the course of drug treatment may not necessarily be related to the pharmacologic effects of the drug. For example, psychological distress often improves with the simple reassurances of a medical caregiver. Many disorders remit spontaneously, so "feeling better" may be the result of coincidence rather than medication. Therefore, it is important to identify unambiguously the nature and expected time course of clinical improvements caused by the pharmacologic effects of the medications.

In clinical practice, a person's subjective impression of a beneficial drug effect is the single most consistent indicator of future response to that drug. Assessments of clinical outcome in randomized, double-blind, placebo-controlled clinical trials rely on quantitative psychiatric rating scales, such as the Brief Psychiatric Rating Scale, Positive and Negative Syndrome Scale, Montgomery–Asberg Depression

Rating Scale, Hamilton Rating Scale for Depression, Hamilton Anxiety Rating Scale, or Global Assessment of Functioning Scale.

Therapeutic Trials.   A common question a patient typically asks is, "How long do I need to take the medication?" Patients can be given a reasonable explanation of the probabilities but told that it is best to first see if the medication works for them and whether the adverse effects are acceptable. Any more definitive discussion of duration of treatment can be held for when the degree of success is clear. Even patients with a philosophical aversion to the use of psychotropic drugs may elect to stay on medication indefinitely if the magnitude of improvement is great.

Treatment is conceptually broken down into three phases: the initial therapeutic trial, the continuation, and the maintenance phase. The initial period of treatment should last at least 4 to 6 weeks because of the delay in therapeutic effects that characterizes most classes of psychotropic drugs. The required duration of a "therapeutic trial" of a drug should be discussed at the outset of treatment so the patient does not have unrealistic expectations of an immediate improvement in symptoms. Unfortunately, patients are more likely to experience adverse effects in the course of pharmacotherapy earlier than any relief from their disorder. In some cases, medication may even exacerbate some symptoms. Patients should be counseled that a poor initial reaction to medication is not an indicator of the ultimate outcome of treatment. For instance, many patients with panic disorder develop jitteriness or an increase in panic attacks after starting on tricyclic or SSRI treatment. Benzodiazepine agonists are an exception to the rule that there is a delay in clinical onset. In most cases, their hypnotic and antianxiety effects are evident immediately.

Ongoing use of medication does not provide absolute protection against relapse. However, continuation therapy may provide significant protective effects against relapse.

Possible Reasons for Therapeutic Failures

The failure of a specific drug trial should prompt the clinician to consider a number of possibilities.

First, was the original diagnosis correct? This consideration should include the possibility of an undiagnosed coexisting disorder or illicit drug or alcohol abuse.

Second, did the person take the drug as directed?

Third, was the drug administered in sufficient dosage for an appropriate period of time? Persons can have varying drug absorption and metabolic rates for the same drug, and, if available, plasma drug concentrations should be obtained to assess this variable.

Fourth, did the drug's adverse effects produce signs and symptoms unrelated to the original disease? If so, did these effects counteract any therapeutic response? Antipsychotic drugs, for example, can produce akinesia, which resembles psychotic withdrawal; akathisia and neuroleptic malignant syndrome resemble increased psychotic agitation. SSRIs can produce fatigue, insomnia, and emotional blunting, symptoms that resemble manifestations of depression.

Fifth, did a pharmacokinetic or pharmacodynamic interaction with another drug the person was taking reduce the efficacy of the psychotherapeutic drug?

Regardless of optimal drug selection and use, some patients fail to respond to repeated trials of medication.

Poorly understood is the phenomenon of drug "poop out," in which patients who have been taking a drug for long periods of time, with good effect, suddenly have a return of symptoms. A number of possibilities have been suggested as causing loss of therapeutic effect. These include the following:

- Pharmacodynamic or pharmacokinetic tolerance (tachyphylaxis)
- Side effects (apathy, anhedonia, and emotional blunting)
- Onset of a comorbid medical disorder
- Increase in disease severity or change in disease pathogenesis (progression)
- Depletion of effector substance
- Serum drug levels that have drifted below or above that drug's therapeutic window
- Accumulation of detrimental metabolites
- Initial misdiagnosis
- Loss of placebo response
- Lack of bioequivalence when compared to a generic version

Strategies for Increasing Efficacy

The most fruitful initial strategy for increasing the efficacy of a psychotherapeutic drug is to review whether the drug is being taken correctly. A fresh clinical evaluation of the psychiatric symptoms and the rationale of the drug therapy is one of the psychopharmacologist's most valuable tools for revealing previously unappreciated impediments to drug efficacy.

Adding a drug with another indication is termed *augmentation*. Augmentation often entails use of a drug that is not primarily considered a psychotropic, though more recently many psychiatric drugs have been approved for augmentation. One example is the addition of atypical antipsychotic aripiprazole (Abilify) to an SSRI for treatment-resistant major depressive disorder. Moreover, it is common while treating depression to add thyroid hormone to an approved antidepressant.

In a typical scenario where augmentation may be deemed necessary, a patient has little or no response to a medication, so the physician adds a second agent to induce a better response. In some cases, the use of multiple medications is the rule. For example, almost all patients with bipolar disorder take more than one psychotropic agent. Combination treatment with drugs that treat depression has long been held as preferable in patients with psychotic depression. Similarly, SSRIs typically produce partial improvement in patients with OCD, so the addition of a serotonin–dopamine antagonist (SDA) may be helpful.

In addition, drugs may be combined to counteract side effects, to treat specific symptoms, and as a temporary measure to transition from one drug to another. It is common practice to add a new agent without the discontinuation of a prior drug, particularly when the first drug has provided partial benefit. This can be done as part of a plan to transition from an agent that is not producing a satisfactory response or as an attempt to maintain the patient on combined therapy.

One limitation of augmentation is increased noncompliance and adverse effects, and the clinician may not be able to determine whether it was the second drug alone or the combination of drugs that resulted in a therapeutic success or a particular adverse effect. Combining drugs can create a broad-spectrum effect and change the ratio of metabolites.

The merits of going to a single drug with a different pharmacologic profile include a lower risk of drug–drug interactions, simplicity, and lower cost. It is less burdensome to take one medication than two or three and is less likely to meet resistance from the patient. Many patients are ambivalent about taking even one medication, let alone two.

Combined Psychotherapy and Pharmacotherapy

Many patients are best treated with a combination of medication and psychotherapy. In many cases, the results of combined therapy are superior to those of either type of therapy alone. For example, pharmacotherapy alleviates the depression that often interferes with the introspection and focus that are needed for psychotherapy. Conversely, patients who are engaged in ongoing therapy are more likely to continue taking medication.

Duration of Treatment

Use of the Correct Dosage.   Subtherapeutic dosages and incomplete trials should not be prescribed solely to assuage the clinician's anxiety about the development of adverse effects. The prescription of drugs for mental disorders must be made by a knowledgeable practitioner and requires continuous clinical observation. Treatment response and the emergence of adverse effects must be monitored closely. The dosage of the drug must be adjusted accordingly, and appropriate treatments for emergent adverse effects must be instituted as quickly as possible.

Long-Term Maintenance Therapy.   Persons with mood, anxiety, and schizophrenic disorders live with an increased risk for relapse into illness at virtually any phase of their lives. Although some patients discontinue treatment because drugs are ineffective or poorly tolerated, many patients stop their medication because they are feeling well. This might be the result of effective treatment or simply naturally occurring remission. Clinicians should anticipate and alert persons to the natural variations of psychiatric illnesses. For example, a person who has taken medication to treat an acute psychotic episode may soon thereafter experience a relatively symptom-free period and may then impulsively discontinue taking the medication without informing their physician.

Long-term data show that persons who stop their medications after resolution of an acute episode of mental illness markedly increase their risk of relapse during the subsequent year compared with persons who remain on maintenance drug therapy. The fact is that most psychiatric disorders are chronic or recurrent. With disorders such as bipolar disorder, schizophrenia, or depression associated with suicide attempts, the consequences of relapse can be severe.

Treating clinicians are obliged to provide continuous educational review and reinforcement of the importance of taking medication. By comparing psychiatric illnesses with common chronic medical conditions, such as hypertension and diabetes mellitus, clinicians can help patients to understand that psychotropic drugs do not cure the disorders but rather keep their manifestations from causing distress or disability.

Special Populations

Children

Other than attention deficit hyperactivity disorder (ADHD) or irritability associated with autism spectrum disorder and OCD, commonly used psychotropic drugs have no labeling for pediatric use. When drugs are used to treat children and adolescents, results are extrapolated from adult studies. This should be done with caution. For example, the smaller volume of distribution suggests the use of lower dosages than in adults, but children's higher rate of metabolism indicates that higher ratios of milligrams of drug to kilograms of body weight might be required.

In practice, it is best to begin with a small dose and to increase it until clinical effects are observed. However, the clinician may use adult doses in children if they are effective and the adverse effects are acceptable.

Geriatric Patients

Cardiac rhythm disturbances, hypotension, cognitive disturbances, and falls are major concerns when treating geriatric persons. Elderly people may also metabolize drugs slowly (Table 1-8) and thus require low doses of medication. Another

TABLE 1-8: Pharmacokinetics and Aging

Phase	Change	Effect
Absorption	Gastric pH increases Decreased surface villi Decreased gastric motility and delayed gastric emptying Intestinal perfusion decreases	Absorption is slowed but just as complete
Distribution	Total body water and lean body mass decrease Increased total body fat, more marked in women than in men	Vd increases for lipid-soluble drugs, decreases for water-soluble drugs
	Albumin decreased, γ-globulin increased, α-1-acid glycoprotein unchanged	The free or unbound percentage of albumin-bound drugs increases
Metabolism	Renal: renal blood flow and glomerular filtration rates decrease Hepatic: decreased enzyme activity and perfusion	Decreased metabolism leads to prolonged half-lives, if Vd remains the same
Total body weight	Decreases	Think on an mg/kg basis
Receptor sensitivity	May increase	Increased effect

Vd, volume of distribution.
Reprinted with permission from the *Concise Guide to Somatic Therapies in Psychiatry*, Laurence.

concern is that geriatric persons often take other medications, thereby requiring clinicians to consider the possible drug interactions.

In practice, clinicians should begin treating geriatric persons with low doses, usually about one-half the usual dose. The dose should be raised in small amounts, more slowly than for middle-aged adults, until either a clinical benefit is achieved, or an unacceptable adverse effect presents itself. Although many geriatric persons require low doses of medication, many others require the usual adult dose.

Pregnant and Nursing Women

Physicians who are considering the use of psychotropic drugs during pregnancy should weigh known risks or the lack of available information against the risks of nontreatment. The basic rule is to avoid administering any drug to a woman who is pregnant (particularly during the first trimester) or who is breastfeeding a child, unless the mother's mental disorder is severe. In 2014, the FDA announced that it was replacing its previous classification system for safety of specific drug use during pregnancy. The new system removes the pregnancy letter categories A, B, C, D, and X, and combines sections pertaining to pregnancy and lactation. It is now required that drug labels be updated when information becomes outdated.

If a drug associated with the risk of birth defects needs to be used during pregnancy, the risks and benefits of the treatment, as well as therapeutic abortion, should be discussed. The most teratogenic psychotropic drugs are valproate (Depakote, Depakene); carbamazepine; and, to a lesser degree, lithium. Valproate exposure is associated with a significant risk of spina bifida and midline craniofacial abnormalities. Carbamazepine exposure is associated with similar midline defects. Prophylactic folic acid supplementation may reduce the risk of spina bifida. Lithium exposure during pregnancy is associated with a small risk of Ebstein anomaly, a serious congenital heart defect that can result in severe cardiac symptoms or even death.

The administration of psychotherapeutic drugs at or near delivery may cause neonatal sedation and respiratory depression, possibly requiring mechanical ventilatory support, or physical dependence on the drug, requiring detoxification and the treatment of a withdrawal syndrome.

Virtually all psychotropic drugs are secreted in the milk of nursing mothers.

Persons with Hepatic or Renal Insufficiency

Persons with hepatocellular insufficiency of any cause, including cirrhosis, hepatitis, metabolic disorders, and bile duct obstruction, are at risk of accumulating elevated concentrations of hepatically metabolized drugs. Drugs that are excreted by the kidneys may accumulate to toxic concentrations in persons with renal insufficiency of any cause, including atherosclerosis, nephrosis, nephritis, infiltrative disorders, and outflow obstruction. The presence of hepatocellular or renal insufficiency requires administration of a reduced dosage, usually half of the recommended dosage for healthy persons. Clinicians should be particularly alert to signs and symptoms of adverse drug effects in persons with hepatic or renal disorders. If available, monitoring of plasma drug concentrations may help guide dosage adjustments.

Persons with Other Medical Illnesses

Medical disorders should be ruled out as the cause of psychiatric symptoms. Considerations in the use of psychotropic drugs in medically ill persons include a potentially increased sensitivity to the drug's adverse effects, either increased or decreased metabolism and excretion of the drug, and interactions with other medications. As with children and geriatric persons, the most reasonable clinical practice is to begin with a low dose, increase it slowly, and watch for both clinical and adverse effects. Special caution is needed with potential drug–disease interactions. Patients with diabetes, for example, should not be routinely treated with drugs such as mirtazapine, clozapine, or olanzapine (Zyprexa), which risk causing weight gain, or drugs such as olanzapine or valproate, which cause insulin resistance. However, in case they are used, risks and benefits should be discussed and regular monitoring as well as coordination with the patient's physicians is necessary. Patients with seizure disorders should not receive bupropion, maprotiline (Ludiomil), or clomipramine (Anafranil), which lower the seizure threshold.

Laboratory Monitoring

It is recommended that prior to the use of any psychotropic drugs, baseline tests (Table 1-9) should be performed. Specific tests to monitor blood levels and metabolic parameters should be done on individual-based cases, depending on the class of drugs being utilized. However, serious complications of treatment with certain drugs can be prevented through laboratory monitoring of either plasma drug concentrations or laboratory indicators of organ dysfunction. Apart from drugs that require monitoring, laboratory testing and therapeutic blood monitoring should be based on clinical circumstances. Lithium and clozapine treatment requires ongoing monitoring. Given the increased use of antidepressant and atypical antipsychotic drugs in combination, it is prudent to obtain baseline and follow-up electrocardiography (EKG) studies. Further information on monitoring is found in the chapter in which each drug is discussed.

TABLE 1-9: Laboratory Monitoring Prior to Psychotropic Medication
Complete blood count
Liver function test
Electrolytes, glucose, and kidney function
Thyroid function tests
Lipid profile
HgA1c
Vitamin B12
Folate

α-Adrenergic Receptor Ligands

2

Generic Name	Trade Name	Adverse Effects	Drug Interactions	CYP Interactions
Clonidine	Catapres, Kapvay	Sedation, dizziness, GI symptoms, hypotension, insomnia	CNS, TRI	3A4
Guanfacine	Tenex, Intuniv	Sedation, dizziness, GI symptoms, hypotension, insomnia	CNS, TRI	2D6
Dexmedetomidine	Precedex, Igalmi	Sedation, dizziness, hypotension, cardiac arrhythmia	QT, CNS	2A6, 1A2, 2E1, 2D6, 2C19
Yohimbine	N/A	Agitation, cardiac arrhythmia, tremor, headache, dizziness, GI symptoms	Stimulants	2D6, 3A4
Prazosin	Minipress	Dizziness, sedation, GI symptoms	None	N/A

Introduction

This chapter covers alpha-2–adrenergic receptor agonists, including clonidine, guanfacine, and dexmedetomidine; the alpha-2–adrenergic receptor antagonist yohimbine; and the alpha-1–adrenergic receptor antagonist prazosin (see Table 2-1).

Adrenergic receptors are divided into alpha (α) and beta (β) receptors. α Receptors are further subdivided into α_1 (postsynaptic) and α_2 (pre and postsynaptic) receptors (see Table 2-2). They are again divided into subtypes α_{1A}, α_{1B}, and α_{1D}; and subtypes α_{2A}, α_{2B}, and α_{2C}. Beta receptors are divided into β_1, β_2, and β_3 subtypes. α_2-adrenergic receptors play an inhibitory role in the central and peripheral nervous systems and α_2-arenergic agonists have been used to treat numerous medical conditions such as opioid, benzodiazepine, and alcohol withdrawal;

TABLE 2-1: Ligands' Effects at Adrenergic Receptors	
Drug	Action
Clonidine	α-2–adrenergic receptor agonist
Guanfacine	Selective α-2A–adrenergic receptor agonist
Dexmedetomidine	α-2–adrenergic receptor agonist
Yohimbine	α-2–adrenergic receptor antagonist
Prazosin	α-1–adrenergic receptor antagonist

TABLE 2-2: Function of α_1-Adrenergic and α_2-Adrenergic Receptors			
Receptor Type	Systemic Function	Specific Tissue	Action
α_1-adrenergic receptor	Genitourinary stimulation, vasoconstriction, gland secretion, GI muscle relaxation, glycogenolysis	Heart	Ramps up contraction force
		Pilomotor smooth muscle	Stiffens hair
		Prostate	Contraction
		Pupillary dilator muscle	Contraction (dilation)
		Vascular smooth muscle	Contraction
α_2-adrenergic receptor	Decreased central sympathetic outflow	Adrenergic and cholinergic nerve terminals	Inhibits release of transmitters
		Fat cells	Lipolysis inhibition
		Platelets	Aggregation
		Postsynaptic neurons (CNS)	Multiple actions
		Vascular smooth muscle	Contraction

hypertension; panic disorder; and symptoms associated with posttraumatic stress disorder (PTSD) and attention deficit hyperactivity disorder (ADHD). Though modulators of these receptors are indicated for numerous medical conditions, this chapter will focus only on psychiatric indications.

α_2-Adrenergic Receptor Agonists

Clonidine (Catapres) is an α_2-adrenergic receptor agonist that affects plasma norepinephrine (inhibitory role) and other neurotransmitters. More recently, guanfacine (Tenex), another α_2-adrenergic receptor agonist, has been preferentially used because its differential affinity for certain α_2-adrenergic receptor subtypes results in less sedation and hypotension. Clonidine extended release (Kapvay) and guanfacine extended release (Intuniv) are approved by the Food and Drug Administration (FDA) for the treatment of ADHD as monotherapy and as adjunctive therapy to stimulant medication in children and adults. These agents are also used as adjuncts to stimulants to enhance therapeutic effects. In addition, clonidine is also used as a soporific in pediatric population considering its α_{2B} receptor activity.

Immediate-release clonidine and guanfacine are FDA approved only for the treatment of hypertension as monotherapy or in combination with other antihypertensive medications. These drugs have also been studied in and used to treat neurologic and psychiatric conditions, other than ADHD. These include Tourette syndrome (TS) and other tic disorders, opiate and alcohol withdrawal, and PTSD.

Dexmedetomidine is an α_2-adrenergic receptor agonist. A recent formulation sold under the trade name Igalmi and administered as a sublingual film was recently approved by the FDA to treat acute agitation associated with schizophrenia or bipolar I or II disorder.

Prazosin (Minipress) is an α_1-postsynaptic antagonist and sympatholytic. It reduces blood pressure (BP) through vasodilation. Prazosin has been used in treating sleep disorders associated with PTSD though recent studies suggest no additional advantage compared to placebo.

CLONIDINE AND GUANFACINE

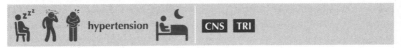

Pharmacologic Actions

Both clonidine and guanfacine are agonists on presynaptic α_2-adrenergic receptors and inhibit sympathetic outflow, causing vasodilation of blood vessels and lowering BP. The agonist effects of clonidine and guanfacine on presynaptic α_2-adrenergic receptors in the sympathetic nuclei of the brain result in a decrease in the amount of norepinephrine released from the presynaptic nerve terminals. This serves generally to reset the body's sympathetic tone at a lower level and decrease arousal. Guanfacine is more selective at α_{2A} with no α_{2B} activity and less potent than clonidine. Immediate-release clonidine and guanfacine are well absorbed from the gastrointestinal tract and reach peak plasma levels 1 to 3 hours after oral administration. The half-life of clonidine is 6 to 20 hours and that of guanfacine is 10 to 30 hours.

Therapeutic Indications

There is recent interest in the use of guanfacine for the same indications that respond to clonidine due to guanfacine's longer half-life and relative lack of sedative effects.

Withdrawal from Opioids, Alcohol, or Nicotine

Clonidine and guanfacine are effective in reducing the autonomic symptoms of rapid opioid withdrawal (e.g., hypertension, tachycardia, dilated pupils, sweating, lacrimation, and rhinorrhea) but not the associated subjective sensations. Clonidine administration (0.1 to 0.2 mg two to four times a day) is initiated before detoxification and is then tapered off over 1 to 2 weeks.

Clonidine and guanfacine can reduce symptoms of alcohol withdrawal, including anxiety, diarrhea, and tachycardia. Clonidine and guanfacine can reduce craving, anxiety, and the irritability symptoms of nicotine withdrawal. The transdermal patch formulation of clonidine is associated with better long-term compliance for the purpose of detoxification than the tablet formulation.

Tourette Disorder

Clonidine and guanfacine are effective drugs for the treatment of Tourette disorder. Most clinicians begin treatment for Tourette disorder with the standard dopamine receptor antagonists, such as haloperidol (Haldol) and serotonin–dopamine antagonists, such as risperidone (Risperdal) and olanzapine (Zyprexa). However, if concerned about the adverse effects of these drugs, the clinician may begin treatment with clonidine or guanfacine. The starting dose of clonidine for children is 0.05 mg a day; it can be increased to 0.3 mg a day in divided doses. Up to 3 months are needed before the beneficial effects of clonidine can be seen in patients with Tourette disorder. The response rate has been reported to be up to 70%.

α-Adrenergic Receptor Ligands

Other Tic Disorders

Clonidine and guanfacine reduce the frequency and severity of tics in persons with tic disorder with or without comorbid ADHD.

Hyperactivity and Aggression in Children

Clonidine and guanfacine can be useful alternatives for the treatment of ADHD. They are used in place of sympathomimetics and antidepressants, which may produce paradoxical worsening of hyperactivity in some children with intellectual disability, aggression, or features on the spectrum of autism. Clonidine and guanfacine can improve mood, reduce activity level, and improve social adaptation. Some impaired children may respond favorably to clonidine, but others may simply become sedated. The starting dose is 0.05 mg a day; it can be raised to 0.3 mg a day in divided doses. The efficacy of clonidine and guanfacine for control of hyperactivity and aggression often diminishes over several months of use.

Clonidine and guanfacine can be combined with methylphenidate (Ritalin) or dextroamphetamine (Dexedrine) to treat hyperactivity and inattentiveness, respectively. A small number of cases have been reported of sudden death of children taking clonidine together with methylphenidate; however, it has not been conclusively demonstrated that these medications contributed to these deaths. The clinician should explain to the family that the efficacy and safety of this combination have not been investigated in controlled trials. Periodic cardiovascular assessments, including vital signs and electrocardiograms, are warranted if this combination is used.

Posttraumatic Stress Disorder

Acute exacerbations of PTSD may be associated with hyperadrenergic symptoms such as hyperarousal, exaggerated startle response, insomnia, vivid nightmares, tachycardia, agitation, hypertension, and perspiration. Preliminary reports suggest that these symptoms may respond to the use of clonidine or, especially for overnight benefit, to the use of guanfacine. At this time studies are mixed and are yet to demonstrate that guanfacine and clonidine produce significant improvement in PTSD symptoms.

Precautions and Adverse Reactions

The most common adverse effects associated with clonidine are dry mouth and eyes, fatigue, sedation, dizziness, nausea, hypotension, and constipation, which result in discontinuation of therapy by about 10% of all persons taking the drug. Some persons also experience sexual dysfunction, which may include decreased libido or impotence in men. Tolerance may develop to these adverse effects. A similar but milder adverse profile is seen with guanfacine, especially in doses of 3 mg or more per day. Clonidine and guanfacine should not be taken by adults with BP below 90/60 mm Hg or with cardiac arrhythmias, especially bradycardia. Development of bradycardia warrants gradual, tapered discontinuation of the drug. Clonidine in particular is associated with sedation, and tolerance does not usually develop to this adverse effect. Uncommon central nervous system (CNS) adverse effects of clonidine include insomnia, anxiety, and depression; rare CNS adverse effects include vivid dreams, nightmares, and hallucinations. Fluid retention associated with clonidine treatment can be treated with diuretics.

The transdermal patch formulation of clonidine may cause local skin irritation, which can be minimized by rotating the sites of application.

Use in Pregnancy and Lactation

There are limited controlled data on clonidine in human pregnancy, so risk cannot be ruled out. It falls into pregnancy category C. The drug passes the placental barrier, possibly lowering the fetal heart rate. It should not be used while breast-feeding. Guanfacine, while not linked to any specific birth defects, is not well studied and should also be avoided during pregnancy and by nursing mothers. Guanfacine is a pregnancy category B drug.

Overdose

Persons who take an overdose of clonidine may present with coma and constricted pupils, symptoms similar to those of an opioid overdose. Other symptoms of overdose are decreased BP, pulse, and respiratory rate. Guanfacine overdose produces a milder version of these symptoms. Elderly persons are more sensitive to the drug than are younger adults. Children are susceptible to the same adverse effects as are adults.

Withdrawal

Abrupt discontinuation of clonidine can cause anxiety, restlessness, perspiration, tremor, abdominal pain, palpitations, headache, and a dramatic increase in BP. These symptoms may appear about 20 hours after the last dose, and these may be observed if one or two doses are skipped. A similar set of symptoms occasionally occurs 2 to 4 days after discontinuation of guanfacine, but the usual course is a gradual return to baseline BP over 2 to 4 days. Because of the possibility of discontinuation symptoms, dosages of clonidine and guanfacine should be tapered slowly.

Drug Interactions

Clonidine and guanfacine cause sedation, especially early in therapy, and when administered with other centrally active depressants, such as barbiturates, alcohol, and benzodiazepines, the potential for additive sedative effects should be considered. Dose reduction may be required in patients receiving agents that interfere with atrioventricular (AV) node and sinus node conduction such as β-blockers, calcium channel blockers, and digitalis. This combination increases the risk of AV block and bradycardia. Clonidine should not be given with tricyclic antidepressants, which can inhibit the hypotensive effects of clonidine.

Laboratory Interferences

No known laboratory interferences are associated with the use of clonidine or guanfacine.

Dosage and Clinical Guidelines

Clonidine is available in 0.1-, 0.2-, and 0.3-mg tablets, 0.1- and 0.2-mg extended-release tablets. The usual starting dosage for the immediate release is 0.1 mg

α-Adrenergic Receptor Ligands

orally twice a day; the dosage can be raised by 0.1 mg a day to an appropriate level (up to 1.2 mg/day). Clonidine must always be tapered when it is discontinued to avoid rebound hypertension, which may occur about 20 hours after the last clonidine dose. A weekly transdermal formulation of clonidine is available at doses of 0.1, 0.2, and 0.3 mg/day. The usual starting dosage is the 0.1-mg-a-day patch, which is changed each week for adults and every 5 days for children; the dose can be increased, as needed, every 1 to 2 weeks. Transition from the oral to the transdermal formulations should be accomplished gradually by overlapping them for 3 to 4 days.

Guanfacine is available in 1- and 2-mg tablets. The usual starting dose is 1 mg before sleep, and this can be increased to 2 mg before sleep after 3 to 4 weeks, if necessary. Regardless of the indication for which clonidine or guanfacine is being used, the drug should be withheld if a person becomes hypotensive (BP below 90/60 mm Hg).

Extended-release guanfacine should be dosed once daily. Tablets should not be crushed, chewed, or broken before swallowing because this will increase the rate of guanfacine release. It should not be administered with high-fat meals, due to increases in peak plasma levels. The extended-release formulation should not be substituted for immediate-release guanfacine tablets on an mg-per-mg basis, because of differing pharmacokinetic profiles. If switching from immediate-release guanfacine, discontinue that treatment, and titrate with extended-release guanfacine according to the following recommended schedule:

1. Begin at a dose of 1 mg/day and adjust in increments of no more than 1 mg/wk, for both monotherapy and adjunctive therapy to a psychostimulant.
2. Maintain the dose within the range of 1 mg to 4 mg once daily, depending on clinical response and tolerability, for both monotherapy and adjunctive therapy to a psychostimulant. In clinical trials, patients were randomized or dose optimized to doses of 1, 2, 3, or 4 mg and received extended-release guanfacine once daily in the morning in monotherapy trials and once daily in the morning or evening in the adjunctive therapy trial.
3. In monotherapy trials, clinically relevant improvements were observed beginning at doses in the range 0.05 to 0.08 mg/kg once daily. Efficacy increased with increasing weight-adjusted dose (mg/kg). If well tolerated, doses up to 0.12 mg/kg once daily may provide additional benefit. Doses above 4 mg/day have not been systematically studied in controlled clinical trials.
4. In the adjunctive trial, the majority of subjects reached optimal doses in the 0.05 to 0.12 mg/kg/day range.

In clinical trials, there were dose-related and exposure-related risks for several clinically significant adverse reactions (e.g., hypotension, bradycardia, sedative events). Thus, consideration should be given to dosing an extended-release preparation of guanfacine on an mg/kg basis in order to balance the exposure-related potential benefits and risks of treatment. The safety of clonidine in pregnancy is uncertain, and well-controlled studies of risks to the fetus do not exist. Studies of guanfacine in humans have shown no evidence of risk to the fetus.

DEXMEDETOMIDINE

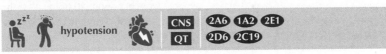

Dexmedetomidine (Precedex, Igalmi) is an α_2-adrenergic receptor agonist that has long been used to induce sedation prior to surgical procedures or intubation and was oftentimes used off-label to induce sedation in psychiatric patients.

Pharmacokinetics

Following sublingual or buccal administration, dexmedetomidine has a bioavailability of 72% and 82%, respectively, and an average protein binding of 94%. Mean maximal concentration is reached approximately 2 hours after administration. Dexmedetomidine is extensively metabolized, with very little of the parent compound be excreted unchanged in either urine or feces. Metabolization is primarily mediated via cytochrome P450 isoenzyme CYP2A6, with CYP1A2, CYP2E1, CYP2D6, and CYP2C19 playing minor roles. Mean terminal elimination half-life is 2.8 hours. Clearance values are lower in patients with hepatic impairment, but not significantly different in patients with renal impairment.

Indications

As of spring 2022, a formulation of dexmedetomidine marketed under the name Igalmi was approved by the FDA to treat acute agitation associated with schizophrenia or bipolar I or II disorder. Igalmi is administered as a sublingual or buccal film. The safety and effectiveness of Igalmi has not been established beyond 24 hours after the first dose.

Precautions and Adverse Effects

Adverse effects associated with dexmedetomidine include dose-dependent hypotension, bradycardia, and QT interval prolongation. Less serious side effects observed during clinical trials included somnolence, paresthesia or hypoesthesia oral, dizziness, dry mouth, nausea, and abdominal discomfort. Risk of bradycardia and/or hypotension is notably higher when a higher dosage than recommended is administered.

Dexmedetomidine should be used with caution in patients with hepatic impairment (see Dosage and Clinical Guidelines).

Pregnancy and Lactation

Dexmedetomidine is labeled a pregnancy category C drug. Adverse developmental effects were observed in animal models at doses less than or equal to the maximum recommended human dose. Available evidence suggests that dexmedetomidine may be excreted in human milk. Consequently, pregnant and nursing women should avoid the use of dexmedetomidine unless the benefits outweigh potential risks.

α-Adrenergic Receptor Ligands

Patient Population	Agitation Severity	Initial Dose (mcg)	Optional Second or Third Doses (mcg)	Maximum Recommended Total Daily Dosage (mcg)
Adult	Mild or moderate	120	60	240
	Severe	180	90	360
Patients with mild hepatic impairment	Mild or moderate	90	60	210
	Severe	120	60	240
Patients with severe hepatic impairment	Mild or moderate	60	60	180
	Severe	90	60	210
Patients ≥65 years of age	Mild, moderate, or severe	120	60	240

TABLE 2-3: Dosage Recommendation for Igalmi

Drug Interactions

Dexmedetomidine may prolong QT intervals, so other drugs that prolong QT intervals could increase the risk of cardiac arrhythmia. Concomitant use with sedatives, anesthetics, hypnotics, and opioids could lead to additive CNS depressant effects.

Laboratory Interferences

No known laboratory interferences are associated with dexmedetomidine use.

Dosage and Clinical Guidelines

Igalmi is the sole dexmedetomidine formulation indicated for psychiatric use. It is administered as a sublingual or buccal film and comes in strengths of 120 mcg and 180 mcg. Film strips can be cut in half with scissors to produce doses of 60 mcg and 90 mcg. Patients should place film under their tongue or behind lower lip, and then let it dissolve. Patients should not eat or drink for 1 hour after administration. For dosing guidelines, see Table 2-3.

α_2-Adrenergic Receptor Antagonists

YOHIMBINE

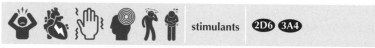 stimulants 2D6 3A4

Yohimbine is an α_2-adrenergic receptor antagonist that is available without a prescription as a nutritional supplement. It is derived from an alkaloid found in *Rubiaceae* and related trees and in the *Rauwolfia serpentina* plant. It has been studied and is promoted as a treatment for both idiopathic and medication-induced erectile disorder and as a "fat burner." There is not sufficient evidence supporting its effectiveness for either of these roles.

Precautions

The side effects of yohimbine include anxiety, elevated BP and heart rate, increased psychomotor activity, irritability, tremor, headache, skin flushing, dizziness, urinary frequency, nausea, vomiting, and sweating. Yohimbine should be used judiciously in psychiatric patients because it may have an adverse effect on their mental status. Patients with panic disorder show heightened sensitivity to yohimbine and experience increased anxiety, increased BP, and increased plasma 3-methoxy-4-hydroxyphenylglycol (MHPG).

Yohimbine should be used with caution in female patients and should not be used in patients with renal disease, cardiac disease, glaucoma, or a history of gastric or duodenal ulcer.

Pregnancy and Lactation

Yohimbine was never assigned to a pregnancy category under the old FDA classification system and animal studies have not been done. Due to the lack of controlled data, yohimbine should not be used during pregnancy and lactation.

Drug Interactions

Yohimbine blocks the effects of clonidine, guanfacine, and other α_2-receptor agonists.

Laboratory Interferences

No known laboratory interferences are associated with yohimbine use.

Dosage and Clinical Guidelines

Yohimbine is available in 5.4-mg tablets. The dosage of yohimbine when used in the treatment of erectile disorder is approximately 18 mg a day, given in dosages that range from 2.7 to 5.4 mg three times a day. In the event of significant adverse effects, dosage should first be reduced and then gradually increased again. Yohimbine should be used judiciously in psychiatric patients because it may have an adverse effect on their mental status.

Other α_2-Adrenergic Receptor Antagonists

Other α_2-adrenergic antagonists include mirtazapine (Remeron) and mianserin (Tolvon), which will be discussed in Chapters 25 and 37, respectively.

α_1-Adrenergic Receptor Antagonists

PRAZOSIN

Prazosin (Minipress) is a quinazoline derivative used as an antihypertensive. It is an α_1-adrenergic receptor antagonist as opposed to the drugs mentioned above, which are α_2-blockers.

Pharmacologic Actions

The exact mechanism of the hypotensive action of prazosin is unknown, particularly its suggested effects in nightmare suppression, though recent studies tend to refute the earlier analysis. Prazosin causes a decrease in total peripheral resistance that is related to its action as an α_1-adrenergic receptor antagonist. BP is lowered in both the supine and standing positions. This effect is most pronounced on the diastolic BP. After oral administration, human plasma concentrations reach a peak at about 3 hours with a plasma half-life of 2 to 3 hours. The drug is highly bound to plasma protein. Tolerance has not been observed to develop with long-term therapy.

Therapeutic Action

Prazosin is used in psychiatry to suppress nightmares, particularly those associated with PTSD. Of note, nightmares return when the drug is discontinued; and as mentioned above, its efficacy has been questioned in light of the recent studies.

Precautions and Adverse Reactions

During clinical trials and subsequent marketing experience, the most frequent reactions were dizziness, 10.3%; headache, 7.8%; drowsiness, 7.6%; lack of energy, 6.9%; weakness, 6.5%; palpitations, 5.3%; and nausea, 4.9%. In most instances, side effects disappeared with continued therapy or have been tolerated with no decrease in dose of drug.

Use in Pregnancy and Lactation

Prazosin should not be used in nursing mothers or during pregnancy.

Drug Interactions

No adverse drug interactions have been reported.

Laboratory Interferences

None reported.

Dosage and Clinical Guidelines

The drug is supplied in 1-, 2-, and 5-mg capsules and a nasal spray. The therapeutic dosages most commonly used have ranged from 6 to 15 mg daily, given in divided doses. Doses higher than 20 mg do not increase efficacy. When adding a diuretic or other antihypertensive agent, the dose should be reduced to 1 or 2 mg three times a day and retitration is then carried out. Concomitant use with a PDE-5 inhibitor can result in additive BP-lowering effects and symptomatic hypotension; therefore, PDE-5 inhibitor therapy should be initiated at the lowest dose in patients taking prazosin.

Table 2-4 provides a summary of α_2-adrenergic receptor agonists used in psychiatry.

TABLE 2-4: Other α_2-Adrenergic Receptor Agonists Used in Psychiatry[a]

Drug	Preparations	Usual Child Starting Dosage	Usual Child Dosage Range	Usual Adult Starting Dosage	Usual Adult Dosage
Clonidine tablets (Catapres)	0.1, 0.2, 0.3 mg	0.05 mg a day	Up to 0.3-mg-a-day tablets in divided doses	0.1–0.2 mg two to four times a day (0.2–0.8 mg a day)	0.3–1.2 mg a day two to three times a day (1.2 mg a day maximal dosage)
Clonidine transdermal system (Catapres-TTS)	0.1, 0.2, 0.3 mg/day	0.05 mg a day	Up to 0.3 mg a day patch every 5 days (0.5 mg a day every 5 days maximal dosage)	0.1 mg a day every 7 days	0.1 mg a day patch per week 0.6 mg a day every 7 days
Clonidine extended release (Kapvay)	0.1- and 0.2-mg tablets	0.1 mg a day	Up to 0.2 mg twice a day	0.1 mg twice a day	0.2 mg twice a day
Guanfacine (Tenex)	1- and 2-mg tablets	1 mg a day at bedtime	1–2 mg a day at bedtime (3 mg a day maximal dosage)	1 mg a day at bedtime	1–2 mg at bedtime (3 mg a day maximal dosage)
Guanfacine extended release (Intuniv)	1-, 2-, 3-, 4-mg tablets	1 mg a day	1–4 mg a day	1 mg a day	0.005–0.12 mg/kg/day (1–7 mg a day maximal dose)

[a]Dosages for medical indications, such as hypertension, vary.

α-Adrenergic Receptor Ligands

3 β-Adrenergic Receptor Antagonists

Generic Name	Trade Name	Adverse Effects	Drug Interactions	CYP Interactions
Propranolol	Inderal	Hypotension, bradycardia, GI symptoms	antipsychotics, anticonvulsants, MAOI, theophylline, levothyroxine sodium	2D6
Metoprolol	Lopressor, Toprol XL	Hypotension, bradycardia, GI symptoms	antipsychotics, anticonvulsants, MAOI, theophylline, levothyroxine sodium	3A4, 2B6, 2C9
Atenolol	Tenormin	Hypotension, bradycardia, GI symptoms	antipsychotics, anticonvulsants, MAOI, theophylline, levothyroxine sodium	1A2
Nadolol	Corgard	Hypotension, bradycardia, GI symptoms	antipsychotics, anticonvulsants, MAOI, theophylline, levothyroxine sodium	N/A
Pindolol	Visken	Hypotension, bradycardia, GI symptoms	antipsychotics, anticonvulsants, MAOI, theophylline, levothyroxine sodium	N/A
Labetalol	Normodyne, Trandate	Hypotension, bradycardia, GI symptoms	antipsychotics, anticonvulsants, MAOI, theophylline, levothyroxine sodium	N/A

Introduction

β-Adrenergic receptor antagonists ("β-blockers") are most frequently used in cardiovascular diseases and bind to β-adrenergic receptors, which are ubiquitously distributed throughout the body, including the heart, lung, autonomic nervous system (ANS), and central nervous system (CNS). They inhibit the binding of epinephrine and norepinephrine and can be nonselective (block β_1-adrenergic and β_2-adrenergic receptors) or selective (block β_1-adrenergic receptors only). These agents are used for treating heart failure, angina, hypertension, and arrhythmias.

Though not currently approved by the Food and Drug Administration (FDA) for any psychiatric disorder, these drugs have been used to treat disparate psychiatric conditions such as performance anxiety, posttraumatic stress disorder (PTSD), panic attacks, major depressive disorder, aggressive and violent behavior, behavioral symptoms associated with dementia, alcohol and cocaine withdrawal, lithium-induced postural tremor, antipsychotic-induced akathisia, and migraine. The five β-adrenergic receptor antagonists most frequently studied for psychiatric application are propranolol (Inderal), metoprolol (Lopressor, Toprol XL), atenolol (Tenormin), nadolol (Corgard), and pindolol (Visken).

Pharmacologic Actions

Pharmacokinetics

β-Adrenergic receptor antagonists differ with regard to pharmacokinetic properties, including lipophilicities, metabolic routes, β-receptor selectivity, and half-lives (Table 3-1). Absorption of the β-receptor antagonists from the gastrointestinal tract is variable. The agents that are most soluble in lipids (i.e., are lipophilic), such as propranolol, are most likely to cross the blood–brain barrier and enter the brain; those agents that are least lipophilic, like atenolol, are less likely to enter the brain. When CNS effects are desired, a lipophilic drug may be preferred; when only peripheral effects are desired, a less lipophilic drug may be indicated. Drugs with high lipophilicity may lead to negative effects (see Table 3-1).

Pharmacodynamics

Whereas propranolol, nadolol, pindolol, and labetalol (Normodyne, Trandate) have essentially equal potency at both the β_1- and β_2-receptors, metoprolol and atenolol have greater affinity for the β_1-receptor than for the β_2-receptor. Relative β_1-selectivity confers few pulmonary and vascular effects of these drugs, although they must be used with caution in persons with asthma because the drugs retain some activity at the β_2-receptors.

Pindolol has sympathomimetic effects in addition to its β-antagonist effects, which has permitted its use for augmentation of antidepressant drugs. Pindolol, propranolol, and nadolol possess some antagonist activity at the serotonin 5-HT$_{1A}$ receptors.

Therapeutic Indications

At this time, no β-adrenergic receptor antagonists have been approved by the Food and Drug Administration (FDA) for the treatment of any psychiatric disorders. However, these drugs have been used off-label with success for the disorders below.

Anxiety Disorders, Obsessive-Compulsive Disorder, and PTSD

Propranolol is useful for the treatment of social phobia, primarily of the performance type (e.g., disabling anxiety before a musical performance). Data are also available for its use in treatment of panic disorder, PTSD, obsessive-compulsive disorder (OCD), and generalized anxiety disorder. In social phobia, the common treatment approach is to take 10 to 40 mg of propranolol 20 to 30 minutes before the anxiety-provoking situation. The β-receptor antagonists are less effective for the treatment of panic disorder than are benzodiazepines or selective serotonin reuptake inhibitors (SSRIs). Some evidence suggests that β-blockers work to decrease the physical symptoms of hyperarousal in PTSD or anxiety in OCD (e.g., tachycardia, hyperventilation), thereby providing relief to the psychiatric symptoms.

Lithium-Induced Postural Tremor

β-Adrenergic receptor antagonists are beneficial for lithium-induced postural tremor and other medication-induced postural tremors—for example, those induced

TABLE 3-1: β-Adrenergic Receptor Antagonist Drugs Used in Psychiatry

Drug	Trade Name	Protein Binding (%)	Lipophilic	ISA	Metabolism	Receptor Selectivity	Half-Life (hours)	Usual Starting Dosage (mg)	Usual Maximal Dosage (mg)
Atenolol (Tenormin)	Tenormin	6–16	No		Renal	$\beta_1 > \beta_2$	6–9	50 QD	50–100 QD
Metoprolol (Lopressor)	Lopressor	5–10	Yes		Hepatic	$\beta_1 > \beta_2$	3–4	50 BID	75–150 BID
Nadolol (Corgard)	Corgard	30	No		Renal	$\beta_1 = \beta_2$	14–24	40 QD	80–240 QD
Propranolol (Inderal)	Inderal	>90	Yes		Hepatic	$\beta_1 = \beta_2$	3–6	10–20 BID/TID	80–140 TID
Pindolol (Visken)	Visken	40	Yes	Minimal	Hepatic	$\beta_1 > \beta_2$	3–4	5 TID/QID	60 BID/TID

ISA, intrinsic sympathomimetic activity; QD, once a day; BID, two times a day; TID, three times a day.

by tricyclic antidepressants (TCAs) and valproate (Depakene). The initial approach to this movement disorder includes lowering the dose of lithium, eliminating aggravating factors (such as caffeine), and administering lithium at bedtime. If these interventions are inadequate, propranolol in the range of 20 to 160 mg a day given two or three times daily is generally effective for the treatment of lithium-induced postural tremor.

Neuroleptic-Induced Acute Akathisia

Many studies have shown that β-receptor antagonists can be effective in the treatment of neuroleptic-induced acute akathisia. They are generally more effective for this indication than are anticholinergics and benzodiazepines. The β-receptor antagonists are not effective in the treatment of such neuroleptic-induced movement disorders as acute dystonia and parkinsonism.

Aggression and Violent Behavior

β-Adrenergic receptor antagonists may be effective in reducing the num ber of aggressive and violent outbursts in persons with impulse disorders, schizophrenia, and aggression associated with brain injury. This includes traumatic brain injuries, tumors, anoxic injury, encephalitis, alcohol-related injuries (e.g., Wernicke–Korsakoff syndrome), and degenerative disorders (e.g., Huntington disease).

Alcohol Withdrawal

Propranolol is reported to be useful as an adjuvant to benzodiazepines but not as a sole agent in the treatment of alcohol withdrawal. The following dose schedule is suggested: no propranolol for a pulse rate below 50 beats/min; 50 mg propranolol for a pulse rate between 50 and 79 beats/min; and 100 mg propranolol for a pulse rate of 80 beats/min or above.

Antidepressant Augmentation

Pindolol has been studied as augmentation to hasten the antidepressant effects of SSRIs, tricyclic drugs, and electroconvulsive therapy. Evidence of its effectiveness in this role is not well established. Historically, β-adrenergic receptor antagonists have been associated with depressive symptoms, but recent data does not support this hypothesis. Patients with ischemic heart disease (IHD) are more prone to depression and are also regularly prescribed β-blockers which may induce fatigue, tiredness, and unusual dreams that may be misinterpreted as depression. However, this needs to be further clarified in controlled trials.

Other Disorders

β-Adrenergic receptor antagonists have also been used in some cases of anxiety-induced stuttering (Table 3-2).

Precautions and Adverse Reactions

β-Adrenergic receptor antagonists are contraindicated for use in people with asthma, insulin-dependent diabetes, congestive heart failure, significant vascular disease, persistent angina, and hyperthyroidism. The contraindication in diabetic

TABLE 3-2: Psychiatric Uses for β-Adrenergic Receptor Antagonists
Definitely effective
Performance anxiety
Lithium-induced tremor
Neuroleptic-induced akathisia
Migraine prophylaxis
Obsessive-compulsive disorder (OCD)
Symptoms associated with posttraumatic stress disorder (PTSD)
Probably effective
Adjunctive therapy for alcohol withdrawal and other substance-related disorders
Adjunctive therapy for aggressive or violent behavior
Stuttering
Possibly effective
Antipsychotic augmentation
Antidepressant augmentation

persons is due to the drugs' interference with the normal physiological response to hypoglycemia. β-Blockers can worsen atrioventricular (AV) conduction defects and lead to complete AV heart block and death. If the clinician decides that the risk-to-benefit ratio warrants a trial in a person with one of these coexisting medical conditions, a β_1-adrenergic receptor selective agent should be the first choice, and the patient should be monitored.

The most common adverse effects of β-adrenergic receptor antagonists are hypotension and bradycardia. In persons at risk for these adverse effects, a test dosage of 20 mg a day of propranolol can be given to assess reaction to the drug. Nausea, vomiting, diarrhea, and constipation can also be caused by treatment with these agents. β-Blockers may blunt cognition in some people. Serious CNS adverse effects (e.g., agitation, confusion, and hallucinations) are rare. Common CNS adverse effects include sleep disorders, fatigue, nightmares, and fall risk. Table 3-3 lists the possible adverse effects of β-receptor antagonists.

Use in Pregnancy and Lactation

There are no proven risks associated with use of β-receptor antagonists during pregnancy and lactation. However, there have been reports of possible fetal growth retardation when these drugs are used early in pregnancy. Furthermore, β-blockers are excreted in breast milk and should be administered with caution to nursing women. Most β-blockers fall under Pregnancy Letter Category C except for atenolol, which is Pregnancy Letter Category D.

Drug Interactions

Concomitant administration of propranolol results in increases in plasma concentrations of antipsychotics, anticonvulsants, theophylline (Theo-Dur, Slo-Bid), and levothyroxine sodium (Synthroid). Other β-adrenergic receptor antagonists may have similar effects. β-Adrenergic receptor antagonists that are eliminated by the kidneys may have similar effects on drugs that are also eliminated by the

TABLE 3-3: Adverse Effects and Toxicity of β-Adrenergic Receptor Antagonists
Cardiovascular
Hypotension
Bradycardia
Congestive heart failure (in patients with compromised myocardial function)
Respiratory
Asthma (less risk with β_1-selective drugs)
Metabolic
Worsened hypoglycemia in diabetic patients on insulin or oral agents
Gastrointestinal
Nausea
Diarrhea
Abdominal pain
Sexual function
Impotence
Neuropsychiatric
Lassitude
Fatigue
Dysphoria
Insomnia
Vivid nightmares
Depression (rare)
Psychosis (rare)
Other (rare)
Raynaud phenomenon
Peyronie disease
Withdrawal syndrome
Rebound worsening of pre-existing angina pectoris when β-adrenergic receptor antagonists are discontinued

renal route. Barbiturates, phenytoin (Dilantin), and cigarette smoking increase the elimination of β-blockers that are metabolized by the liver. Several reports have associated hypertensive crises and bradycardia with the coadministration of β-adrenergic receptor antagonists and monoamine oxidase inhibitors (MAOIs). Depressed myocardial contractility and AV nodal conduction can occur from concomitant administration of β-blockers and calcium channel inhibitors.

Laboratory Interferences

β-Adrenergic receptor antagonists do not interfere with standard laboratory tests.

Dosage and Clinical Guidelines

Propranolol is available in 10-, 20-, 40-, 60-, 80-, and 90-mg tablets; 4-, 8-, and 80-mg/mL solutions; and 60-, 80-, 120-, and 160-mg sustained-release capsules.

Nadolol is available in 20-, 40-, 80-, 120-, and 160-mg tablets.

Pindolol is available in 5- and 10-mg tablets.

Metoprolol is available in 50- and 100-mg tablets and 50-, 100-, and 200-mg sustained-release tablets.

Atenolol is available in 25-, 50-, and 100-mg tablets.

Acebutolol is available in 200- and 400-mg capsules.

For the treatment of chronic disorders, propranolol administration is usually initiated at 10 mg by mouth three times a day or 20 mg by mouth twice daily. The dosage can be raised from 20 to 30 mg a day until a therapeutic effect emerges. The dosage should be leveled off at the appropriate range for the disorder under treatment. The treatment of aggressive behavior sometimes requires dosages up to 80 mg a day, and therapeutic effects may not be seen until the person has been receiving the maximal dosage for 4 to 8 weeks. For the treatment of social phobia, primarily the performance type, the patient should take 10 to 40 mg of propranolol 20 to 30 minutes before the performance.

Pulse and blood pressure (BP) readings should be taken regularly, and the drug should be withheld if the pulse rate is below 50 beats/min or the systolic BP is below 90 mm Hg. The drug should be temporarily discontinued if it produces severe dizziness, ataxia, or wheezing. Treatment with β-receptor antagonists should never be discontinued abruptly. Propranolol should be tapered by 60 mg a day until a dosage of 60 mg a day is reached, after which, the drug should be tapered by 10 to 20 mg a day every 3 or 4 days.

The clinical guidelines for the other drugs listed in this chapter are similar to propranolol, taking into consideration the different doses used. For example, if propranolol is prescribed initially at the lowest available dose (e.g., 10 mg), then metoprolol should be prescribed at its lowest available dose (e.g., 50 mg).

Anticholinergic Agents

4

Generic Name	Trade Name	Adverse Effects	Drug Interactions	CYP Interactions
Benztropine	Cogentin	Anticholinergic Effects	DRA, TRI/TET, SSRI, MAOI	N/A
Biperiden	Akineton	Anticholinergic Effects	DRA, TRI/TET, SSRI, MAOI	2D6
Ethopropazine	Parsidol	Anticholinergic Effects	DRA, TRI/TET, SSRI, MAOI	N/A
Orphenadrine	Norflex, Disipal	Anticholinergic Effects	DRA, TRI/TET, SSRI, MAOI	2B6, 3A4, 2E1, 1A2, 2D6
Procyclidine hydrochloride	Kemadrin	Anticholinergic Effects	DRA, TRI/TET, SSRI, MAOI	N/A
Scopolamine	N/A	Anticholinergic Effects	DRA, TRI/TET, SSRI, MAOI	3A4
Trihexyphenidyl	Artane, Trihexane, Trihexy-5	Anticholinergic Effects	DRA, TRI/TET, SSRI, MAOI	N/A

Introduction

Anticholinergic drugs inhibit the binding of acetylcholine to acetylcholine/
cholinergic receptors located in the peripheral nervous system and central nervous
system (CNS). There are two kinds of cholinergic receptors, nicotinic and muscarinic. Only drugs that act as antagonists at the latter have applications in the field of
psychiatry, where they are used to treat medication-induced movement disorders,
particularly neuroleptic-induced parkinsonism, neuroleptic-induced acute dystonia,
and medication-induced postural tremor. In addition, they have wide-ranging effects
across the body and can also be used to treat asthma, chronic obstructive pulmonary
disease, nausea, vomiting, motion sickness, urinary incontinence, excessive sweating, overactive bladder, tremors of Parkinson disease, as well as depression.

Pharmacologic Actions

All anticholinergic drugs are well absorbed from the gastrointestinal (GI) tract
after oral administration and are sufficiently lipophilic to pass the blood–brain
barrier and enter the CNS. Trihexyphenidyl (Artane) and benztropine (Cogentin)
reach peak plasma concentrations in 2 to 3 hours after oral administration, and
their duration of action is 1 to 12 hours. Benztropine is absorbed equally rapidly
by intramuscular (IM) and intravenous (IV) administration. IM administration is
preferred because of its low risk for adverse effects.

   All six anticholinergic drugs listed (Table 4-1) in this section block muscarinic acetylcholine receptors, of which there are five subtypes (M1 to M5). Benztropine also has some antihistaminergic effects and can be used to treat allergies.
None of the available anticholinergic drugs have any effects on the nicotinic

45

					Short-Term Intramuscular or Intravenous Dosage
Generic Name	Brand Name	Tablet Size	Injectable	Usual Daily Oral Dosage	
Benztropine	Cogentin	0.5, 1, 2 mg	1 mg/mL	1–4 mg one to three times	1–2 mg
Biperiden	Akineton	2 mg	5 mg/mL	2 mg one to three times	2 mg
Ethopropazine	Parsidol	10, 50 mg	—	50–100 mg one to three times	—
Orphenadrine	Norflex, Disipal	100 mg	30 mg/mL	50–100 mg three times	60 mg IV given over 5 minutes
Procyclidine hydrochloride	Kemadrin	5 mg	—	2, 5–5 mg three times	—
Trihexyphenidyl	Artane, Trihexane, Trihexy-5	2, 5 mg elixir 2 mg/5 mL	—	2–5 mg two to four times	—

TABLE 4-1: Anticholinergic Drugs Commonly Used in Psychiatry

IV, intravenous.

acetylcholine receptors. Of these drugs, trihexyphenidyl is the most stimulating agent, perhaps acting through dopaminergic neurons, and benztropine is the least stimulating and thus is least associated with abuse potential.

Therapeutic Indications

The primary indication for the use of anticholinergics in psychiatric practice is for the treatment of *neuroleptic-induced parkinsonism*, which is characterized by tremor, rigidity, cogwheeling, bradykinesia, sialorrhea, stooped posture, and festination. Neuroleptic-induced parkinsonism is most common in elderly persons and women. It is most frequently seen with high-potency dopamine receptor antagonists (DRAs), for example, haloperidol (Haldol). The onset of symptoms usually occurs after 2 or 3 weeks of treatment. The incidence of neuroleptic-induced parkinsonism is lower with the second-generation antipsychotic drugs, also referred to as serotonin–dopamine antagonists (SDAs). All available anticholinergics are equally effective in the treatment of parkinsonian symptoms.

Another common indication is for the treatment of *neuroleptic-induced acute dystonia*, which is most common in young men and is commonly associated with high-potency DRAs (e.g., haloperidol). The syndrome often occurs early in the course of treatment and most commonly affects the muscles of the neck, tongue, face, and back. Anticholinergic drugs are effective both in the short-term treatment of dystonia and in prophylaxis against neuroleptic-induced acute dystonia.

Off-Label Uses

Treatment of Akathisia

Akathisia is characterized by a subjective and objective sense of restlessness, anxiety, and agitation. Although a trial of anticholinergics for the treatment of neuroleptic-induced acute akathisia is reasonable, these drugs are not generally considered as effective as the β-adrenergic receptor antagonists, the benzodiazepines, and clonidine (Catapres). Therefore, they should be considered as second-line therapies when first-line agents are contraindicated or fail to show efficacy.

Biperiden

Limited research suggests that biperiden may reduce incidence and intensity of spontaneous epileptic seizures following traumatic brain injury.

Scopolamine

Several studies have found that scopolamine may be used off-label in treating unipolar and bipolar depression, as well as anxiety. These findings indicate that effects are more pronounced in females. Unfortunately, the long-term effects of the treatment have not been adequately studied. Scopolamine and atropine treatment may reduce cravings for nicotine in individuals who have quit smoking, though the evidence of efficacy is wanting.

Trihexyphenidyl

Use of trihexyphenidyl has been associated with symptom improvement in psychotic depression. A small, open-label and single-blind study series found that patients with refractory posttraumatic stress disorder (PTSD)-related nightmares and flashbacks responded very well to treatment with trihexyphenidyl.

Precautions and Adverse Reactions

The adverse effects of the anticholinergic drugs result from blockade of muscarinic acetylcholine receptors. The most common side effects are shown in Table 4-2. Anticholinergics are occasionally used as drugs of abuse because of their mild mood-elevating properties, and this is most notable with

TABLE 4-2: Common Side Effects Associated with Anticholinergic Drugs
Dizziness
Drowsiness
Confusion
Increased heart rate
Dry mouth
Decreased sweating
Blurred vision
Dry eyes
Constipation
Urinary retention
Flushed appearance
Hallucinations
Heart rhythm disturbance

trihexyphenidyl. Clinicians should be vigilant when patients specifically ask for trihexyphenidyl prescription, especially in those with a history of substance abuse. Patients should also be cautioned to refrain from alcohol use, as such combination may lead to unconsciousness or even death.

In addition, exercise caution when prescribing anticholinergics to patients with prostatic hypertrophy, myasthenia gravis, Alzheimer disease, urinary retention, and narrow-angle glaucoma. Heat exhaustion may occur in those exercising especially during hot weather or those indulging in long hot baths.

Moreover, anticholinergics should be avoided in patients with urinary retention, bowel obstruction, ulcerative colitis, myasthenia gravis, and severe heart disease.

Caution is required in the elderly, especially in those with cognitive impairment, dementia, or delirium. Studies have shown a 54% higher risk of developing dementia in patients treated for 3 years or more. Elderly patients may also be on multiple medicines with anticholinergic properties as well as over-the-counter (OTC) products that may increase risk of sedation, confusion, and constipation. Consequently, use of anticholinergics should be avoided in this population.

The most serious adverse effect associated with anticholinergic toxicity is anticholinergic toxidrome (a portmanteau of toxicity and syndrome), which can be characterized by the following collection of similes:

- Hot as a desert: Hyperthermia
- Dry as a bone: Dry mouth, dry eyes, decreased sweating, urinary retention
- Red as a beet: Flushing
- Blind as a bat: Blurred vision
- Mad as a hatter: Confusion, delirium

Additional signs and symptoms are listed in Table 4-3.

TABLE 4-3: Signs and Symptoms of Anticholinergic Toxidrome
Mild Toxicity • Fever • Skin flushing • Dilated pupils • Blurred vision • Agitation • Tachycardia • Dry mouth • Decreased sweating
Moderate Toxicity • Hyperthermia • Delirium • Hypertension • Urinary retention
Severe Toxicity • Seizures • Hypotension • Rhabdomyolysis • Coma

Intoxication can be diagnosed and treated with physostigmine (Antilirium, Eserine), an inhibitor of anticholinesterase, 1 to 2 mg IV (1 mg every 2 minutes) or IM every 30 or 60 minutes. Treatment with physostigmine should be used only in severe cases and only when emergency cardiac monitoring and life-support services are available because physostigmine can lead to severe hypotension and bronchial constriction. In most cases, discontinuation of all anticholinergics will suffice.

Use in Pregnancy and Lactation

The safety of these medicines has not been established, and though there are no proven risks associated with use of anticholinergics during pregnancy and lactation caution is advised because of possible cases of neonatal paralytic ileus and of decreases in milk production.

Drug Interactions

The most common drug–drug interactions with the anticholinergics occur when they are co-administered with psychotropics that also have high anticholinergic activity, such as DRAs, tricyclic and tetracyclic drugs, SSRIs (fluoxetine, paroxetine), and monoamine oxidase inhibitors (MAOIs). Many other prescription drugs and OTC cold preparations also induce significant anticholinergic activity. The coadministration of those drugs can result in a life-threatening anticholinergic intoxication syndrome. Anticholinergic drugs can also delay gastric emptying, thereby decreasing the absorption of drugs that are broken down in the stomach and usually absorbed in the duodenum (e.g., levodopa [Larodopa] and DRAs).

Laboratory Interferences

No known laboratory interferences have been associated with anticholinergics.

Dosage and Clinical Guidelines

The three most commonly used anticholinergic drugs within the purview of this chapter, trihexyphenidyl (Artane), benztropine (Cogentin), and procyclidine (Kemadrin), are available in a range of preparations (Table 4-1).

Neuroleptic-Induced Parkinsonism

For the treatment of neuroleptic-induced parkinsonism, the equivalent of 1 to 3 mg of benztropine should be given one to two times daily. It should be administered for 4 to 8 weeks, and then it should be discontinued to assess whether the person still requires the drug. Anticholinergic drugs should be tapered over a period of 1 to 2 weeks.

Treatment with anticholinergics as prophylaxis against the development of neuroleptic-induced parkinsonism is uncommon because the onset of symptoms is usually sufficiently mild and gradual to allow the clinician to initiate treatment only after it is clearly necessary. In young men, prophylaxis may be indicated, however, especially if a high-potency DRA is being used. The clinician should attempt to discontinue the antiparkinsonian agent in 4 to 6 weeks to assess whether its continued use is necessary.

Neuroleptic-Induced Acute Dystonia

For the short-term treatment and prophylaxis of neuroleptic-induced acute dystonia, 1 to 2 mg of benztropine or its equivalent in another drug should be given IM. The dose can be repeated in 20 to 30 minutes, as needed. If the person still does not improve in another 20 to 30 minutes, a benzodiazepine (e.g., 1 mg IM or IV lorazepam [Ativan]) should be given. Laryngeal dystonia is a medical emergency and should be treated with benztropine, up to 4 mg in a 10-minute period, followed by 1 to 2 mg of lorazepam, administered slowly by the IV route.

Prophylaxis against dystonia is indicated in persons who have had one episode or in persons at high risk (young men taking high-potency DRAs). Prophylactic treatment is given for 4 to 8 weeks and then gradually tapered over 1 to 2 weeks to allow assessment of its continued need. The prophylactic use of anticholinergics in persons requiring antipsychotic drugs has largely become a moot issue because of the availability of SDAs, which are relatively free of parkinsonian effects.

Akathisia

As mentioned, anticholinergics are not the drugs of choice for this akathisia. β-Adrenergic receptor antagonists (Chapter 3), benzodiazepines (Chapter 8), or clonidine (Chapter 2) are preferable drugs to try initially.

Anticonvulsants

5

Generic Name	Trade Name	Adverse Effects	Drug Interactions	CYP Interactions
Gabapentin	Neurontin	Agitation, sedation, paranoia, mood swings	Antacids	N/A
Topiramate	Topamax	Arrhythmia, dizziness, memory impairment, sedation, cognitive problems	Anticonvulsants, carbonic anhydrase inhibitors	3A4, 2C19
Tiagabine	Gabitril	Agitation, GI symptoms, confusion	Anticonvulsants	3A
Levetiracetam	Keppra	Agitation, memory impairment, dizziness, sedation, mood swings, paranoia, GI symptoms, headache	None	N/A
Zonisamide	Zonegran	GI symptoms, dizziness, sedation, mood swings, memory impairment, skin rash, headache	Carbonic anhydrase inhibitors	3A
Pregabalin	Lyrica	GI symptoms, sedation, memory impairment, paranoia, weight gain, seizures, headache	None	N/A
Phenytoin	Dilantin	Confusion, dizziness, sedation, GI symptoms, headache	CNS	2C9, 2C19, 1A2, 2A6, 2B6, 2C8, 2D6, 2E1, 3A4, 3A5, 3A7

Anticonvulsants

Introduction

Many of the anticonvulsants or antiepileptic drugs (AEDs) described in this chapter were initially developed to treat epilepsy but have been found to have beneficial effects in psychiatric disorders. These include specifically bipolar affective disorders though have also been used for other conditions including alcohol and benzodiazepine withdrawal, affective disorder, panic and anxiety disorders, schizophrenia, and dementia. They may also be used as skeletal muscle relaxants and to treat neurogenic pain besides numerous off-label uses. The 11 anticonvulsants have different mechanisms of action (MOA) but grouped together specific MOA include increasing γ-aminobutyric acid (GABAergic) function and decreasing glutamatergic function. Other MOAs include reducing neuronal hyperexcitability by altering sodium and calcium channels.

This chapter includes six anticonvulsants that are sometimes used in treating psychiatric disorders: gabapentin (Neurontin), topiramate (Topamax), tiagabine (Gabitril), levetiracetam (Keppra), zonisamide (Zonegran), and pregabalin (Lyrica), as well as one of the first used anticonvulsants, phenytoin (Dilantin). Additional drugs that are classified as anticonvulsants or demonstrated some efficacy will be discussed in later chapters. These include carbamazepine (Tegretol) and oxcarbazepine (Trileptal), which will be discussed in Chapter 15; cannabidiol (Epidiolex) in Chapter 14; lamotrigine (Lamictal) in Chapter 20; and valproate (Depakene, Depakote) in Chapter 38.

In 2008, the U.S. Food and Drug Administration (FDA) issued a warning (not a "black box" warning) that anticonvulsant drugs may increase the risk of suicidal ideation or behavior in some persons compared with placebo. This continues to be somewhat controversial, as clinical trials have revealed that the relative risk for suicidality is higher in patients with epilepsy compared with those with psychiatric disorders. Some published data has corroborated the FDA's warning but noted that the extent of the risk of suicidality appears to be very low and clearly outweighed by the benefits of the medication.

This risk may only be relevant when used to treat epilepsy. Other published data has found that anticonvulsants may have a protective effect on suicidal thoughts in bipolar disorder. Still, considering the inherent increased risk of suicide in persons with bipolar disorder, clinicians should be aware of these warnings.

GABAPENTIN

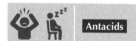

Antacids

Gabapentin was first approved for use by the FDA in 1993 to treat epilepsy in adult patients and pediatric patients aged 3 years and older. It was also found to have sedative effects that were useful in some psychiatric disorders, especially insomnia, and to be beneficial in reducing neuropathic pain and is currently indicated for the treatment of postherpetic neuralgia and as adjunctive therapy for partial seizures.

Pharmacologic Actions

Gabapentin circulates in the blood largely unbound and is not appreciably metabolized in humans. It is less than 3% protein bound and is eliminated unchanged by renal excretion and can be removed by hemodialysis. Food only moderately affects the rate and extent of absorption. Clearance is decreased in elderly persons, requiring dosage adjustments. Gabapentin elimination half-life is 5 to 7 hours.

Gabapentin appears to increase GABA synthesis but has no direct effect on GABA receptors and may inhibit glutamate synthesis. It increases human whole blood serotonin concentrations and modulates calcium channels to reduce monoamine release. It has antiseizure as well as antispastic activity and antinociceptive effects in pain.

Therapeutic Indications

In neurology, gabapentin is used for the treatment of both general and partial seizures. It is effective in reducing the pain of postherpetic neuralgia and other pain syndromes associated with diabetic neuropathy, neuropathic cancer pain, fibromyalgia, meralgia paresthetica, amputation, and headache. It has been found to be effective in some cases of chronic pruritus and in treating nerve pain associated with shingles. Gabapentin is also indicated for the treatment of restless leg syndrome. In psychiatry, gabapentin is used for anxiety and as a hypnotic agent because of its sedating effects.

Off-Label Uses

Gabapentin is used to ease anxiety symptoms (generalized anxiety, social phobia, and panic attacks)., The antianxiety effect may be particularly useful in patients with substance use and may reduce the need for self-medication with alcohol, improve social interaction as well as decrease in panic attacks. Gabapentin is also frequently used as a hypnotic in patients who may be at risk of benzodiazepine abuse but not as a main intervention in mania or treatment-resistant mood disorders, even if it may improve mood by reducing anxiety. Still, some bipolar patients have benefited when gabapentin is used adjunctively with mood stabilizers though this may be related to improved sleep. Similarly, patients with trauma- and stressor-related disorders like posttraumatic stress disorder (PTSD) may experience improved sleep with gabapentin.

Limited evidence from open-label trials indicates that gabapentin may decrease cravings for alcohol in some patients and could be used to treat other substance use disorders, most likely as an adjunctive medication.

Gabapentin is also used to treat cocaine withdrawal, diabetic neuropathy, and tremors in multiple sclerosis.

Precautions and Adverse Reactions

Adverse effects are typically mild and dose related (see Table 5-1). Overdose (over 4.5 g) has been associated with diplopia, slurred speech, lethargy, and diarrhea, but all patients recovered.

Anticonvulsants

TABLE 5-1: Common Side Effects Associated with Anticonvulsants

Drug	Side Effects	
Gabapentin	Aggression[a] Anxiety[a] Ataxia Blurred vision Clumsiness Crying[a] Depression[a] Difficulty concentrating[a] Daytime drowsiness Delusions Diarrhea Diplopia Eye movements (uncontrolled, often back-and-forth or rolling in nature)	Fatigue Flu-like symptoms Hoarseness Hyperactivity[a] Irascibility[a] Lethargy Mood swings[a] Pain (joints, muscles, lower back, side) Paranoia[a] Restlessness[a] Slurred speech Swelling in extremities Trembling Unusual sense of well-being[a] Unusual weakness

(continued)

TABLE 5-1: Common Side Effects Associated with Anticonvulsants (*Continued*)

Drug	Side Effects	
Topiramate	Anorexia Anxiety Arrhythmia Blurred vision Burning sensation Cognitive problems Dizziness Dysgeusia Eye redness Eye movements (uncontrolled, often back-and-forth or rolling in nature)	Increased eye pressure Memory problems Menstrual problems Paresthesia Renal calculi formation Somnolence Speech or language problems Unsteady gait and/or lack of ambulatory coordination Unusual weakness
Tiagabine	Abnormal cognition Aggression Anxiety Confusion Depression Difficulty concentrating Dizziness Drowsiness Fatigue Increased appetite Irritability Nausea	Painful and/or frequent urination Pruritus Somnolence Sleep difficulties Speech of language problems Status epilepticus Stomach pain Unsteady gait and/or lack of ambulatory coordination Unusual weakness
Levetiracetam	Aggression Anxiety Apathy Ataxia Blurred vision Chills Congestion Cough Depersonalization Depression Dizziness Diarrhea Difficulty swallowing Disorientation Drowsiness Dry mouth Eye irritation Fever Hallucinations Headache Hoarseness Irascibility Irregular heartbeat Irritability Joint pain Loss of appetite	Loss of strength Memory problems Mood swings Nausea Numbness (around mouth, feet and hands) Painful or difficult urination Pain (joints, muscles, lower back, side) Paranoia Personality change Restlessness Rhinorrhea Shivering Skin color changes Sleep troubles Sore throat Sweating Swollen glands in neck with tenderness Unexplained sobbing Unusual sense of well-being Voice changes Vomiting Weakness

TABLE 5-1: Common Side Effects Associated with Anticonvulsants (Continued)	
Drug	Side Effects
Zonisamide	Abdominal pain / Anhedonia / Anxiety / Apathy / Diarrhea / Difficulty concentrating / Dizziness / Diplopia / Discouragement / Drowsiness / Headache Irritability / Loss of appetite / Malaise / Memory problems / Mood swings / Nausea / Restlessness / Troubled sleep / Unsteady gait and/or lack of ambulatory coordination / Unusual weakness
Pregabalin	Blurred vision / Breathing problems / Chest tightness / Clumsiness / Cold sweats / Confusion / Constipation / Cough (productive) / Difficulty urinating / Drowsiness / Dry mouth / Fever / Headache / Hoarseness Increased appetite / Memory problems / Pain (chest, muscles, side, back) / Paranoia / Paresthesia / Rapid weight gain / Seizures / Speech or language difficulties / Twitching / Unsteady gait and/or lack of ambulatory coordination / Unusual weakness
Phenytoin	Blisters / Bruising / Chest pain / Confusion / Constipation / Difficulty swallowing or breathing / Dizziness / Drowsiness / Dysgeusia / Eye movements (uncontrolled, often back-and-forth or rolling in nature) / Flu-like symptoms / Gum overgrowth / Headache / Hives / Irregular heartbeat / Jaundice Lip enlargement / Loss of appetite / Nausea / New hair growth / Pain or curving of the penis / Pain in the upper right abdomen / Red or purple bumps on skin / Shortness of breath / Sleep problems / Slurred speech / Swelling of the eyes, face, lips, throat, tongue / Swollen glands / Twitching / Unsteady gait and/or lack of ambulatory coordination / Vomiting

aMore common in children.

Anticonvulsants

Use in Pregnancy and Lactation

Gabapentin is classified as a pregnancy category C drug. Risk to the fetus has not been ruled out since the drug is excreted in breast milk. It is best to avoid gabapentin in pregnant women and nursing mothers.

Drug Interactions

The bioavailability of gabapentin may decrease by as much as 20% when administered with antacids. In general, there are no drug interactions. Chronic use does not interfere with lithium administration.

Laboratory Interferences

Gabapentin does not interfere with any laboratory tests, although spontaneous reports of false-positive or positive drug toxicology screenings for amphetamines, barbiturates, benzodiazepines, and marijuana have been reported.

Dosages and Clinical Guidelines

Gabapentin is well tolerated, and the dosage can be increased to the maintenance range within a few days. A general approach for treatment of seizures is to start with 300 mg on the first day of treatment, increase to 600 mg on day 2, 900 mg on day 3, and subsequently increase up to 1,800 mg per day in divided doses as needed to relieve symptoms. Final total daily doses tend to be between 1,200 and 2,400 mg per day but occasionally results can be achieved with dosages as low as 200 to 300 mg per day, especially in elderly persons. Sedation is usually the limiting factor in determining the dosage. Some patients have taken dosages as high as 4,800 mg per day without significant adverse effects.

For anxiety-related condition, it is recommended to start low and go slow to avoid dizziness and excessive sedation and adjust dose as tolerance to these effects buildup. Starting dose can be between 100 and 300 mg once or twice a day and can be adjusted accordingly. Most patients may require 300 to 400 mg once or twice a day. Patients should be warned about using alcohol, driving or combining medications with sedative effects. Hypnotic doses usually range between 600 and 800 mg at bedtime.

Gabapentin is available as 100-, 300-, and 400-mg capsules and as 600- and 800-mg tablets. A 250-mg/5-mL oral solution is also available. Other formulations include extended-release gabapentin enacarbil (Horizant), available as 300 and 600 mg extended-release tablet.

Although abrupt discontinuation of gabapentin does not cause withdrawal effects, use of all anticonvulsant drugs should be gradually tapered.

TOPIRAMATE

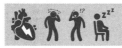 Anticonvulsants carbonic anhydrase inhibitors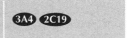

Topiramate (Topamax) was developed as a second-generation antiepileptic drug and was found useful in migraine prevention, treatment of obesity, bulimia, binge eating, and alcohol dependence. It was approved by the FDA in 1996 for the treatment of epilepsy and migraine disorder.

Pharmacologic Actions

Topiramate has GABAergic effects and increases cerebral GABA in humans. It has 80% oral bioavailability and is not significantly altered by food. Topiramate is 15% protein bound, and about 70% of the drug is eliminated by renal excretion. With renal insufficiency, topiramate clearance decreases about 50%, so the dosage needs to be decreased. It has a half-life of approximately 24 hours.

Therapeutic Indications

Topiramate is used primarily as an antiepileptic medication and has been found to be superior to placebo as monotherapy in patients with seizure disorders in adults and children aged 2 years and older. Topiramate has also been approved for adjunctive therapy in both adults and pediatric patients 2 years and older with primary generalized onset tonic–clonic seizures, partial-onset seizures, and Lennox–Gastaut syndrome. It is also used in the prevention of migraine.

Off-Label Uses

Topiramate has been used for smoking cessation, substance use disorder, pain syndromes (e.g., low back pain), cluster headache prevention, PTSD, essential tremor, and Prader–Willi syndrome. There is limited evidence suggesting that topiramate may be effective at treating tic disorders like Tourette syndrome. Self-mutilating behavior may be decreased in borderline personality disorder, but it is of little or no benefit in the treatment of psychotic disorders. Clinical evidence of its utility in treating bipolar disorder is weak at best.

Coadministration of topiramate with selective serotonin reuptake inhibitors (SSRIs) may potentiate the efficacy of the latter in the treatment of obsessive-compulsive disorder and major depressive disorder.

The drug has also been associated with weight loss, particularly to counteract the weight gain caused by many psychotropic drugs. Clinicians should be aware that there is an association with some cognitive problems and calcium phosphate kidney stones with high doses. Topiramate has also been used to promote weight loss and in the treatment of bulimia and binge-eating disorder as both monotherapy and as a combination of phentermine and topiramate, which is marketed under the brand name Qsymia. Topiramate is also used in combination with bupropion (Wellbutrin). The combination of phentermine-topiramate (Qsymia) is FDA approved for the treatment of obesity and overweight patients with weight-related comorbidities.

Precautions and Adverse Reactions

The most common adverse effects of topiramate are noted in Table 5-1. In general, 10% of patients may report cognitive problems. Patients may have difficulty with attention, concentration, and particularly struggle with word finding difficulty and appear to be dose related. Slow-dose escalation or dose reduction may alleviate these issues.

In many cases, the adverse effects are mild to moderate and can be attenuated by decreasing the dose. No deaths have been reported during overdose. The drug affects acid–base balance (low serum bicarbonate), which can be associated with cardiac arrhythmias, and the formation of renal calculi in about 1.5% of cases. Patients taking the drug should be encouraged to drink plenty of fluids.

Use in Pregnancy and Lactation

Topiramate is a pregnancy category D drug because its use during the first trimester is associated with an increased risk of oral clefts. Topiramate should be avoided during pregnancy and while breastfeeding, as it is carried in breast milk.

Anticonvulsants

Drug Interactions

Topiramate has few drug interactions with other anticonvulsant drugs. Topiramate may increase phenytoin concentrations up to 25% and valproic acid up to 11%; it does not affect the concentration of carbamazepine, phenobarbital (Luminal), or primidone (Mysoline). Topiramate concentrations are decreased by 40% to 48% with concomitant administration of carbamazepine or phenytoin. Topiramate should not be combined with other carbonic anhydrase inhibitors, such as acetazol-amide (Diamox) or dichlorphenamide (Daranide), because this could increase the risk of nephrolithiasis or heat-related problems (oligohydrosis and hyperthermia).

Laboratory Interferences

Topiramate does not interfere with any laboratory tests.

Dosages and Clinical Guidelines

Topiramate is available as unscored 25-, 100-, and 200-mg tablets. To reduce the risk of adverse cognitive and sedative effects, topiramate dosage for epilepsy is titrated gradually over 8 weeks to a maximum of 200 mg twice a day. Off-label topiramate is typically used for weight loss. Considering the cognitive side effects particularly with rapid titration, it is essential that the dose be increased gradually. It is recommended that topiramate dosage begin at 25 mg at bedtime and increase by no more than 25 mg weekly as necessary and titrated to 100 mg nightly. Final doses in efforts to promote weight loss are often between 150 and 200 mg per day. It can be given at bedtime to take advantage of topiramate's sedative effects though cognitive adverse effects may be the limiting factor. Doses higher than 400 mg are not associated with increased efficacy.

Further details on dosage guidelines for the treatment of weight loss will be discussed in Chapter 41.

Persons with renal insufficiency should reduce doses by half.

TIAGABINE

       Anticonvulsants

Tiagabine was introduced as a treatment for epilepsy in 1997 and was found to have efficacy in some psychiatric conditions, including acute mania. However, safety concerns along with a lack of controlled data have limited the use of tiagabine in disorders other than epilepsy.

Pharmacologic Actions

Tiagabine is well absorbed with a bioavailability of about 90% and is extensively (96%) bound to plasma proteins. Tiagabine is a CYP3A substrate and is extensively transformed into inactive 5-oxo-tiagabine and glucuronide metabolites, with only 2% being excreted unchanged in the urine. The remainder is excreted as metabolites in the feces (65%) and the urine (25%). Tiagabine blocks uptake of the inhibitory amino acid neurotransmitter GABA into neurons and glia, enhancing the inhibitory action of GABA at both $GABA_A$ and $GABA_B$ receptors, putatively yielding anticonvulsant and antinociceptive effects, respectively. It has mild blocking effects on histamine 1 (H_1), serotonin type 1B ($5\text{-}HT_{1B}$), benzodiazepine, and chloride channel receptors.

Therapeutic Indications

Tiagabine is indicated for the treatment of partial seizures as an adjunctive therapy in adults and children 12 years of age and older. It is rarely used for psychiatric disorders.

Off-Label Uses

Tiagabine may be used to treat generalized anxiety disorder, panic disorder, insomnia, and neuropathic pain. Limited data suggests tiagabine may be more effective in the treatment of PTSD in females than in males.

Precautions and Adverse Reactions

Tiagabine may cause withdrawal seizures, cognitive or neuropsychiatric problems (impaired concentration, speech or language problems, somnolence, and fatigue), status epilepticus, and sudden unexpected death in epilepsy (see Table 5-1). Acute oral overdoses of tiagabine have been associated with seizures, status epilepticus, coma, ataxia, confusion, somnolence, drowsiness, impaired speech, agitation, lethargy, myoclonus, stupor, tremors, disorientation, vomiting, hostility, temporary paralysis, and respiratory depression. Deaths have been reported in polydrug overdoses involving tiagabine. Cases of serious rash may occur, including Stevens–Johnson syndrome.

Use in Pregnancy and Lactation

Tiagabine is classified as a pregnancy category C drug. It has been linked to fetal loss and teratogenicity has been demonstrated in animals, and therefore should not be given to pregnant women. As the drug is excreted in breast milk, use of tiagabine in nursing mothers should be avoided.

Laboratory Tests

Tiagabine does not interfere with any laboratory tests.

Dosage and Administration

Tiagabine should not be rapidly loaded or rapidly initiated because of the risk of serious adverse effects. In adults and adolescents 12 years of age or older with epilepsy who are also taking enzyme inducers, tiagabine should be initiated at 4 mg per day and increased weekly by 4 mg per day during the first month and then increased weekly by 4 to 8 mg per day for weeks 5 and 6, yielding 24 to 32 mg per day administered in two to four divided doses by week 6.

In adults (but not adolescents), tiagabine doses may be further increased weekly by 4 to 8 mg per day to as high as 56 mg per day. Plasma concentrations in epilepsy patients commonly range between 20 and 100 ng/mL but do not appear to be systematically related to antiseizure effects and thus are not routinely monitored.

LEVETIRACETAM

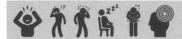

Initially developed as a nootropic (memory enhancing) drug, levetiracetam proved to be a potent anticonvulsant and received FDA approval as a treatment for partial seizures in 2000. It has been used to treat acute mania and anxiety and to augment antidepressant drug therapy.

Pharmacologic Actions

The central nervous system (CNS) effects of levetiracetam are not well understood, but it appears to indirectly enhance GABA inhibition. It is rapidly and completely absorbed, and peak concentrations are reached in 1 hour. Food delays the rate of absorption and decreases the amount of absorption. Levetiracetam is not significantly plasma protein bound and is not metabolized through the hepatic CYP system. Its metabolism involves hydrolysis of the acetamide group. Serum concentrations are not correlated with therapeutic effects.

Therapeutic Indications

Levetiracetam's major indication is for the treatment in convulsive disorders, including partial onset seizures (adults and children 4 years of age and older), myoclonic seizures (adults and adolescents 12 years of age and older), and tonic–clonic seizures in adults and children 6 years of age and older with idiopathic generalized epilepsy. It is sometimes used off-label for status epilepticus and seizure prophylaxis in subarachnoid hemorrhage.

Off-Label Uses

Levetiracetam has been used off label to treat neuropathic pain and migraine prophylaxis. In psychiatry, it has been used for acute mania, as an add-on treatment for major depression, and as an anxiolytic agent. Some evidence suggests that it may be effective as an add-on treatment for rapid cycling bipolar disorder.

Precautions and Adverse Reactions

The most common side effects of levetiracetam include drowsiness, dizziness, ataxia, diplopia, memory impairment, apathy, paresthesia, and hallucinations. A more robust listing of side effects can be found in Table 5-1. Some patients develop behavioral disturbances during treatment, and recent studies suggest worsening of depression, agitation, and other mood symptoms. Suicidal patients may become agitated. Clinicians should remain vigilant about these symptoms.

Use in Pregnancy and Lactation

Levetiracetam is classified as a pregnancy category C drug. Though there are no proven risks associated with use of levetiracetam during pregnancy, risks cannot be ruled out. Similarly, even though small amounts of the medication pass into breast milk, it should not be used when breastfeeding.

Drug Interactions

There are few if any interactions with other drugs, including other anticonvulsants. There is no interaction with lithium.

Laboratory Interferences

No laboratory interferences have been reported.

Dosages and Clinical Guidelines

The drug is available as 250-, 500-, 750-, and 1,000-mg tablets; 500-mg extended-release tablets; a 100-mg/mL oral solution; and a 100-mg/mL intravenous solution. In epilepsy, the typical adult daily dose is 1,000 mg.

In view of its renal clearance, dosages should be reduced in patients with impaired renal function.

ZONISAMIDE

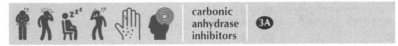

carbonic anhydrase inhibitors **3A**

Zonisamide is a 1,2 benzisoxazole derivative indicated for the treatment of seizure disorders. Zonisamide has also been found to be useful in bipolar disorder, obesity, and binge-eating disorder.

Pharmacologic Actions

Following oral administration, zonisamide is rapidly absorbed and evenly distributed with maximum concentrations occurring within 2 and 5 hours. Zonisamide is metabolized by the hepatic CYP4503A system, so enzyme-inducing agents, such as carbamazepine, alcohol, and phenobarbital, increase the clearance and reduce the availability of the drug. Zonisamide does not affect the metabolism of other drugs. It has a long half-life of 60 hours, so it can be dosed once daily, preferably at nighttime. Zonisamide blocks sodium channels and may weakly potentiate dopamine and serotonin activity. It also inhibits carbonic anhydrase. Some evidence suggests that it may block calcium channels and could inhibit glutamate release.

Therapeutic Indications

Zonisamide was approved for use as an adjunctive therapy in the treatment of generalized seizure disorders and in refractory partial seizures in patients 16 years of age and older. Some evidence suggests that it may be useful in the treatment of simple partial seizures, complex partial seizures, infantile seizures, myoclonic seizures, progressive myoclonic epilepsy, and Lennox–Gastaut syndrome.

Off-Label Uses

Some evidence suggests that zonisamide may be used to treat neuropathic pain. In psychiatry, controlled studies found zonisamide to be of use in obesity and binge-eating disorder. For more information about zonisamide and weight loss, see Chapter 41.

Uncontrolled trials have found it useful as a treatment in acute phases of bipolar disorder, particularly mania; however, further studies are warranted for this indication. Some studies report improvement in Parkinson disease symptoms when zonisamide is added to existing treatment regimens. Zonisamide may also be an effective therapy in the treatment of head tremors, essential tremors, as well as neuropathic pain,

Precautions and Adverse Reactions

Zonisamide is a sulfonamide and thus may cause severe rash (Stevens–Johnson syndrome) and blood dyscrasias, although these events are rare. About 4% of patients develop kidney stones. The most common side effects are drowsiness, cognitive impairment, insomnia, ataxia, nystagmus, paresthesia, speech abnormalities, constipation, diarrhea, nausea, and dry mouth. Weight loss is also a common side effect, which has been exploited as a therapy for patients who have gained weight during treatment with psychotropics and have ongoing difficulty controlling their eating. Additional side effects are listed in Table 5-1.

Use in Pregnancy and Lactation

Zonisamide is listed as a pregnancy category C drug and should not be used in pregnant women or breastfeeding mothers. Fetal abnormalities or embryofetal deaths have been reported in animal tests at doses and maternal plasma levels similar to or less than human therapeutic concentrations.

Drug Interactions

Zonisamide does not inhibit CYP450 isoenzymes and does not instigate drug interactions. It is important not to combine carbonic anhydrase inhibitors with zonisamide because of an increased risk of nephrolithiasis related to increased blood levels of urea.

Laboratory Interferences

Zonisamide can elevate hepatic alkaline phosphatase and increase blood urea nitrogen and creatinine.

Dosages and Clinical Guidelines

Zonisamide is available in 100- and 200-mg capsules. In epilepsy, the dosage range is 100 to 400 mg per day, with side effects becoming more pronounced at doses above 300 mg. Because of its long half-life, zonisamide can be given once a day.

PREGABALIN

Pregabalin was approved by the FDA for use in treating partial-onset seizures in patients 4 years of age and older, as well as neuropathic pain, postherpetic neuralgia, and fibromyalgia. It is pharmacologically similar to gabapentin and is

believed to work by inhibiting the release of excess excitatory neurotransmitters. It increases neuronal GABA levels, and its binding affinity is six times greater than that of gabapentin.

Pharmacologic Actions

Pregabalin exhibits linear pharmacokinetics. It is extremely and rapidly absorbed in proportion to its dose. The time to maximal plasma concentration is about 1 hour and that to steady state is within 24 to 48 hours. Pregabalin demonstrates high bioavailability, and it has a mean elimination half-life of about 6.5 hours. Food does not affect absorption. Pregabalin does not bind to plasma proteins and is excreted virtually unchanged (<2% metabolism) by the kidneys. It is not subjected to hepatic metabolism and does not induce or inhibit liver enzymes such as the CYP450 system. Dose reduction may be necessary in patients with creatinine clearance (CrCl) less than 60 mL per minute. Daily doses should be further reduced by approximately 50% for each additional 50% decrease in CrCl. Pregabalin is highly cleared by hemodialysis, so additional doses may be needed for patients on chronic hemodialysis treatment after each hemodialysis treatment.

Though pregabalin is structurally similar to GABA, it does not directly bind to GABA-A or GABA-B receptors. It targets $\alpha_2\delta$ subunits of voltage-gated calcium channels and reduces the release of excitatory neurotransmitters. This is believed to account for the analgesic and anticonvulsant effects of the drug.

Therapeutic Indications

Pregabalin is approved for the management of diabetic peripheral neuropathy, neuropathic pain associated with spinal cord injury, postherpetic neuralgia, fibromyalgia, and as an adjunctive treatment for partial onset seizures.

Off-Label Uses

Pregabalin has multiple off-label uses for chronic pain conditions, chronic pruritus, chronic cough, and restless leg syndrome. In the field of psychiatry, it has been found to be of benefit to some patients with generalized anxiety disorder. In studies, no consistent dose–response relationship was found, although 300 mg of pregabalin per day was more effective than 150 or 450 mg. Some patients with panic disorder or social anxiety disorder may benefit from pregabalin, but little evidence supports its routine use in treating persons with these disorders. Pregabalin may be a promising candidate for patients with insomnia struggling with hypnotic withdrawal. There is limited evidence to support the use of pregabalin to treat other forms of insomnia or bipolar disorder.

Precautions and Adverse Reactions

The most common adverse events associated with pregabalin use are dizziness, somnolence, blurred vision, peripheral edema, amnesia or loss of memory, and tremors. Additional side effects are listed in Table 5-1. Pregabalin potentiates the sedating effects of alcohol, antihistamines, benzodiazepines, and other CNS depressants. It remains to be seen if pregabalin is associated with benzodiazepine-type withdrawal symptoms.

Anticonvulsants

TABLE 5-2: Dosage Adjustment for Patients with Reduced Creatine Clearance	
Creatine Clearance Range	Dosage Adjustment
30–60 mL/min	50% recommended daily dose
15–30 mL/min	25% recommended daily dose
≤15 mL/min	8–16% recommended daily dose

Use in Pregnancy and Lactation

Prenatal pregabalin use is associated with an increased risk of major birth defects. These include heart defects and CNS abnormalities. Consequently, pregabalin has been labeled a pregnancy category C drug and should not be used by individuals who are pregnant or nursing.

Drug Interactions

In view of the absence of hepatic metabolism, pregabalin lacks metabolic drug interactions.

Laboratory Interferences

There are no effects on laboratory tests.

Dosage and Clinical Guidelines

The recommended dose for postherpetic neuralgia is 50 or 100 mg orally three times a day. The recommended dose for diabetic peripheral neuropathy is 100 to 200 mg orally three times a day. Patients with fibromyalgia may require up to 450 to 600 mg per day given in divided doses. Pregabalin is available as 25-, 50-, 75-, 100-, 150-, 200-, 225-, and 300-mg capsules. Dosages should be adjusted for patients with reduced creatine clearance (see Table 5-2) for those who are undergoing hemodialysis (see Table 5-3).

PHENYTOIN

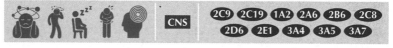

Phenytoin sodium (Dilantin) is an antiepileptic drug that is related to barbiturates in chemical structure and has been in use since the 1950s. It is indicated for the

TABLE 5-3: Supplemental Dosage for Patients Undergoing Hemodialysis	
QD Regimen of Pregabalin	Supplemental Dose
25 mg	25 or 50 mg
25–50 mg	50 or 75 mg
50–75 mg	75 or 100 mg
75 mg	100 or 150 mg

control of generalized tonic–clonic (grand mal) and complex partial (psychomotor, temporal lobe) seizures, as well as the prevention and treatment of seizures occurring during or after neurosurgery. Studies have shown comparable efficacy of phenytoin to other anticonvulsants in bipolar disorder, but clinicians should take into account the danger of numerous severe side effects with the medication. These include gingival hyperplasia, leukopenia, or anemia, as well as the danger of toxicity caused by nonlinear pharmacokinetics.

Pharmacologic Action

Similar to other anticonvulsants, phenytoin causes blockade of voltage-activated sodium channels. In addition to acting as an anticonvulsant, it is also efficacious as an antimanic agent. The plasma half-life after oral administration averages 22 hours, with a range of 7 to 42 hours. Steady-state therapeutic levels are achieved at least 7 to 10 days (5 to 7 half-lives) after initiation of therapy with recommended doses of 300 mg per day. Serum level should be obtained at least 5 to 7 half-lives after treatment initiation. Phenytoin is excreted in the bile, which is then reabsorbed from the intestinal tract and excreted in the urine. Urinary excretion of phenytoin occurs partly with glomerular filtration and by tubular secretion. Small incremental doses of phenytoin may increase the half-life and produce very substantial increases in serum levels. Patients should adhere strictly to the prescribed dosage, and serial monitoring of phenytoin levels is recommended.

Therapeutic Indications

Though it has been around for decades, it continues to be a widely used medication that is currently indicated for generalized tonic–clonic (grand mal) and complex partial (psychomotor, temporal lobe) seizures. In the past, phenytoin was used as an antiarrhythmic and to treat toxicity secondary to digoxin and tricyclic antidepressants but is not routinely used for this purpose at this time.

Off-Label Uses

Phenytoin has been used to treat anxiety and as a mood stabilizer in the treatment of acute mania in bipolar disorder. Phenytoin may also be effective in the treatment of trigeminal neuralgia.

Precautions and Adverse Reactions

The most common adverse reactions reported with phenytoin therapy are usually dose related and include nystagmus, ataxia, slurred speech, decreased coordination, and mental confusion. Other side effects include dizziness, insomnia, transient nervousness, motor twitching, and headaches. There have been rare reports of phenytoin-induced dyskinesias, similar to those induced by phenothiazine and other neuroleptic drugs. More serious side effects include thrombocytopenia, leukopenia, agranulocytosis, and pancytopenia with or without bone marrow suppression. A rare condition associated with intravenous phenytoin use is known as purple glove syndrome (PGS), which often presents with edema, pain, and discoloration that spreads to the distal limb.

A number of reports have suggested the development of lymphadenopathy (local or generalized), including benign lymph node hyperplasia, pseudolymphoma,

lymphoma, and Hodgkin disease. Hyperglycemia has been reported, and it may also increase the serum glucose level in diabetic patients. Individuals with folate deficiency may suffer drug-induced gingival enlargement. Additional side effects are listed in Table 5-1.

Use in Pregnancy and Lactation

There is positive evidence that prenatal exposure to phenytoin may increase the risks for birth defects. The most severe is fetal hydantoin syndrome, which is characterized by mental and physical birth defects. In addition to congenital malformations, newborns exposed to phenytoin in utero may develop a potentially life-threatening bleeding disorder related to decreased levels of vitamin K–dependent clotting factors. Deficiencies in vitamins K and D, as well as folate, may cause megaloblastic anemia. Consequently, phenytoin is listed as a pregnancy category D drug and should not be taken by individuals who are pregnant, planning to become pregnant, or nursing.

Drug Interactions

Acute alcohol intake, amiodarone, chlordiazepoxide, cimetidine, diazepam, disulfiram, estrogens, fluoxetine, H_2-antagonists, isoniazid, methylphenidate, phenothiazines, salicylates, and trazodone may increase phenytoin serum levels. Drugs that may lower phenytoin levels include carbamazepine, chronic alcohol abuse, and reserpine.

Laboratory Interferences

Phenytoin may decrease serum concentrations of thyroxine. It may cause increased serum levels of glucose, alkaline phosphatase, and γ-glutamyl transpeptidase.

Dosage and Clinical Guidelines

Patients may be started on one 100-mg extended oral capsule three times daily and the dosage then adjusted to suit individual requirements. Patients may then be switched to once-a-day daily dosing, which is more convenient. In this case, extended-release capsules may be used. Serial monitoring of phenytoin levels is recommended, and the normal range is usually 10 to 20 mcg/mL.

Antihistamines

6

Generic Name	Trade Name	Adverse Effects	Drug Interactions	CYP Interactions
Diphenhydramine	Benadryl	Sedation, dizziness, hypotension, GI symptoms, headache	Anticholinergics, CNS, DRA, TRI/TET	2D6, 1A2
Hydroxyzine	Atarax, Vistaril	Sedation, dizziness, hypotension, GI symptoms, headache	Anticholinergics, CNS, DRA, TRI/TET	3A4, 3A5
Promethazine	Phenergan	Sedation, dizziness, hypotension, GI symptoms, headache	Anticholinergics, CNS, DRA, TRI/TET	2D6
Cyproheptadine	Periactin	Sedation, dizziness, hypotension, GI symptoms, headache	Anticholinergics, CNS, DRA, TRI/TET	3A4

Introduction

Antihistamines have a long history of being used to treat psychiatric disorders as well as to counteract side effects of various psychotropics, particularly those that target histamine H_1 receptors, which are expressed on vascular endothelial cells, the heart, in smooth muscles, and throughout the central nervous system (CNS). While some first- and second-generation antihistamines are known to cause sedation or cardiac adverse events such as sinus tachycardia, reflex tachycardia, and supraventricular arrhythmias, many of the recently developed antihistamines (e.g., fexofenadine [Allegra], loratadine [Claritin], desloratadine [Clarinex], cetirizine [Zyrtec]) carry less risk of adverse cardiac events. However, these so-called third-generation antihistamines are not commonly used in psychiatric practice.

Within the field of psychiatry, antihistamines are used off-label to treat neuroleptic-induced parkinsonism and neuroleptic-induced acute dystonia. In addition, some of them can be substituted for conventional hypnotics and anxiolytics. The newer H_2-receptor antagonists, such as cimetidine (Tagamet), work primarily on gastric mucosa, inhibiting gastric secretion. Both cimetidine and ranitidine have also been shown to reduce appetite and weight in overweight individuals, as well as those with type II diabetes mellitus. However, the data is conflicted, and these are not routinely used for such purposes.

The antihistamines most commonly used in psychiatry are listed in Table 6-1. Table 6-2 lists antihistamines not used in psychiatry but may cause psychiatric adverse effects or lead to drug–drug interactions.

TABLE 6-1: Antihistamines Commonly Used in Psychiatry

Generic Name	Trade Name	Duration of Action (hours)
Diphenhydramine	Benadryl	4–6
Hydroxyzine	Atarax, Vistaril	6–24
Promethazine	Phenergan	4–6
Cyproheptadine	Periactin	4–6

Pharmacologic Actions

The H_1 antagonists used in psychiatry should not be considered interchangeable. All are well absorbed from the gastrointestinal (GI) tract following oral administration but are metabolized by different cytochrome P450 isoenzymes, which could lead to interaction with other medications.

Diphenhydramine is primarily metabolized by CYP2D6 and, to a lesser extent, CYP1A2, CYP2C9, and CYP2C19 isoenzymes. It is excreted in the urine and has a half-life of 2.4 to 9.3 hours. **Hydroxyzine** is metabolized by CYP3A4 and CYP3A5 isoenzymes, primarily excreted in urine (approximately 70% of which is unchanged from the active metabolite, cetirizine), and has a significant degree of variation in half-life (14 to 25 hours), depending on the patient. In children, it tends to be shorter (approximately 7 hours). **Promethazine** is metabolized by CYP2D6 isoenzymes, has a half-life of 12 to 15 hours, and very little is excreted in urine unchanged. **Cyproheptadine** is metabolized by CYP3A4 isoenzymes and has a terminal half-life of 8 hours. Approximately 20% is excreted in feces and 40% is excreted in urine.

The antiparkinsonian effects of intramuscular (IM) diphenhydramine have their onset in 15 to 30 minutes, while the sedative effects peak within 1 to 3 hours. The sedative effects of hydroxyzine and promethazine begin after 20 to 60 minutes and last for 4 to 6 hours. Because all three drugs are metabolized in the liver, persons with hepatic disease, such as cirrhosis, may attain high plasma concentrations with long-term administration.

Activation of H_1 receptors stimulates wakefulness; therefore, receptor antagonism causes sedation. All four agents also possess some antimuscarinic cholinergic activity. Cyproheptadine is unique among the drugs because it has both potent antihistamine and serotonin $5\text{-}HT_2$ receptor antagonist properties.

TABLE 6-2: Other Antihistamines

Class	Generic Name	Trade Name
Third-generation antihistamines	Cetirizine	Zyrtec
	Loratadine	Claritin
	Fexofenadine	Allegra
H_2-receptor antagonists	Nizatidine	Axid
	Famotidine	Pepcid
	Ranitidine	Zantac
	Cimetidine	Tagamet

TABLE 6-3: Uses for Antihistamines

H₁ Antihistamines	H₂ Antihistamines
Common: • Allergic conjunctivitis • Allergic rhinitis • Anaphylaxis • Angioedema • Cold symptoms • Drug hypersensitivity • Food allergies • Hives • Insect bites/stings • Nausea/vomiting • Pruritus • Seasonal allergies • Skin rashes	Common: • Duodenal or gastric ulcers • Gastroesophageal reflux disease (GERD) • Heartburn • Indigestion • Zollinger–Ellison syndrome
Less common: • Anorexia • Anxiety • Bone pain • Depression • Headaches • Insomnia • Motion sickness • Parkinsonism • Vertigo	

Indications

At this time, only hydroxyzine is indicated for the treatment of numerous psychiatric symptoms. It provides symptomatic relief from anxiety and is also used as an adjunct treatment in organic conditions that may cause anxiety, though its efficacy has not been assessed for long-term use as an anxiolytic agent. It is also used for insomnia, nausea, vomiting, itching, and allergies.

Off-Label Psychiatric Uses

An outline of some of the uses for antihistamines can be found in Table 6-3. Antihistamines are relatively safe hypnotics but are not superior to the benzodiazepines in terms of efficacy and safety. In addition, antihistamines have not been proven effective for long-term use as anxiolytics; therefore, benzodiazepines, buspirone (BuSpar), and selective serotonin reuptake inhibitors (SSRIs) continue to be the preferred treatments.

Diphenhydramine has been shown to be useful as a treatment for neuroleptic-induced parkinsonism, neuroleptic-induced acute dystonia, and neuroleptic-induced akathisia. It can also be used as an alternative to anticholinergics and amantadine for these purposes.

Cyproheptadine is sometimes used to treat impaired orgasms, especially delayed orgasm resulting from treatment with serotonergic drugs. Since it promotes weight gain, cyproheptadine may also be of some use in the treatment of eating disorders, such as anorexia nervosa. Cyproheptadine can also reduce recurrent nightmares with posttraumatic themes. In addition, the antiserotonergic activity of cyproheptadine may counteract the serotonin syndrome caused by concomitant use of multiple serotonin-activating drugs, such as SSRIs and monoamine oxidase inhibitors. Some evidence suggests that cyproheptadine can reduce the frequency and intensity of migraine headaches.

Precautions and Adverse Reactions

Antihistamines are commonly associated with sedation, dizziness, and hypotension, all of which can be severe in elderly persons, who are also likely to experience the anticholinergic effects of those drugs. This may lead to confusion, disorientation, and cognitive problems which may be exacerbated in older patients who concomitantly may also be on other medicines with anticholinergic effects. Paradoxical excitement or agitation is an adverse effect seen in a small number of patients. These combined effects may lead to delirium and long-term use is associated with cognitive decline and risk of dementia. In addition, poor motor coordination may result in accidents; therefore, patients should be warned about driving and operating dangerous machinery. Other common adverse effects include epigastric distress, nausea, vomiting, diarrhea, and constipation. For a more complete list of side effects, see Table 6-4.

Because of anticholinergic activity, some people experience dry mouth, urinary retention, blurred vision, and constipation. Consequently, antihistamines should be used only at very low doses, if at all, by persons with narrow-angle glaucoma or obstructive GI, prostate, or bladder conditions. A central anticholinergic syndrome with psychosis may be induced by either cyproheptadine or diphenhydramine. The use of cyproheptadine in some persons has been associated with weight gain, which may contribute to its reported efficacy in some persons with anorexia nervosa.

Promethazine contains a black box warning that the drug should not be used in patients younger than 2 years of age secondary to risk of fatal respiratory depression.

TABLE 6-4: Common Side Effects Associated with Antihistamine Use		
First-Generation Antihistamines	Second-Generation Antihistamines	H₂ Antihistamines
Blurred vision	Abdominal discomfort	Breast swelling/tenderness
Constipation	Cough	Confusion
Dizziness	Drowsiness	Dizziness
Drowsiness	Headache	Drowsiness
Dry mouth	Nausea	Headache
Dry eyes	Sore throat	Joint/muscle pain
Headache	Vomiting	
Low blood pressure		
Mucous thickening in airways		
Tachycardia		
Urinary retention		

In addition to the above adverse effects, antihistamines have some potential for abuse. The coadministration of antihistamines and opioids can increase the euphoria experienced by persons with substance dependence. Overdoses of antihistamines can be fatal.

Use in Pregnancy and Lactation

Because of some potential for teratogenicity, pregnant women should avoid the use of antihistamines. Antihistamines are excreted in breast milk, so they should only be used by nursing mothers if deemed necessary. Diphenhydramine and cyproheptadine are classified as pregnancy category B drugs, while hydroxyzine and promethazine are classified as pregnancy category C drugs.

Drug Interactions

The sedative property of antihistamines can be additive with other CNS depressants, such as alcohol, other sedative-hypnotic drugs, and many psychotropic drugs, including tricyclic drugs and dopamine receptor antagonists (DRAs). Anticholinergic activity can also be additive with that of other anticholinergic drugs and may sometimes result in severe anticholinergic symptoms or intoxication.

Laboratory Interferences

H_1 antagonists may eliminate the wheal and induration that form the basis of allergy skin tests. Promethazine may interfere with pregnancy tests and may increase blood glucose concentrations. Diphenhydramine may yield a false-positive urine test result for phencyclidine (PCP). Hydroxyzine use can falsely elevate the results of certain tests for urinary 17-hydroxycorticosteroids.

Dosage and Clinical Guidelines

Antihistamines are available in a variety of preparations (Table 6-5). IM injections should be given deep into the muscle because superficial administration can cause local irritation. This is especially true with promethazine, which can cause gangrene if administered incorrectly.

Intravenous (IV) administration of 25 to 50 mg of diphenhydramine is an effective treatment for neuroleptic-induced acute dystonia, which may resolve immediately. Treatment with 25 mg three times a day—up to 50 mg four times a day, if necessary—can be used to treat neuroleptic-induced parkinsonism, akinesia, and buccal movements. Diphenhydramine can be used as a hypnotic at a 50-mg dose for mild transient insomnia. Doses of 100 mg have not been shown to be superior to doses of 50 mg, but they produce more anticholinergic effects.

Hydroxyzine is most commonly used as a short-term anxiolytic. Hydroxyzine should not be given IV considering it is irritating to the blood vessels. Dosages of 50 to 100 mg given orally four times a day for long-term treatment or 50 to 100 mg IM every 4 to 6 hours for short-term treatment are usually effective.

SSRI-induced anorgasmia may be reversed sometimes with 4 to 16 mg a day of cyproheptadine taken by mouth 1 or 2 hours before anticipated sexual activity. A number of case reports and small studies have also reported that

TABLE 6-5: Dosage and Administration of Common Histamine Antagonists

Medication	Route	Preparation	Common Dosage
Diphenhydramine (Benadryl)	PO	Capsules and tablets: 25 mg, 50 mg Liquid: 12.5 mg/5.0 mL	Adults: 25–50 mg three to four times per day Children: 5 mg/kg three to four times per day, not to exceed 300 mg/day
	Deep IM or IV	Solution: 10 or 50 mg/mL	Same as oral
Hydroxyzine Hydrochloride (Atarax)	PO	Tablets: 10, 25, 50, and 100 mg Syrup: 10 mg/5 mL	Adults: 50–100 mg three to four times daily Children younger than 6 years of age: 2 mg/kg/day in divided doses Children older than 6 years of age: 12.5–25.0 mg three to four times daily
	IM	Solution: 25 or 50 mg/mL	Same as oral
Pamoate (Vistaril)	PO	Suspension: 25 mg/mL Capsules: 25, 50, and 100 mg	Same as dosages for hydrochloride
Promethazine (Phenergan)	PO	Tablets: 15.2, 25.0, and 50.0 mg Syrup: 3.25 mg/5 mL	Adults: 50–100 mg three to four times daily for sedation Children: 12.5–25.0 mg at night for sedation
	Rectal	Suppositories: 12.5, 25.0, and 50.0 mg	
	IM	Solution: 25 and 50 mg/mL	
Cyproheptadine (Periactin)	PO	Tablets: 4 mg Syrup: 2 mg/5 mL	Adults: 4–20 mg/day. Children 2–7 years of age: 2 mg two to three times daily (maximum, 12 mg/day). Children 7–14 years of age: 4 mg two to three times daily (maximum of 16 mg/day)

IM, intramuscular; IV, intravenous; PO, oral.

cyproheptadine may be of some use in the treatment of eating disorders, such as anorexia nervosa. Cyproheptadine is available in 4-mg tablets and a 2-mg/5-mL solution.

Clinicians should be aware that children and elderly patients are more sensitive to the effects of antihistamines than are younger and healthy adults.

Barbiturates and Similarly Acting Drugs

7

Generic Name	Trade Name	Adverse Effects	Drug Interactions	CYP Interactions
Aprobarbital	Alurate	Confusion, sedation, agitation, respiratory depression	CNS	3A4
Butabarbital	Butisol	Confusion, sedation, agitation, respiratory depression	CNS	N/A
Mephobarbital	Mebaral	Confusion, sedation, agitation, respiratory depression	CNS	2C19, 2B6
Methohexital	Brevital	Confusion, sedation, agitation, respiratory depression	CNS	N/A
Pentobarbital	Nembutal	Confusion, sedation, agitation, respiratory depression	CNS	2C19, 2A6, 3A4
Phenobarbital	Luminal	Confusion, sedation, agitation, respiratory depression	CNS	2C19, 2C9, 2E1, 2B6, 2C8, 3A4, 1A2, 3A5, 1A1, 2C18, 3A7
Secobarbital	Seconal	Confusion, sedation, agitation, respiratory depression	CNS	1A2, 2C19, 2C8, 2C9
Paraldehyde	N/A	Confusion, sedation, GI symptoms	CNS, disulfiram	N/A
Meprobamate	N/A	Confusion, sedation, coma	CNS	N/A
Chloral hydrate	Nortec	Confusion, sedation, coma	CNS, warfarin	N/A

Introduction

Barbiturates have long been used in psychiatry because of their depressive effects on the central nervous system (CNS). They are effective hypnotics, sedatives, and anxiolytics that became widely used between the 1920s and 1950s, though use dates back to 1903 when the first drug of this class, barbital (Veronal), became commercially available as a sleep agent. It was followed by phenobarbital (Luminal) in 1912, amobarbital (Amytal) in 1923, secobarbital (Seconal) in 1929, pentobarbital (Nembutal) in 1930, and thiopental (Pentothal) in the early 1930s. Many others have been synthesized, but only a handful has been used clinically (Table 7-1).

Many problems are associated with these drugs, including high abuse and addiction potential, a narrow therapeutic range with low therapeutic index, and unfavorable side effects. The use of barbiturates and similar compounds such as meprobamate (Miltown) has practically been eliminated by the benzodiazepines and hypnotics, such as zolpidem (Ambien), eszopiclone (Lunesta), and zaleplon (Sonata), which have a lower abuse potential and a higher therapeutic index than the barbiturates. Nevertheless, barbiturates still have an important role in the treatment of certain mental and convulsive disorders.

TABLE 7-1: Barbiturate Dosages (Adult)

Drug	Trade Name	Available Preparations	Hypnotic Dose Range	Anticonvulsant Dose Range
Amobarbital	Amytal	200 mg	50–300 mg	65–500 mg IV
Aprobarbital	Alurate	40-mg/5-mL elixir	40–120 mg	Not established
Butabarbital	Butisol	15-, 30-, and 50-mg tablets, 30-mg/5-mL elixir	45–120 mg	Not established
Mephobarbital	Mebaral	32-, 50-, and 100-mg tablets	100–200 mg	200–600 mg
Methohexital	Brevital	500 mg/50 cc	1 mg/kg for electroconvulsive therapy	Not established
Pentobarbital	Nembutal	50- and 100-mg capsules, 50-mg/mL injection or elixir 30-, 60-, 120-, and 200-mg suppository	100–200 mg	100 mg IV, each minute up to 500 mg
Phenobarbital	Luminal	Tablets range from 15–100 mg, 20-mg/5-mL elixir 30- to 130-mg/mL injection	30–150 mg	100–300 mg IV, up to 600 mg/day
Secobarbital	Seconal	100-mg capsule, 50-mg/mL injection	100 mg	5.5 mg/kg IV

IV, intravenous.

Since all barbiturates have a similar pharmacologic profile, they will be described as a group. Nonbarbiturate drugs will then follow.

Pharmacologic Actions

Though the parent compound of all barbiturates, barbituric acid, is poorly absorbed and produces negligible clinical effects, the barbiturates are well absorbed after oral administration. The binding of barbiturates to plasma proteins is high, but lipid solubility varies. The individual barbiturates are metabolized by the liver and excreted by the kidneys. The half-lives of specific barbiturates range from 1 to 120 hours (see Table 7-2). The barbiturates may also induce hepatic enzymes (CYP450), thereby reducing the levels of both the barbiturate and any other concurrently administered drugs metabolized by the liver. The mechanism of action of barbiturates involves the γ-aminobutyric acid (GABA) receptor–benzodiazepine receptor–chloride ion channel complex.

Therapeutic Indications

Electroconvulsive Therapy

Methohexital (Brevital) is commonly used as an anesthetic agent for electroconvulsive therapy (ECT). It has lower cardiac risks than other barbiturate anesthetics. Used intravenously (IV), methohexital produces rapid unconsciousness, and because of its rapid redistribution, it has a brief duration of action (5 to 7 minutes).

TABLE 7-2: Half Lives of Barbiturate Drugs		
Drug	Trade Name	Half-Life
Amobarbital	Amytal	15–40 hours
Aprobarbital	Alurate	14–40 hours
Butabarbital	Butisol	100 hours
Mephobarbital	Mebaral	34 hours
Methohexital	Brevital	2–6 hours
Pentobarbital	Nembutal	15–50 hours
Phenobarbital	Luminal	37–140 hours
Secobarbital	Seconal	15–40 hours

Typical dosing for ECT is 0.7 to 1.2 mg/kg. Methohexital can also be used to abort prolonged seizures in ECT or to limit postictal agitation.

Seizures

Phenobarbital (Solfoton, Luminal), the most commonly used barbiturate for treatment of seizures, has indications for the treatment of generalized tonic–clonic and simple partial seizures. Parenteral barbiturates are used in the emergency management of seizures independent of cause. IV phenobarbital should be administered slowly at 10 to 20 mg/kg for status epilepticus.

Sleep

The barbiturates reduce sleep latency and the number of awakenings during sleep, although tolerance to these effects generally develops within 2 weeks. Discontinuation of barbiturates often leads to rebound increases on electroencephalographic measures of sleep and a worsening of the insomnia.

Anxiety

The barbiturates are effective at reducing general anxiety or apprehension prior to a procedure (particularly complex surgery). However, benzodiazepines can produce similar effect with less potential for abuse and have a higher therapeutic index.

Narcoanalysis

Amobarbital (Amytal) has been used historically as a diagnostic aid in a number of clinical conditions, including conversion reactions, catatonia, hysterical stupor, and unexplained muteness, and to differentiate stupor of depression, schizophrenia, and structural brain lesions. While not commonly used for this purpose any longer, barbiturates were once described as "truth serums" because their analgesic, anxiolytic, and soporific effects were believed to grant patients access to repressed memories or to render them incapable of constructing false narratives.

Because of the risk of laryngospasm with IV amobarbital, diazepam has become the drug of choice on the rare occasion that narcoanalysis is performed.

Withdrawal from Sedative-Hypnotics

Barbiturates are sometimes used to determine the extent of tolerance to barbiturates or other hypnotics to guide detoxification. After intoxication has resolved, a test dose of pentobarbital (200 mg) is given orally. One hour later, the patient is examined. Tolerance and dose requirements are determined by the degree to which the patient is affected. If the patient is not sedated, another 100 mg of pentobarbital can be administered every 2 hours, up to three times (maximum, 500 mg over 6 hours). The amount needed for mild intoxication corresponds to the approximate daily dose of barbiturate used. Phenobarbital (30 mg) may then be substituted for each 100 mg of pentobarbital. This daily dose requirement can be administered in divided doses and gradually tapered by 10% a day, with adjustments made according to withdrawal signs.

Precautions and Adverse Reactions

Some adverse effects of barbiturates are similar to those of benzodiazepines, including paradoxical dysphoria, hyperactivity, and cognitive disorganization. Rare adverse effects associated with barbiturate use include the development of Stevens–Johnson syndrome, megaloblastic anemia, and neutropenia.

Prior to the advent of benzodiazepines, the widespread use of barbiturates as hypnotics and anxiolytics made them the most common cause of acute porphyria reactions. Severe attacks of porphyria have decreased largely because barbiturates are now seldom used and are contraindicated in patients with the disease.

A major difference between the barbiturates and the benzodiazepines is the low therapeutic index of the barbiturates. An overdose of barbiturates can easily prove fatal. In addition to narrow therapeutic indexes, the barbiturates are associated with a significant risk of abuse potential and the development of tolerance and dependence. Barbiturate intoxication is similar to acute ethanol intoxication and is manifested by confusion, drowsiness, irritability, hyporeflexia or areflexia, ataxia, and nystagmus. These drugs were commonly abused in the past, but their availability on illicit markets has diminished significantly because they have been supplanted by benzodiazepines. However, individuals can still develop barbiturate addiction, the symptoms and signs of which are noted in Table 7-3. The

TABLE 7-3: Signs and Symptoms of Barbiturate Intoxication and Abuse	
Agitation	Impaired judgment
Bradycardia	Inability to urinate
Clumsiness	Irritability
Concentration problems	Mood swings
Confusion	Respiratory arrest
Delusions	Respiratory depression
Depression	Shallow breathing
Dilated pupils	Slowed pulse
Dizziness	Sluggishness
Double vision	Slurred speech
Drowsiness	Unsatisfying sleep
Hallucinations	Unusual excitement
Hypotension	Vision problems

TABLE 7-4: Signs and Symptoms of Barbiturate Withdrawal	
Agitation	Irritability
Anxiety	Mood swings
Confusion	Nausea
Convulsions	Seizures
Delirium	Sleep disturbances
Fever	Tremors
Hallucinations	Vomiting
Hypotension	Weakness

symptoms of barbiturate withdrawal are similar to, but more severe than those of benzodiazepine withdrawal and are described in Table 7-4).

Ten times the daily dose (approximately 1 g) of most barbiturates causes severe toxicity; 2–10 g generally proves fatal. Manifestations of barbiturate intoxication may include delirium, confusion, excitement, headache, CNS, and respiratory depression ranging from somnolence to coma. Other adverse reactions include Cheyne–Stokes respiration, shock, miosis, oliguria, tachycardia, hypotension, hypothermia, irritability, hyporeflexia or areflexia, ataxia, and nystagmus.

Treatment of overdose includes induction of emesis or lavage, activated charcoal, and saline cathartics; supportive treatment, including maintaining airway and respiration and treating shock as needed; maintaining vital signs and fluid balance; alkalinizing the urine which increases excretion; forced diuresis if renal function is normal; or hemodialysis in severe cases.

Barbiturates should be used with caution by patients with a history of substance abuse, depression, diabetes, hepatic impairment, renal disease, severe anemia, pain, hyperthyroidism, or hypoadrenalism. Barbiturates are also contraindicated in patients with acute intermittent porphyria, impaired respiratory drive, or limited respiratory reserve.

Use in Pregnancy and Lactation

Because of some evidence of teratogenicity, barbiturates should not be used by pregnant women or women who are breastfeeding. They are classified as pregnancy category D drugs.

Drug Interactions

The primary area for concern about drug interactions is the potentially dangerous effects of respiratory depression. Barbiturates should be used with great caution with other prescribed CNS drugs (including antipsychotic and antidepressant drugs) and nonprescribed CNS agents (e.g., alcohol). Caution must also be exercised when prescribing barbiturates to patients who are taking other drugs that are metabolized in the liver, especially cardiac drugs and anticonvulsants. Because individual patients have a wide range of sensitivities to barbiturate-induced enzyme induction, it is not possible to predict the degree to which the metabolism of concurrently administered medications may be affected. Drugs that have their metabolism enhanced by barbiturate administration include opioids, antiarrhythmic agents, antibiotics, anticoagulants, anticonvulsants, antidepressants, β-adrenergic receptor antagonists, dopamine receptor antagonists, contraceptives, and immunosuppressants.

Laboratory Interferences

No known laboratory interferences are associated with the administration of barbiturates.

Dose and Clinical Guidelines

Barbiturates and other drugs described later begin to act within 1 to 2 hours of administration. The doses of barbiturates vary, and treatment should begin with low doses that are increased to achieve a clinical effect. Children and older people are more sensitive to the effects of barbiturates than are young adults. The most commonly used barbiturates are available in a variety of dose forms. Barbiturates with half-lives in the 15 to 40-hour range are preferable because long-acting drugs tend to accumulate in the body. Clinicians should instruct patients clearly about the adverse effects and the potential for dependence associated with barbiturates.

Although determining plasma concentrations of barbiturates is rarely necessary in psychiatry, monitoring of phenobarbital concentrations is a standard practice when the drug is used as an anticonvulsant. The therapeutic blood concentrations for phenobarbital in this indication range from 15 to 40 mg/L, although some patients may experience significant adverse effects in that range.

Barbiturates are contained in combination products with which the clinician should be familiar.

Other Similarly Acting Drugs

A number of agents that act similarly to the barbiturates have been used in the treatment of anxiety and insomnia. Three such available drugs are paraldehyde (Paral), meprobamate, and chloral hydrate (Noctec). These drugs are rarely used because of their abuse potential and potential toxic effects. Use of meprobamate has been discontinued in the European Union and Canada.

PARALDEHYDE

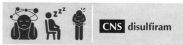

CNS disulfiram

Paraldehyde is a cyclic ether that was first observed in 1835 by German chemist Justus von Liebig and was first used in 1882 as a hypnotic. It has also been used to treat epilepsy, alcohol withdrawal symptoms, and delirium tremens. Because of its low therapeutic index, it has largely been supplanted by the benzodiazepines and other anticonvulsants.

Pharmacologic Actions

Paraldehyde is rapidly absorbed from the gastrointestinal (GI) tract and from intramuscular (IM) injections. It is primarily metabolized to acetaldehyde by the liver, and unmetabolized drug is expired by the lungs. Reported half-lives range from 3.4 to 9.8 hours. The onset of action is 15 to 30 minutes.

Therapeutic Indications

Paraldehyde is not indicated as an anxiolytic or a hypnotic and has little place in current psychopharmacology. It is occasionally used to treat status epilepticus.

Precautions and Adverse Reactions

Paraldehyde frequently causes foul breath because of expired unmetabolized drug. It can inflame pulmonary capillaries and cause coughing. It can also cause local thrombophlebitis with IV use. Patients may experience nausea and vomiting with oral use. Overdose leads to metabolic acidosis and decreases renal output. Paraldehyde is a Schedule IV drug and there is risk of abuse among individuals with a history of substance use disorders.

Use in Pregnancy and Lactation

Paraldehyde is classified as s pregnancy category C drug and should not be used during pregnancy or lactation.

Drug Interactions

Disulfiram (Antabuse) inhibits acetaldehyde dehydrogenase and reduces metabolism of paraldehyde, leading to possible toxic concentration of paraldehyde. Paraldehyde has addictive sedating effects in combination with other CNS depressants such as alcohol or benzodiazepines.

Laboratory Interferences

Paraldehyde can interfere with the metyrapone, phentolamine, and urinary 17-hydroxycorticosteroid tests.

Dosing and Clinical Guidelines

Paraldehyde is available in 30-mL vials for oral, IV, or rectal use. For seizures in adults, up to 12 mL (diluted to a 10% solution) can be administered by gastric tube every 4 hours. For children, the oral dose is 0.3 mg/kg.

MEPROBAMATE

Meprobamate, a carbamate, was introduced shortly before the benzodiazepines, specifically to treat anxiety. It is also used for muscle relaxant effects. During the 1950s and 1960s, the drug was marketed as a minor tranquilizer under the tradename Milltown and became ubiquitous in the United States. In 1957, one-third of all prescriptions written were for the drug. By the 1960s, use of meprobamate had declined due to the introduction of benzodiazepines and the realization that meprobamate was actually a sedative (not a tranquilizer) and had a relatively high potential for abuse. In 2012, marketing authorization in the EU for meprobamate was rescinded. Canada withdrew marketing authorization for the drug in 2013.

Pharmacologic Actions

Meprobamate is rapidly absorbed from the GI tract and from IM injections. It is primarily metabolized by the liver, and a small portion is excreted unchanged in urine. The plasma half-life is approximately 10 hours.

Therapeutic Indications

Meprobamate is indicated for short-term treatment of anxiety disorders. It has also been used as a hypnotic and is prescribed as a muscle relaxant. Its use is now uncommon.

Precautions and Adverse Reactions

Meprobamate can cause CNS depression and death in overdose and carries the risk of abuse by patients with drug or alcohol dependence. Abrupt cessation after long-term use can lead to withdrawal syndrome, including seizures and hallucinations. Meprobamate can exacerbate acute intermittent porphyria. Other rare side effects include hypersensitivity reactions, wheezing, hives, paradoxical excitement, and leukopenia. It should not be used in patients with hepatic compromise.

Use in Pregnancy and Lactation

Meprobamate is a pregnancy category D drug. An increased risk of congenital malformations, especially when used in the first trimester, has been suggested, and it is secreted in breastmilk. Therefore, use during pregnancy or nursing is not recommended.

Drug Interactions

Meprobamate has additive sedating effects in combination with other CNS depressants, such as alcohol, barbiturates, or benzodiazepines.

Laboratory Interferences

Meprobamate can interfere with the metyrapone, phentolamine, and urinary 17-hydroxycorticosteroid tests.

Dosing and Clinical Guidelines

Meprobamate is available in 200-, 400-, and 600-mg tablets; 200- and 400-mg extended-release capsules; and various combinations. For example, a combination of aspirin and meprobamate is available that contains 325 mg of aspirin and 200 mg of meprobamate for oral use. For adults, the usual dose is 400 to 800 mg twice daily. Elderly patients and children aged 6 to 12 years require half the adult dose.

CHLORAL HYDRATE

 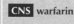 CNS warfarin

Chloral hydrate is a hypnotic agent that is only rarely used in psychiatry because numerous safer options, such as benzodiazepines, are available. It was discovered in 1832 by German chemist Justus von Liebig and it was frequently used throughout the late nineteenth and early twentieth centuries by medical professionals and members of the general public to induce sedation. Chloral hydrate has a long history of illicit use, most famously by the bartender Mickey Finn, who would lace patrons' drinks with the drug, and then rob them once they were incapacitated. Following Finn's arrest and conviction, drugging an unsuspecting individual became commonly known as "slipping someone a mickey."

Pharmacologic Actions

Chloral hydrate is well absorbed in the GI tract. The parent compound is metabolized within minutes by the liver to the active metabolite trichloroethanol, which has a half-life of 8 to 11 hours. A dose of chloral hydrate induces sleep within 30 to 60 minutes, and one may remain asleep for 4 to 8 hours. It probably potentiates GABAergic neurotransmission, which suppresses neuronal excitability.

Therapeutic Indications

Chloral hydrate is not currently available as an FDA-approved product.

Off-Label Uses

Chloral hydrate is approved for use in the United Kingdom, Canada, Australia, Abu Dhabi, and Hong Kong. The major indication for chloral hydrate is to induce sleep. It should be used for no more than 2 or 3 days because longer-term treatment is associated with an increased incidence and severity of adverse effects. Tolerance develops to the hypnotic effects of chloral hydrate after 2 weeks of treatment. The benzodiazepines are superior to chloral hydrate for all psychiatric uses.

Precautions and Adverse Reactions

Chloral hydrate has adverse effects on the CNS, GI system, and skin. High doses (>4 g) may be associated with stupor, confusion, ataxia, falls, or coma. The GI effects include nonspecific irritation, nausea, vomiting, flatulence, and an unpleasant taste. With long-term use and overdose, gastritis and gastric ulceration can develop. In addition to the development of tolerance, dependence on chloral hydrate can occur, with symptoms like those of alcohol dependence. With a lethal dose between 5,000 and 10,000 mg, chloral hydrate is a particularly poor choice for potentially suicidal persons.

Use in Pregnancy and Lactation

Chloral hydrate should not be prescribed to pregnant women and can pass through the breast milk and harm the infant.

Drug Interactions

Because of metabolic interference, chloral hydrate should be strictly avoided with alcohol, a notorious concoction known as a *Mickey Finn* or a mickey (see above). Chloral hydrate may displace warfarin (Coumadin) from plasma proteins and enhance anticoagulant activity; therefore, this combination should also be avoided.

Laboratory Interferences

Chloral hydrate administration can lead to false-positive results for urine glucose determinations that use cupric sulfate (e.g., Clinitest) but not in tests that use glucose oxidase (e.g., Clinistix and Tes-Tape). Chloral hydrate can also interfere with the determination of urinary catecholamines in 17-hydroxycorticosteroids.

Dosing and Clinical Guidelines

Chloral hydrate is available in 500-mg capsules; 500-mg/5-mL solution; and 324-, 500-, and 648-mg rectal suppositories. The standard dose of chloral hydrate is 500 to 2,000 mg at bedtime. Because the drug is a GI irritant, it should be administered with excess water, milk, other liquids, or antacids to decrease gastric irritation.

PROPOFOL

Propofol (Diprivan) is a $GABA_A$ agonist that is used as an anesthetic. It induces presynaptic release of GABA and dopamine (the latter possibility through an action on $GABA_B$ receptors) and is a partial agonist at dopamine D_2 and NMDA receptors. Because of propofol's solubility in lipids, it crosses the blood–brain barrier readily and induces anesthesia in less than 1 minute. Rapid redistribution out of the CNS results in offset of action within 3 to 8 minutes after the infusion is discontinued. It is well tolerated when used for conscious sedation, but it has a potential for acute adverse effects, including respiratory depression, apnea, and bradyarrhythmia. Prolonged infusion can cause acidosis and mitochondrial myopathies. The carrier used for the infusion is a soybean emulsion that can be a culture medium for various organisms. The carrier also can impair macrophage function and cause hematologic and lipid abnormalities and anaphylactic reactions.

There is limited evidence that high-dose propofol treatment could be used in patients with treatment-resistant depression who are otherwise healthy in a manner like ketamine. Preliminary studies have also found that propofol and a combination of propofol and remifentanil before ECT have been shown to prolong seizure duration and reduce recovery time.

ETOMIDATE

Etomidate is a carboxylated imidazole that acts at the β_2 and β_3 subunits of the $GABA_A$ receptor. It has a rapid onset (1 minute) and short duration (less than 5 minutes) of action. The propylene glycol vehicle has been linked to hyperosmolar metabolic acidosis. It has both proconvulsant and anticonvulsant properties, and it inhibits cortisol release, with possible adverse consequences after long-term use.

Preliminary research indicates that etomidate may prolong seizure duration when administered before ECT and may improve therapeutic responses to ECT when seizure length is too short.

Benzodiazepines and Drugs Acting on GABA Receptors

8

Generic Name	Trade Name	Adverse Effects	Drug Interactions	CYP Interactions
Diazepam	Valium	Sedation	CNS, clozapine, cimetidine, disulfiram, isoniazid, estrogen, oral contraceptives	3A4, 2C19
Clonazepam	Klonopin	Sedation	CNS, lithium, clozapine	3A4, 2E1
Alprazolam	Xanax	Sedation, weight gain	CNS, clozapine, nefazodone, fluvoxamine, carbamazepine	3A7, 3A4, 2C9, 3A5
Lorazepam	Ativan	Sedation	CNS, clozapine	3A4
Oxazepam	Serax	Sedation	CNS, clozapine	N/A
Chlordiazepoxide	Librium	Sedation	CNS, clozapine, cimetidine, disulfiram, isoniazid, estrogen, oral contraceptives	3A4
Clorazepate	Tranxene	Sedation	CNS, clozapine, cimetidine, disulfiram, isoniazid, estrogen, oral contraceptives	3A4
Midazolam	Versed	Sedation	CNS, clozapine	3A4
Flurazepam	Dalmane	Sedation	CNS, clozapine, cimetidine, disulfiram, isoniazid, estrogen, oral contraceptives	3A4, 2E1, 2A6
Temazepam	Restoril	Sedation	CNS, clozapine	N/A
Triazolam	Halcion	Sedation, memory impairment, agitation	CNS, clozapine, nefazodone, fluvoxamine	3A7, 3A4, 2C8, 3A5
Estazolam	ProSom	Sedation	CNS, clozapine	3A4
Quazepam	Doral	Sedation	CNS, clozapine	2C19, 2C9, 3A4, 2B6
Zolpidem	Ambien	Sedation, dizziness	CNS, clozapine	3A4, 1A2, 2C9, 2C19, 2D6
Zaleplon	Sonata	Sedation, dizziness	CNS, clozapine, cimetidine, rifampin, phenytoin, carbamazepine, phenobarbital	3A4, 3A5, 3A7
Eszopiclone	Lunesta	Sedation, confusion	CNS, clozapine	3A4, 2C8, 2E1

(continued)

Generic Name	Trade Name	Adverse Effects	Drug Interactions	CYP Interactions
Flumazenil	Romazicon	GI symptoms, dizziness, agitation, seizures, memory impairment, headache	None	N/A
Suvorexant	Belsomra	Sedation, dizziness	CNS, azole antifungals, protease inhibitors, conivaptan, nefazodone	3A, 2C19
Lemborexant	Dayvigo	Sedation	CNS, azole antifungals, anticonvulsants, nefazodone	3A4, 3A5, 2B6
Brexanolone	Zulresso	Sedation, dizziness, loss of consciousness	CNS, antidepressants, levomethadyl acetate, sodium oxybate	N/A

Introduction

Benzodiazepines are a class of drugs that were developed in the 1950s. The first benzodiazepine to be introduced was chlordiazepoxide (Librium), in 1959. This was followed 4 years later with the release of diazepam (Valium) in 1963. Since then, dozens of benzodiazepines and drugs that act on benzodiazepine receptors have been synthesized and marketed around the world. This class of drugs has a superior safety profile and are well-tolerated in the majority of patients, allowing them to supplant older antianxiety and hypnotic medications, such as the barbiturates and meprobamate (Miltown).

Though they are still commonly prescribed, many benzodiazepines are not available in the United States, and some have been discontinued due to lack of regular use. Table 8-1 provides a list of the currently available benzodiazepines in the United States.

All benzodiazepines share a similar molecular structure and have a similar effect on receptors that have been termed benzodiazepine receptors, which in turn modulate γ-aminobutyric acid (GABA) activity. Several drugs that do not target benzodiazepine receptors, including zolpidem (Ambien), zaleplon (Sonata), and eszopiclone (Lunesta)—the so-called "Z drugs"—are discussed in this chapter because their clinical effects result from binding domains located close to benzodiazepine receptors. Flumazenil (Romazicon), a benzodiazepine receptor antagonist used to reverse benzodiazepine-induced sedation and in emergency care of benzodiazepine overdosage, is also covered here.

Because benzodiazepines have a rapid anxiolytic sedative effect, they are most commonly used for acute treatment of insomnia, anxiety, agitation, or anxiety associated with any psychiatric disorder. Benzodiazepines are also used as anesthetics, anticonvulsants, and muscle relaxants and as the preferred treatment for catatonia. Remimazolam (Byfavo) was also recently approved for use by the Food and Drug Administration for the induction and maintaining of procedural sedation for procedures lasting 30 minutes or less and currently has no approved psychiatric uses. Because of the risk of psychological and physical dependence associated with long-term use of benzodiazepines, ongoing assessment should be

TABLE 8-1: Preparations and Doses of Medications Acting on the Benzodiazepine Receptor Available in the United States

Medication	Brand Name	Dose Equivalent	Usual Adult Dose (mg)	How Supplied
Diazepam	Valium	5	2.5–40.0	2-, 5-, and 10-mg tablets 15-mg slow-release tablets
Clonazepam	Klonopin	0.25	0.5–4.0	0.5-, 1.0-, and 2.0-mg tablets
Alprazolam	Xanax	0.5	0.5–6.0	0.25-, 0.5-, 1.0-, and 2.0-mg tablets 1.5-mg sustained-release tablet
Lorazepam	Ativan	1	0.5–6.0	0.5-, 1.0-, and 2.0-mg tablets 4 mg/mL parenteral
	Loreev XR		1.5–18	1-, 1.5-, 2-, and 3-mg extended-release capsules
Oxazepam	Serax	15	15–120	7.5-, 10.0-, 15.0-, and 30.0-mg capsules 15-mg tablets
Chlordiazepoxide	Librium	25	10–100	5-, 10-, and 25-mg capsules and tablets
Clorazepate	Tranxene	7.5	15–60	3.75-, 7.50-, and 15.0-mg tablets 11.25- and 22.50-mg slow-release tablets
Midazolam	Versed	0.25	1–50	5 mg/mL parenteral 1-, 2-, 5-, and 10-mL vials
Flurazepam	Dalmane	15	15–30	15- and 30-mg capsules
Temazepam	Restoril	15	7.5–30.0	7.5-, 15.0-, and 30.0-mg capsules
Triazolam	Halcion	0.125	0.125–0.250	0.125- and 0.250-mg tablets
Estazolam	ProSom	1	1–2	1- and 2-mg tablets
Quazepam	Doral	5	7.5–15.0	7.5- and 15.0-mg tablets
Zolpidem	Ambien	10	5–10	5- and 10-mg tablets
	Ambien CR	5	6.25–12.5	6.25- and 12.5-mg tablets
Zaleplon	Sonata	10	5–20	5- and 10-mg capsules
Eszopiclone	Lunesta	1	1–3	1-, 2-, and 3-mg tablets
Flumazenil	Romazicon	0.05	0.2–0.5 per min	0.1 mg/mL
5- and 10-mL vials				
Remimazolam	Byfavo		7.5–15	20-mg vial, equivalent to 27.2 mg remimazolam besylate

made as to the continued clinical need for these drugs in treating patients. In most patients, given the nature of their disorders, it is often best if benzodiazepine agents are used in conjunction with psychotherapy and in cases where alternative agents have been tried and proven ineffective or poorly tolerated. In many forms of chronic anxiety disorders, antidepressant drugs such as the selective serotonin reuptake inhibitors (SSRIs) and serotonin–norepinephrine reuptake inhibitors (SNRIs) are now used as primary treatments, with benzodiazepines used as adjuncts. Benzodiazepine abuse is rare and usually only found in patients who abuse multiple prescription and recreational drugs.

γ-Hydroxybutyrate (GHB; Xyrem) is also an agonist at the $GABA_A$ receptor, where it binds to specific GHB receptors. It is notoriously used in small doses as a recreational drug to induce euphoria and in larger doses as a "date-rape" drug, as it can lead to extreme grogginess and loss of consciousness, as well as significantly impair memory in the period following consumption.

Pharmacologic Actions

All benzodiazepines except clorazepate (Tranxene) and remimazolam are completely absorbed after oral administration and reach peak serum levels within 30 minutes to 2 hours. Metabolism of clorazepate in the stomach converts it to desmethyldiazepam, which is then completely absorbed. Remimazolam, an ultra-short acting benzodiazepine, is administered intravenously and is completely absorbed in the gastrointestinal (GI) system.

The absorption, the attainment of peak concentrations, and the onset of action are quickest for remimazolam, followed by diazepam (Valium), lorazepam (Ativan, Loreev XR), alprazolam (Xanax), triazolam (Halcion), and estazolam (ProSom). Except for remimazolam, the rapid onset of effects is important to persons who take a single dose of a benzodiazepine to calm an episodic burst of anxiety or to fall asleep rapidly. Several benzodiazepines are effective after intravenous (IV) injection, but only lorazepam and midazolam (Versed) have rapid and reliable absorption after intramuscular (IM) administration.

Diazepam, chlordiazepoxide, clonazepam (Klonopin), clorazepate, flurazepam (Dalmane), and quazepam (Doral) have plasma half-lives of 30 hours to more than 100 hours and are technically described as long-acting benzodiazepines. The plasma half-lives of these compounds can be as high as 200 hours in persons whose metabolism is genetically slow. Because the attainment of steady-state plasma concentrations of the drugs can take up to 2 weeks, persons may experience symptoms and signs of toxicity after only 7 to 10 days of treatment with a dosage that seemed initially to be in the therapeutic range.

Clinically, half-life alone does not necessarily determine the duration of therapeutic action for most benzodiazepines. The fact that all benzodiazepines are lipid soluble to varying degrees means that benzodiazepines and their active metabolites bind to plasma proteins. The extent of this binding is proportional to their lipid solubility. The amount of protein binding varies from 70% to 99%. Distribution, onset, and termination of action after a single dose are thus largely determined by benzodiazepine lipid solubility, not elimination half-life. Preparations with high lipid solubility, such as diazepam and alprazolam, are absorbed rapidly from the gastrointestinal (GI) tract and distribute rapidly to the brain by passive diffusion along a concentration gradient, resulting in a rapid onset of action. However, as the concentration of the medication increases in the brain and decreases in the bloodstream, the concentration gradient reverses itself, and these medications leave the brain rapidly, resulting in fast cessation of drug effect.

Drugs with longer elimination half-lives, such as diazepam, may remain in the bloodstream for a substantially longer period of time than their actual pharmacologic action at benzodiazepine receptors because the concentration in the brain decreases rapidly below the level necessary for a noticeable effect. In contrast, lorazepam, which has a shorter elimination half-life than diazepam but is less lipid soluble, has a slower onset of action after a single dose because the drug is absorbed and enters the brain more slowly. However, the duration of action after a single dose is longer because it takes longer for lorazepam to leave the brain and for brain levels to decrease below the concentration that produces an effect. In chronic dosing, some of these differences are not as apparent because brain levels are in equilibrium with higher and more consistent steady-state blood levels, but additional doses still produce a more rapid but briefer action with diazepam than with lorazepam. Benzodiazepines are distributed widely in adipose tissue. As a result, medications may persist in the body after discontinuation longer than would be predicted from their elimination half-lives. In addition, the dynamic half-life (i.e., duration of action on the receptor) may be longer than the elimination half-life.

The advantages of long half-life drugs over short half-life drugs include less frequent dosing, less variation in plasma concentration, and less severe withdrawal phenomena. The disadvantages include drug accumulation, increased risk of daytime psychomotor impairment, and increased daytime sedation.

The half-lives of lorazepam, oxazepam (Serax), temazepam (Restoril), and estazolam are between 8 and 30 hours. Alprazolam has a half-life of 10 to 15 hours, and triazolam has the shortest half-life (2 to 3 hours) of all the orally administered benzodiazepines. Rebound insomnia and anterograde amnesia are thought to be more of a problem with the short–half-life drugs than with the long–half-life drugs.

Because administration of medications more frequently than the elimination half-life leads to drug accumulation, medications such as diazepam and flurazepam accumulate with daily dosing, eventually resulting in increased daytime sedation.

Some benzodiazepines (e.g., oxazepam) are conjugated directly by glucuronidation and are excreted. Most benzodiazepines are oxidized first by CYP3A4 and CYP2C19, often to active metabolites. These metabolites may then be hydroxylated to another active metabolite. For example, diazepam is oxidized to desmethyldiazepam, which, in turn, is hydroxylated to produce oxazepam. These products undergo glucuronidation to inactive metabolites. A number of benzodiazepines (e.g., diazepam, chlordiazepoxide) have the same active metabolite (desmethyldiazepam), which has an elimination half-life of more than 120 hours. Flurazepam (Dalmane), a lipid-soluble benzodiazepine used as a hypnotic that has a short elimination half-life, has an active metabolite (desalkylflurazepam) with a half-life greater than 100 hours. This is another reason that the duration of action of a benzodiazepine may not correspond to the half-life of the parent drug.

Zaleplon, zolpidem, and eszopiclone are structurally distinct and vary in their binding to the GABA receptor subunits. Benzodiazepines activate all three specific GABA–benzodiazepine (GABA–BZ) binding sites of the $GABA_A$-receptor, which opens chloride channels and reduces the rate of neuronal and muscle firing. Zolpidem, zaleplon, and eszopiclone have selectivity for certain subunits of the GABA receptor. This may account for their selective sedative effects and relative lack of muscle relaxant and anticonvulsant effects.

Zolpidem, zaleplon, and eszopiclone are rapidly and well absorbed after oral administration, although absorption can be delayed by as much as 1 hour if they are taken with food. Zolpidem reaches peak plasma concentrations in 1.6 hours and has a half-life of 2.6 hours. Zaleplon reaches peak plasma concentrations in 1 hour and has a half-life of 1 hour. If taken immediately after a high-fat or heavy meal, the peak is delayed by approximately 1 hour, reducing the effects of eszopiclone on sleep onset. The terminal-phase elimination half-life is approximately 6 hours in healthy adults. Eszopiclone is weakly bound to plasma protein (52% to 59%).

The rapid metabolism and lack of active metabolites of zolpidem, zaleplon, and eszopiclone avoid the accumulation of plasma concentrations compared to the long-term use of benzodiazepines.

Flumazenil is a benzodiazepine antagonist that can reverse the binding of benzodiazepine agonists and is used to negate the effects of benzodiazepines, particularly during an overdose. Following oral administration, flumazenil is rapidly absorbed with peak concentrations being achieved within 20 to 90 minutes. Terminal half-life is 40 to 80 minutes and is almost completely metabolized by the liver and excreted within 72 hours (90% to 95% in urine and 5% to 10% in feces). Onset of action is typically 1 to 2 minutes, with an 80% response occurring within 3 minutes of administration. Peak effect is reached within 6 to 10 minutes and duration ranges between 19 and 50 minutes, depending on dose and the plasma concentration of benzodiazepines.

Therapeutic Indications

For a brief list of FDA-approved indications and off-label uses of benzodiazepines, see Table 8-2.

Insomnia

Insomnia is oftentimes a symptom of a physical or a psychiatric disorder, so clinicians should not prescribe hypnotics for more than 7 to 10 consecutive days without conducting a thorough investigation into why the patient is having difficulty sleeping. That said, many patients have long-standing sleep difficulties and can benefit greatly from long-term use of hypnotic agents.

Temazepam, flurazepam, estazolam, quazepam, and triazolam are benzodiazepines with a sole indication for insomnia. Zolpidem, zaleplon, and eszopiclone are also indicated only for insomnia. Although these "Z drugs" are not usually associated with rebound insomnia after the discontinuation of their use for short periods, some patients experience increased sleep difficulties the first few nights after discontinuing their use. Use of zolpidem, zaleplon, and eszopiclone for periods longer than 1 month is not associated with the delayed emergence of adverse effects. No development of tolerance to any parameter of sleep measurement was observed over 6 months in clinical trials of eszopiclone.

Flurazepam, temazepam, quazepam, estazolam, and triazolam are approved for use as hypnotics. The benzodiazepine hypnotics differ principally in their

TABLE 8-2: Indications and Off-Label Uses of Benzodiazepines

Medication	Brand Name	FDA Indications	Off-Label Uses
Diazepam	Valium	Anxiety disorders, procedure-related anxiety, alcohol withdrawal syndrome, spasms, status epilepticus, seizures	Spasticity for children with cerebral palsy
Clonazepam	Klonopin	Seizure disorders, panic disorder	Acute mania, restless leg syndrome, insomnia, tardive dyskinesia, akathisia, rapid eye movement disorder, bruxism
Alprazolam	Xanax	Anxiety disorders, panic disorders with and without agoraphobia	Insomnia, premenstrual dysphoric disorder (PMDD), depression
Lorazepam	Ativan	Short-term relief of symptoms associated with anxiety disorders, anxiety-associated insomnia, procedure-related anxiety, status epilepticus	Alcohol withdrawal syndrome, insomnia, panic disorder, delirium, psychogenic catatonia, antiemetic following or prior to chemotherapy, tranquilization of agitated patients
Oxazepam	Serax	Anxiety disorders, alcohol withdrawal syndrome	Insomnia, sleep terrors, posttraumatic stress disorder (PTSD), social phobia, catatonia, confusional arousal, premenstrual dysphoric disorder
Chlordiazepoxide	Librium	Anxiety disorders, alcohol withdrawal syndrome	Catatonia, social phobia, insomnia, PTSD, PMDD
Clorazepate	Tranxene	Anxiety disorders, alcohol withdrawal syndrome, seizures	
Midazolam	Versed	For sedation, anxiolysis and amnesia prior to induction of anesthesia; seizures; status epilepticus	Behavioral or psychological disturbances in geriatric populations
Flurazepam	Dalmane	Insomnia	
Temazepam	Restoril	Short-term insomnia	
Triazolam	Halcion	Short-term insomnia	Procedure-related anxiety
Estazolam	ProSom	Short-term insomnia	
Quazepam	Doral	Short-term insomnia	
Zolpidem	Ambien	Short-term Insomnia	Traumatic brain injury, Parkinson disease, dystonia, prolonged disorders of consciousness
Zaleplon	Sonata	Short-term insomnia	Alzheimer-related sleep difficulties
Eszopiclone	Lunesta	Insomnia	
Flumazenil	Romazicon	Benzodiazepine overdose, reversal of postoperative benzodiazepine sedation	Alcohol withdrawal syndrome, cannabis intoxication, baclofen intoxication, hepatic encephalopathy
Remimazolam	Byfavo	Induction and maintenance of procedural sedation in adults undergoing surgical procedures lasting 30 minutes or less	

half-lives. Flurazepam has the longest half-life, while triazolam has the shortest. Flurazepam may be associated with minor cognitive impairment on the day after its administration, and triazolam may be associated with mild rebound anxiety and anterograde amnesia. Quazepam may be associated with daytime impairment when used for a long time. Temazepam or estazolam may be a reasonable compromise for most adults. Estazolam produces rapid onset of sleep and a hypnotic effect for 6 to 8 hours.

GHB is approved for the treatment of narcolepsy and improves slow-wave sleep. GHB also has the capacity both to reduce drug craving and to induce dependence, abuse, and absence seizures as a result of complex actions on tegmental dopaminergic systems.

Several other benzodiazepines are used off-label to treat insomnia, including chlordiazepoxide, oxazepam, lorazepam, clonazepam, and alprazolam. Zaleplon may be useful in treating sleep difficulties among patients with Alzheimer disease.

Anxiety Disorders

Generalized Anxiety Disorder.   Benzodiazepines like diazepam, alprazolam, lorazepam, oxazepam, chlordiazepoxide, and clorazepate are highly effective for the relief of anxiety associated with generalized anxiety disorder. Most persons should be treated for a predetermined, specific, and relatively brief period. However, because generalized anxiety disorder is a chronic disorder with a high rate of recurrence, some persons with generalized anxiety disorder may warrant long-term maintenance treatment with benzodiazepines.

Panic Disorder.   Alprazolam and clonazepam, both high-potency benzodiazepines, are commonly used medications for panic disorder with or without agoraphobia. Although SSRIs are also indicated for treatment of panic disorder, benzodiazepines have the advantage of working quickly and not causing significant sexual dysfunction and weight gain. However, SSRIs are still often preferred because they target common comorbid conditions, such as depression or obsessive-compulsive disorder. Benzodiazepines and SSRIs can be initiated together to treat acute panic symptoms. Use of the benzodiazepine can be tapered after 3 to 4 weeks, as the therapeutic benefits of the SSRI will have taken effect.

Lorazepam has been shown to be effective for panic disorder, as well, but is not currently indicated for this use.

Social Phobia.   Clonazepam has been shown to be an effective treatment for social phobia. In addition, several other benzodiazepines (e.g., diazepam) have been used as adjunctive medications for treatment of social phobia. Additionally, chlordiazepoxide and oxazepam have been used off-label to treat this condition.

Other Anxiety Disorders.   Benzodiazepines are used adjunctively for treatment of adjustment disorder with anxiety, pathologic anxiety associated with life events (e.g., after an accident), and obsessive-compulsive disorder. Benzodiazepines like diazepam, lorazepam, and midazolam are also regularly used to relieve procedure-related anxiety, particularly before major surgeries. Midazolam may also induce sedation and amnesia prior to induction of anesthesia.

Triazolam has been used off-label to quell procedure-related anxiety.

Anxiety Associated with Depression. Depressed patients often experience significant anxiety, and antidepressant drugs may cause initial exacerbation of these symptoms. Accordingly, benzodiazepines are indicated for the treatment of anxiety associated with depression. Use of alprazolam in the treatment of depression is not uncommon, but evidence to support its efficacy is inconclusive.

Anxiety-Induced Insomnia. In addition to treating both anxiety and insomnia, lorazepam is specifically indicated for the use of treating anxiety-induced insomnia.

Spasticity and Seizures

Benzodiazepines are indicated for adjunctive use in the treatment of skeletal muscle spasms due to local pathology, upper motor neuron disorders, athetosis, stiff person syndrome, and tetanus. Diazepam, clonazepam, and midazolam are indicated for use in treating seizure disorders, and are often useful adjuncts when treating these disorders, particularly for those who are resistant to standard treatments. Diazepam, lorazepam, clorazepate, and midazolam are also indicated for use in treating status epilepticus.

Diazepam may be used off-label for treating spasticity in children with cerebral palsy.

Alcohol Withdrawal Syndrome

Diazepam, oxazepam, chlordiazepoxide, and clorazepate are used to manage the symptoms of alcohol withdrawal. Lorazepam may also be used off-label to treat these symptoms. Flumazenil may also be effective at treating alcohol withdrawal syndromes, particularly in patients who are exhibiting signs of concomitant benzodiazepine abuse.

Off-Label Uses

Bipolar I and II Disorders

Clonazepam, lorazepam, and alprazolam are effective in the management of acute manic episodes and as an adjuvant to maintenance therapy in lieu of antipsychotics. As an adjuvant to lithium (Eskalith) or lamotrigine (Lamictal), clonazepam may increase intervals between mood cycles and fewer depressive episodes. Benzodiazepines may help patients with bipolar disorder sleep better.

Akathisia

The first-line drug for akathisia is most commonly a β-adrenergic receptor antagonist. However, benzodiazepines are also effective in treating some patients with akathisia, particularly clonazepam.

Catatonia

Lorazepam, sometimes in low doses (less than 5 mg per day), and at other times in very high doses (12 mg per day or more), is regularly used to treat acute catatonia, which is more frequently associated with bipolar disorder than with schizophrenia. Other benzodiazepines, particularly oxazepam and chlordiazepoxide, have also been said to be helpful. However, there are no valid controlled trials of benzodiazepines in catatonia. Of note, chronic catatonia does not respond as well to benzodiazepines. The definitive treatment for catatonia is electroconvulsive therapy.

Parkinson Disease

A small number of persons with idiopathic Parkinson disease respond to long-term use of zolpidem with reduced bradykinesia and rigidity. Zolpidem dosages of 10 mg four times daily may be tolerated without sedation for several years.

Posttraumatic Stress Disorder

There is limited evidence to support the use of benzodiazepines in the treatment of posttraumatic stress disorder (PTSD), though some patients may experience short-term relief from specific symptoms.

Other Psychiatric Indications

The benzodiazepines (especially IM lorazepam) are used to manage substance induced and psychotic agitation in the emergency department. Benzodiazepines have been used instead of amobarbital (Amytal) for drug-assisted interviewing. Some benzodiazepines, particularly alprazolam, oxazepam, and chlordiazepoxide have been used to treat premenstrual dysphoric disorder.

Additionally, clonazepam may be effective at treating tardive dyskinesia, restless leg syndrome, rapid eye movement behavior disorder, and bruxism.

Oxazepam may be effective at treating sleep disorders, including sleep terrors and confusional arousal. Midazolam has been shown to be effective in quelling behavioral or psychological disturbances in geriatric populations, though more studies are needed to confirm how well tolerated its use is among this population.

Subsedative doses of zolpidem have been shown to help patients recover from stroke, traumatic brain injury, and hypoxia. There is also some evidence that zolpidem may restore brain function in patients currently in vegetative state following traumatic brain injury after having been treated for several months, particularly if the injury affected nonbrainstem areas. There is limited evidence to support its use in chronic disorders of consciousness, too. However, these benefits are far from universal.

Precautions and Adverse Reactions

The most common adverse effect of the benzodiazepines is drowsiness, which occurs in about 10% of all persons. Because of this adverse effect, persons should be advised to be careful while driving or using dangerous machinery when taking the drugs. Drowsiness can be present several hours after waking following the use of benzodiazepines to treat insomnia. This is known as residual daytime sedation. Some persons also experience ataxia (fewer than 2%) and dizziness (less than 1%). These symptoms can result in falls and hip fractures, especially in elderly persons.

The most serious adverse effects of the benzodiazepines occur when other sedative substances, such as alcohol, are taken concurrently. These combinations can result in marked drowsiness, disinhibition, or even respiratory depression.

Infrequently, benzodiazepine receptor agonists cause mild cognitive deficits that may impair job performance. Persons taking benzodiazepine receptor agonists should be advised to exercise additional caution when driving or operating dangerous machinery.

High-potency benzodiazepines, especially triazolam, can cause anterograde amnesia. A paradoxical increase in aggression has been reported in persons with preexisting brain damage. Allergic reactions to the drugs are rare, but a few studies report maculopapular rashes and generalized itching. The symptoms of benzodiazepine intoxication include confusion, slurred speech, ataxia, drowsiness, dyspnea, and hyporeflexia.

Triazolam has received significant attention in the media because of an alleged association with serious aggressive behavioral manifestations. Therefore, the manufacturer recommends that the drug be used for no more than 10 days for treatment of insomnia and that physicians carefully evaluate the emergence of any abnormal thinking or behavioral changes in persons treated with triazolam and take into consideration all potential causes. Triazolam was banned in Great Britain in 1991.

Zolpidem (Ambien) has also been associated with automatic behavior and amnesia. Some complex behaviors, including driving and eating, have been reported.

Persons with hepatic disease and elderly persons are particularly likely to have adverse effects and toxicity from the benzodiazepines, including hepatic coma, especially when the drugs are administered repeatedly or in high dosages. Benzodiazepines can produce clinically significant impairment of respiration in persons with chronic obstructive pulmonary disease and sleep apnea. Alprazolam may exert a direct appetite stimulant effect and may cause weight gain. The benzodiazepines should be used with caution by persons with a history of substance abuse, cognitive disorders, renal disease, hepatic disease, porphyria, central nervous system (CNS) depression, or myasthenia gravis.

Zolpidem and zaleplon are generally well tolerated. At zolpidem dosages of 10 mg per day and zaleplon dosages above 10 mg per day, a small number of persons will experience dizziness, drowsiness, dyspepsia, or diarrhea. The dosage of zolpidem and zaleplon should be reduced in elderly persons and persons with hepatic impairment.

In rare cases, zolpidem may cause hallucinations and behavioral changes. The coadministration of zolpidem and SSRIs may extend the duration of hallucinations in susceptible patients.

Eszopiclone exhibits a dose–response relationship in elderly adults for the side effects of pain, dry mouth, and unpleasant taste.

Use in Pregnancy and Lactation

The benzodiazepines are commonly used during pregnancy and there is some positive evidence of fetal risk, including preterm delivery, floppy infant syndrome, and low birth weight but these risks may not outweigh the potential benefits of the drug. Consequently, most benzodiazepines are classified as pregnancy category D drugs. The drugs are secreted in the breast milk and are therefore contraindicated for use by nursing mothers.

Tolerance, Dependence, and Withdrawal

When benzodiazepines are used for short periods (1 to 2 weeks) in moderate dosages, they usually cause no significant tolerance, dependence, or withdrawal effects. The short-acting benzodiazepines (e.g., triazolam) may be an exception to this rule because some persons have reported increased anxiety the day after taking a single dose of the drug and then stopping its use. Some persons also report a tolerance for the anxiolytic effects of benzodiazepines and require increased doses to maintain the clinical remission of symptoms.

The appearance of a withdrawal syndrome, also called a discontinuation syndrome, depends on the length of time the person has been taking a benzodiazepine, the dosage the person has been taking, the rate at which the drug is tapered, and the half-life of the compound. Benzodiazepine withdrawal syndrome consists of anxiety, nervousness, diaphoresis, restlessness, irritability, fatigue, light-headedness, tremor, insomnia, and weakness (Table 8-3). Abrupt discontinuation of benzodiazepines, particularly those with short half-lives, is associated with severe withdrawal symptoms, which may include depression, paranoia, delirium, and seizures. These severe symptoms are more likely to occur if flumazenil is used for rapid reversal of the benzodiazepine receptor agonist effects. Some features of the syndrome may occur in as many as 90% of persons treated with the drugs. The development of a severe withdrawal syndrome is seen only in persons who have taken high dosages for long periods. The appearance of the syndrome may be delayed for 1 or 2 weeks in persons who had been taking benzodiazepines with long half-lives. Alprazolam seems to be particularly associated with an immediate and severe withdrawal syndrome and should be tapered gradually.

When the medication is to be discontinued, the drug must be tapered slowly, typically at a rate of 25% of the original dose every 2 weeks with at least one interval in dose reduction (see Table 8-4); otherwise, recurrence or rebound of symptoms is likely. Monitoring of any withdrawal symptoms (possibly with a standardized rating scale) and psychological support of the person are helpful in the successful accomplishment of benzodiazepine discontinuation. Concurrent use of carbamazepine (Tegretol) during benzodiazepine discontinuation has been reported to permit a more rapid and better-tolerated withdrawal than does a gradual taper alone. The dosage range of carbamazepine used to facilitate withdrawal is 400 to 500 mg a day. Some clinicians report difficulty in tapering and discontinuing alprazolam, especially in persons who have been receiving high dosages for

TABLE 8-3: Signs and Symptoms of Benzodiazepine Withdrawal

Anxiety	Tremor
Irritability	Depersonalization
Insomnia	Hyperesthesia
Hyperacusis	Myoclonus
Nausea	Delirium
Difficulty concentrating	Seizures

TABLE 8-4: Example of a Benzodiazepine Tapering Schedule		
Time	Action	Dosage
Week 0	No action	40 mg/day
Week 1	Decrease dose by 5 mg	35 mg/day
Week 2	Decrease dose by 5 mg	30 mg/day (75% of original dose)
Week 3	Decrease dose by 5 mg	25 mg/day
Week 4	Decrease dose by 5 mg	20 mg/day (50% of original dose)
Week 5–8	Hold dose	20 mg/day
Week 9–10	Decrease dose by 5 mg	15 mg/day
Week 11–12	Decrease dose by 5 mg	10 mg/day (25% of original dose)
Week 13–14	Decrease dose by 5 mg	5 mg/day
Week 15	Decrease dose by 5 mg	0 mg

long periods. There have been reports of successful discontinuation of alprazolam by switching to clonazepam, which is then gradually withdrawn.

Zolpidem and zaleplon can produce a mild withdrawal syndrome lasting 1 day after prolonged use at higher therapeutic dosages. Rarely, a person taking zolpidem has self-titrated up the daily dosage to 30 to 40 mg a day. Abrupt discontinuation of such a high dosage of zolpidem may cause withdrawal symptoms for 4 or more days. Tolerance does not develop to the sedative effects of zolpidem and zaleplon.

Drug Interactions

The most common and potentially serious benzodiazepine receptor agonist interaction is excessive sedation and respiratory depression occurring when benzodiazepines, zolpidem, or zaleplon are administered concomitantly with other CNS depressants, such as alcohol, barbiturates, tricyclic and tetracyclic drugs, dopamine receptor antagonists, opioids, and antihistamines. Ataxia and dysarthria may be likely to occur when lithium, antipsychotics, and clonazepam are combined. The combination of benzodiazepines and clozapine (Clozaril) has been reported to cause delirium and should be avoided. Cimetidine (Tagamet), disulfiram (Antabuse), isoniazid, estrogen, and oral contraceptives increase the plasma concentrations of diazepam, chlordiazepoxide, clorazepate, and flurazepam. Cimetidine increases the plasma concentrations of zaleplon. The plasma concentrations of triazolam and alprazolam are increased to potentially toxic concentrations by nefazodone (Serzone) and fluvoxamine (Luvox). The manufacturer of nefazodone recommends that the dosage of triazolam be lowered by 75% and the dosage of alprazolam lowered by 50% when given concomitantly with nefazodone. However, antacids may reduce GI absorption of benzodiazepines.

Over-the-counter preparations of kava plant, advertised as a "natural tranquilizer," can potentiate the action of benzodiazepine receptor agonists through synergistic overactivation of GABA receptors. Carbamazepine can lower the plasma concentration of alprazolam. Antacids and food may decrease the plasma concentrations of benzodiazepines, and smoking may increase the metabolism of benzodiazepines. Rifampin (Rifadin), phenytoin (Dilantin), carbamazepine, and phenobarbital (Solfoton, Luminal) significantly increase the metabolism of zaleplon. The benzodiazepines may increase the plasma concentrations of phenytoin and digoxin (Lanoxin). The SSRIs may prolong and exacerbate the severity of zolpidem-induced hallucinations. Deaths have been reported when parental lorazepam is given with parental olanzapine.

The CYP3A4 and CYP2E1 enzymes are involved in the metabolism of eszopiclone. Eszopiclone did not show any inhibitory potential on CYP450 1A2, 2A6, 2C9, 2C19, 2D6, 2E1, and 3A4 in cryopreserved human hepatocytes. Coadministration of 3 mg of eszopiclone to subjects receiving 400 mg of ketoconazole, a potent inhibitor of CYP3A4, resulted in a 2.2-fold increase in exposure to eszopiclone.

Laboratory Interferences

No known laboratory interferences are associated with the use of the benzodiazepines, zolpidem, and zaleplon.

Dosage and Clinical Guidelines

The clinical decision to treat an anxious person with a benzodiazepine should be carefully considered, and medical causes of anxiety (e.g., thyroid dysfunction, caffeinism, and prescription medications) should first be ruled out. Benzodiazepine use should be started at a low dosage, and the person should be instructed regarding the drug's sedative properties and abuse potential. An estimated length of therapy should be decided at the beginning of therapy, and the need for continued therapy should be reevaluated at least monthly because of the problems associated with long-term use. However, certain persons with anxiety disorders are unresponsive to treatments other than benzodiazepines in long-term use.

Benzodiazepines are available in a wide range of formulations. Clonazepam is available in a wafer formulation that facilitates its use in patients who have trouble swallowing pills. Alprazolam and lorazepam (Loreev XR) are available in extended-release forms, which reduces the frequency of dosing. For example, patients taking Loreev XR only need to take one dose in the morning rather than three divided doses of the nonextended release over the course of the day. Some benzodiazepines are more potent than others in that one compound requires a relatively smaller dosage than another compound to achieve the same effect. For example, clonazepam requires 0.25 mg to achieve the same effect as 5 mg of diazepam; thus, clonazepam is considered a high-potency benzodiazepine. Conversely, oxazepam has an approximate dosage equivalence of 15 mg and is a low-potency drug.

Zaleplon is available in 5- and 10-mg capsules. A single 10-mg dose is the usual adult dose. The dose can be increased to a maximum of 20 mg as tolerated. A single dose of zaleplon can be expected to provide 4 hours of sleep with minimal residual impairment. For persons older than age 65 or persons with hepatic impairment, an initial dose of 5 mg is advised.

Eszopiclone is available in 1-, 2-, and 3-mg tablets. The starting dose should not exceed 1 mg in patients with severe hepatic impairment or those taking potent CYP3A4 inhibitors. The recommended dosing to improve sleep onset or maintenance is 2 or 3 mg for adult patients (ages 18 to 64 years) and 2 mg for older adult patients (ages 65 years and older). The 1-mg dose is for sleep onset in older adult patients whose primary complaint is difficulty falling asleep.

Table 8-1 lists preparations and doses of medications discussed in this chapter.

FLUMAZENIL

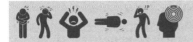

Benzodiazepine Overdosage

Flumazenil is used to reverse the adverse psychomotor, amnestic, and sedative effects of benzodiazepine receptor agonists, including benzodiazepines, zolpidem, and zaleplon. Flumazenil is administered via IV and has a half-life of 7 to 15 minutes. The most common adverse effects of flumazenil are nausea, vomiting, dizziness, agitation, emotional lability, cutaneous vasodilation, injection-site pain, fatigue, impaired vision, and headache. The most common serious adverse effect associated with the use of flumazenil is the precipitation of seizures, which is especially likely to occur in persons with seizure disorders, those who are physically dependent on benzodiazepines, and those who have ingested large quantities of benzodiazepines. Flumazenil alone may impair memory retrieval.

In mixed drug overdosage, the toxic effects (e.g., seizures and cardiac arrhythmias) of other drugs (e.g., tricyclic antidepressants) may emerge with the reversal of the benzodiazepine effects of flumazenil. For example, seizures caused by an overdosage of tricyclic antidepressants may have been partially suppressed in a person who had also taken an overdosage of benzodiazepines. With flumazenil treatment, the tricyclic-induced seizures or cardiac arrhythmias may appear and result in a fatal outcome.

For the initial management of a known or suspected benzodiazepine overdosage, the recommended initial dosage of flumazenil is 0.2 mg (2 mL) administered IV over 30 seconds. If the desired consciousness is not obtained after 30 seconds, a further dose of 0.3 mg (3 mL) can be administered over 30 seconds. Further doses of 0.5 mg (5 mL) can be administered over 30 seconds at 1-minute intervals up to a cumulative dose of 3.0 mg. The clinician should not rush the administration of flumazenil. A secure airway and IV access should be established before the administration of the drug. Persons should be awakened gradually.

Most persons with a benzodiazepine overdose respond to a cumulative dose of 1 to 3 mg of flumazenil; doses above 3 mg of flumazenil do not reliably produce additional effects. If a person has not responded 5 minutes after receiving a cumulative dose of 5 mg of flumazenil, the major cause of sedation is probably not benzodiazepine receptor agonists, and additional flumazenil is unlikely to have an effect.

Sedation can return in 1% to 3% of persons treated with flumazenil. It can be prevented or treated by giving repeated dosages of flumazenil at 20-minute intervals. For repeat treatment, no more than 1 mg (given as 0.5 mg a minute) should be given at any one time, and no more than 3 mg should be given in any 1 hour.

Flumazenil Off-Label Uses

Flumazenil has been used to treat alcohol withdrawal syndrome, cannabis intoxication, and baclofen intoxication, but does not reverse the effects of ethanol, barbiturates, or opioids. It has also shown some efficacy in the treatment of hepatic encephalopathy.

OREXIN ANTAGONISTS—SUVOREXANT (BELSOMRA) AND LEMBOREXANT (DAYVIGO)

Suvorexant (Belsomra) and lemborexant (Dayvigo) are dual orexin receptor antagonists currently indicated for the treatment of insomnia. In this respect, these medications differ from other commonly prescribed sleep aids that cause sleepiness by enhancing GABA or melatonin activity.

Suvorexant was approved for use by the FDA in 2014, while lemborexant was approved in 2019. Both drugs block orexin, a molecule that functions in the brain to keep people awake and alert, and the effects are oftentimes felt immediately. Peak plasma concentration is achieved in 2 hours for suvorexant and ranges from 1 to 3 hours for lemborexant. The half-lives of the former have been estimated to be 9.0 ± 7.2 hours at 10 mg and 10.8 ± 3.6 hours at 50 mg, while mean half-life for the latter is 17 hours for 5 mg and 19 hours for 10 mg. Both drugs are metabolized by CYP3A isoenzymes, while CYP2C19 plays a minor role in the metabolism of suvorexant. Residual daytime sedation was the most reported side effect and is more common in females than males. This effect appears to be related to dose. Both drugs are classified as pregnancy category C drugs, as no well-controlled studies have been conducted on how they affect nursing or pregnant individuals.

The FDA has approved suvorexant in four different strengths: 5, 10, 15, and 20 mg. The recommended dose to start is 10 mg taken 30 minutes prior to bedtime and at least 7 hours before planned wake time. The maximum recommended dosage is 20 mg. Lemborexant has been approved in two different strengths, 5- and 10-mg tablets. The recommended dose to start is 5 mg taken 30 minutes prior to bedtime and at least 7 hours before planned wake time. Dosage may be increased to 10 mg based on clinical response and tolerability. Individuals with moderate hepatic impairment should not take more 5 mg of lemborexant and is not recommended for use in patients with severe hepatic impairment.

BREXANOLONE

 CNS antidepressants

Brexanolone is an antidepressant used in postpartum depression but is mentioned here since its mechanism of action involves GABA receptor modulation.

Brexanolone (Zulresso) is the first drug to be granted FDA approval for the treatment of postpartum depression. The FDA granted brexanolone Breakthrough Therapy Designation because postpartum depression is a severe condition affecting between 10% and 20% of women worldwide that presents with significant depressive symptoms following delivery. Comorbid anxiety is common.

Pharmacologic Actions

Brexanolone has a very low bioavailability of <5% with protein binding greater than 99%. The drug is extensively metabolized via keto-reduction, glucuronidation, and sulfation, and <1% of the parent compound was recovered unchanged in urine. It is eliminated through feces (47%) and urine (42%). The terminal half-life of brexanolone is approximately 9 hours. Major metabolites are not pharmacologically active.

The mechanism of action of brexanolone is unknown. It is an aqueous formulation of allopregnanolone, a metabolite of progesterone. Allopregnanolone is an endogenous neuroactive steroid that serves as a positive allosteric modulator at $GABA_A$ receptors.

Therapeutic Indications

Brexanolone is indicated for postpartum depression.

Precautions and Adverse Events

There is a black box warning for brexanolone because patients treated with the drug may develop excessive sedation or sudden loss of consciousness. Consequently, brexanolone is only available through a restricted program called the Zulresso Risk Evaluation and Mitigation Strategy (ZULRESSO REMS).

Common side effects associated with use included sedation, dizziness, dry mouth, flushing, loss of consciousness, diarrhea, oropharyngeal pain, dyspepsia, and tachycardia. Overdosage may result in loss of consciousness, sedation, and respiratory challenges.

Use in Pregnancy and Lactation

No controlled studies have determined the potential risks to fetal development if brexanolone is used during pregnancy, though other drugs that cause GABAergic inhibition have been shown to cause harm. At this time, brexanolone has not been assigned to a pregnancy category.

The relative infant dose is very low (between 1% and 2% of the maternal weight-adjusted dosage). Available data does not suggest a significant risk to breastfed infants, though risk cannot be ruled out.

Drug Interactions

Excessive sedation and respiratory depression may occur when used with other CNS depressants, such as alcohol, barbiturates, tricyclic and tetracyclic drugs, dopamine receptor antagonists, opioids, and antihistamines. Antidepressants may also lead to increased risk of sedation-related events.

Benzodiazepines and Drugs Acting on GABA Receptors

Dosage and Clinical Guidelines

Brexanolone is supplied in vials as a concentrated solution requiring dilution before administration via infusion. The diluted product can be kept in infusion bags at room temperature for 12 hours but under refrigerated conditions for up to 96 hours. Administration will require at least five infusion bags. Additional bags will be required for patients weighing >90 kg.

Brexanolone is administered over the course of 60 hours as follows:

- 0 to 4 hours: 30 mcg/kg/h
- 4 to 24 hours: Increase dosage to 60 mcg/kg/h
- 24 to 52 hours: Increase dosage to 90 mcg/kg/h; if the patient cannot tolerate the 90 mcg/kg/h dosage, return to 60 mcg/kg/h dosage
- 52 to 56 hours: Decrease dosage to 60 mcg/kg/h
- 56 to 60 hours: Decrease dosage to 30 mcg/kg/h

Bupropion

9

venlafaxine, lithium, fluoxetine, MAOI
dopamine agonists, dopamine receptor
antagonists

2B6
2D6

Introduction

Bupropion (Wellbutrin, Wellbutrin SR, Wellbutrin XL, Zyban) is one of the most commonly prescribed antidepressant drugs on the market and inhibits the reuptake of norepinephrine, dopamine, and, to a far lesser extent, serotonin. As it only acts weakly upon the serotonin system, its side-effect profile is characterized by minimal risks of sexual dysfunction and sedation and with modest weight loss during acute and long-term treatment. No withdrawal syndrome has been linked to the discontinuation of bupropion.

Although increasingly used as first-line monotherapy, a significant percentage of bupropion use occurs as add-on therapy to other antidepressants, usually SSRIs. Bupropion is also a nicotinic acetylcholine receptor antagonist and has thus been marketed under the name Zyban for use in smoking cessation regimens, so clinicians should not combine these two formulations as this may increase the risk of adverse effects, particularly seizures. A bupropion/naltrexone combination (Contrave) is FDA approved for weight loss. Bupropion also has the unique clinical distinction of being the only antidepressant approved by the FDA as a proven treatment for seasonal affective disorder (SAD).

Pharmacologic Actions

Three formulations of bupropion are available: immediate release (taken three times daily), sustained release (taken twice daily), and extended release (taken once daily). The different versions of the drug contain the same active ingredient but differ in their pharmacokinetics and dosing. There have been reports of inconsistencies in bioequivalence between various branded and generic versions of bupropion. Any changes with this drug in tolerability or clinical efficacy in a patient who had been doing well should prompt an inquiry about whether these changes correspond to a switch to a new formulation.

Immediate-release bupropion is well absorbed from the gastrointestinal (GI) tract. Peak plasma concentrations are usually reached within 2 hours of oral administration, while peak levels of the sustained-release version are seen after 3 hours. The mean half-life of the compound is 12 hours with a range of 8 to 40 hours. Peak levels of extended-release bupropion occur 5 hours after ingestion. This provides a longer time to maximum plasma concentration (t_{max}) but comparable peak and trough plasma concentrations. The 24-hour exposure occurring after administration of the extended-release version of 300 mg once daily is equivalent to that provided by sustained release of 150 mg twice daily.

101

Clinically, this permits the drug to be taken once a day in the morning. Plasma levels are also reduced in the evening, making it less likely for some patients to experience treatment-related insomnia. Bupropion is almost exclusively metabolized by cytochrome P450 CYP2B6 isoenzymes, while its major metabolites are CYP2D6 inhibitors.

The mechanism of action for the antidepressant effects of bupropion is presumed to involve the inhibition of dopamine and norepinephrine reuptake. Bupropion binds to the dopamine transporter in the brain. The effects of bupropion on smoking cessation may be related to its effects on dopamine reward pathways and antagonistic activity at nicotinic acetylcholine receptors. Recent evidence has found that bupropion acts upon the serotonin system by inhibiting serotonin-induced currents in 5-HT_{3A} and 5-HT_{3AB} receptors.

Therapeutic Indications

Depression

Although overshadowed by the SSRIs as first-line treatment for major depression, the therapeutic efficacy of bupropion in depression is well established in both outpatient and inpatient settings. Observed rates of response and remission are comparable to those seen with the SSRIs. Bupropion has been found to prevent seasonal major depressive episodes in patients with a history of seasonal pattern or affective disorder.

Smoking Cessation

Marketed under the brand name Zyban, bupropion is indicated for use in combination with behavioral modification programs for smoking cessation. It is intended to be used in patients who are highly motivated and who receive some form of structured behavioral support. Bupropion is most effective when combined with nicotine substitutes (Nicoderm, Nicotrol).

Off-Label Uses

Attention-Deficit/Hyperactivity Disorder

Bupropion is used as a second-line agent, after the sympathomimetics, for treatment of attention-deficit/hyperactivity disorder (ADHD) in adults and pediatric patients. It has not been compared with proven ADHD medications such as methylphenidate (Ritalin), amphetamine/dextroamphetamine (Adderall), or atomoxetine (Strattera) for childhood and adult ADHD. Bupropion is an appropriate choice for persons with comorbid ADHD and depression or persons with comorbid ADHD, conduct disorder, or substance abuse. It may also be considered for use in patients who develop tics when treated with psychostimulants or have an aversion to such drugs.

Bipolar Disorders

Bupropion is less likely than tricyclic antidepressants to precipitate mania in persons with bipolar I disorder and less likely than other antidepressants to exacerbate or induce rapid cycling bipolar II disorder. However, the evidence about use of bupropion in the treatment of patients with bipolar disorder is limited.

Cocaine Detoxification

Bupropion may be associated with a euphoric feeling; thus, it may be contra-indicated in persons with histories of substance abuse. However, because of its dopaminergic effects, bupropion has been explored as a treatment to reduce the cravings for cocaine in persons who have withdrawn from the substance. Results have been inconclusive, with some patients showing a reduction in drug craving and others finding their cravings increased.

Hypoactive Sexual Desire Disorder

Bupropion is often added to drugs such as SSRIs to counteract sexual side effects and may be helpful as a treatment for nondepressed individuals with hypoactive sexual desire disorder. Bupropion may improve sexual arousal, orgasm comple-tion, and sexual satisfaction.

Neuropathic Pain

Bupropion sustained release at a dosage of 150 to 300 mg/day may be effective at treating neuropathic pain in some patients.

Weight Loss

Although bupropion can cause modest weight loss, it can produce clinically significant weight loss when combined with naltrexone. Naltrexone is an opi-oid receptor antagonist. The fixed-dose combination medicine is sold under the brand name Contrave as an extended-release 8/90-mg tablet. It is labeled as an adjunct to increased physical activity and reduced calorie diet. This treatment is covered in greater depth in Chapter 41.

Precautions and Adverse Reactions

Bupropion's most common side effects include headache, insomnia, dry mouth, tremor, and nausea. Restlessness, agitation, weight loss, and irritability may also occur. Patients with severe anxiety or panic disorder should not be prescribed bupropion. Most likely because of its potentiating effects on dopaminergic neu-rotransmission, bupropion can cause psychotic symptoms, including hallucina-tions, delusions, and catatonia, as well as delirium. Bupropion exerts indirect sympathomimetic activity, producing positive inotropic effects in human myo-cardium, an effect that may reflect catecholamine release. Some patients may experience cognitive impairment, most notably word finding difficulties though it is a rare side effect.

Despite these adverse reactions, bupropion does not produce many of the side effects associated with other antidepressants. These side effects include sig-nificant drug-induced orthostatic hypotension, weight gain, daytime drowsiness, and anticholinergic effects. Hypertension may occur in some patients, but bupro-pion causes no other significant cardiovascular or clinical laboratory changes.

Concern about seizure has deterred some physicians from prescribing bupro-pion. However, the risk of seizure is dose dependent. Studies show that at dos-ages of 300 mg a day or less of sustained-release bupropion, the incidence of seizures is 0.05%, which is no worse than the incidence of seizures with other antidepressants. The risk of seizures increases to about 0.1% with dosages of 400 mg a day. In addition, anorexia can increase the risk for seizures, which may be worsened by taking bupropion. Clinicians should carefully evaluate patients with prior history of eating disorders since bupropion has been found to increase seizure risk in patients with a prior diagnosis of bulimia or anorexia.

Changes in electroencephalographic (EEG) waveforms have been reported to be associated with bupropion use. About 20% of individuals treated with bupropion exhibit spike waves, sharp waves, and focal slowing. The likelihood of females having sharp waves is higher than males. The presence of these waveforms in individuals taking a medication known to lower the seizure threshold may be a risk factor for developing seizures. Other risk factors for seizures include a history of seizures, use of alcohol, recent benzodiazepine withdrawal, organic brain disease, head trauma, or pretreatment epileptiform discharges on EEG. Any of these predisposing factors are reason to use extreme caution when administering bupropion.

Few deaths have been reported after overdoses of bupropion. Poor outcomes are associated with cases of huge doses and mixed-drug overdoses. Seizures occur in about one-third of all overdoses and are dose dependent, with those having seizures ingesting a significantly higher median dose. Fatalities can involve uncontrollable seizures, sinus bradycardia, and cardiac arrest. Symptoms of poisoning most often involve seizures, sinus tachycardia, hypertension, GI symptoms, hallucinations, and agitation. All seizures are typically brief and self-limited. In general, however, bupropion is safer in overdose cases than are other antidepressants, except perhaps SSRIs.

Use in Pregnancy and Lactation

There is insufficient information about the safety of bupropion use in pregnancy and is classified as a pregnancy category C drug. It is excreted in breast milk. Potential benefits may warrant use among nursing women.

Drug Interactions

Given the fact that bupropion is frequently combined with SSRIs or venlafaxine, potential interactions are significant. Bupropion has been found to have an effect on the pharmacokinetics of venlafaxine. One study noted a significant increase in venlafaxine levels and a consequent decrease in its main metabolite O-desmethylvenlafaxine during combined treatment with sustained-release bupropion. Bupropion hydroxylation is weakly inhibited by venlafaxine. No significant changes in plasma levels of the SSRIs paroxetine and fluoxetine have been reported. However, some case reports indicate that the combination of bupropion and fluoxetine (Prozac) may be associated with panic, delirium, or seizures. Bupropion in combination with lithium (Eskalith) may rarely cause seizures and increase the risk of lithium neurotoxicity.

Because of possibility of inducing a hypertensive crisis, bupropion should not be used concurrently with monoamine oxidase inhibitors (MAOIs). At least 14 days should pass after the discontinuation of an MAOI before initiating treatment with bupropion. In some cases, the addition of bupropion may permit persons taking antiparkinsonian medications to lower the doses of their dopaminergic drugs. However, delirium, psychotic symptoms, and dyskinetic movements may be associated with the coadministration of bupropion and dopaminergic agents such as levodopa (Larodopa), pergolide (Permax), ropinirole (Requip), pramipexole (Mirapex), amantadine (Symmetrel), and bromocriptine (Parlodel). Sinus bradycardia may occur when bupropion is combined with metoprolol.

Carbamazepine (Tegretol) may decrease plasma concentrations of bupropion, and bupropion may increase plasma concentrations of valproic acid (Depakene).

In vitro biotransformation studies of bupropion have found that formation of a major active metabolite, hydroxybupropion, is mediated by CYP2B6. Bupropion has a significant inhibitory effect on CYP2D6.

Laboratory Interferences

A report has appeared indicating that bupropion may give a false-positive result on urinary amphetamine screens. No other reports have appeared of laboratory interferences clearly associated with bupropion treatment. Clinically nonsignificant changes in the electrocardiogram (premature beats and nonspecific ST-T changes) and decreases in the white blood cell count (by about 10%) have been reported in a small number of persons.

Dosage and Clinical Guidelines

Immediate-release bupropion is available in 75-, 100-, and 150-mg tablets. Sustained-release bupropion is available in 100-, 150-, 200-, and 300-mg tablets. Extended-release bupropion comes in 150- and 300-mg strengths. Dosing guidelines are covered below and in Table 9-1.

Initiation of immediate-release bupropion in the average adult person should be 100 mg orally twice a day. On the fourth day of treatment, the dosage can

TABLE 9-1: Bupropion Dosage Guidelines and Titration Schedule

Formulation	Initial Dose	Maintenance Dose	Maximum Dose	Titration Schedule
Immediate-release tablet	100 mg BID	100–150 mg TID	450 mg/day; 150 mg per dose	Initial dose for at least 3 days before maintenance dose; maintenance dose should not be increased for several weeks and only if medication is well tolerated.
Sustained-release tablet	150 mg QD	200 mg BID or 300 mg in morning and 100 mg in afternoon	400 mg/day; 300 mg per dose	Initial dose for at least 3 days; dose can then be increased to 150 mg BID; titrate to 200 mg BID after several weeks if needed. Administer at least 8 h apart.
Extended-release tablet	150 mg QD	300 mg QD	450 mg/day	Initial dose for no less than 4 days; titrate to target dose based on patient tolerance and response.

QD, once per day; BID, twice per day; TID, three times per day.

be increased to 100 mg three times a day. Because 300 mg is the recommended dose, the person should be maintained on this dose for several weeks before increasing it further. The maximum dosage, 450 mg a day, should be given as 150 mg three times a day. Because of the risk of seizures, increases in dose should never exceed 100 mg in a 3-day period; a single dose of immediate-release bupropion should never exceed 150 mg, and the total daily dosage should not exceed 450 mg. The maximum of 400 mg of the sustained-release version should be used as a twice-a-day regimen of either 200 mg twice daily or 300 mg in the morning and 100 mg in the afternoon. A starting dosage of the sustained-release version, 150 mg once a day, can be increased to 150 mg twice a day after 4 days. Then, 200 mg twice a day may be used. A single dose of sustained-release bupropion should never exceed 300 mg. The maximum dosage is 200 mg twice a day of the immediate-release or sustained-release formulations. An advantage of the extended-release preparation is that the dosage can be given all at once in the morning. The initial dosage of 150 mg once per day can be increased to 300 mg once per day after no less than 4 days. Further titration should be gradual and based on patient tolerance and response to the medication. After appropriate titration, a maximum dose of 450 mg can be given all at once in the morning.

For smoking cessation, the patient should start taking 150 mg of sustained-release bupropion a day 10 to 14 days before quitting smoking. On the fourth day, the dosage should be increased to 150 mg twice daily. Treatment generally lasts 7 to 12 weeks.

Buspirone

10

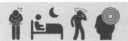 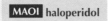 MAOI haloperidol 3A4 2D6 3A5

Introduction

Buspirone hydrochloride (BuSpar), an azapirone, is approved for the treatment of generalized anxiety disorder (GAD). Chemically distinct from other psychotropic agents, buspirone has a high affinity for 5-HT$_{1A}$ serotonin receptors, acting as an agonist or partial agonist, and moderate affinity for the D$_2$ dopamine receptor, acting as both an agonist and an antagonist. Unlike many other medications for GAD, buspirone does not possess anticonvulsant or muscle relaxant effects.

Initially approved by the Food and Drug Administration (FDA) in 1986, buspirone was initially anticipated to be a better alternative to the benzodiazepines since buspirone is not sedating, does not possess potential for dependence and abuse, and does not have adverse cognitive and psychomotor effects. However, while it has these safety and tolerability advantages, combined evidence reveals that it is not more effective than benzodiazepines in the treatment of GAD. Rather than being used as a monotherapy, many patients have benefitted from the addition of buspirone to their antidepressant regimen. Its use in this adjunctive role probably is more common than its use as an anxiolytic.

Pharmacologic Actions

Buspirone is well absorbed from the gastrointestinal tract, but absorption is delayed by food ingestion. Peak plasma levels are achieved 40 to 90 minutes after oral administration. At doses of 10 to 40 mg, single-dose linear pharmacokinetics are observed. Nonlinear pharmacokinetics are observed after multiple doses. Because of its short half-life (2 to 11 hours), buspirone is dosed three times daily. Buspirone undergoes first-pass metabolism primary by cytochrome P450 CYP3A4 isoenzymes, and to a lesser extent by CYP2D6 and CYP3A5 isoenzymes. An active metabolite of buspirone, 1-pyrimidinylpiperazine (1-PP), is about 20% less potent than buspirone but is up to 30% more concentrated in the brain than the parent compound. The elimination half-life of 1-PP is 6 hours. Buspirone is primarily excreted in urine, but fecal excretion may account for between 18% and 38% of the dose.

Patients may not observe any noticeable effect of treatment with buspirone for 1 to 4 weeks after starting the medication. Clinicians are advised to stress that the drug is slow acting to avoid noncompliance.

Buspirone has no effect on the γ-aminobutyric acid (GABA)-associated chloride ion channel or the serotonin reuptake transporter, both of which are targets of other drugs that are effective in GAD. Buspirone's primary mechanism of action is via activity at 5-HT$_{1A}$ and dopamine type 2 (D$_2$) receptors, although the significance of the effects at these receptors is unknown. It is a 5-HT$_{1A}$ partial agonist and has lower affinities for several other serotonin receptors (5-HT$_{2A}$, 5-HT$_{2B}$, 5-HT$_{2C}$, 5-HT$_6$, and 5-HT$_7$). At D$_2$ receptors, it has properties of both an agonist and an antagonist. Buspirone is also antagonist at D$_3$ and D$_4$ receptors.

Therapeutic Indications

Generalized Anxiety Disorder

Buspirone is a narrow-spectrum antianxiety agent with demonstrated efficacy only in the treatment of GAD. In contrast to the SSRIs or venlafaxine (Effexor), buspirone is not effective in the treatment of panic disorder, obsessive-compulsive disorder (OCD), or social phobia. Buspirone, however, has an advantage over these agents in that it does not typically cause sexual dysfunction or weight gain. It has little efficacy as an intervention for acute anxiety, as its anxiolytic effects can take weeks until they are experienced. The full benefit of buspirone is evident only at dosages above 30 mg a day, sometimes for upward of 4 weeks.

Some evidence suggests that compared with benzodiazepines, buspirone is generally more effective for symptoms of anger and hostility, equally effective for psychic symptoms of anxiety, and less effective for somatic symptoms of anxiety. If an immediate response is needed, patients can be started on a benzodiazepine and then withdrawn from the drug after buspirone's effects begin. Sometimes the sedative effects of benzodiazepines, which are not found with buspirone, are desirable; however, these sedative effects may cause impaired motor performance and cognitive deficits. Unlike benzodiazepines, buspirone lacks any euphoric effect.

Off-Label Uses

Many other clinical uses of buspirone have been reported, but most have not been confirmed in controlled trials. Because buspirone does not act on the GABA–chloride ion channel complex, the drug is not recommended for the treatment of withdrawal from benzodiazepines, alcohol, or sedative-hypnotic drugs, except as treatment of comorbid anxiety symptoms.

Depression

Evidence of the efficacy of high-dosage buspirone (30 to 90 mg a day) for depressive disorders is mixed. Buspirone appears to have weak antidepressant activity, which has led to its use as an augmenting agent in patients who have failed standard antidepressant therapy. In a large study, buspirone augmentation of SSRIs worked as well as other commonly used strategies.

Obsessive-Compulsive Disorder

Buspirone is sometimes used to augment SSRIs in the treatment of OCD. Evidence to support its use as a monotherapy, however, is weak at best.

Posttraumatic Stress Disorder

There are reports that buspirone may be beneficial for increased arousal and flashbacks associated with posttraumatic stress disorder (PTSD). Additionally, its good safety profile and low potential for abuse and withdrawal symptoms make it a promising alternative to benzodiazepines. However, more clinical trials are needed to confirm efficacy.

Other

Scattered trials suggest that buspirone reduces aggression and anxiety in persons with organic brain disease or traumatic brain injury. It is also used for SSRI-induced bruxism and sexual dysfunction, nicotine craving, and attention deficit hyperactivity disorder.

Precautions and Adverse Reactions

Buspirone does not cause weight gain, sexual dysfunction, discontinuation symptoms, or significant sleep disturbance. It does not produce sedation or cognitive and psychomotor impairment. The most common adverse effects of buspirone are headache, nausea, dizziness, and (rarely) insomnia. Some persons may report a minor feeling of restlessness, although that symptom may reflect an incompletely treated anxiety disorder. No deaths have been reported from overdoses of buspirone, and the median lethal dose is estimated to be 160 to 550 times the recommended daily dose. Buspirone should be used with caution by persons with hepatic and renal impairment, though buspirone can be used safely by the elderly.

Use in Pregnancy and Lactation

There is no evidence that pregnant women and nursing mothers taking buspirone have an increased risk of adverse effects on the newborn. It is classified as a pregnancy category B drug.

Drug Interactions

The coadministration of buspirone and haloperidol (Haldol) results in increased blood concentrations of haloperidol. Buspirone should not be used with monoamine oxidase inhibitors (MAOIs) to avoid hypertensive episodes, and a 2-week washout period should pass between the discontinuation of MAOI use and the initiation of treatment with buspirone. Drugs or foods that inhibit CYP3A4 (e.g., erythromycin (E-mycin), itraconazole (Sporanox), nefazodone (Serzone), and grapefruit juice) increase buspirone plasma concentrations.

Laboratory Interferences

Single doses of buspirone can cause transient elevations in growth hormone, prolactin, and cortisol concentrations, although the effects are not clinically significant.

Dosage and Clinical Guidelines

Buspirone is available in single-scored 5- and 10-mg tablets and triple-scored 15- and 30-mg tablets; treatment is usually initiated with either 5 mg orally three times daily or 7.5 mg orally twice daily. The dosage can be raised by 5 mg every 2 to 4 days to the usual dosage range of 15 to 60 mg a day.

Buspirone

Buspirone should not be used in patients with past hypersensitivity to the drug, in cases of diabetes-associated metabolic acidosis, or in patients with severely compromised liver and/or renal function.

Switching from a Benzodiazepine to Buspirone

Buspirone is not cross-tolerant with benzodiazepines, barbiturates, or alcohol. A common clinical problem, therefore, is how to initiate buspirone therapy in a patient who is currently taking benzodiazepines.

There are two alternatives. First, the clinician can start buspirone treatment gradually while the benzodiazepine is being withdrawn. Second, the clinician can start buspirone treatment and bring the patient up to a therapeutic dosage for 2 to 3 weeks while they are still receiving the regular dosage of the benzodiazepine, and then slowly taper the benzodiazepine dosage.

Patients who have received benzodiazepines in the past, especially in recent months, may find that buspirone is not as effective as the benzodiazepines in the treatment of their anxiety. This might be explained by the absence of the immediacy and mildly euphoric and sedative effects of benzodiazepines. The coadministration of buspirone and benzodiazepines may be effective in the treatment of persons with anxiety disorders who have not responded to treatment with either drug alone.

Calcium Channel Inhibitors 11

Generic Name	Trade Name	Adverse Effects	Drug Interactions	CYP Interactions
Verapamil	Calan	Dizziness, tachycardia, GI symptoms, hypotension, bradycardia, headache	Alcohol, β-adrenergic receptor antagonists, hypotensives, antiarrhythmics	2C8, 3A4, 3A5
Nifedipine	Procardia, Adalat	Dizziness, tachycardia, GI symptoms, headache	β-Adrenergic receptor antagonists, anticonvulsants, hypotensives, antiarrhythmics	3A4, 2D6, 1A2, 2A6, 2C8, 1A1, 2B6, 2E1, 2C9, 3A5
Nimodipine	Nimotop	Dizziness, tachycardia, GI symptoms, headache	β-Adrenergic receptor antagonists, hypotensives, antiarrhythmics	3A4
Isradipine	DynaCirc	Dizziness, tachycardia, GI symptoms, headache	Cimetidine, rifampicin	3A4
Amlodipine	Norvasc, Lotrel	Dizziness, tachycardia, GI symptoms, EPS, headache	Hypertensives, dantrolene, idelalisib, nefazodone, ivacaftor, simvastatin	3A4, 1A1, 2B6, 3A5, 2C8, 2D6
Diltiazem	Cartia XT, Tiazac	Dizziness, tachycardia, GI symptoms, hypotension, bradycardia, tremors, headache	β-Adrenergic receptor antagonists, benzodiazepines, carbamazepine, digoxin, fingolimod	3A4, 2D6, 3A5, 3A7, 2C19, 2C8

Introduction

Calcium channel inhibitors, also known as calcium channel blockers (CCBs), are medications that limit body's use of calcium, an essential mineral. Outside the field of psychiatry, they are regularly prescribed to treat high blood pressure, arrhythmias, angina, and several other cardiac diseases. CCBs have been shown to attenuate symptoms associated with bipolar disorder and to help stabilize mood, since elevated basal and stimulated free intracellular calcium ion (Ca^{2+}) activity is associated with bipolar disorder.

Research has shown that intracellular Ca^{2+} regulates the activity of multiple neurotransmitters, such as serotonin and dopamine, thereby accounting for its role as a treatment in mood disorders. CCBs are frequently used as antimanic agents for persons who are refractory to, or cannot tolerate, treatment with first-line mood-stabilizing agents, such as lithium (Eskalith), carbamazepine (Tegretol), and divalproex (Depakote). They have also been shown to be useful in treating ultradian or ultrarapid cycling bipolar disorder (mood cycling in less than 24 hours). Calcium channel inhibitors include nifedipine (Procardia,

111

Adalat), nimodipine (Nimotop), isradipine (DynaCirc), amlodipine (Norvasc, Lotrel), nicardipine (Cardene), nisoldipine (Sular), nitrendipine (Baypress), verapamil (Calan), clevidipine (Cleviprex), diltiazem (Cartia XT, Tiazac), and felodipine (Plendil).

Though they have been used to treat bipolar disorder for over 30 years, CCBs have never become an established therapeutic approach for any psychiatric condition. However, interest in their potential has increased within the last decade, largely due to two genome-wide findings implicating genes encoding L-type voltage-gated calcium channel subunits as susceptibility genes for bipolar disorder, schizophrenia, major depressive disorder, attention deficit hyperactivity disorder, and autism. Nimodipine probably has greater potential for psychiatric applications, because it crosses the blood–brain barrier more readily than verapamil and it acts on T- as well as L-type channels.

Pharmacologic Actions

The calcium channel inhibitors are nearly completely absorbed after oral use, with significant first-pass hepatic metabolism. For nimodipine, this occurs largely via cytochrome P-450 CYP3A4 isoenzymes. Verapamil is metabolized via CYP2C8, CYP3A4, and CYP3A5. Considerable intra- and interindividual variations are seen in the plasma concentrations of the drugs after a single dose. Peak plasma levels of most of these agents are achieved within 30 minutes, though amlodipine does not reach peak plasma levels for about 6 hours. The half-life of verapamil after the first dose is 2 to 8 hours; it increases from 5 to 12 hours after the first few days of therapy. The half-lives of the other CCBs range from 1 to 2 hours for nimodipine and isradipine, while amlodipine's half-life ranges from 30 to 50 hours (Table 11-1).

The primary mechanism of action of CCBs in bipolar disorder has not been fully elucidated. The calcium channel inhibitors discussed in this section inhibit the influx of calcium into neurons through L-type (long-acting) voltage-dependent calcium channels.

TABLE 11-1: Half-Lives, Dosages, and Effectiveness of Selected Calcium Channel Inhibitors in Psychiatric Disorders

	Verapamil (Calan, Isoptin)	Nimodipine (Nimotop)	Isradipine (DynaCirc)	Amlodipine (Norvasc)
Half-life	Short (5–12 hours)	Short (1–2 hours)	Short (1–2 hours)	Long (30–50 hours)
Starting dosage	40 mg TID	30 mg TID	2.5 mg BID	5 mg HS
Peak daily dosage	360 mg	240–450 mg	20 mg	10–15 mg
Antimanic	++	++	++	a
Antidepressant	±	+	+	a
Antiultradian[b]	±	++	++	a

[a]No systematic studies, only case reports.
[b]Rapid cycling bipolar disorder.
BID, twice a day; HS, half strength; TID, three times a day.
Table adapted from Robert M. Post, MD.

Indications

Calcium channel inhibitors have been used to treat medical conditions such as angina, hypertension, migraine headaches, Raynaud phenomenon, esophageal spasm, premature labor, and headache. Verapamil has antiarrhythmic activity and has been used to treat supraventricular arrhythmias.

Off-Label Psychiatric Uses

Bipolar Disorder

Nimodipine and verapamil have been demonstrated to be effective as maintenance therapy in persons with bipolar illness. Patients who respond to lithium appear to also respond to treatment with verapamil. Nimodipine may be useful for ultradian cycling and recurrent brief depression. The clinician should begin treatment with a short-acting drug, such as nimodipine (or possibly isradipine), beginning with a low dosage and increasing the dosage every 4 to 5 days until a clinical response is seen or adverse effects appear. When symptoms are controlled, a longer-acting drug, such as amlodipine, can be substituted as maintenance therapy. Failure to respond to verapamil does not exclude a favorable response to one of the other drugs. Verapamil has been shown to prevent antidepressant-induced mania. The CCBs can be combined with other agents, such as carbamazepine, in patients who are partial responders to monotherapy.

Other Psychiatric Indications

Nifedipine is used to treat hypertensive crises associated with the use of monoamine oxidase inhibitors. Isradipine may reduce the subjective response to methamphetamine. There is also some evidence to support the use of CCBs in the treatment of Tourette disorder, Huntington disease, panic disorder, intermittent explosive disorder, and tardive dyskinesia. Verapamil has been used as a prophylactic treatment for cluster headaches at a minimum dosage of 240 mg per day.

Precautions and Adverse Reactions

The most common adverse effects associated with CCBs are those attributable to vasodilation: dizziness, headache, tachycardia, nausea, dysesthesias, and peripheral edema. Verapamil and diltiazem can cause hypotension, bradycardia, and atrioventricular heart block, which necessitate close monitoring and sometimes discontinuation of the drugs. In all patients with cardiovascular disease, these medications should be used with caution.

Other common adverse effects include constipation, fatigue, rash, coughing, and wheezing. Adverse effects noted with diltiazem include hyperactivity, akathisia, and parkinsonism; with verapamil, delirium, hyperprolactinemia, and galactorrhea; with nimodipine, subjective sense of chest tightness and skin flushing; and with nifedipine, depression.

Use in Pregnancy and Lactation

Though CCBs are classified as pregnancy category C drugs, they are commonly used during pregnancy and nursing to treat hypertension, arrhythmias, and preeclampsia.

Drug Interactions

All CCBs have a potential for drug–drug interactions. The types and risks of these interactions vary by compound. Verapamil raises serum levels of carbamazepine, digoxin, and other CYP3A4 substrates. Verapamil and diltiazem, but not nifedipine, have been reported to precipitate carbamazepine-induced neurotoxicity. Calcium channel inhibitors should not be used by persons taking β-adrenergic receptor antagonists, hypotensives (e.g., diuretics, vasodilators, and angiotensin-converting enzyme inhibitors), or antiarrhythmic drugs (e.g., quinidine and digoxin) without consultation with an internist or cardiologist. Cimetidine (Tagamet) has been reported to increase plasma concentrations of nifedipine and diltiazem.

Some patients who are treated with lithium and calcium channel inhibitors concurrently may be at an increased risk of neurotoxicity and death.

Laboratory Interferences

No known laboratory interferences are associated with the use of calcium channel inhibitors.

Dosage and Clinical Guidelines

Verapamil is available in 40-, 80-, and 120-mg tablets; 120-, 180-, and 240-mg sustained-release tablets; and 100-, 120-, 180-, 200-, 240-, 300-, and 360-mg sustained-release capsules. The starting dosage is 40 mg orally three times a day and can be increased in increments every 4 to 5 days up to 80 to 120 mg three times a day. The patient's blood pressure, pulse, and electrocardiogram (in patients older than 40 years old or with a history of cardiac illness) should be routinely monitored.

Nifedipine is available in 10- and 20-mg capsules, as well as 30-, 60-, and 90-mg extended-release tablets. Administration should be started at 10 mg orally three or four times a day and can be increased up to a maximum dosage of 120 mg a day.

Nimodipine is available in 30-mg capsules. It has been used at 60 mg every 4 hours for ultra–rapid-cycling bipolar disorder. Daily doses of up to 630 mg have been reported but only for brief periods of time.

Isradipine is available in 2.5- and 5-mg capsules, with a maximum of 20 mg/day. An extended-release formulation of isradipine has been discontinued.

Amlodipine is available in 2.5-, 5-, and 10-mg tablets. Administration should start at 5 mg once at night and can be increased to a maximum dosage of 10 to 15 mg a day.

Diltiazem is available in 30-, 60-, 90-, and 120-mg tablets; 60-, 90-, 120-, 180-, 240-, 300-, and 360-mg extended-release capsules; and 60-, 90-, 120-, 180-, 240-, 300-, and 360-mg extended-release tablets. Administration should start with 30 mg orally four times a day and can be increased up to a maximum of 360 mg a day.

Elderly persons are more sensitive to CCBs than younger adults. No specific information is available regarding the use of the agents for children.

Cannabis

Introduction

Cannabis has been used recreationally, medicinally, and for industrial purposes throughout the world for millennia. There are hundreds of constituents within the plant, including more than 150 compounds known as cannabinoids, the most abundant of which are Δ9-tetrahydrocannabinol (THC) and cannabidiol (CBD)—the former being psychoactive and an intoxicant, the latter being psychoactive but not an intoxicant. Subsequent chapters will discuss the pharmacology of THC and CBD. This chapter will explore the science of the plant, the legal distinction between hemp and marijuana, and provide an overview of the endocannabinoid system (ECS)—an endogenous biochemical communication and regulatory system that is influenced by endogenous cannabinoids like N-arachidonoylethanolamide (more commonly known as anandamide) and 2-arachidonoylglycerol (2-AG), and phytocannabinoids like THC and CBD.

Cannabis—The Plant

"Cannabis" is the umbrella term for all plants of the genus *Cannabis*. All cannabis are dioecious (see Fig. 12-1 and Fig. 12-2) and follow a four-stage lifecycle: germination, seedling, vegetative, and flowering. In addition to looking different and having different functional anatomy, the two sexes of the plant produce vastly

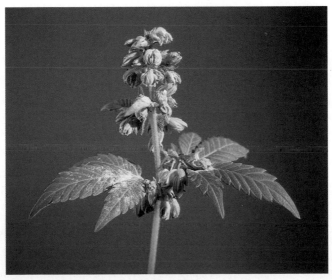

FIGURE 12-1 A flowering male cannabis plant.

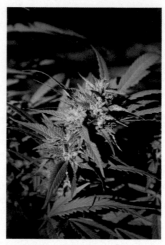

FIGURE 12-2 A flowering female cannabis plant.

dissimilar amounts of trichomes, which are small glandular structures that grow on the stalks, leaves, and flowers of male and female plants (see Fig. 12-3 and Fig. 12-4). Female plants produce far more trichomes than males, with the highest concentrations appearing on the unpollinated flowers of female cannabis plants.

These trichomes synthesize, store, and secrete the vast majority of the secondary metabolites that produce cannabis' therapeutic and intoxicating effects (see Table 12-1). Some of these secondary metabolites are compounds that are commonly found throughout the plant world. Terpenes and flavonoids,

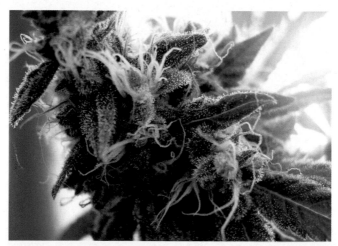

FIGURE 12-3 Trichomes give cannabis a frosted appearance when seen from afar.

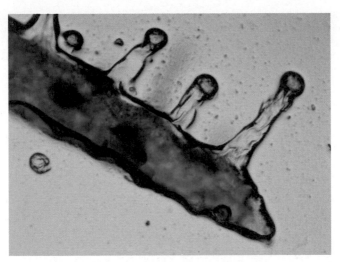

FIGURE 12-4 Close up, glandular trichomes have the appearance of enoki mushrooms.

TABLE 12-1: Commonly Found Constituents of Commercial Cannabis

Constituent	Type	Structure
Δ9-Tetrahy-drocannabinol (THC)	Phytocanna-binoid	
Δ9-Tetrahydro-cannabinolic acid (THCA)	Phytocanna-binoid	
Δ9-Tetrahydro-cannabivarin (THCV)	Phytocanna-binoid	

(continued)

TABLE 12-1: Commonly Found Constituents of Commercial Cannabis (*continued*)

Constituent	Type	Structure
Δ9-Tetrahydro-cannabivarinic acid (THCVA)	Phytocanna-binoid	
Δ8-letrahy-drocannabinol (Δ8-THC)	Phytocanna-binoid	
Cannabidiol (CBD)	Phytocanna-binoid	
Cannabidiolic acid (CBDA)	Phytocanna-binoid	

TABLE 12-1: Commonly Found Constituents of Commercial Cannabis (*continued*)		
Constituent	Type	Structure
Cannabigerol (CBG)	Phytocanna-binoid	
Cannabig-erolic acid (CBGA)	Phytocanna-binoid	
Cannabi-chromene (CBC)	Phytocanna-binoid	
Cannabi-chromenic acid (CBCA)	Phytocanna-binoid	

(*continued*)

Cannabis

TABLE 12-1: Commonly Found Constituents of Commercial Cannabis (*continued*)

Constituent	Type	Structure
Cannabinol (CBN)	Phytocanna-binoid	
Cannabidiolic acid (CBNA)	Phytocanna-binoid	
β-Myrcene	Terpene	
Limonene	Terpene	
Linalool	Terpene	
Pinene	Terpene	(α-pinene left; β-pinene right)
β-Caryophyl-lene	Terpene	
Humulene	Terpene	

Constituent	Type	Structure
Nerolidol	Terpene	
Borneol	Terpene	
Δ-3-Carene	Terpene	
Terpinolene	Terpene	
Cannflavin A	Flavonoid	
Cannflavin B	Flavonoid	

TABLE 12-1: Commonly Found Constituents of Commercial Cannabis (continued)

Cannabis

for example, are responsible for giving fruits, vegetables, and flowers their distinctive smells and tastes.

There are also metabolites that are rarely produced in plants besides cannabis. These compounds are known as phytocannabinoids (often shortened to cannabinoids), which follow several synthetic pathways, the most common of which is illustrated in Figure 12-5. These phytocannabinoids exert their therapeutic or intoxicating effects on users directly or indirectly via the ECS, which is found in all vertebrates.

Phytocannabinoids

Cannabis is not the only plant that produces phytocannabinoids. These compounds have also been found in cacao, black pepper, echinacea, and broccoli—typically

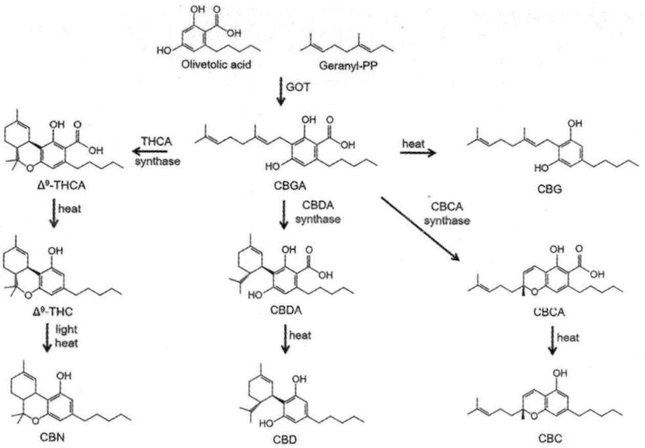

FIGURE 12-5 Tetrahydrocannabinolic acid (THCA), cannabidiolic acid (CBDA), and cannabichromenic acid (CBCA) have the same precursor—cannabigerolic acid (CBGA), which is formed through the synthesis of olivetolic acid and geranyl pyrophosphate. The level of THCA, CBDA, or CBCA a plant will eventually produce appears to be mediated by the level of THCA synthase, CBDA synthase, or CBCA synthase available, something that is regulated by a plant's genetics. Decarboxylation of CBGA, THCA, CBDA, and CBCA leads to the formation of cannabigerol (CBG), tetrahydrocannabinol (THC), cannabinol (CBD), and cannabichromene (CBC), respectively.

in only trace amounts. Even within cannabis, the vast majority of the more than 150 phytocannabinoids occur in only very small concentrations with the exception of cannabidiolic acid (CBDA) and tetrahydrocannabinolic acid (THCA), which are the two most abundant phytocannabinoids in virtually all commercial varieties of hemp and marijuana. CBDA and THCA are only converted to CBD and Δ9-THC, respectively, via decarboxylation either during storage, under alkaline conditions, or upon heating.

Decarboxylation is necessary to convert nonintoxicating THCA to cannabis' primary intoxicant, THC. Other phytocannabinoids that have been shown to cause intoxication include the following:

- Δ8-THC (often marketed as "Delta 8 THC")
- Δ10-THC (often marketed as "Delta 10 THC")
- Tetrahydrocannabivarin (THCV)
- Cannabinol (CBN)
- Δ9-Tetrahydrocannabiphorol (THCP)

Δ8-THC, Δ10-THC, THCV, and CBN are significantly less potent than THC, while THCP is far more potent. Though few phytocannabinoids produce intoxication, several are believed to have therapeutic properties (see Table 12-2). Research into the clinical applications of these compounds is ongoing and most clinical studies have focused on CBD and THC.

Hemp and Marijuana

In addition to being the primary intoxicant found in cannabis, as well as one of the most important therapeutic compounds produced by the plant, THC is also important from a legal perspective in the United States. While hemp has been grown by myriad cultures throughout the world for thousands of years and was

TABLE 12-2: Potential Therapeutic Applications of Minor Cannabinoids and Terpenes

Compound	Reputed Therapeutic Effect	Reference
Tetrahydrocannabivarin (THCV)	Weight loss, decrease in body fat	Cawthorne et al. (2007); Riedel et al. (2009)
	Anticonvulsant	Hill et al. (2010)
	Hyperalgesia suppressant and anti-inflammatory	Bolognini et al. (2010)
Tetrahydrocannabinolic acid (THCA)	Antinausea and antiemetic	Rock et al. (2013)
	Parkinson disease treatment	Moldzio et al. (2012)
	Anticancer	Moreno-Sanz (2016)
Cannabidiolic acid (CBDA)	Antiemetic	Moreno-Sanz (2016); Rock & Parker (2013)
Cannabidivarin (CBDV)	Antinausea and antiemetic	Rock, Sticht & Parker (2014)
	Anticonvulsant	Williams, Jones & Whalley (2014)
Cannabigerol (CBG)	Muscle relaxant	Banerjee, Snyder & Mechoulam (1975)
	Analgesic and antierythemic	Evans (1991)
	Antifungal	ElSohly et al. (1981)
	Anticancer	Baek et al. (1998); Ligresti et al. (2006)
	Antidepressant and antihypertensive agent	Maor, Gallily & Mechoulam (2006); Musty & Deyo (2006)
	Psoriasis treatment	Wilkinson & Williamson (2007)
	Analgesic and antidepressant	Cascio et al. (2010); Formukong, Evans & Evans (1988)
Cannabichromene (CBC)	Analgesic and anti-inflammatory	Cascio & Pertwee (2014), Davis & Hatoum (1983); Maione et al. (2011)
	Neuroprotective	Shinjyo & Di Marzo (2013)
	Anti-inflammatory	DeLong et al. (2010)
Cannabinol (CBN)	Psoriasis treatment	Wilkinson & Williamson (2007)
	Burn treatment	Qin et al. (2008); Russo (2014)
	Bone formation	Scutt & Williamson (2017)
	Breast cancer treatment	Holland, Allen & Arnold (2008)

Cannabis

(continued)

TABLE 12-2: Potential Therapeutic Applications of Minor Cannabinoids and Terpenes (*continued*)

Compound	Reputed Therapeutic Effect	Reference
β-Myrcene	Analgesic	Rao, Menezes & Viana (1990); Paula-Freire et al. (2013)
	Anticancer	De-Oliveira, Ribeiro-Pinto, & Paumgartten (1997)
	Anti-inflammatory	Lorenzetti et al. (1991)
	Antiosteoarthritic	Rufino et al. (2015)
	Antiulcer	Bonamin et al. (2014)
	Neuroprotective	Ciftci, Oztanir & Cetin (2014)
	Sedative, muscle relaxant	do Vale et al. (2002)
Limonene	Acne treatment	Kim et al. (2008)
	Antibiotic	Onawunmi, Yisak & Ogunlana (1984)
	Anticancer	Vigushin et al. (1998); Miller et al. (2013)
	Anti-inflammatory	d'Alessio et al. (2013)
	Anxiolytic	Carvalho-Freitas and Costa (2002); Costa CARA et al. (2013)
	Dermatophytosis treatment	Sanguinetti, et al. (2007); Singh et al. (2010)
	Gastroesophageal reflux	Harris (2010)
	Hyperalgesia treatment	Piccinelli et al. (2017)
	Immunostimulant	Komori et al. (1995)
Linalool	Analgesic	Peana et al. (2006)
	Anticancer	Han et al. (2016)
	Anticonvulsant	Elisabetsky, Marschner, & Souza (1995); Ismail (2006)
	Antidepressant	McPartland & Russo (2001)
	Antileishmanial	do Socorro et al. (2003); Kim et al. (2007)
	Antinociceptive	Batista et al. (2008)
	Anxiolytic	Russo (2001, 2011)
	Burn treatment	Gattefosse (1993)
	Local anesthetic	Ghelardini et al. (1999); Re et al. (2000)
	Sedative	Buchbauer et al. (1993)
Pinene	Antibiotic	Kose et al. (2010); Kovac et al. (2015)
	Anti-inflammatory	Gil et al. (1989)
	Anxiolytic	Kasuya et al. (2015)
	Bronchodilator	Falk et al. (1990)
	Memory booster	Perry et al. (2000)
	Antibiotic	Rivas da Silva et al. (2012)

TABLE 12-2: Potential Therapeutic Applications of Minor Cannabinoids and Terpenes (*continued*)

Compound	Reputed Therapeutic Effect	Reference
β-caryophyllene	Anti-inflammatory	Gertsch (2008); Bento et al. (2011)
	Antimalarial	Campbell et al. (1997)
	Antinociceptive	Katsuyama et al. (2013); Paula-Freire et al. (2014)
	Gastric cytoprotective	Russo (2011)
Humulene (α-humulene/ α-caryophyllene)	Anticancer	Legault & Pichette (2007)
Nerolidol	Antileishmanial	Arruda et al. (2005)
	Antimalarial	Lopes et al. (1999); Rodrigues Goulart et al. (2004)
	Dermatophytosis treatment	Langenheim (1994)
	Sedative	Binet et al. (1972); Lapczynski et al. (2008)
	Skin penetrant	Cornwell & Barry (1994)
Borneol	Anti-inflammatory	Almeida et al. (2013)
	Antinociceptive	Almeida et al. (2013)
Δ-3-carene	Osteoporosis treatment	Jeong et al. (2008)
Terpinolene	Anticancer	Okumura et al. (2012)
	Antioxidant	Grassmann et al. (2005)
	Sedative	Ito & Ito (2013)

used for industrial and medicinal purposes, THC-rich cannabis has been used in parts of Asia and Africa for recreational, ceremonial, and medicinal purposes. It was rarely used as an intoxicant by Europeans in the Americas until the late 19th and early 20th centuries.

Regulatory History—20th Century

During the 1920s and 30s, "marijuana" became associated with jazz music, bohemians, Black artists, and newly arrived immigrants from Latin America. Consequently, its use was demonized in the press and by federal agencies like the Federal Bureau of Narcotics. At the same time, the hemp industry shrank into obsolescence. Subsequently, the federal government passed the Marihuana Tax Act of 1937, which effectively eradicated the legal cannabis industry. After gaining popularity in the 1950s and 1960s by multiple counter-cultural movements, its use was further criminalized. Furthermore, after the passage of the Controlled Substances Act of 1970, it was placed on the list of Schedule I drugs—that is, drugs with no currently accepted medical use and a high potential for abuse. This severely impeded research into the potential therapeutic utility

TABLE 12-3: Schedule of Cannabis-Based Drugs

Drug Name	Trade Name	Schedule (Year Approved by FDA)	Indications
Dronabinol (synthetic THC)	Marinol	Schedule III (1985)	HIV/AIDS-induced anorexia and chemotherapy-induced nausea and vomiting
Dronabinol (synthetic THC)	Syndros	Schedule II (2017)	HIV/AIDS-induced anorexia and chemotherapy-induced nausea and vomiting
Nabilone (synthetic THC)	Cesamet	Schedule II (1985)	Chemotherapy-induced nausea and vomiting
Cannabidiol	Epidiolex	Schedule V (2018)	Seizures associated with: Lennox–Gastaut Syndrome Dravet Syndrome Tuberous sclerosis complex (2020)
Nabiximols (formulation consisting of THC, CBD, and minor constituents)	Sativex	Not available in the United States; available in over 25 countries, including European Union members and Canada	Spasticity and neuropathic pain associated with multiple sclerosis

CBD, cannabidiol; FDA, Food and Drug Administration; THC, tetrahydrocannabinol.

of cannabis in the United States and began the modern war on drugs. Despite these impediments, multiple formulations containing cannabinoids have been approved by the Food and Drug Administration (FDA) or similar agencies in other nations (see Table 12-3).

Regulatory History—21st Century

Though several states decriminalized its possession, legalized medical programs for cannabis, or allowed for adult-use programs, there was no legal distinction between hemp and marijuana at the federal level until the 2014 Farm Bill was passed. According to this law, if the amount of THC content does not exceed 0.3% by dry weight, it is legally considered hemp while a cannabis plant that exceeds 0.3% THC by dry weight, is legally considered marijuana. The 2018 Farm Bill affirmed the legal distinction between hemp and marijuana based on THC concentration and removed hemp from the list of controlled substances. However, marijuana is still considered a Schedule I drug by the federal government.

The legislation allowed states to create hemp markets and federally legalized CBD, a nonintoxicating compound found in both marijuana and hemp. Products containing hemp-derived CBD are now widely available to consumers and are not subject to regulation by the FDA. Though marijuana remains illegal at the federal level, and THC is still a Schedule I drug in all formulations except for those approved by the FDA, several states have legalized the adult use of products containing high levels of THC and dozens of states have created medical marijuana programs that facilitate the cultivation and distribution of products containing marijuana or high concentrations of THC. Since marijuana remains a Schedule I drug, medical professionals are not allowed to prescribe it—they may only recommend it in states with medical marijuana programs.

Sativa and Indica

While there is an explicit distinction between hemp and marijuana, even if it is a legal construct, there is far less clarity with respect to the number of species within the genus, though there are often said to be three (see Fig. 12-6):

* *Cannabis sativa:* Historically grown in northern latitudes and East Asia. Sativa varieties include those that produce high-quality fibers, those that produce high seed yields, and those that produce significant levels of trichomes. Sativa plants are tall and have narrow leaves.

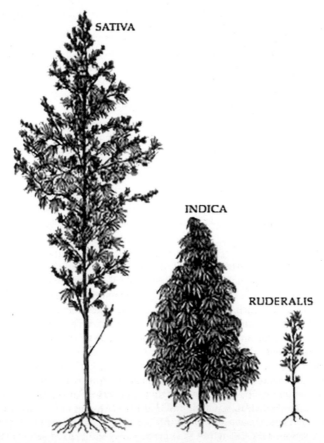

FIGURE 12-6 An illustration depicting the three varieties of cannabis: sativa, indica, and ruderalis.

- *Cannabis indica:* Historically grown in South Asia, indica plants produced significantly higher levels of trichomes than sativa varieties and low-quality fibers. Indica plants are shorter, bushier, and produce broad leaves.
- *Cannabis ruderalis:* A feral, weedy variety of cannabis found in northern areas that produces neither high levels of THC nor high-quality fibers.

Some argue that each of these was a distinct species prior to the 20th century. Others claim that C. sativa has always been the sole species of the genus *Cannabis*, and that the aforementioned distinctions are just variations (i.e., *C. sativa vars. sativa, C. sativa var. indica,* and *C. sativa var. ruderalis*). Nonetheless, due to interbreeding, particularly among commercially available varietals, any genetically significant taxologic distinction has been lost. Furthermore, the amount of trichomes created by sativa plants can now rival the amount of trichomes created by indica plants, so the distinction between the two is no longer relevant with respect to cannabinoid concentration. A "strain" of sativa may have identical CBD and THC concentrations as a "strain" of indica.

Despite extensive interbreeding, the words "sativa" and "indica" are still very important within the world of cannabis, and dispensaries will often organize their inventory of strains under three groupings, sativa, indica, and hybrid, because users report a notable difference in subjective effects. Indica is said to have a more narcotic effect that eases pain while promoting rest and relaxation. Sativa is said to offer similar pain relief but makes users more social. Many feel it calms their anxiety and improves their ability to engage with others.

These subjective effects are believed to be mediated by the hundreds of minor cannabinoids, flavonoids, and terpenes found in trace amounts through a phenomenon known as the entourage effect. Even though many of these molecules may not occur in high concentrations, they do seem to have an effect when they appear in conjunction with other compounds found in cannabis. Patients may not notice these effects when prescribed FDA formulations that solely contain synthetic THC (as is the case with nabilone and dronabinol).

The Endocannabinoid System

The endocannabinoid system, or ECS, is a wide-ranging biochemical communication and regulatory system that is primarily found in the central nervous system (CNS) and peripheral nervous system, the immune system, and virtually every organ system among vertebrates. Its role has been characterized as being one of the body's mechanisms for maintaining physiologic homeostasis. It is composed of receptors, ligands known as endocannabinoids, and enzymes that synthesize endocannabinoids and degrade both endocannabinoids and phyto-cannabinoids.

The first cannabinoid receptor, known as CB1, was discovered in the late 1980s. Activation of CB1 by either full agonists or partial agonists (such as THC, Δ8-THC, Δ10-THC, THCV, CBN, or THCP) leads to the kind of intoxication associated with marijuana use. They are also the most abundant G protein-coupled receptors (GPCRs) in the CNS, and they play a role in regulating memory, executive functions, coordination, time perception, appetite, pain, and the pleasure pathways in the brain (see Table 12-4). Their abundance in the CNS is one

TABLE 12-4: Distribution of CB1 in the Nervous System

Brain Part	Dense	Moderate	Low
Cerebrum:	• Primary somatosensory cortex (layers II, III, and VI) • Cingulate cortex (layer II) • Entorhinal cortex (layers II and IV) • Piriform cortex (layer III) • Frontal lobe (associational cortical regions) • Hippocampus (fields CA1, CA2, and CA3; subicular complex) • Outer molecular layer of dentate gyrus • Olfactory bulb (ependymal and subependymal layers) • Anterior olfactory nucleus • Olfactory tract • Anterior commissure (olfactory fibers) • Amygdala nucleus • Basal ganglia (internal portion of the globus pallidus, putamen, caudate nucleus, striatonigral pathway, and entopeduncular nucleus)	• Somatosensory cortex (layer V) • Temporal association cortex • Secondary somatosensory cortex • Supplementary motor cortex • Visual cortex • Auditory cortex • Inner polymorphic layer of dentate gyrus • Basal forebrain • Basal ganglia (external portion of the globus pallidus, ventral pallidum, and claustrum)	• Somatosensory cortex (layer IV) • Primary motor cortex • Granule cell layer of dentate gyrus • Olfactory tubercle • Basal ganglia (nucleus accumbens)
Cerebellum:	All regions		
Diencephalon:		• Thalamus (anterior, dorsomedial, and intralaminar nuclei) • Stria terminalis • Epithalamus (habenular nucleus) • Hypothalamus (lateral and paraventricular nuclei) • Infundibular stem	• Thalamus (medial geniculate, lateral geniculate, ventral posterior, and ventral lateral nuclei) • Subthalamic nucleus
Brain stem:	• Substantia nigra (pars reticulata) • Periaqueductal gray (PAG) • Gray matter around the fourth ventricle • Spinal trigeminal nucleus and spinal tract of the trigeminal nucleus	• Solitary nucleus • Nucleus ambiguous • Inferior olivary nucleus	• Ventral tegmental area • Substantia nigra (pars compacta)
Spinal Cord.	• Dorsal horn • Lamina X • Dorsal root ganglions	• Deep dorsal horn • Thoracic intermediolateral nucleus	

of the reasons why there are far more studies on cannabinoids for neurologic disorders than most other areas of medicine.

The discovery of the CB1 receptor was soon followed by the discovery of a second cannabinoid receptor, called CB2, which is highly expressed throughout the immune system, particularly in B cells, natural killer cells, monocytes, neutrophils, CD8 lymphocytes, CD4 lymphocytes, and glial cells within the CNS. Many researchers believe that cannabinoids that target CB2 receptors could be used to treat autoimmune disorders, and several synthetic cannabinoids have since been developed that selectively bind with CB2 receptors but are inactive at CB1, and therefore do not produce intoxication.

Beyond the immune system, CB2 receptors are expressed in specific sub-populations of neurons in the cerebrum, the cerebellum, the brain stem, and the diencephalon—which is involved in many crucial bodily functions including coordinating with the endocrine system to release hormones, relaying sensory and motor signals to the cerebral cortex, and regulating circadian rhythms (see Table 12-5). CB2 receptors are also found within the neuroimmune system in microglia, astrocytes, and oligodendrocytes. Evidence suggests these receptors could serve as therapeutic targets for several neurodegenerative disorders and to potentially counteract neuroinflammation in general.

TABLE 12-5: Distribution of CB2 in the Nervous System

Brain Part	Dense	Moderate	Low
Cerebrum:	• Orbital cortex (layers III and V) • Visual cortex (layers III and V) • Auditory cortex (layers III and V) • Motor cortex (layers III and V) • Piriform cortex (layers III and V) • Islands of Calleja • Hippocampus (pyramidal neurons in fields CA2 and CA3) • Anterior olfactory nucleus • Amygdala nucleus • Basal ganglia (striatum nucleus)		
Cerebellum:	• Purkinje cells • Granule cells	• Purkinje dendrites in the molecular layer	
Diencephalon:	• Thalmus (ventral posterior, lateral posterior, posterior, and paracentral nuclei)	• Thalmus (lateral geniculate nucleus)	• Thalamus (paraventricular and mediodorsal nuclei) • Hypothalamus (ventromedial and arcuate nuclei)
Brain stem:	• Dorsal cochlear nucleus • Facial motor nucleus	• Substantia nigra (pars reticulata) • Periaqueductal gray (PAG) • Inferior colliculus • Interpeduncular, paratrochlear and red nuclei • Lateral lemniscus (paralemniscal and dorsal nuclei) • Pontine nucleus • Medial and lateral vestibular nuclei • Parvocellular reticular nucleus • Spinal tract of the trigeminal nucleus	

After CB2 receptors came the discovery of two ligands that are partial ago-nists at both CBRs: N-arachidonoylethanolamide (more commonly known as anandamide, which is based on the Sanskrit word for bliss, Ananda) and 2-AG.

Evidence has more recently emerged that the ECS includes additional GPCRs, with candidates including GPR55, GPR119, and GPR18, though this remains controversial. Similarly, many terpenes, phytocannabinoids, and endo-cannabinoids have demonstrated activity at receptors well beyond the ECS indicating crosstalk between multiple systems (see Table 12-6). For example,

TABLE 12-6: Phytocannabinoid Receptor Activity

Phytocannabinoid	Receptor	Activity
Δ9-Tetrahydrocannabinol (THC)	CB_1	Agonist
	CB_2	Agonist
	GPR18	Agonist
	GPR55	Agonist/antagonist
	PPARγ	Agonist
	TRPA1	Agonist
	TRPA8	Agonist
	TRPM8	Antagonist
	TRPV2	Agonist
	TRPV3	Agonist
	TRPV4	Agonist
	$5\text{-}HT_{3A}$	Antagonist
	β-adrenoceptor	Potentiator
	μ-opioid	Negative allosteric modulator
	δ-opioid	Negative allosteric modulator
Cannabidiol (CBD)	Adenosine (A_1)	Agonist
	Adenosine (A_{2A})	Agonist
	CB_1	Antagonist/allosteric modulator
	CB_2	Inverse agonist/antagonist
	Dopamine 2 (D2)	Partial agonist
	GPR3	Inverse agonist
	GPR6	Inverse agonist
	GPR12	Inverse agonist
	GPR55	Antagonist
	PPARγ	Agonist
	TRPA1	Agonist
	TRPM8	Antagonist
	TRPV1	Agonist
	TRPV2	Agonist
	TRPV3	Agonist
	$5\text{-}HT_{1A}$	Agonist

(continued)

Cannabis

TABLE 12-6: Phytocannabinoid Receptor Activity (*continued*)		
Phytocannabinoid	Receptor	Activity
Cannabigerol (CBG)	CB_1	Agonist/antagonist
	CB_2	Agonist
	TRPA1	Agonist
	TRPM8	Antagonist
	TRPV1	Agonist
	TRPV2	Agonist
	TRPV3	Agonist
	TRPV4	Agonist
	TRPV8	Antagonist
	$5\text{-}HT_{1A}$	Antagonist
	α-adrenoceptor	Agonist
Cannabichromene (CBC)	CB_1	Agonist
	CB_2	Agonist
	TRPA1	Agonist
	TRPM8	Antagonist
Cannabinol (CBN)	CB_1	Agonist
	CB_2	Agonist
	TRPA1	Agonist
	TRPM8	Antagonist
	TRPV2	Agonist
	TRPV4	Agonist
Tetrahydrocannabivarin (THCV)	CB_1	Agonist/antagonist
	CB_2	Agonist
	TRPA1	Agonist
	TRPM8	Antagonist
	TRPV1	Agonist
	TRPV2	Agonist
	TRPV3	Agonist
	TRPV4	Agonist
Tetrahydrocannabinol acid A (THCA-A)	CB1	Agonist
	CB2	Agonist
	TRPA1	Agonist
	TRPM8	Antagonist
	TRPV2	Agonist

TABLE 12-6: Phytocannabinoid Receptor Activity *(continued)*		
Phytocannabinoid	Receptor	Activity
Cannabidivarin (CBDV)	TRPA1	Agonist
	TRPM8	Antagonist
	TRPV1	Agonist
	TRPV2	Agonist
	TRPV4	Agonist
Cannabidiolic acid (CBDA)	GPR55	Agonist
	TRPA1	Agonist
	TRPM8	Antagonist
	TRPV1	Agonist
	5-HT$_{1A}$	Agonist

anandamide has been shown to bind to transient receptor potential (TRP) channels, particularly the vanilloid receptor 1 (also known as the capsaicin receptor and best known for its function in nociceptive pathways detecting noxious heat and pain), as well as peroxisome proliferator–activated receptors (which are ligand-activated transcription factors that are involved in regulating glucose and lipid homeostasis, inflammation, proliferation, and differentiation).

Endocannabinoid System Signaling

Perhaps the most distinguishing feature of the ECS is that endocannabinoids like 2-AG and anandamide are synthesized on demand in the postsynaptic neuron following physiologic and pathologic stimuli, and then travel across the synaptic cleft to the presynaptic neuron to modulate signal transduction pathways. This makes them retrograde neuromodulators.

At CB1, anandamide and 2-AG inhibit the excessive release of excitatory neurotransmitters, particularly glutamate. At CB2, endocannabinoids suppress proinflammatory cytokine and chemokine release. This mechanism of action helps to explain cannabis' anti-inflammatory and immunomodulatory effects. Some researchers have even proposed that selective CB2 agonists could mitigate the phenomenon known as cytokine storm. In essence, a properly functioning ECS is meant to behave a bit like a braking system or a dimmer switch to prevent hyperactive signaling that can lead to cell damage and to maintain physiologic homeostasis.

There is also a growing body of evidence indicating that CB1 receptors play a very important role in neuronal migration, which is why cannabis use, especially the use of cannabis that is extremely high in THC, should be discouraged in adolescents, young adults under the age of 25, and pregnant or breastfeeding women.

Cannabis and the ECS

Ongoing research into the extent of the ECS has indicated that many cannabinoids and terpenes interact with CB1 and CB2 receptors either directly or indirectly. THC, for example, is a partial agonist at both CB1 and CB2 receptors, while CBD is believed to be a negative allosteric modulator at CB1 and possibly only a weak agonist at CB2. CBD has also been shown to inhibit fatty acid amide hydrolase, or FAAH, which breaks down anandamide. By disrupting the breakdown of anandamide, this allows the molecule to stay active for longer periods.

While endocannabinoids naturally degrade very quickly, phytocannabinoids, such as THC and CBD, may remain active for several hours depending on route of administration. Beyond providing a more prolonged therapeutic effect in the suppression of excitatory neurotransmitter release or leukocyte proliferation, it is also why exogenous CB1 agonists produce intoxicating effects, whereas endogenous agonists do not.

CBD and THC, as well as the dozens of other minor cannabinoids and terpenes that appear in commercially available cannabis, are also active at several additional receptor sites (see Table 12-6). This complex interplay between myriad receptors may explain not only the variation in subjective experience following the use of different samples of cannabis, but also differences in action that are of a clinical nature. In other words, as cannabis science improves, research may find that specific varieties of cannabis are better at treating specific conditions due to their unique cannabinoid and terpene profiles.

Conclusion

To summarize, the ECS should be understood as a network involved in maintaining physiologic homeostasis. When homeostasis is disrupted in the CNS or immune system, a healthy ECS is supposed to act as a dimmer switch and bring the system back into harmony. In instances when the ECS is incapable of correcting these disruptions on its own, cannabis appears to offer additional support.

The two following chapters will explore how THC and CBD interact with the ECS, as well as their indications, pharmacokinetics, and pharmacodynamics. Some of the minor cannabinoids show similar activity and research is ongoing into just how many have therapeutic potential. We're just starting to gain an understanding of their individual pharmacology and we may soon come to learn that some of these minor cannabinoids have unique therapeutic properties that act through the ECS or beyond.

Marijuana

13

Generic Name	Trade Name	Adverse Effects	Drug Interactions	CYP Interactions
Marijuana	N/A	GI symptoms, paranoia, dizziness, drowsiness, confusion, tachycardia, headache	CNS, lithium, sympathomimetics, TRI/TET, cyclosporine, warfarin, ritonavir, amphotericin B	2C9, 3A4, 2C19, 1A1, 1A2, 1B1, 2B6, 2C8, 2E1, 2D6, 3A5, 3A7
Dronabinol	Marinol	GI symptoms, paranoia, dizziness, drowsiness, confusion, tachycardia, headache	CNS, lithium, sympathomimetics, TRI/TFT, cyclosporine, warfarin, ritonavir, amphotericin B	2C9, 3A4, 2C19, 1A2, 2B6, 2D6, 1A1, 3A5, 3A7, 1B1, 2A6
Nabilone	Cesamet	GI symptoms, paranoia, dizziness, drowsiness, confusion, tachycardia, headache	CNS, lithium, sympathomimetics, TRI/TET, cyclosporine, warfarin, ritonavir, amphotericin B	2C9, 3A4, 2C8, 2E1

Introduction

Cannabis sativa plants that contain high levels of Δ9-tetrahydrocannabinol (THC) and preparations of dried plant material (typically the female cannabis flower) have been referred to as marijuana since the 19th century. As noted in Chapter 12, this distinction was only recently codified by the federal government following the passage of the Farm Bill of 2014, which defined cannabis that contains concentrations exceeding 0.3% THC by dry weight as marijuana. Since 1996, more than three dozen states and the District of Columbia have created medical cannabis programs, legalized the recreational use of cannabis, or both. Restrictions in these states vary significantly, both with regard to who is allowed access to these formulations and what levels of THC are lawful. THC is the most abundant phytocannabinoid in drug-type cannabis, as well as the most well-studied cannabinoid.

This chapter will focus on the pharmacology of marijuana and specifically THC, the primary intoxicant and therapeutic compound in marijuana as well as the two Food and Drug Administration (FDA)-approved cannabinoids, dronabinol (a synthetic form of THC), and nabilone. Cannabidiol (CBD) will be covered in the following chapter.

MEDICAL MARIJUANA

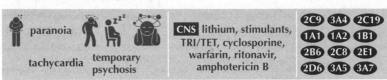

paranoia

tachycardia temporary psychosis

CNS lithium, stimulants, TRI/TET, cyclosporine, warfarin, ritonavir, amphotericin B

2C9 3A4 2C19
1A1 1A2 1B1
2B6 2C8 2E1
2D6 3A5 3A7

Marijuana should not be considered a single or uniform drug unless it is administered as one of two formulations that have been approved by the FDA. These are dronabinol and nabilone, which produce subjective and therapeutic effects that are similar to the primary active intoxicant in cannabis, Δ9-THC. Beyond variations in cannabinoid content (especially levels of CBD and THC), marijuana that is purchased legally at a dispensary may come in a wide variety of forms and strengths, making a straightforward pharmacokinetic or pharmacodynamic profile impossible, especially with respect to the absorption, metabolism, and route of administration of THC.

It is highly advised that cannabis-naive patients avoid formulations that contain more than 10 mg of THC per dose/serving or cannabis flower that contains excessive levels of THC (>20%). Patients should be advised that edible forms of cannabis often take upwards of 2 hours to take effect and that in all circumstances it is best to start low and go slow to avoid unwanted adverse events or unpleasant levels of intoxication.

Pharmacokinetics

Onset of action, peak plasma levels, and even the bioavailability of THC can be affected by route of administration (see Tables 13-1 and 13-2), as well as intrapersonal and interpersonal factors. For example, smoking cannabis may result in rapid onset of action, but upwards of 30% of available phytocannabinoids may be lost due to pyrolysis and even more may be cast off as side-stream smoke. Meanwhile, plasma concentrations of THC and its metabolites can vary depending on route of administration, which may also have an impact on pharmacokinetics and the subjective experience of patients, since THC is converted into 11-hydroxy-Δ9-tetrahydrocannabinol (11-OH-THC) and 11-nor-9-carboxy-Δ9-tetrahydrocannbinol (THC-COOH) following first-pass metabolism. Of note, 11-OH-THC produces a greater level of intoxication than its parent compound. When cannabis is smoked, 11-OH-THC plasma concentrations may only reach 10% of THC plasma concentrations. However, when administered orally, 11-OH-THC plasma concentrations can vary from 50% to 100% of THC plasma

TABLE 13-1: Pharmacokinetics of Various Routes of Administration of THC		
Route of Administration	Peak Plasma Levels	Bioavailability
Inhalation	3–10 minutes	18–50%
Oral	60–120 minutes	4–12%
Sublingual	90–120 minutes	4–20%

TABLE 13-2: Strengths and Weaknesses of Various Routes of Administration of THC

Route of Administration	Onset (minutes)	Duration (hours)	Strength	Weakness
Inhalation	0–5	1–3	• Rapid onset • Easy titration • Good safety record, especially for vaporized flower	• Respiratory irritation • Pungent smell, especially smokable flower • Risk of adverse pulmonary/cardiovascular side effects
Oral/enteric	60–120	6–8	• Long duration of action • More palatable than other options	• Slow onset • Increased variability in effect • Increased psychoactive effects from 11-OH-THC following first-pass metabolism
Sublingual	15–20	2–3	• Easy titration • Intermediate duration of action	• Intermediate onset (15–20 minutes) • Increased psychoactive effects from 11-OH-THC if swallowed

concentrations. Bioavailability may be additionally enhanced following oral administration if patients eat a meal that is high in fat, as THC is highly lipophilic. Meanwhile, sublingual administration bypasses hepatic metabolism and provides therapeutic action more quickly compared to when THC is taken orally but less quickly than when it is smoked or vaped.

These kinds of variations can make proper dosing difficult, so clinicians should advise patients to start low and go slow when using marijuana for the first time or titrating their dose.

Distribution

THC is rapidly distributed into organs that are well vascularized (i.e., lung, heart, brain, liver) and accumulates in adipose tissue upon repeated use.

Elimination and Excretion

Between 80% and 90% of a single dose of THC is eliminated within 5 days, 65% through feces (predominately as the metabolite 11-OH-THC) and approximately 20% through urine (as the metabolite THC-COOH glucuronide conjugates). Metabolites may be detectable in frequent users for several weeks upon cessation.

Pharmacodynamics

Mechanism of Action

THC interacts with the endocannabinoid system (ECS), a signaling network consisting of endogenous ligands, breakdown enzymes, two cannabinoid receptors (CB1 and CB2), and several other receptors located throughout the body (a more detailed examination of the ECS can be found in Chapter 12). THC is a CB1 partial agonist and can behave as either an agonist or antagonist at CB2 receptors and has approximately an equal affinity for both CB1 and

CB2 receptors. CB1 receptors are located throughout the central nervous system (CNS) on presynaptic terminals (see Table 12-4), mediate the release of excitatory and inhibitory neurotransmitters (serotonin, dopamine, and glutamate), and modulate ion channels. The effects on mood, perception, emotion, and cognition often associated with cannabis use are due to the activation of CB1 receptors. Activation of CB1 receptors in the CNS also leads to antinociception, catalepsy, suppression of locomotor activity, and hypothermia. Low or moderate doses of THC can also stimulate appetite (hyperphagia) while higher doses can reduce appetite (hypophagia).

CB2 receptors in the periphery are located mainly in the immune system (bone marrow, mast cells, natural killer cells, polymorphonuclear neutrophils, spleen, thymus, tonsils, and T and B lymphocytes) and modulate immune cell migration and the release of cytokines. Within the CNS, CB2 receptors are also found within the neuroimmune system in microglia, astrocytes, and oligodendrocytes, as well as on the presynaptic terminals of specific neuron types (see Table 12-5). There is some hope that these receptors could serve as therapeutic targets for several neurodegenerative disorders and to potentially counteract neuroinflammation in general. Trauma and inflammation increase CB2 expression indicating that CB2 receptors play an immunomodulatory role.

THC also interacts with several other receptors (see Table 13-3), including orphan G-protein receptors (GPR18 and GPR55); 5-HT3A receptors; and transient receptor potential (TRP) channels. What potential therapeutic role these receptors play is currently unclear.

TABLE 13-3: Observed Receptor Activity of THC	
Receptor	Activity
CB_1	Agonist
CB_2	Agonist
GPR18	Agonist
GPR55	Agonist/antagonist
PPARγ	Agonist
TRPA1	Agonist
TRPA8	Agonist
TRPM8	Antagonist
TRPV2	Agonist
TRPV3	Agonist
TRPV4	Agonist
5-HT_{3A}	Antagonist
β-Adrenoceptor	Potentiator
μ-Opioid	Negative allosteric modulator
δ-Opioid	Negative allosteric modulator

Therapeutic Index

Beyond the wide variety of types of products that qualify as medical marijuana, it is also highly idiosyncratic, and effective doses can vary from patient to patient. Fortunately, cannabis has a high therapeutic index, and it has been estimated that a lethal dose of THC is at least 1,000 times greater than an effective dose.

Tolerance, Dependence, and Withdrawal

Frequent cannabis users may develop a tolerance to cannabis. Frequent and heavy users may also develop dependence, as well as cannabis use disorder, which the Diagnostic and Statistical Manual of Mental Disorders, Fifth Edition (DSM-5) describes as being characterized by cravings for cannabis and withdrawal symptoms upon cessation that may include anxiety, irritability, restlessness, loss of appetite, headache, and difficulty sleeping, among others.

Therapeutic Indications

At this time, marijuana has not been approved for any indications as it remains a Schedule I drug, and only three cannabinoid-based therapies have received FDA approval: dronabinol (Marinol, Syndros), nabilone (Cesamet), and CBD (Epidiolex), which will be discussed in the next chapter. Dronabinol and nabilone have received FDA approval for use in treating nausea and vomiting associated with cancer chemotherapy for patients who have not responded well to first-line antiemetics (see Table 13-4). Dronabinol has also been approved to treat anorexia/cachexia associated with weight loss in patients with HIV/acquired immune deficiency syndrome (AIDS) and has been used off-label to help patients with obstructive sleep apnea.

TABLE 13-4: Schedules of Cannabis-Based Drugs			
Drug Name	Trade Name	Schedule (Year Approved by FDA)	Indications
Dronabinol (synthetic THC)	Marinol	Schedule III (1985)	HIV/AIDS-induced anorexia and chemotherapy-induced nausea and vomiting
Dronabinol (synthetic THC)	Syndros	Schedule II (2017)	HIV/AIDS-induced anorexia and chemotherapy-induced nausea and vomiting
Nabilone (synthetic THC)	Cesamet	Schedule II (1985)	Chemotherapy-induced nausea and vomiting
Cannabidiol	Epidiolex	Schedule V (2018)	Seizures associated with: Lennox–Gastaut Syndrome Dravet Syndrome Tuberous sclerosis complex (2020)
Nabiximols (formulation consisting of THC, CBD, and minor constituents)	Sativex	Not available in the United States; available in over 25 countries, including EU members and Canada	Spasticity and neuropathic pain associated with multiple sclerosis

Marijuana

State Approved Indications

Depending on the state, medical marijuana may be recommended for dozens of conditions and has shown a great deal of promise as a means of mitigating chronic and neuropathic pain, autoimmune disorders, and spasticity. It may also offer palliative care or some relief for patients enduring end-of-life care. Each state with a medical marijuana program either has a list of qualifying conditions that providers should consult before recommending cannabis or allows eligible medical professionals to use their best judgment when recommending cannabis through states' medical marijuana programs (see Table 13-5).

TABLE 13-5: Potential Qualifying Conditions for Medical Marijuana
Alzheimer disease
Amyotrophic lateral sclerosis (ALS)
Anorexia nervosa
Anxiety
Arnold–Chiari malformation
Arthritis
Autism spectrum disorder
Bulimia
Cachexia
Cancer
Causalgia
Cerebral palsy
Chronic inflammatory demyelinating polyneuropathy
Chronic pancreatitis
Chronic traumatic encephalopathy
Cirrhosis
Colitis
Complex regional pain syndrome
Crohn disease
Cystic fibrosis
Diabetes
Dysmenorrhea
Dystonia
Ehlers–Danlos syndrome
Elevated intraocular pressure
Endometriosis
Epidermolysis bullosa

TABLE 13-5: Potential Qualifying Conditions for Medical Marijuana (*continued*)
Epilepsy
Fibromyalgia
Fibrous dysplasia
Friedrich ataxia
Glaucoma
Hepatitis C
HIV/AIDS
Huntington disease
Hydrocephalus
Hydromyelia
Inclusion body myositis
Interstitial cystitis
Inflammatory bowel disease
Intractable headache syndromes
Irreversible spinal cord injury
Lewy body disease (LBD)
Lupus
Medial arcuate ligament syndrome (MALS)
Migraines
Mitochondrial disease
Muscular dystrophy
Multiple sclerosis
Myasthenia gravis
Myoclonus
Nail-patella syndrome
Neuralgia
Neuro-Behcet autoimmune disease
Neurodegenerative disorders
Neurofibromatosis
Neuropathic pain
Obstructive sleep apnea
Obsessive–compulsive disorder (OCD)
Opioid dependency
Opioid substitution
Osteoarthritis

Marijuana

(*continued*)

TABLE 13-5: Potential Qualifying Conditions for Medical Marijuana (*continued*)
Osteogenesis imperfecta
Parkinson disease
Peripheral neuropathy
Polycystic kidney disease (PKD)
Postconcussion syndrome
Postlaminectomy syndrome
Posttraumatic stress disorder (PTSD)
Psoriasis
Psoriatic arthritis
Reflex sympathetic dystrophy
Residual limb pain
Rheumatoid arthritis
Seizures
Severe or chronic nausea
Severe or chronic pain
Severe and persistent muscle spasms
Sickle cell diseases
Sjogren syndrome
Spasmodic torticollis
Spinal cord diseases
Spinal cord injury
Spinal muscular atrophy
Spinal stenosis
Spinocerebellar ataxia syndrome
Superior canal dehiscence syndrome
Syringomyelia
Tarlov cysts
Tourette syndrome
Traumatic brain injury
Ulcerative colitis
Vulvodynia

Potential Indications and Ongoing Research

Research indicates that marijuana may be effective at improving quality of life for patients and treating several neurologic or psychiatric conditions, including but not limited to nonmotor symptoms associated with Parkinson disease,

TABLE 13-6: Adverse Reactions to Dronabinol		
Rate of Incidence 3–10%	Rate of Incidence 1–3%	Rate of Incidence >1%
• Abnormal thinking • Abdominal pain • Dizziness • Euphoria • Nausea • Paranoia • Somnolence • Vomiting	• Asthenia • Amnesia • Anxiety • Ataxia • Confusion • Depersonalization • Hallucination	• Conjunctivitis • Depression • Diarrhea • Fecal incontinence • Flushing • Hypotension • Myalgia • Nightmares • Speech difficulties • Tinnitus • Vision difficulties

multiple sclerosis (MS), traumatic brain injury, Alzheimer disease and other forms of dementia, amyotrophic lateral sclerosis and other motor neuron diseases, Huntington disease, migraines, obstructive sleep apnea, and Tourette syndrome. However, due to marijuana's status as a Schedule I drug, research into its potential uses has been limited and there is little evidence at this time to support its use for these indications.

Nabiximols (Sativex), which contains THC, CBD, and other cannabinoids, has been approved to treat MS in more than two dozen countries and is currently undergoing advanced phase III trials in the United States.

Precautions and Adverse Events

Commonly reported adverse effects of THC are similar to those reported during use of dronabinol or nabilone (see Tables 13-6 and 13-7, respectively). Paradoxically, THC may on occasion induce nausea or vomiting and in extremely rare cases consistent use with high-THC products may cause cannabis hyperemesis syndrome, which is characterized by cyclic vomiting and nausea that is reportedly eased by hot showers and baths and ceases upon discontinuing marijuana use. As is the case with cigarette smoking, excessive cannabis smoking can adversely impact lung function and cardiovascular health.

TABLE 13-7: Adverse Reactions to Nabilone	
Rate of Incidence >10%	Rate of Incidence <10%
• Vertigo/dizziness • Drowsiness • Dry mouth • Ataxia • Depression • Visual disturbance • Difficulty concentrating • Euphoria • Sleep disturbance	• Dysphoria • Hypotension • Asthenia • Anorexia • Headache • Nausea • Sedation • Disorientation • Depersonalization • Increased appetite

Marijuana

Psychiatric Adverse Reactions

Extremely high doses of THC can induce acute, transient psychotic states and there is an ongoing debate about the role that THC can play in the development of psychotic disorders, such as schizophrenia, especially during adolescent years. Considering the high risk in this age group, research is ongoing to determine the pre-existing factors and numerous studies are exploring the link for causality in the vulnerable population. Clinicians should be cautious when recommending medical marijuana for patients who have a personal or family history of psychotic disorders or if patients are under the age of 25, as THC may disrupt neuronal migration and development.

Hazardous Activities

Patients should not drive or use heavy machinery while under the influence of cannabis.

Risk of Overdose or Abuse

An overdose of medical marijuana will likely result in an unpleasant experience, but the effects will fade in time. As cannabis has a high therapeutic index, risk of ingesting a lethal dosage is extremely low.

Cannabis use disorder is a well-documented phenomenon characterized by cravings for cannabis, as well as withdrawal symptoms upon cessation that may include anxiety, irritability, restlessness, loss of appetite, headache, and difficulty sleeping, among others.

Use in Pregnancy and Lactation

Women who are breastfeeding, pregnant, or actively trying to become pregnant should not use cannabis. While the dangers that marijuana and THC specifically poses to fetuses and breastfeeding infants have not been studied due to ethical concerns, use of nonsynthetic cannabis has been associated with adverse fetal/neonatal outcomes. THC readily crosses the placenta and it has an estimated mean half-life of 17 days in breast milk.

Drug Interactions

THC is metabolized primarily by cytochrome P450 enzymes CYP2C9 and CYP3A4. Drug-induced inhibition of either CYP2C9 or CYP3A4 may result in higher plasma concentrations of THC, which may increase the potential of adverse reactions and excessive THC intoxication. Inducers of these isoenzymes may result in lower plasma concentration of THC. Clinicians should adjust dosages when co-administered with drugs that affect either isoenzyme.

THC may produce an additive effect when taken in conjunction with alcohol, anticholinergics, antihistamines, barbiturates, benzodiazepines, buspirone, lithium, muscle relaxants, opioids, sympathomimetics, and tricyclic antidepressants. Because THC is highly bound to plasma proteins, it may augment the free fraction of co-administered protein-bound drugs (as when taken with amphotericin B, cyclosporine, and warfarin). Co-administration of ritonavir exacerbates the effects of THC.

DRONABINOL

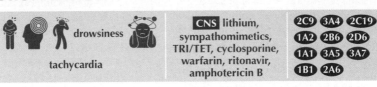

drowsiness

tachycardia

CNS lithium, sympathomimetics, TRI/TET, cyclosporine, warfarin, ritonavir, amphotericin B

2C9 3A4 2C19
1A2 2B6 2D6
1A1 3A5 3A7
1B1 2A6

Dronabinol is a synthetic version of Δ9-THC. It may be administered as Marinol, which is formulated in sesame oil and is dispensed in the form of a capsule, or Syndros, which is clear to amber oral solution administered via oral dosing syringe or enteral feeding tube.

Pharmacokinetics

Absorption

Between 90% and 95% of dronabinol is absorbed after a single oral dose, but only 10% to 20% reaches systemic circulation due to a combination of first-pass hepatic metabolism and high lipid solubility. Concentrations of dronabinol and its major active metabolite, 11-hydroxy-Δ9-tetrahydrocannabinol (11-OH-THC), peak between 0.5 and 4 hours and decline over the course of several days. Plasma concentrations are dose dependent. Food intake, particularly a high-fat/high-calorie meal, delays absorption by about 4 hours and causes a threefold increase in total exposure.

Distribution and Bioavailability

Dronabinol has a high protein binding of 97% with apparent volume of distribution of approximately 10 L/kg.

Elimination

The initial half-life of dronabinol is approximately 4 hours and the terminal half-life ranges from 25 to 36 hours.

Metabolism

Dronabinol undergoes extensive first-pass hepatic metabolism, with CYP2C9 and CYP3A4 being the primary enzymes.

Excretion

Dronabinol and its metabolites are excreted in both feces and urine, though biliary excretion is the primary route of elimination. Low levels of dronabinol metabolites may continue to be excreted in urine and feces for up to 5 weeks.

Pharmacodynamics

Mechanism of Action

Dronabinol has a complex set of effects on the CNS via the ECS, particularly at CB1 receptors.

Marijuana

Dose-Response Curve

The onset of action of dronabinol is approximately 0.5 to 1 hour, with peak subjective effects occurring within 2 to 4 hours. Psychoactive effects typically abate after 4 to 6 hours. Dronabinol may stimulate appetite for up to 24 hours after administration.

Tolerance, Dependence, and Withdrawal

Tolerance to dronabinol develops quickly and is readily reversible. Continued administration of dronabinol may lead to dependency or addiction and withdrawal following cessation. Withdrawal symptoms may include anxiety, irritability, restlessness, loss of appetite, headache, and difficulty sleeping, among others.

Therapeutic Indications

There are two indications for dronabinol:

1. Anorexia associated with weight loss in patients with AIDS.
2. Nausea and vomiting associated with cancer chemotherapy in patients who have failed to respond to other antiemetic treatments.

Precautions and Adverse Events

Some of the most common adverse effects to dronabinol, as well as marijuana, can be found in Table 13-6. The most frequently reported adverse experiences involved the CNS, especially during the first 2 weeks of use. These include euphoria, confusion, fast heartbeat (tachycardia), and severe dizziness.

Psychiatric Adverse Reactions

Like marijuana, dronabinol may exacerbate existing psychiatric conditions such as schizophrenia, bipolar disorder, and depression. Clinicians should screen patients for existing psychiatric conditions before initiating treatment with dronabinol and use of the drug should be avoided in patients with a history of mental illness and those who have a personal or family history of psychotic disorders or if patients are under the age of 25. If use of the drug cannot be avoided, clinicians should monitor patients for new or worsening symptoms. In addition, clinicians should avoid concomitant use of dronabinol with other drugs associated with similar psychiatric effects.

Hazardous Activities

Patients should not drive or use heavy machinery while using dronabinol.

Risk of Abuse and Dependence

Dronabinol is a Schedule III drug and may pose a potential risk of abuse. Though this risk may be quite low, continued administration of dronabinol may lead to dependency or addiction. With long-term use, symptoms of dependence may appear within 12 hours of discontinuation (e.g., irritability, insomnia, and restlessness). Most symptoms dissipate after 48 hours of discontinuation, though some patients have reported sleep disturbances for several weeks following treatment.

Use in Pregnancy and Lactation

Women who are breastfeeding, pregnant, or actively trying to become pregnant should not use cannabis or FDA-approved formulations of THC, including dronabinol.

Drug Interactions

Dronabinol is metabolized by CYP2C9 and CYP3A4 isoenzymes, and inhibition of either CYP will result in higher plasma concentrations of dronabinol. Clinicians may need to adjust dosages when co-administered with an inhibitor or inducer of either isoenzyme. Dronabinol is highly protein bound and may displace and increase the free portion of other highly protein-bound drugs (e.g., warfarin, cyclosporine, amphotericin B).

Dosing and Clinical Guidelines

Dronabinol is available in 2.5-, 5-, and 10-mg capsules, as well as in an oral solution with a 5 mg/mL dose. When treating anorexia, the starting dosage should be 2.5 mg twice daily approximately 1 hour before lunch and dinner. If patients do not experience an increase in appetite, the dosage can be gradually increased but should not exceed a dosage of 10 mg twice daily. When treating chemotherapy-induced nausea and vomiting, body surface area based dosing can be helpful in optimizing dosage. The dosage should start at 5 mg/m^2 and be administered 1 to 3 hours before chemotherapy and repeat every 2 to 4 following for a total of 4 to 6 doses per day. The maximum dosage is 15 mg/m^2 four to six times per day.

Geriatric Use

Elderly patients with dementia may experience exacerbated CNS effects of somnolence or dizziness, thereby increasing the risk of injury from a fall. Clinicians should be advised to exercise caution with dose selection when initiating treatment.

NABILONE

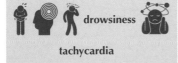 drowsiness, tachycardia

CNS lithium, sympathomimetics, TRI/TET, cyclosporine, warfarin, ritonavir, amphotericin B

 2C9 3A4 2C8 2E1

Nabilone is a synthetic cannabinoid that is similar to Δ9-THC. It is administered via capsule and each capsule contains 1 mg of nabilone.

Pharmacokinetics

Absorption

Data indicates that nabilone is completely absorbed in the gastrointestinal tract when administered orally. Following the administration of a 2 mg dose, peak plasma concentrations of 2 ng/mL were reached within 2.0 hours.

Distribution

Nabilone has an apparent volume of distribution of approximately 12.5 L/kg.

Bioavailability

The bioavailability of nabilone is not available at this time.

Metabolism

The precise information regarding the metabolism of nabilone and the accumulation of its metabolites is not currently available, though available evidence suggests that at least one nabilone metabolite has a terminal elimination half-life that exceeds that of the parent compound.

At least two metabolic pathways associated with the biotransformation of nabilone have been confirmed, and two metabolites, one an isomeric carbinol metabolite and one an isomeric diol metabolite, have been identified. As is the case with other cannabinoids, particularly THC and CBD, evidence indicates that there is extensive metabolism by multiple cytochrome P450 enzyme isoforms.

Elimination

Plasma half-life for nabilone and its metabolites was found to be 2 hours and 35 hours, respectively. Food intake did not significantly alter the rate of absorption.

Excretion

Within 7 days, approximately 67% of intravenously administered nabilone was eliminated through feces and 22% was eliminated through urine. Of the 67% excreted in feces, approximately 5% was unchanged nabilone and 16% was a carbinol metabolite. Following oral administration, 60% was eliminated through feces and 24% was eliminated through urine.

Pharmacodynamics

Mechanism of Action

Nabilone has a complex set of effects on the CNS via the ECS, particularly at CB1 receptors.

Dose-Response Curve

Nabilone has a high degree of interpatient variability, and patients should be supervised during initial use and following dose adjustments. The onset of action of nabilone is approximately 1 to 1.5 hours and may persist for 8 to 12 hours.

Tolerance, Dependence, and Withdrawal

Tolerance to nabilone develops quickly and is readily reversible. Continued administration of nabilone may lead to dependency or addiction. A clinical trial that lasted 5 days produced no evidence of withdrawal symptoms following discontinuance. Longer periods of use may lead to withdrawal symptoms that include anxiety, irritability, restlessness, loss of appetite, headache, and difficulty sleeping.

Therapeutic Indications

Nabilone is indicated for nausea and vomiting associated with cancer chemotherapy in patients who have failed to respond to other antiemetic treatments.

Precautions and Adverse Reactions

The most common adverse effects of nabilone are drowsiness, vertigo, dry mouth, euphoria, ataxia, headache, and difficulty concentrating. Additional adverse reactions are noted in Table 13-7. Nabilone may affect the CNS, which may cause feelings of dizziness, drowsiness, euphoria, anxiety, ataxia, disorientation, depression, hallucinations, and even psychosis. It may also cause tachycardia and hypotension. Some of these effects may be exacerbated by other drugs, particularly alcohol, hypnotics, sedatives, or other psychoactive substances.

Psychiatric Adverse Reactions

Nabilone may exacerbate existing psychiatric conditions such as schizophrenia, bipolar disorder, and depression. Clinicians should screen patients for existing psychiatric conditions before initiating treatment with dronabinol and use of the drug should be avoided in patients with a history of mental illness and those who have a personal or family history of psychotic disorders or if patients are under the age of 25. If use of the drug cannot be avoided, clinicians should monitor patients for new or worsening symptoms. In addition, clinicians should avoid concomitant use of nabilone with other drugs associated with similar psychiatric effects.

Hazardous Activities

Patients should not drive or use heavy machinery while using nabilone.

Risk of Abuse and Dependence

Nabilone is a Schedule II drug and may pose a potential risk of abuse.

Pregnant and Nursing Women

There is limited information on the effects of nabilone during pregnancy or while breastfeeding, but it is recommended that nursing women, pregnant women, or women who plan to become pregnant be prescribed nabilone.

Drug Interactions

Nabilone is highly bound to plasma proteins and may displace other protein-bound drugs, requiring adjustment of dosage. Nabilone has not been shown to significantly inhibit CYP1A2, CYP2A6, CYP2C19, CYP2D6, or CYP3A4; had a weak inhibitory effect on CYP2E1 and CYP3A4; and had a moderate inhibitory effect on CYP2C8 and CYP2C9. When co-administered with other drugs, nabilone is unlikely to interfere with P450-mediated degradation.

Dosage and Clinical Guidelines

Nabilone marketed under the name Cesamet is administered orally and is available in capsule formulation containing 1 mg of nabilone. Treatment with 1 or 2 mg of nabilone may be administered two to three times daily during each cycle of chemotherapy. Nabilone can be administered either 1 to 3 hours prior to chemotherapy or taken the night before with the maximum daily dose of 6 mg/day administered in three divided doses (t.i.d). If necessary, nabilone may be administered up to 48 hours following the last dose of each cycle of chemotherapy.

Geriatric Use

Clinicians should exercise caution before prescribing nabilone to elderly patients, as they may be more sensitive to its psychotropic and cardiovascular effects.

Cannabidiol (CBD)

  CNS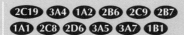

Introduction

Cannabidiol (CBD) is one of the more than 150 phytocannabinoids found in the plant *Cannabis sativa L.*, which is legally defined in the United States as either marijuana (0.3% Δ9-tetrahydrocannabinol [THC] by dry weight or more) or hemp (less than 0.3% THC by dry weight). CBD occurs in relatively low concentrations in marijuana, but in high concentrations in industrial hemp. While the use of CBD has become widespread in recent years as an over-the-counter treatment for a host of conditions ranging from insomnia to chronic pain associated with inflammatory conditions like arthritis, it is currently only indicated for use in treating rare forms of epilepsy—including Lennox–Gastaut syndrome and Dravet syndrome, as well as seizures associated with tuberous sclerosis complex—under the name Epidiolex.

Pharmacology

CBD is one of the phytocannabinoids found in cannabis. It is found in herbal cannabis and in a myriad of products. The sole formulation of CBD approved by the Food and Drug Administration (FDA) is Epidiolex, which is a clear, colorless to slightly yellow solution that contains CBD at a concentration of 100 mg/mL. It is administered orally via a calibrated oral syringe.

Pharmacokinetics

In patients, CBD exhibits an increase in exposure that is less than dose proportional over the range of 5 to 20 mg/kg/day. Peak plasma levels and bioavailability of CBD depend on the route of administration in a manner that is very similar to THC (see Table 14-1).

Absorption. When taken orally, maximum plasma concentration (Tmax) occurs between 2.5 and 5 hours, and food, particularly a high-fat/high-calorie meal,

TABLE 14-1: Pharmacokinetics of Various Routes of Administration of CBD		
Route of Administration	Peak Plasma Levels	Bioavailability
Inhalation	3–10 minutes	11–45%
Oral	2.5–5 hours	13–19%
Sublingual	1.64–4.2 hours	13–19%

151

increases the maximum serum concentration (Cmax) fivefold, and area under the concentration-time curve from time zero extrapolated to infinity (AUCinf) by four-fold. Inhaled CBD can reach peak blood plasma levels in as little as 3 minutes while sublingual administration falls between these two extremes.

Bioavailability.   The bioavailability of CBD depends on the route of adminis-tration and has been estimated to be 13% to 19% when administered orally or sublingually or in the range of 11% to 45% when inhaled. The extremely wide range in the latter is due to the numerous variables in smoking dynamics.

Distribution.   In healthy volunteers, CBD and its metabolites exhibit in vitro protein binding >94%.

Metabolism.   CBD is metabolized primarily by cytochrome P450 enzyme (CYP) system, specifically CYP2C19 and CYP3A4 enzymes, as well as UGT1A7, UGT1A9, and UGT2B7 isoforms. The two primary metabolites of CBD are 7-hydroxy-cannabidiol (7-OH-CBD) and 7-carboxy-cannabidiol (7-COOH-CBD), both of which may have anti-inflammatory properties.

Elimination.   The half-life of CBD in plasma is between 56 and 61 hours after twice-a-day dosing for 7 days, with a plasma clearance of 1,111 L/hour following a single dose 1.1 times the maximum recommended daily dosage of 1,500 mg.

Excretion.   The majority of CBD is excreted through feces, with only minor renal clearance.

Pharmacodynamics

Mechanism of Action.   The precise mechanism of action of CBD is unknown and its anticonvulsant effects are not due to its interaction with cannabinoid receptors. It is likely that the anticonvulsant effects are due to the cumulative effects arising from the modulation of Gamma-aminobutyric (GABA) channels and its activity at other sites. CBD has been shown to be active at transient receptor potential (TRP) channels (see Table 14-2), acts as an agonist at sero-tonin (5-HT1A) receptors, a partial agonist at dopamine (D2) receptors, and has been shown to enhance the signaling of adenosine and glycine receptors. CBD is also believed to be an antagonist at orphan G-protein–coupled receptor 55 (GPR55) at nanomolar to micromolar concentrations.

Unlike THC, CBD does not cause intoxication, though it can be consid-ered psychotropic because of its anxiolytic and stimulating effects. Also, unlike THC, CBD appears to indirectly interact with cannabinoid receptor 1 (CB1) and cannabinoid receptor 2 (CB2). Moreover, it acts as a negative allosteric modulator at CB1 and CB2 receptors and may antagonize both CB receptors when administered with THC, thereby attenuating some of the unpleasant effects of THC or the THC metabolite 11-hydrodxy-Δ9-tetrahy-drocannbinol (11-OH-THC), particularly, anxiety, tachycardia, sedation, and hunger. CBD also inhibits first-pass metabolism of THC and can reduce plasma levels of the THC metabolite 11-OH-THC, which is significantly more potent than its parent compound.

| TABLE 14-2: Observed Receptor Activity ||
Receptor	Activity
Adenosine (A₁)	Agonist
Adenosine (A₂ₐ)	Agonist
CB₁	Antagonist/allosteric modulator
CB₂	Inverse agonist/antagonist
Dopamine 2 (D2)	Partial agonist
GPR3	Inverse agonist
GPR6	Inverse agonist
GPR12	Inverse agonist
GPR55	Antagonist
PPARγ	Agonist
TRPA1	Agonist
TRPM8	Antagonist
TRPV1	Agonist
TRPV2	Agonist
TRPV3	Agonist
5-HT₁ₐ	Agonist

Therapeutic Index. The therapeutic index of CBD is very high. Doses of 50 mg/kg/day have been well tolerated.

Tolerance, Dependence, and Withdrawal. Frequent users of CBD do not appear to develop tolerance or dependence, nor do they experience withdrawal upon cessation.

Therapeutic Indications

The CBD formulation Epidiolex is currently indicated to treat rare forms of epilepsy, including Lennox–Gastaut syndrome and Dravet syndrome, as well as seizures associated with tuberous sclerosis complex. CBD is believed to have myriad additional therapeutic properties, including acting as an analgesic, anticonvulsive, anti-inflammatory, antioxidant, antipsychotic, and neuroprotective agent (see Table 14-3). Some evidence suggests that CBD may also be capable of penetrating cell membranes and could boost natural intracellular defenses against viruses, particularly interferon signaling pathways. Clinical studies to examine the veracity of these claims and others are ongoing.

Precautions and Adverse Events

CBD has an extremely good safety profile and most side effects associated with its use are minor and disappear upon cessation. They include decreased

TABLE 14-3: Selected Therapeutic Applications of CBD	
Observed Effect	Selected References
Addiction treatment	Russo (2011)
Analgesic	Petzke et al. (2016); Boychuk et al. (2015)
Anticancer	Ligresti et al. (2006); McAllister et al. (2011); Shrivastava et al. (2011)
Anticonvulsant	Pertwee (2008); Jones et al. (2010)
Antidepressant	El-alfy et al. (2010); Hsiao et al. (2012); Shoval et al. (2016)
Anti-inflammatory	Malfait et al. (2000); Hayakawa et al. (2007); Ribeiro et al. (2012, 2015)
Antinausea	Parker et al. (2002); Rock et al. (2008)
Antioxidant	Hampson et al. (1998)
Anxiolytic	Russo et al. (2005)
Graft-v-host disease treatment	Yeshurun et al. (2015)
Neuroprotective	De Lago & Fernández-Ruiz (2007); Hofmann & Frazier (2013); Martin-Moreno et al. (2011); Scuderi et al. (2009)

appetite, diarrhea, fatigue, poor sleep quality, and somnolence. Weight loss has been reported among individuals who have been prescribed large doses (20 mg/kg/day) of Epidiolex. CBD has also been associated with decreases in hemoglobin and hematocrit, as well as increases in serum creatine and transaminases.

As CBD may cause drowsiness in some individuals, the operation of cars or heavy machinery should be avoided until the patient understands how specific formulations of CBD make them feel.

Risk of Overdose and Abuse

Patients receiving daily doses of 750 mg of CBD for 4 weeks did not show signs or symptoms of withdrawal following drug discontinuation. Administration of CBD at doses of 750, 1,500, and 4,500 mg in the fasting state produced positive subjective measures within the accepted placebo range. The results of these studies suggest that CBD does not produce physical dependence and that the risk of abuse is low.

Hepatocellular Injury

Dose-related elevations in liver transaminases (alanine aminotransferase [ALT] or aspartate aminotransferase [AST]) may occur with CBD and elevations of three times the upper limit of normal (ULN) without elevated bilirubin and without an alternative explanation are potential indications of severe liver injury. Of note, these elevations occurred primarily early and within the first 2 months of treatment though there have been cases up to 18 months after initiation. Concomitant administration with valproate and clobazam may increase the risk of transaminase elevation and dose adjustment or discontinuation of valproate or clobazam may be necessary. Seventeen percent of patients had transaminase elevations compared to 1% on placebo.

Baseline Measurement and Monitoring

Baseline transaminase levels are strong indicators of subsequent elevations. Clinicians should obtain baseline serum transaminases (ALT and AST) prior to initiation of CBD and subsequently be tested at 1 month, 3 months, 6 months, and as clinically indicated after the initiation of CBD.

Levels should also be obtained 1 month following any adjustment to dosage or introduction of medications known to impact liver function. Consider more frequent monitoring if the patient is taking valproate or clobazam, or if they have elevated liver enzymes at baseline.

In two-thirds of cases, liver transaminase levels returned to normal following either the discontinuance of CBD or a reduction in dosage. In one-third of cases, liver transaminase levels returned to normal without altering dosage.

Clinicians should be vigilant and monitor patients for signs and symptoms of liver dysfunction (nausea, jaundice, vomiting, fatigue, anorexia, etc.), and accordingly suspend or discontinue CBD treatment and measure serum transaminase and total bilirubin. CBD treatment should be discontinued in patients with elevations of liver transaminases three times the ULN or bilirubin levels greater than two times the ULN, as well as in patients with elevations of liver transaminases five times the ULN.

Use in Pregnancy and Lactation

Women who are breastfeeding, pregnant, or actively trying to become pregnant should not use cannabis or CBD. While the dangers that CBD poses to fetuses and breastfeeding infants have not been studied due to ethical concerns, research has shown that CBD readily crosses the placenta, and it is believed to be transmitted to infants through breast milk. Until relevant data is produced on the subject, it is not recommended that pregnant or nursing women consume CBD.

Drug Interactions

CBD is metabolized by cytochrome P450 enzymes CYP3A4 and CYP2C19 and, to a lesser extent, CYP2C8 and CYP2C9. Caution is advised when CBD is co-administered with drugs that use these pathways or with substrates of UDP-glucuronosyltransferases UGT1A9 and UGT2B7.

Dosage and Clinical Guidelines

Epidiolex is a solution that contains CBD at a concentration of 100 mg/mL. A starting dosage of 2.5 mg/kg twice daily is recommended and may be increased to 5 mg/kg twice daily after 1 week. Patients who continue to experience seizures may benefit from an increase to the maximum recommended dose of 10 mg/kg twice daily. Increased dosages may result in a concomitant rise in adverse reactions. When discontinuing use, dosages should be gradually diminished, since increased seizure frequency may occur if cessation is abrupt.

Guidance on Quality Assurance of CBD

It should be noted that many CBD products are not subject to the same level of scrutiny and testing as medications that have received FDA approval and that CBD is not technically a dietary supplement. Patients should be advised only to purchase CBD products that have undergone rigorous quality assurance.

Pediatric Use

CBD has been shown to be safe and effective for the treatment of seizures in patients 2 years of age and older.

Carbamazepine and Oxcarbazepine

15

Generic Name	Trade Name	Adverse Effects	Drug Interactions	CYP Interactions
Carbamazepine	Tegretol	GI symptoms, sedation, rash	See Table 15-1	3A4, 2C8, 3A5, 2B6
Oxcarbazepine	Trileptal	GI symptoms, sedation	Alcohol, benzodiazepines, oral contraceptives	3A4, 3A5, 2C19

Introduction

Carbamazepine (Tegretol) and oxcarbazepine (Trileptal) share a similar chemistry and structure but are used to treat different conditions. Oxcarbazepine is a structural analog of carbamazepine but has a different metabolic pathway. Carbamazepine is indicated for the treatment of epilepsy but is also recognized in most guidelines as a first- or second-line mood stabilizer useful in the treatment and prevention of both phases of bipolar affective disorder. A long-acting sustained release formulation (Equetro) was approved by the Food and Drug Administration (FDA) for the treatment of acute mania in 2002. It is structurally similar to the tricyclic antidepressant imipramine (Tofranil) but has a very different clinical spectrum of efficacy.

Oxcarbazepine is a 10-keto derivative of carbamazepine that is classified as an anticonvulsant and voltage-sensitive sodium channel antagonist. It is approved for use in treating partial seizures in adults and children aged 4 to 16 years with epilepsy. Though oxcarbazepine is not FDA approved for the treatment of acute mania, many clinicians use it as a treatment for patients with bipolar disorder. At least one study has suggested better efficacy of oxcarbazepine in less severe mania compared with more severe mania, while carbamazepine is effective in severe forms of mania.

TABLE 15-1: Adverse Events Associated with Carbamazepine	
Dosage-Related Adverse Effects	**Idiosyncratic Adverse Effects**
Double or blurred vision	Agranulocytosis
Vertigo	Stevens–Johnson syndrome
GI disturbances	Aplastic anemia
Task performance impairment	Hepatic failure
Hematologic effects	Rash
	Pancreatitis
GI, gastrointestinal.	

CARBAMAZEPINE

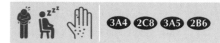

Pharmacologic Actions

Absorption of carbamazepine is slow and unpredictable. Food enhances absorption. Peak plasma concentrations are reached 2 to 8 hours after a single dose, and steady-state levels are reached after 2 to 4 days. It is 70% to 80% protein bound. The half-life of carbamazepine ranges from 18 to 54 hours, with an average of 26 hours. Carbamazepine is mostly metabolized in the liver by cytochrome P450 isoenzyme CYP3A4 and, to a lesser degree, CYP2C8, CYP3A5, and CYP2B6. Metabolism also involves glucuronidation by UGT2B7 enzyme and several other metabolic reactions. With chronic administration, the half-life of carbamazepine decreases to an average of 12 hours because carbamazepine induces its own metabolism, also known as autoinduction. The induction of hepatic enzymes reaches its maximum level after about 3 to 5 weeks of therapy. One of the metabolites of carbamazepine, 10,11-epoxide metabolite, acts as an anticonvulsant though its effect in the treatment of bipolar disorders is unknown. Long-term use of carbamazepine is associated with an increased ratio of the epoxide to the parent molecule. The pharmacokinetics of carbamazepine is different for two long-acting preparations of carbamazepine, each of which uses slightly different technology. One formulation, Tegretol XR, requires food to ensure normal gastrointestinal (GI) transit time. The other preparation, Carbatrol, relies on a combination of intermediate, extended-release, and very slow–release beads, making it suitable for bedtime administration.

The anticonvulsant effects of carbamazepine are thought to be mediated mainly by binding to voltage-dependent sodium channels in the inactive state and prolonging their inactivation. This secondarily reduces voltage-dependent calcium channel activation and, thus, synaptic transmission. Additional effects include reduction of currents through N-methyl-D-aspartate (NMDA) glutamate-receptor channels, competitive antagonism of adenosine A_1–receptors, and potentiation of central nervous system (CNS) catecholamine neurotransmission. Whether any or all of these mechanisms also result in mood stabilization is not known.

Therapeutic Indications

Bipolar Disorder

Acute Mania.   The acute antimanic effects of carbamazepine are typically evident within the first several days of treatment. About 50% to 70% of all persons respond within 2 to 3 weeks of initiation. Studies suggest that carbamazepine may be especially effective in persons who are not responsive to lithium, such as persons with dysphoric mania, rapid cycling, or a negative family history of mood disorders. The antimanic effects of carbamazepine can be, and often are, augmented by concomitant administration of lithium (Eskalith), valproic acid (Depakene), thyroid hormones, dopamine receptor antagonists (DRAs), or serotonin–dopamine antagonists (SDAs). Some persons may respond to carbamazepine but not lithium or valproic acid and vice versa.

Mixed Manic-Depressive Episodes. A regular feature of bipolar disorder observed in approximately 40% of patients, mixed episodes are associated with more severe symptomology and outcome, largely because they are so difficult to treat. A study involving 94 patients treated with carbamazepine while experiencing a mixed episode saw significant improvement compared to placebo group ($n = 98$). A second study involving 120 patients experiencing a mixed episode also showed significant improvement over 3 weeks, while the placebo group ($n = 115$) experienced minor improvement over the same period.

Prophylaxis. Carbamazepine is effective in preventing relapses, particularly among patients with bipolar II disorder, schizoaffective disorder, and dysphoric mania.

Off-Label Uses

Acute Depression

A subgroup of treatment-refractory patients with acute depression responds well to carbamazepine. Patients with more severe episodic and less chronic depression also seem to be better responders to carbamazepine. Nevertheless, carbamazepine remains an alternative drug for depressed persons who have not responded to conventional treatments, including electroconvulsive therapy (ECT).

Other Disorders

Carbamazepine helps to control symptoms associated with acute alcohol withdrawal, although benzodiazepines are more effective in this population. Carbamazepine has been suggested as a treatment for anxiety, panic disorder, and the paroxysmal recurrent component of posttraumatic stress disorder (PTSD). Uncontrolled studies suggest that carbamazepine is effective in controlling impulsive, aggressive behavior in nonpsychotic persons of all ages, including children and elderly persons. Carbamazepine is also effective in controlling nonacute agitation and aggressive behavior in patients with schizophrenia and schizoaffective disorder. Persons with prominent positive symptoms (e.g., hallucinations) may be likely to respond, as are persons who display impulsive aggressive outbursts.

Carbamazepine has also been used off-label to treat neuropathic and nociceptive pain, as well as diabetes insipidus.

Precautions and Adverse Reactions

Carbamazepine is relatively well tolerated. Mild GI (nausea, vomiting, gastric distress, constipation, diarrhea, and anorexia) and CNS (ataxia, drowsiness) side effects are the most common. The severity of these adverse effects is reduced if the dosage of carbamazepine is increased slowly and kept at the minimal effective plasma concentration. In contrast to lithium and valproate (other drugs used to manage bipolar disorder), carbamazepine does not appear to cause weight gain. Because of the phenomena of autoinduction, with consequent reductions in carbamazepine concentrations, side-effect tolerability may improve over time.

Most of the adverse effects of carbamazepine are correlated with plasma concentrations above 9 µg/mL. *The rarest but most serious adverse effects of carbamazepine are blood dyscrasias, hepatitis, and serious skin reactions* (Table 15-1).

Blood Dyscrasias

The drug's hematologic effects are not dose related. Severe blood dyscrasias (aplastic anemia, agranulocytosis) occur in about 1 in 125,000 persons treated with carbamazepine. There does not appear to be a correlation between the degree of benign white blood cell (WBC) suppression (leukopenia), which is seen in 1% to 2% of persons, and the emergence of life-threatening blood dyscrasias. Persons should be warned that the emergence of such symptoms as fever, sore throat, rash, petechiae, bruising, and easy bleeding can potentially herald a serious dyscrasia, and the person should seek medical evaluation immediately. Routine hematologic monitoring in carbamazepine-treated persons is recommended at 3, 6, 9, and 12 months. If there is no significant evidence of bone marrow suppression by that time, many experts would reduce the interval of monitoring. However, even assiduous monitoring may fail to detect severe blood dyscrasias before they cause symptoms.

Hepatitis and Cholestasis

Within the first few weeks of therapy, carbamazepine can cause both hepatitis associated with increases in liver enzymes, particularly transaminases, and cholestasis associated with elevated bilirubin and alkaline phosphatase. Mild transaminase elevations warrant observation only, but persistent elevations more than three times the upper limit of normal levels indicate the need to discontinue the drug. Hepatitis can recur if the drug is reintroduced to the person and can result in death.

Dermatologic Effects

About 10% to 15% of persons treated with carbamazepine develop a benign maculopapular rash within the first 3 weeks of treatment. Stopping the medication usually leads to resolution of the rash. Some patients may experience life-threatening dermatologic syndromes, including exfoliative dermatitis, erythema multiforme, Stevens–Johnson syndrome, and toxic epidermal necrolysis. The possible emergence of these serious dermatologic problems causes most clinicians to discontinue carbamazepine use in people who develop any type of rash. The risk of drug rash is about equal between valproic acid and carbamazepine in the first 2 months of use but is subsequently much higher for carbamazepine. If carbamazepine seems to be the only effective drug for a person who has a benign rash with carbamazepine treatment, a retrial of the drug can be undertaken. Many patients can be rechallenged without reemergence of the rash. Pretreatment with prednisone (40 mg a day) may suppress the rash, although other symptoms of an allergic reaction (e.g., fever and pneumonitis) may develop even with steroid pretreatment.

Renal Effects

Carbamazepine is occasionally used to treat diabetes insipidus not associated with lithium use. This activity results from direct or indirect effects on the vasopressin receptor. It may also lead to the development of hyponatremia and water intoxication in some patients, particularly elderly persons, or when used in high doses.

Other Adverse Effects

Carbamazepine decreases cardiac conduction (although less than the tricyclic drugs do) and can thus exacerbate pre-existing cardiac disease. Carbamazepine should be used with caution in persons with glaucoma, prostatic hypertrophy, diabetes, or a history of alcohol abuse. Carbamazepine occasionally activates vasopressin receptor function, which results in a condition resembling the syndrome of secretion of inappropriate antidiuretic hormone, characterized by hyponatremia and, rarely, water intoxication. This is the opposite of the renal effects of lithium (i.e., nephrogenic diabetes insipidus). However, augmentation of lithium with carbamazepine does not reverse the lithium effect. Emergence of confusion, severe weakness, or headache in a person taking carbamazepine should prompt measurement of serum electrolytes.

Carbamazepine use rarely elicits an immune hypersensitivity response consisting of fever, rash, eosinophilia, and possibly fatal myocarditis.

Use in Pregnancy and Lactation

Carbamazepine is classified as a pregnancy category D drug. Cleft palate, fingernail hypoplasia, microcephaly, and spina bifida in infants may be associated with the maternal use of carbamazepine during pregnancy. Therefore, pregnant women should not use carbamazepine unless absolutely necessary. All women with childbearing potential should take 1 to 4 mg of folic acid daily even if they are not trying to conceive. Carbamazepine is secreted in breast milk and should be avoided by nursing mothers.

Drug Interactions

Carbamazepine decreases serum concentrations of numerous drugs as a result of prominent induction of hepatic CYP3A4 (Table 15-2). Monitoring for a decrease in clinical effects is frequently indicated. Carbamazepine can decrease the blood concentrations of oral contraceptives, resulting in breakthrough bleeding and uncertain prophylaxis against pregnancy. Carbamazepine should not be administered with monoamine oxidase inhibitors (MAOIs), which should be discontinued at least 2 weeks before initiating treatment with carbamazepine. Grapefruit juice inhibits the hepatic metabolism of carbamazepine. When carbamazepine

TABLE 15-2: Carbamazepine–Drug Interactions

Effect of Carbamazepine on Plasma Concentrations of Concomitant Agents	Agents That May Affect Carbamazepine Plasma Concentrations
Carbamazepine may decrease drug plasma concentration of	Agents that may increase carbamazepine plasma concentration
Acetaminophen	Allopurinol
Alprazolam	Cimetidine
Amitriptyline	Clarithromycin

(continued)

TABLE 15-2: Carbamazepine–Drug Interactions (continued)

Effect of Carbamazepine on Plasma Concentrations of Concomitant Agents	Agents That May Affect Carbamazepine Plasma Concentrations
Bupropion	Danazol
Clomipramine	Diltiazem
Clonazepam	Erythromycin
Clozapine	Fluoxetine
Cyclosporine	Fluvoxamine
Desipramine	Gemfibrozil
Dicumarol	Itraconazole
Doxepin	Ketoconazole
Doxycycline	Isoniazid[a]
Ethosuximide	Itraconazole
Felbamate	Lamotrigine
Fentanyl	Loratadine
Fluphenazine	Macrolides
Haloperidol	Nefazodone
Hormonal contraceptives	Nicotinamide
Imipramine	Propoxyphene
Lamotrigine	Terfenadine
Methadone	Troleandomycin
Methsuximide	Valproate[a]
Methylprednisolone	Verapamil
Nimodipine	Viloxazine
Pancuronium	*Drugs that may decrease carbamazepine plasma concentrations*
Phensuximide	Carbamazepine (autoinduction)
Phenytoin	Cisplatin
Primidone	Doxorubicin HCl
Theophylline	Felbamate
Valproate	Phenobarbital
Warfarin	Phenytoin
Carbamazepine may increase drug plasma concentrations of	Primidone
Clomipramine	Rifampin[b]
Phenytoin	Theophylline
Primidone	Valproate

[a]Increased concentrations of the active 10,11-epoxide.
[b]Decreased concentrations of carbamazepine and increased concentrations of the 10,11-epoxide.
Table by Carlos A. Zarate, Jr, MD and Mauricio Tohen, MD.

and valproate are used in combination, the dosage of carbamazepine should be decreased because valproate displaces carbamazepine binding on proteins, and the dosage of valproate may need to be increased.

Laboratory Interferences

Circulating levels of thyroxine and triiodothyronine are associated with a decrease in thyroid-stimulating hormone and may be associated with treatment. Carbamazepine is also associated with an increase in total serum cholesterol, primarily by increasing high-density lipoproteins. The thyroid and cholesterol effects are not clinically significant. Carbamazepine may interfere with the dexamethasone suppression test and may also cause false-positive pregnancy test results.

Dosing and Administration

The target dose for antimanic activity is 1,200 mg a day, although this varies considerably. Immediate-release carbamazepine needs to be taken three or four times a day, which leads to lapses in compliance. Extended-release formulations are thus preferred because they can be taken once or twice a day. One form of extended-release carbamazepine, Carbatrol, comes as 100-, 200-, and 300-mg capsules. Another form called Equetro is identical to Carbetrol and is marketed as a treatment for bipolar disorder. These capsules contain tiny beads with three different types of coatings and dissolve at different times. Capsules should not be crushed or chewed. The contents can be sprinkled over food, however, without affecting the extended-release qualities. This formulation can be taken either with or without meals, though the rate of absorption is faster when it is given with a high-fat meal. The entire daily dose can be given at bedtime.

Another extended-release form of carbamazepine, Tegretol XR, uses a different drug-delivery system than Carbatrol. It is available in 100-, 200-, and 300-mg tablets.

Pre-existing hematologic, hepatic, and cardiac diseases can be relative contraindications for carbamazepine treatment. Persons with hepatic disease require only one-third to one-half the usual dosage; the clinician should be cautious about raising the dosage in such persons and should do so only slowly and gradually. The laboratory examination should include a complete blood count with platelet count, liver function tests, serum electrolytes, and an electrocardiogram in persons older than 40 years of age or with a pre-existing cardiac disease. An electroencephalogram is not necessary before the initiation of treatment, but it may be helpful in some cases for the documentation of objective changes correlated with clinical improvement. See Table 15-3 for a brief user's guide to carbamazepine in bipolar disorder.

Routine Laboratory Monitoring

Serum levels for antimanic efficacy have not been established. The anticonvulsant blood concentration range for carbamazepine is 4 to 12 µg/mL, and this range should be reached before determining that carbamazepine is not effective in the treatment of a mood disorder. A clinically insignificant suppression of the WBC count commonly occurs during carbamazepine treatment. This benign decrease can be reversed by adding lithium, which enhances colony-stimulating factor.

TABLE 15-3: Carbamazepine in Bipolar Illness: A Brief User's Guide

1. Start with low (200 mg) bedtime dose in depression or euthymia; higher doses (600–800 mg/day in divided doses) in manic inpatients.
2. Carbamazepine extended-release preparation may be taken once daily, at bedtime.
3. Titrate slowly to the individual's response or side-effect threshold.
4. Hepatic enzyme CYP450 (3A4) induction and autoinduction occurring 2 to 3 weeks; slightly higher doses may be needed or tolerated at that time.
5. Warn regarding benign rash, which occurs in 5–10% of those taking the drug; progression to rare, severe rash is unpredictable, so the drug should be discontinued if any rash develops.
6. Benign white blood cell count decreases occur regularly (usually inconsequential).
7. Rarely, agranulocytosis and aplastic anemia may develop (several per million new exposures); warn regarding appearance of fever, sore throat, petechiae, and bleeding gums and to check with physician to obtain an immediate complete blood cell count.
8. Use adequate birth control methods, including higher dosage forms of estrogen (as carbamazepine lowers estrogen levels).
9. Avoid carbamazepine in pregnancy (spina bifida occurs in 0.5%; other severe adverse outcomes occur in about 8%).
10. Some people will respond well to carbamazepine and not to other mood stabilizers (lithium) or anticonvulsants (valproic acid).
11. Combination treatment often required to maintain remission and prevent loss of effect via tolerance.
12. Major drug interactions associated with increases in carbamazepine and potential toxicity from 3A4 enzyme inhibition include calcium channel blockers (isradipine and verapamil); erythromycin and related macrolide antibiotics; and valproate.

Potential serious hematologic effects of carbamazepine, such as pancytopenia, agranulocytosis, and aplastic anemia, occur in about 1 in 125,000 patients.

Complete laboratory blood assessments may be performed every 2 weeks for the first 2 months of treatment and quarterly thereafter, but the FDA has revised the package insert for carbamazepine to suggest that blood monitoring be performed at the discretion of the physician. Patients should be informed that fever, sore throat, rash, petechiae, bruising, or unusual bleeding may indicate a hematologic problem and should prompt immediate notification of a physician. This approach is probably more effective than is frequent blood monitoring during long-term treatment.

It has also been suggested that liver and renal function tests be conducted quarterly, although the benefit of conducting tests this frequently has been questioned. It seems reasonable, however, to assess hematologic status, along with liver and renal functions whenever a routine examination of the person is being conducted. A monitoring protocol is listed in Table 15-4.

TABLE 15-4: Laboratory Monitoring of Carbamazepine for Adult Psychiatric Disorders

	Baseline	Weekly to Stability	Monthly for 6 Months	6–12 Months
CBC	+	+	+	+
Bilirubin.	+		+	+
Alanine aminotransferase	+		+	+
Aspartate aminotransferase	+		+	+
Alkaline phosphatase	+		+	+
Carbamazepine level	+	+		+
CBC, complete blood count.				

Carbamazepine treatment should be discontinued and a consult with a hematologist should be obtained if the following laboratory values are found: a total WBC count below 3,000/mm³, erythrocytes below 4.0×10^6/mm³, neutrophils below 1,500/mm³, hematocrit less than 32%, hemoglobin less than 11 g/100 mL, platelet count below 100,000/mm³, reticulocyte count below 0.3%, and a serum iron concentration below 150 mg/100 mL.

OXCARBAZEPINE

 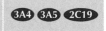 alcohol, benzodiazepines, oral contraceptives 3A4 3A5 2C19

Although structurally related to carbamazepine, the usefulness of oxcarbazepine as a treatment for mania has not been established in controlled trials. It is currently only indicated for use in treating seizures.

Pharmacologic Actions

Absorption is rapid and unaffected by food. Peak concentrations occur after about 45 minutes. The elimination half-life of the parent compound is 2 hours, which remains stable over long-term treatment. The monohydroxide metabolite of oxcarbazepine has a half-life of 9 hours. Most of the drug's anticonvulsant activity is presumed to result from this monohydroxy derivative.

Oxcarbazepine's mechanism of action is mediated through the inhibition of glutamate release and because it binds to sodium channels, thereby limiting repetitive neuronal firing.

Off-Label Psychiatric Uses

There is weak evidence to support the use of oxcarbazepine as a mood stabilizer in the treatment of bipolar disorder—especially acute manic episodes—both as monotherapy and add-on therapy. Given its similar structure and less severe adverse effect profile when compared to carbamazepine, it may be suitable for patients who had difficulty tolerating carbamazepine.

Precautions and Adverse Effects

The adverse effect profile of oxcarbazepine is milder than carbamazepine, even if the two are structurally and chemically similar. The most common side effects are sedation and nausea. Less frequent side effects are cognitive impairment, ataxia, diplopia, nystagmus, dizziness, and tremor. In contrast to carbamazepine, oxcarbazepine does not have an increased risk of serious blood dyscrasias, so hematologic monitoring is not necessary. The frequency of benign rash is lower than observed with carbamazepine, and serious rashes are extremely rare. However, about 25% to 30% of patients who develop an allergic rash while taking carbamazepine also develop a rash with oxcarbazepine. Oxcarbazepine is more likely to cause hyponatremia than carbamazepine. Approximately 3% to 5% of patients taking oxcarbazepine develop this side effect. It is advisable to obtain serum sodium concentrations early in the course of treatment because hyponatremia may be clinically silent. In severe cases, confusion and seizure may occur.

Use in Pregnancy and Lactation

There is very little information about the safety of oxcarbazepine among individuals who are pregnant or nursing, though it is known that the drug does pass into breast milk. Consequently, oxcarbazepine has been classified as a pregnancy category C drug.

Drug Interactions

Drugs such as phenobarbital and alcohol, which induce CYP34A, increase the clearance and reduce oxcarbazepine concentrations. Oxcarbazepine induces CYP3A4/5 and inhibits CYP2C19, which may affect the metabolism of drugs that use that pathway. Women taking oral contraceptives should be told to consult with their gynecologists because oxcarbazepine may reduce concentrations of their contraceptive and thus decrease its efficacy.

Dosing and Administration

Oxcarbazepine dosing for bipolar disorder has not been established. It is available in 150-, 300-, and 600-mg tablets. In the treatment of epilepsy, the dose range may vary from 150 to 2,400 mg per day given in divided doses twice a day. In clinical trials for mania, the doses typically used were from 900 to 1,200 mg per day with a starting dose of 150 or 300 mg at night. Oxcarbazepine is also available in an extended-release form (Oxteller ER), taken once a day on an empty stomach. It is available as 150-, 300-, and 600-mg tablets.

Cholinesterase Inhibitors, Memantine, and Aducanumab

16

Generic Name	Trade Name	Adverse Effects	Drug Interactions	CYP Interactions
Donepezil	Aricept	GI symptoms, cardiac arrhythmia	TRI	2D6, 3A4
Rivastigmine	Exelon	GI symptoms, dizziness, sedation, headache	TRI	N/A
Galantamine	Reminyl, Razadyne	dizziness, GI symptoms, headache	TRI	2D6, 3A4
Memantine	Namenda	Dizziness, headache	hydrochlorothiazide triamterene, cimetidine, ranitidine, quinidine, nicotine	2A6, 2C19, 2B6
Aducanumab	Aduhelm	Confusion, dizziness, headache	None	N/A

Introduction

For many years, the only medications approved by the Food and Drug Administration (FDA) for the treatment of Alzheimer disease (AD) and other dementias were cholinesterase inhibitors—donepezil (Aricept), rivastigmine (Exelon), galantamine (Reminyl, Razadyne)—and memantine (Namenda), an N-methyl-D-aspartate (NMDA) receptor antagonist that was approved for monotherapy in 2003. In 2014, a fixed combination of donepezil and memantine (Namzaric) was approved by the FDA (Table 16-1). This has changed with the controversial 2021 approval of aducanumab (Aduhelm), which is an amyloid beta–directed monoclonal antibody.

Originally, cholinesterase inhibitors were indicated only for mild to moderately ill patients with AD. Recently, their indication has expanded to include patients with moderate to severe AD (especially in conjunction with memantine) and patients with dementia associated with Parkinson disease (PD). Cholinesterase inhibitors reduce the inactivation of the neurotransmitter acetylcholine and, thus, potentiate cholinergic neurotransmission, which in turn produces a modest improvement in memory and goal-directed thought.

Tacrine (Cognex), the first cholinesterase inhibitor to be introduced, is no longer available because of its multiple daily dosing regimens, its potential for hepatotoxicity, and the consequent need for frequent laboratory monitoring.

TABLE 16-1: Medications Used in Neurocognitive Disorders

Drug (Brand)	Formulation	Indications	Starting Dose	Titration	Dosage Range
Tacrine (Cognex)	10-, 20-, 30-, 40-mg capsules	Mild to moderate AD dementia	10 mg 4 times a day	Increase by 10 mg 4 times a day (40 mg total daily) every 4 weeks	40–160 mg daily with 4 times a day dosing
Donepezil (Aricept)	5-, 10-, 23-mg tablets 5-, 10-mg disintegrated tablets	Mild to moderate and severe AD dementia	5 mg daily	Increase to 10 mg after 4 weeks. Increase to 23 mg daily after 3 months	10–23 mg daily
Rivastigmine (Exelon, Exelon Patch)	1.5-, 3-, 4.5-, 6-mg oral solution 4.6-, 9.5-, 13.3-mg transdermal patch	Mild to moderate AD dementia Major neurocognitive disorder due to Parkinson disease	4 mg twice a day 8 mg daily extended release	By 1.5 mg twice a day every 4 weeks. Increase to 9.5 mg in 4 weeks and then to 13.3 mg after 4 weeks for transdermal patch	3–6 mg daily for oral preparation. 4.6–13.3 mg daily for transdermal patch
Galantamine (Razadyne, Razadyne ER)	4-, 8-, 12-mg tablets 8-, 16-, 24-mg extended-release capsules 4-mg/mL oral solution	Mild to moderate AD dementia	1.5 mg twice a day 4.6-mg transdermal patch	Increase by 4 mg twice a day every 4 weeks. Increase by 8 mg every 4 weeks for extended release	4–12 mg in divided doses for oral preparation. 8–24 mg daily for extended release
Memantine (Namenda, Namenda XR)	5-, 10-mg tablets 7-, 14-, 21-, 28-mg extended-release capsules 10-mg/5-mL oral solution	Moderate to severe AD dementia	5 mg daily 7-mg extended-release formula	By 5 mg daily in weekly intervals. Increase by 7 mg daily extended-release formula	10–20 mg daily in divided dose for oral preparation. 7–28 mg daily for extended release
Memantine XR and donepezil combination (Namzaric)	14-mg memantine ER/10-mg donepezil capsules 28-mg memantine ER/10-mg donepezil capsules	Moderate to severe Alzheimer disease when patient already stabilized on memantine ER and donepezil	14-mg memantine ER/10-mg donepezil daily 28-mg memantine ER/10-mg donepezil daily in severe renal impairment		

Borrowed from Sadock BJ, Sadock VA, Kaplan HI, eds. *Kaplan & Sadock's Comprehensive Textbook of Psychiatry*. 10th ed. Lippincott Williams & Wilkins; 2017.

Cholinesterase Inhibitors

Pharmacologic Actions

Donepezil is absorbed completely from the gastrointestinal (GI) tract. Peak plasma concentrations are reached 3 to 4 hours after oral dosing. The half-life of donepezil is 70 hours in elderly persons, and it is taken only once daily. Steady-state levels are achieved within about 2 weeks. The presence of stable alcoholic cirrhosis reduces clearance of donepezil by 20%. Donepezil undergoes extensive metabolism via both CYP2D6 and 3A4 isoenzymes.

Rivastigmine is rapidly and completely absorbed from the GI tract and reaches peak plasma concentrations in 1 hour, but this is delayed by up to 90 minutes if rivastigmine is taken with food. The half-life of rivastigmine is 1 hour, but because it remains bound to cholinesterases, a single dose is therapeutically active for 10 hours. It is taken twice daily. Rivastigmine is primarily metabolized via cholinesterase-mediated hydrolysis, with minimal involvement of the cytochrome P450 system.

Galantamine is an alkaloid similar to codeine and is extracted from daffodils of the plant *Galanthus nivalis*. It is readily absorbed following oral administration with maximum concentrations reached in 0.5 to 2 hours. Food decreases the maximum concentration by 25%. The elimination half-life of galantamine is approximately 6 hours. Galantamine undergoes extensive metabolism via both CYP2D6 and 3A4 isozymes.

The primary mechanism of action of cholinesterase inhibitors is the reversible, nonacylating inhibition of acetylcholinesterase and butyrylcholinesterase; the enzymes that catabolize acetylcholine in the central nervous system (CNS). The enzyme inhibition increases synaptic concentrations of acetylcholine, especially in the hippocampus and cerebral cortex. Donepezil's favorable side-effect profile appears to correlate with its lack of inhibition of cholinesterases in the GI tract. Rivastigmine appears to have somewhat more peripheral activity than donepezil and is thus more likely to cause GI adverse effects than is donepezil.

Therapeutic Indications

Cholinesterase inhibitors are effective for the treatment of mild to moderate cognitive impairment in dementia seen in AD. In long-term use, they slow the progression of memory loss and diminish apathy, depression, hallucinations, anxiety, euphoria, and purposeless motor behaviors. Functional autonomy is less well preserved. Some patients note immediate improvement in memory, mood, psychotic symptoms, and interpersonal skills. Others note little initial benefit but are able to retain their cognitive and adaptive faculties at a relatively stable level for many months. A practical benefit of cholinesterase inhibitor use is that it can reduce or at least delay the need for nursing home placement.

Rivastigmine is also indicated for mild to moderate dementia associated with PD, and that it may reduce the risk of falls and improve gait stability in patients with PD.

Off-Label Uses

Donepezil and galantamine may be beneficial for patients with PD and Lewy body disease and for the treatment of cognitive deficits caused by traumatic brain

TABLE 16-2: Potential Off-Label Uses for Galantamine

Monotherapy	Combination Therapy	Accompanying Medication(s)
Cognitive dysfunction associated with bipolar disorder	Alzheimer disease	Memantine
Cognitive impairment associated with electroconvulsive therapy	Autism spectrum disorder symptoms in children	Risperidone
Cognitive impairment related to Lewy body disease	Cognitive impairment associated with electroconvulsive therapy	Memantine
Cognitive impairment related to traumatic brain injury	Cognitive impairment related to traumatic brain injury	Memantine
Dementia associated with Down syndrome	Cognitive, negative, and positive symptoms of schizophrenia	Antipsychotics and memantine
Dementia associated with multiple sclerosis		
Dementia associated with Parkinson disease		
Frontotemporal dementia		
Mixed dementia		
Noncommunicative behavior in autism spectrum disorder		
Organophosphorus poisoning		
Poststroke aphasia		
posttraumatic nerve palsy in oculomotor and trochlear nerves		
Scopolamine toxicity		
Sleep disorders in patients with mild to moderate Alzheimer disease		
Smoking cessation in alcohol-dependent patients		
Vascular dementia		

injury. People with vascular dementia may respond to acetylcholinesterase inhibitors, particularly donepezil. Perioperative rivastigmine may diminish postoperative delirium in older patients. A list of potential off-label uses for galantamine can be found in Table 16-2.

Use of cholinesterase inhibitors to improve cognition by nondemented individuals should be discouraged.

Precautions and Adverse Reactions

Occasionally, cholinesterase inhibitors elicit an idiosyncratic catastrophic reaction, with signs of grief and agitation, which is self-limited after the drug is discontinued.

Donepezil.   Donepezil is generally well tolerated at recommended dosages. Fewer than 3% of persons taking donepezil experience nausea, diarrhea, and vomiting. These mild symptoms are more common with a 10-mg dose than with a 5-mg dose, and when present, they tend to resolve after 3 weeks of continued use. Donepezil may cause weight loss. Donepezil treatment has been infrequently associated with bradyarrhythmia, especially in persons with underlying cardiac disease. A small number of persons experience syncope.

Rivastigmine.   Rivastigmine is generally well tolerated, but recommended dosages may need to be scaled back in the initial period of treatment to limit GI and CNS adverse effects. These mild symptoms are more common at dosages above 6 mg a day, and when present, they tend to resolve after the dosage is lowered. The most common adverse effects associated with rivastigmine are nausea, vomiting, dizziness, headache, diarrhea, abdominal pain, anorexia, fatigue, and somnolence. Rivastigmine may cause weight loss, but it does not appear to cause hepatic, renal, hematologic, or electrolyte abnormalities.

Galantamine.   The most common side effects of galantamine are dizziness, headache, nausea, vomiting, diarrhea, and anorexia. These side effects tend to be mild and transient.

Table 16-3 summarizes the incidence of major adverse side effects associated with each of the cholinesterase inhibitors.

Use in Pregnancy and Lactation.   Since the users of these drugs are not women of childbearing age, their off-label use in that population should be avoided. Data about use in this population are not available. Donepezil and galantamine are classified as pregnancy category C drugs, while rivastigmine has been classified as a pregnancy category B drug.

Drug Interactions

All cholinesterase inhibitors should be used cautiously with drugs that also possess cholinomimetic activity, such as succinylcholine (Anectine) and bethanechol

TABLE 16-3: Incidence (%) of Major Adverse Side Effects with Cholinesterase Inhibitors

Drug	Dose (mg/day)	Nausea	Vomiting	Diarrhea	Dizziness	Muscle Cramps	Insomnia
Donepezil	5	4	3	9	15	9	7
Donepezil	10	17	10	17	13	12	8
Rivastigmine	1–4	14	7	10	15	NR	NR
Rivastigmine	6–12	48	27	17	24	NR	NR
Galantamine	8	5.7	3.6	5	NR	NR	NR
Galantamine	16	13.3	6.1	12.2	NR	NR	NR
Galantamine	24	16.5	9.9	5.5	NR	NR	NR

NR, not reported from clinical trial data; incidence less than 5%.

(Urecholine). The coadministration of cholinesterase inhibitors and drugs that have cholinergic antagonist activity (e.g., tricyclic drugs) is probably counterproductive. Paroxetine (Paxil) has the most marked anticholinergic effects of any of the newer antidepressant and anxiolytic drugs and should be avoided for that reason, as well as its inhibiting effect on the metabolism of some of the cholinesterase inhibitors.

Donepezil undergoes extensive metabolism via both CYP2D6 and 3A4 isozymes. The metabolism of donepezil may be increased by phenytoin (Dilantin), carbamazepine (Tegretol), dexamethasone (Decadron), rifampin (Rifadin), and phenobarbital (Solfoton). Commonly used agents such as paroxetine, ketoconazole (Nizoral), and erythromycin can significantly increase donepezil concentrations. Donepezil is highly protein bound, but it does not displace other protein-bound drugs, such as furosemide (Lasix), digoxin (Lanoxin), or warfarin (Coumadin). Rivastigmine circulates mostly unbound to serum proteins and has no significant drug interactions.

Like donepezil, galantamine is metabolized by both CYP2D6 and 3A4 isozymes and thus may interact with drugs that inhibit these pathways. Paroxetine and ketoconazole should be used with great caution.

Rivastigmine has no known severe interactions with other drugs, but rivastigmine should not be given concomitantly with other cholinomimetics and cholinesterase inhibitors.

Laboratory Interferences

No laboratory interferences have been associated with the use of cholinesterase inhibitors.

Dosage and Clinical Guidelines

Before initiation of cholinesterase inhibitor therapy, potentially treatable causes of dementia should be ruled out and the diagnosis of dementia of the Alzheimer type established.

Donepezil is available in 5- and 10-mg tablets. Treatment should be initiated at 5 mg each night. If well tolerated and of some discernible benefit after 4 weeks, the dosage should be increased to a maintenance dosage of 10 mg each night. Donepezil absorption is unaffected by meals.

Rivastigmine is available in 1.5-, 3-, 4.5-, and 6-mg capsules. The recommended initial dosage is 1.5 mg twice daily for a minimum of 2 weeks, after which, increases of 1.5 mg a day can be made at intervals of at least 2 weeks to a target dosage of 6 mg a day, taken in two equal dosages. If tolerated, the dosage may be further titrated upward to a maximum of 6 mg twice daily. The risk of adverse GI events can be reduced by administration of rivastigmine with food.

Rivastigmine administration can also occur via transdermal patch. Patches are available in 4.6-mg and 9.5-mg doses. An initial dose of 4.6 mg/24 hours can be increased to a maintenance dose of 9.5 mg/24 hours if the initial dose is well tolerated for a minimum of 4 weeks. Weight should be monitored during treatment with the rivastigmine patch.

Galantamine is available in 4-, 8-, and 16-mg tablets. The suggested dose range is 16 to 32 mg per day given twice a day. The higher dose is better tolerated than the lower dose. The initial dosage is 8 mg per day, and after a minimum of 4 weeks, the dose can be raised. All subsequent dosage increases should occur at 4-week intervals and should be based on tolerability.

MEMANTINE

 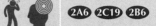

Pharmacologic Actions

Memantine is well absorbed after oral administration with peak concentrations reached in about 3 to 7 hours. Food has no effect on the absorption of memantine. Memantine has linear pharmacokinetics over the therapeutic dose range and has a terminal elimination half-life of about 60 to 80 hours. Plasma protein binding is 45%. Memantine undergoes little metabolism, with the majority (57% to 82%) of an administered dose excreted unchanged in urine; the remainder is converted primarily to three polar metabolites, the N-gludantan conjugate, 6-hydroxy memantine, and 1-nitroso-deaminated memantine. These metabolites possess minimal NMDA receptor antagonist activity.

Memantine is a low- to moderate-affinity NMDA receptor antagonist. It is thought that overexcitation of NMDA receptors by the neurotransmitter glutamate may play a role in AD because glutamate plays an integral role in the neural pathways associated with learning and memory. Excess glutamate overstimulates NMDA receptors to allow too much calcium into nerve cells, leading to the eventual cell death observed in AD. Memantine may protect cells against excess glutamate by partially blocking NMDA receptors associated with abnormal transmission of glutamate while allowing for physiologic transmission associated with normal cell functioning.

Therapeutic Indications

Memantine is the only approved therapy in the United States for moderate to severe AD.

Off-Label Uses

Memantine is frequently used to treat mild to moderate AD, as well as mild to moderate vascular dementia. In addition, memantine may be effective in treating chronic pain and mild cognitive impairment (MCI).

As monotherapy, memantine has been shown to be effective in treating psychiatric disorders such as obsessive–compulsive disorder (OCD), negative symptoms associated with schizophrenia, and bipolar disorder when patients are experiencing manic episodes. As combination therapy, memantine may be effective in treating OCD (in conjunction with selective serotonin reuptake inhibitors), schizophrenia (in conjunction with antipsychotics and galantamine), cognitive impairment associated with either electroconvulsive therapy or traumatic brain injury (in conjunction with galantamine), and catatonia.

Precautions and Adverse Reactions

Memantine is safe and well tolerated. The most common adverse effects are dizziness, headache, constipation, and confusion. The use of memantine in patients with severe renal impairment is not recommended. In a documented case of an overdose with up to 400 mg of memantine, the patient experienced restlessness, psychosis, visual hallucinations, somnolence, stupor, and loss of consciousness. The patient recovered without permanent sequelae.

Use in Pregnancy and Lactation

Memantine has been classified as a pregnancy category B drug. Animal studies have failed to demonstrate a risk to the fetus, but no well-controlled studies have been conducted on pregnant women. Memantine is likely excreted into breast milk, but no studies have been conducted on its effects on infants. Clinicians should only advise nursing mothers to take memantine if the benefits clearly outweigh potential risks.

Drug Interactions

In vitro studies conducted with marker substrates of CYP450 enzymes (CYP1A2, 2A6, 2C9, 2D6, 2E1, and 3A4) showed minimal inhibition of these enzymes by memantine. No pharmacokinetic interactions with drugs metabolized by these enzymes are expected.

Because memantine is eliminated in part by tubular secretion, coadministration of drugs that use the same renal cationic system, including hydrochlorothiazide triamterene (Dyrenium), cimetidine (Tagamet), ranitidine (Zantac), quinidine, and nicotine, could potentially result in altered plasma levels of both agents. Coadministration of memantine and a combination of hydrochlorothiazide and triamterene does not affect the bioavailability of either memantine or triamterene, and the bioavailability of hydrochlorothiazide decreases by 20%.

Urine pH is altered by diet, drugs (e.g., carbonic anhydrase inhibitors, topiramate [Topamax], sodium bicarbonate), and the clinical state of the patient (e.g., renal tubular acidosis or severe infections of the urinary tract). The clearance of memantine is reduced by about 80% under alkaline urine conditions at pH 8. Therefore, alterations of urine pH toward the alkaline condition may lead to an accumulation of the drug with a possible increase in adverse effects. Hence, memantine should be used with caution under these conditions.

Laboratory Interferences

No laboratory interferences have been associated with the use of memantine.

Dosage and Clinical Guidelines

Memantine is available in 5- and 10-mg tablets, with a recommended starting dose of 5 mg daily. The recommended target dose is 20 mg per day. The drug is administered twice daily in separate doses with 5-mg increment increases weekly depending on tolerability. It is also available as 5- and 10-mg extended-release tablets and as 7-, 14-, 21- and 28-mg extended-release capsules.

The combination of donepezil and extended-release memantine is available in fixed doses of 8-mg donepezil/10-mg memantine and 28-mg donepezil/10-mg memantine.

ADUCANUMAB

Aducanumab was approved by the FDA in 2021 to slow the progression of AD and is administered through monthly infusions. It is a recombinant human immunoglobin gamma 1 (IgG1) monoclonal antibody that targets soluble and insoluble forms of amyloid beta peptides, which are the primary components of plaques found in the brains of patients with AD. Amyloid beta plaque is believed to be central to the pathology of AD.

Aducanumab remains controversial because it received accelerated approval from the FDA and clinical trials failed to show improvement in cognition in patients with AD. Moreover, the FDA initially approved aducanumab for the treatment of all stages of AD, but eventually revised the indication to those with MCI or mild dementia due to AD, as was the case with the participants in the drug's phase 3 clinical trial.

Pharmacologic Actions

Aducanumab attains steady-state concentrations after 16 weeks following administration every 4 weeks. Systematic accumulation is 1.7-fold. Mean volume for distribution at steady state is 9.63 L. The drug is expected to be degraded into peptides and amino acids similar to endogenous IgG1. Aducanumab is not expected to undergo renal elimination or to be metabolized in the liver. Terminal half-life is 24.8 days.

Aducanumab targets amyloid beta plaque in the brains of AD patients. It has been shown to reduce levels of plaque at both low doses and high doses. Reductions were observed in a time- and dose-dependent manner through week 222 of one study. Aducanumab also reduced markers of tau pathophysiology

Therapeutic Indications

Aducanumab is indicated for the treatment of MCI due to Alzheimer and mild Alzheimer dementia.

Off-Label Uses

Though aducanumab remains a controversial treatment for AD, some have speculated that it could be used to treat other neurologic conditions where beta-amyloid abnormalities play a role in the pathophysiology of the disease, such as cerebral amyloid angiopathy.

Precautions and Adverse Reactions

There are still significant uncertainties with the use of aducanumab. Of particular concern is the high rate of incidence of brain swelling (amyloid-related imaging abnormalities-edema [ARIA-E]) and small brain bleeding (amyloid-related imaging abnormalities-microhemorrhage [ARIA-H]) reported during clinical trials. Specifically, ARIA-E indicates brain edema or sulcal effusions. The effects of ARIA-E can range from headaches, confusion, vomiting, and nausea to tremor, gait disturbance, and alterations in mental state. ARIA-H refers to cerebral hemorrhages and/or superficial siderosis. Though these conditions are typically temporary, the rate of ARIA (-E or -H) was fourfold higher in patients treated with aducanumab than controls during clinical trials. Incidence was notably higher in carriers of apolipoprotein E ε4 (ApoE ε4).

During these trials, treatment with aducanumab also produced clinical adverse reactions. Symptoms were reported by 24% of patients treated with maintenance dosage of aducanumab compared with 5% of controls. The most common symptoms included headache (13%), confusion/delirium/alterations in mental state (5%), dizziness (4%), visual disturbances (2%), and nausea (2%). Serious symptoms were reported in 0.3% of patients. Of those with serious clinical symptoms, 88% resolved during the period of observation. However, clinical vigilance and monitoring of ARIA is recommended, especially during titration.

Considering the controversy, appropriate patient selection is necessary, and clinicians are advised to follow the following guidelines drafted by an expert panel in 2021.

1. Eligible patients should meet clinical criteria for mild AD-related dementia or MCI due to AD, and cognitive scores on validated scales should corroborate clinical diagnosis. These patients may already be taking cholinesterase inhibitors or memantine.
2. An amyloid PET scan should be conducted, and the scan properly interpreted by a trained radiologist, to confirm amyloid status. Confirmation can also be obtained by measuring cerebrospinal fluid biomarkers.
3. Given the heightened risk of ARIA in carriers of ApoE ε4, genotyping should be discussed with the patient and their family.
4. Within 1 year of initiating aducanumab treatment, a brain magnetic resonance imaging (MRI) should be obtained.
5. The patient's cardiovascular, medical, and psychiatric status should be assessed and deemed stable before initiating treatment. Patients should be excluded from receiving aducanumab if they are pregnant, on anticoagulant medications, or brain MRI revealed evidence of significant cerebrovascular disease.
6. Clinicians should describe the requirements of therapy to ensure patients and their care partners understand what is involved in the administration of the treatment.
7. Clinicians should recognize that they may need to collaborate with or refer to specialists with expertise when making these assessments.

TABLE 16-4: Aducanumab Dosing Schedule	
IV Infusion Every 4 Weeks	Aducanumab Dosage
Infusion 1 and 2	1 mg/kg
Infusion 3 and 4	3 mg/kg
Infusion 5 and 6	6 mg/kg
Subsequent infusions	10 mg/kg

Use in Pregnancy and Lactation

Adequate data on the use of aducanumab in pregnant and nursing mothers do not exist.

Drug Interactions

None.

Laboratory Interferences

No laboratory interferences have been associated with the use of aducanumab.

Dosage and Clinical Guidelines

Aducanumab is a solution available in one of two forms:

- 170 mg/1.7 mL in a single-dose vial
- 300 mg/3 mL in a single-dose vial

It is administered as an IV infusion every 4 weeks and is titrated to a dose of 10 mg/kg over a 6-month period (see Table 16-4 for dosing schedule).

A brain MRI scan from before treatment must be obtained prior to the 7th infusion (first dose at 10 mg/kg) and 12th infusion. If 10 or more new incident microhemorrhages or more than two focal areas of superficial siderosis are observed, treatment may be continued with caution, provided another MRI reveals radiographic stabilization.

If an infusion is missed, resume the dose schedule at the same dose as soon as possible.

Cholinesterase Inhibitors, Memantine, and Aducanumab

17 Disulfiram and Acamprosate

Generic Name	Trade Name	Adverse Effects	Drug Interactions	CYP Interactions
Disulfiram	Antabuse	Fatigue	Alcohol, CNS, TRI, anticoagulants, paraldehyde, phenytoin, caffeine, tetrahydrocannabinol, isoniazid	3A4, 3A5, 2E1
Acamprosate	Campral	GI symptoms, headache	Alcohol, naltrexone	N/A

Introduction

Disulfiram (Antabuse) and acamprosate (Campral) are two of the three medications approved by the Food and Drug Administration to treat alcohol dependence and alcohol use disorder. The third is naltrexone, which will be discussed in Chapter 29.

Disulfiram is now considered a second-line option in the treatment of alcohol use disorder, largely because of the severe physical reactions the drug causes after drinking. Disulfiram's main therapeutic effect is its ability to produce unpleasant and even dangerous symptoms after alcohol intake (also known as disulfiram–alcohol reaction). In the most severe cases, patients who have taken disulfiram may experience respiratory depression, cardiovascular collapse, acute heart failure, convulsions, and loss of consciousness after consuming alcohol. Death may occur in rare cases. Experience has shown, however, that at recommended doses, it is an acceptable and safe medication for dependent drinkers seeking to sustain abstinence.

These potential complications, as well as the development of alternative antialcohol medications, have limited wider use of disulfiram. Unlike disulfiram, acamprosate, the other drug discussed in this chapter, does not produce aversive side effects. Acamprosate is now prescribed more commonly than disulfiram in outpatient settings, but disulfiram is prescribed more often in inpatient settings because it helps facilitate initial abstinence.

Other drugs that are useful in reducing alcohol consumption include naltrexone (ReVia, Trexan), naltrexone long acting (Vivitrol), nalmefene (Revex), topiramate (Topamax), and gabapentin (Neurontin). These agents are discussed in their respective chapters.

DISULFIRAM

 alcohol, CNS TRI anticoagulants, paraldehyde, phenytoin, caffeine, tetrahydrocannabinol, isoniazid

Pharmacologic Actions

Disulfiram is almost completely absorbed from the gastrointestinal (GI) tract after oral administration. Its half-life is estimated to be 60 to 120 hours. Therefore, 1 or 2 weeks may be needed before disulfiram is totally eliminated from the body after the last dose has been taken.

The metabolism of ethanol proceeds through oxidation via alcohol dehydrogenase to the formation of acetaldehyde, which is further metabolized to acetyl-coenzyme A (acetyl-CoA) by aldehyde dehydrogenase. Disulfiram is an aldehyde dehydrogenase inhibitor that interferes with the metabolism of alcohol by producing a marked increase in blood acetaldehyde concentration. The accumulation of acetaldehyde (to a level up to 10 times higher than occurs in the normal metabolism of alcohol) produces a wide array of unpleasant reactions characterized by nausea, throbbing headache, vomiting, hypertension, flushing, sweating, thirst, dyspnea, tachycardia, chest pain, vertigo, and blurred vision. Known as the *disulfiram–alcohol reaction*, it occurs almost immediately after the ingestion of one alcoholic drink and may last from 30 minutes to 2 hours. Many have compared the experience to an extremely bad hangover.

Blood Concentrations in Relation to Action

Plasma concentrations of disulfiram may vary among individuals because of several factors, most notably age and hepatic function. In general, the severity of disulfiram–alcohol reaction has been shown to be proportional to the amount of the ingested disulfiram and alcohol. Nevertheless, disulfiram plasma levels are rarely obtained in clinical practice. The positive correlation between plasma concentrations of alcohol and the intensity of the reaction is described as follows: in sensitive individuals, as little as 5 to 10 mg per 100 mL increase of the plasma alcohol level may produce mild symptoms; fully developed symptoms occur at alcohol levels of 50 mg per 100 mL; and levels as high as 125 to 150 mg per 100 mL result in loss of consciousness and coma.

Therapeutic Indications

The primary indication for disulfiram use is as an aversive conditioning treatment for alcohol dependence. Either the fear of having a disulfiram–alcohol reaction or the memory of having had one is meant to condition the person not to use alcohol. Usually, describing the severity and the unpleasantness of the disulfiram–alcohol reaction graphically enough discourages the person from imbibing alcohol. Disulfiram treatment should be combined with such treatments as psychotherapy, group therapy, and support groups such as Alcoholics Anonymous (AA). Treatment with disulfiram requires careful monitoring because a person can simply decide not to take the medication.

Disulfiram and Acamprosate

Studies examining the efficacy of disulfiram in treating patients with cocaine dependence, comorbid alcohol and cocaine dependence, and comorbid alcohol dependence and posttraumatic stress disorder (PTSD) are ongoing.

Precautions and Adverse Reactions

With Alcohol Consumption

The intensity of the disulfiram–alcohol reaction varies with each person. In extreme cases, it is marked by respiratory depression, cardiovascular collapse, myocardial infarction, convulsions, and even death. Therefore, disulfiram is contraindicated for persons with significant pulmonary or cardiovascular disease. In addition, disulfiram should be used with caution, if at all, by persons with nephritis, brain damage, hypothyroidism, diabetes, hepatic disease, seizures, polydrug dependence, or an abnormal electroencephalogram. Most fatal reactions occur in persons who take more than 500 mg a day of disulfiram and who consume more than 3 oz of alcohol. The treatment of a severe disulfiram–alcohol reaction is primarily supportive to prevent shock. The use of oxygen, intravenous vitamin C, ephedrine, and antihistamines has been reported to aid in recovery.

Without Alcohol Consumption

The adverse effects of disulfiram in the absence of alcohol consumption include fatigue, dermatitis, impotence, optic neuritis, a variety of mental changes, and hepatic damage. A metabolite of disulfiram inhibits dopamine-β-hydroxylase, the enzyme that metabolizes dopamine into norepinephrine and epinephrine, and thus may exacerbate psychosis in persons with psychotic disorders. Catatonic reactions may also occur.

Use in Pregnancy and Lactation

There are no well-controlled studies of disulfiram effects on the fetus or newborn, or whether it crosses into breast milk. Consequently, it is classified as a pregnancy category C drug.

Drug Interactions

Disulfiram increases the blood concentration of diazepam (Valium), paraldehyde, phenytoin (Dilantin), caffeine, tetrahydrocannabinol (the active ingredient in marijuana), barbiturates, anticoagulants, isoniazid (Nydrazid), and tricyclic drugs. Disulfiram should not be administered concomitantly with paraldehyde because paraldehyde is metabolized to acetaldehyde in the liver.

Laboratory Interferences

In rare instances, disulfiram has been reported to interfere with the incorporation of iodine-131 into protein-bound iodine. Disulfiram may reduce urinary concentrations of homovanillic acid, the major metabolite of dopamine, because of its inhibition of dopamine hydroxylase.

Dosage and Clinical Guidelines

Disulfiram is supplied in 250- and 500-mg tablets. The usual initial dosage is 500 mg a day taken by mouth for the first 1 or 2 weeks, followed by a maintenance dosage of 250 mg a day. The dosage should not exceed 500 mg a day. The maintenance dosage range is 125 to 500 mg a day.

Persons taking disulfiram must be instructed that the ingestion of even the smallest amount of alcohol will bring on a disulfiram–alcohol reaction, with all its unpleasant effects. In addition, persons should be warned against ingesting any alcohol-containing preparations, such as cough drops, tonics of any kind, and alcohol-containing foods and sauces. Some reactions have occurred in patients who used alcohol-based lotions, toilet water, colognes, or perfumes and inhaled the fumes; therefore, precautions must be explicit and should include any topically applied preparations containing alcohol, including perfume.

Disulfiram should not be administered until the person has abstained from alcohol for at least 12 hours. Persons should be warned that the disulfiram–alcohol reaction may occur as long as 1 or 2 weeks after the last dose of disulfiram. Persons taking disulfiram should carry identification cards describing the disulfiram–alcohol reaction and listing the name and telephone number of the physician to be called.

ACAMPROSATE

 alcohol, naltrexone

Pharmacologic Actions

Acamprosate has a low oral bioavailability of around 11% and typically reaches maximum concentrations in 6.3 hours. Its half-life is 32 hours, with a complete elimination approximately 96 hours after administration. It is excreted unchanged in urine. Steady-state plasma of 1.5 to 5 μm is typically reached on day 5 of treatment.

Acamprosate's mechanism of action is not fully understood, but it is thought to antagonize neuronal overactivity related to the actions of the excitatory neurotransmitter glutamate. In part, this may result from the modulation of N-methyl-D-aspartate (NMDA) receptor transmission and indirect effects of γ-aminobutyric acid type A (GABA$_A$) receptor transmission.

Indications

Acamprosate is used for treating alcohol-dependent individuals seeking to continue to remain alcohol free after they have stopped drinking. Its efficacy in promoting abstinence has not been demonstrated in persons who have not undergone detoxification and who have not achieved alcohol abstinence before beginning treatment.

Off-Label Uses

Investigations into the utility of acamprosate in treating other substance use disorders and drug dependencies have not produced conclusive results. Similarly, investigations into the use of acamprosate to treat pathologic gambling have not shown clinically significant efficacy. A small ($n = 20$) placebo-controlled study failed to show a reduction in binging episodes among individuals with binge-eating disorder, but did show a reduction in cravings, as well as slight weight loss in the active group compared to the control group.

Precautions and Adverse Effects

Side effects are mostly seen early in treatment and are usually mild and transient in nature. The most common side effects are headache, diarrhea, flatulence, abdominal pain, paresthesias, and various skin reactions. No adverse events occur after abrupt withdrawal of acamprosate, even after long-term use. There is no evidence of addiction to the drug. Patients with severe renal impairment (creatinine clearance of less than 30 mL/minute) should not be given acamprosate.

Use in Pregnancy and Lactation

There are no well-controlled studies of acamprosate effects on pregnant or nursing mothers, but potential risks warrant caution. Acamprosate is a pregnancy category C drug.

Drug Interactions

The pharmacokinetics of acamprosate are unaffected by alcohol, benzodiazepines, or disulfiram. Plasma levels are diminished when paired with food. Coadministration of naltrexone with acamprosate produces an increase in concentrations of acamprosate. No adjustment of dosage is recommended in such patients. The pharmacokinetics of naltrexone and its major metabolite 6-β-naltrexol were unaffected after coadministration with acamprosate. During clinical trials, patients taking acamprosate concomitantly with antidepressants more commonly reported both weight gain and weight loss compared with patients taking either medication alone.

Laboratory Interferences

Acamprosate has not been shown to interfere with commonly done laboratory tests.

Dosage and Clinical Guidelines

It is important to remember that acamprosate should not be used to treat alcohol withdrawal symptoms. It should only be started after the individual has been successfully weaned off alcohol. Patients should show a commitment to remaining abstinent, and treatment should be part of a comprehensive management program that includes counseling or support group attendance. Acamprosate on its own does not lead to abstinence.

Each tablet contains 333 mg of acamprosate calcium, which is equivalent to 300 mg of acamprosate. The dose of acamprosate is different for different patients. The recommended dosage is two 333-mg tablets (each dose should total 666 mg) taken three times daily. Although dosing may be done without regard to meals, dosing at mealtime is suggested as an aid to encourage compliance in patients who regularly eat three meals daily. A lower dose may be effective in some patients. A missed dose should be taken as soon as possible. However, if it is almost time for the next dose, the missed dose should be skipped, and then the regular dosing schedule should be resumed. Doses should not be doubled up.

For patients with moderate renal impairment (creatinine clearance of 30 to 50 mL/minute), a starting dosage of one 333-mg tablet taken three times daily is recommended. People with severe renal insufficiency should not take acamprosate.

Dopamine Receptor Agonists and Precursors

18

Generic Name	Trade Name	Adverse Effects	Drug Interactions	CYP Interactions
Amantadine	Symmetrel	Dizziness, insomnia, agitation, seizures, GI symptoms, skin rash, headache	Anticholinergics, stimulants, MAOI	N/A
Apomorphine	Apokyn, Kynmobi	Cardiac arrhythmia, GI symptoms, dizziness, dystonia, cognitive problems, mood swings, headache	CNS, TRI, MAOI	2B6, 2C8, 3A4, 3A5
Bromocriptine	Parlodel	Cardiac arrhythmia, GI symptoms, dizziness, dystonia, cognitive problems, mood swings, headache	CNS, TRI, MAOI, oral contraceptives	3A4
Cabergoline	Dostinex, Caberlin	Cardiac arrhythmia, GI symptoms, dizziness, dystonia, cognitive problems, mood swings, headache	CNS, TRI, MAOI	3A4
Carbidopa	Lodosyn	Cardiac arrhythmia, GI symptoms, dizziness, dystonia, cognitive problems, mood swings, headache	CNS, TRI, MAOI	N/A
Levodopa (L-Dopa)	Larodopa	Cardiac arrhythmia, GI symptoms, dizziness, dystonia, cognitive problems, mood swings, headache	CNS, TRI, MAOI	N/A
Pramipexole	Mirapex	Loss of consciousness, cardiac arrhythmia, GI symptoms, dizziness, dystonia, cognitive problems, mood swings, headache	CNS, TRI, MAOI, cimetidine	N/A
Ropinirole	Requip	Loss of consciousness, cardiac arrhythmia, GI symptoms, dizziness, dystonia, cognitive problems, mood swings, headache	CNS, TRI, MAOI, oral contraceptives, ciprofloxacin	N/A
Rotigotine	Neupro	Cardiac arrhythmia, GI symptoms, dizziness, dystonia, cognitive problems, mood swings, headache	CNS, TRI, MAOI	3A4, 2D6, 2C19

Introduction

The neurotransmitter dopamine is responsible for a wide variety of bodily functions. Within the central nervous system (CNS), it assists in the regulation of memory, cognition, sleep–wake cycles, and mood. It is also an integral part of brain's reward pathways and plays a major role in addiction. In peripheral tissue, dopamine plays a vital role in the function of the kidneys, pancreas, cardiovascular, and gastrointestinal (GI) systems.

Following the discovery that administration of levodopa (a/k/a L-DOPA), the precursor to dopamine, leads to significant improvement in parkinsonian symptoms, the drug became the first-line pharmacologic treatment for Parkinson disease (PD). However, severe extrapyramidal side effects after long-term administration make the use of levodopa undesirable in younger patients, and researchers began searching for other dopamine receptor agonists (DAs) as adjunctive therapies with levodopa as early as the 1970s. At present, DAs monotherapy is recommended in younger patients to avoid the side effects associated with levodopa.

DAs that have been developed within the last 50 years activate dopamine receptors in the absence of endogenous dopamine and have been widely used to treat idiopathic PD, hyperprolactinemia, certain pituitary tumors (prolactinoma), and restless leg syndrome (RLS). Since dopamine stimulates the heart and increases blood flow to the liver, kidneys, and other organs, low levels of dopamine are associated with low blood pressure and low cardiac output. Dopamine agonist drugs are also administered to treat shock and congestive heart failure.

This class of drugs is subdivided into nonergoline and ergot derivatives.

Nonergoline DAs include apomorphine (Apokyn, Kynmobi), pramipexole (Mirapex), ropinirole (Requip), rotigotine (Neupro), and piribedil, which goes by numerous trade names but is not currently available in the United States. Pramipexole, ropinirole, and rotigotine are Food and Drug Administration (FDA) approved for use in PD and RLS and have been studied as an adjunctive treatment for unipolar and bipolar depression.

The ergot class of DAs includes bromocriptine (Parlodel), cabergoline (Dostinex, Caberlin), lisuride (Dopergin) and pergolide (Permax). Lisuride is no longer available in the United States, while pergolide was withdrawn from U.S. markets in 2007 but is still available to veterinarians. Bromocriptine is FDA approved for use in PD, galactorrhea (due to hyperprolactin conditions), and acromegaly. It is used off-label to treat RLS and neuroleptic malignant syndrome (NMS). Cabergoline is FDA approved for the treatment of hyperprolactinemic disorders, either idiopathic or due to pituitary adenomas.

Amantadine (Symmetrel), an adamantane derivative that was originally developed as an antiviral medication, is FDA approved to treat PD, drug-induced extrapyramidal symptoms (EPS), and influenza A infection. However, it is not technically a dopamine agonist; rather, it blocks reuptake of dopamine and has an agonistic effect on postsynaptic dopamine receptors. It is also used off-label to treat NMS and Cotard syndrome, a psychiatric condition that involves a delusional belief that one is dead.

Other classes of drugs may also exert agonist effects on the dopamine receptor. The wakefulness-promoting agents modafinil (Provigil) and armodafinil (Nuvigil) have complex prodopaminergic activity, including dopamine transporter inhibition, and may also have dopamine (D2) receptor partial agonist effects. These drugs have been FDA approved to improve wakefulness in adult patients with excessive sleepiness associated with narcolepsy, obstructive sleep apnea (OSA), or shift work disorder (SWD). They have been studied as an adjunctive treatment for unipolar and bipolar depression, and attention deficit hyperactivity disorder (ADHD). Modafinil and armodafinil are discussed in Chapter 23.

Pharmacologic Actions

Levodopa is rapidly absorbed after oral administration, and peak plasma levels are reached after 30 to 120 minutes. The half-life of levodopa is 90 minutes. Absorption can be significantly reduced by changes in gastric pH and by ingestion with meals. Coadministration with carbidopa (Lodosyn) under trade names Duopa, Rytary, Parcopa, Sinemet, and Stalevo (which contains carbidopa, levodopa, and entacapone) prevents the breakdown of levodopa in periphery, thereby allowing more of the drug to pass the blood–brain barrier. Pharmacokinetic data about ergoline and nonergoline DAs is varied, as shown in Table 18-1.

After levodopa enters the dopaminergic neurons of the CNS, it is converted into the neurotransmitter dopamine, while both ergoline and nonergoline DAs act on dopamine receptors directly. Levodopa, pramipexole, and ropinirole bind about 20 times more selectively to dopamine D_3 than D_2 receptors; the corresponding ratio for bromocriptine is less than 2:1. Apomorphine binds selectively to D_1 and D_2 receptors, with little affinity for D_3 and D_4 receptors. Rotigotine is a potent agonist at all dopamine receptors, especially D_1, D_2, and D_3 receptors. L-Dopa, pramipexole, and ropinirole have no significant activity at nondopaminergic receptors, but bromocriptine binds to serotonin 5-HT$_1$ and 5-HT$_2$ and α_1-, α_2-, and β-adrenergic receptors. Cabergoline has a high affinity for D_2 and D_3 receptors, as well as 5-HT$_{2B}$ receptors.

Recent studies have indicated that pramipexole has anti-inflammatory properties and decreases concentrations of two inflammatory cytokines—tumor necrosis factor α and interleukin-6—in the substantia nigra of rats.

Therapeutic Indications

Parkinson Disease

Levodopa has been used to treat PD since the 1960s. Unfortunately, its efficacy wanes over time and it causes significant extrapyramidal side effects. Consequently, levodopa is now used once PD symptoms have become difficult to manage with other therapies. A combination of levodopa and carbidopa can enhance the efficacy of levodopa compared to when it is used as monotherapy.

Ergoline DAs including bromocriptine and cabergoline were initially used as adjunctive therapies with levodopa or as monotherapies prior to levodopa use but have fallen into disuse due to a risk of valvular defects and lung fibrosis. Nonergoline DAs, including pramipexole, ropinirole, apomorphine, and rotigotine, are more commonly used in the treatment of PD. Pramipexole and ropinirole are the most frequently prescribed nonergoline DAs in the United States.

Rotigotine, which is administered via transdermal patch, may be useful when treating patients who have difficulty maintaining a drug regimen.

Patients who experience sudden "off" episodes may experience relief with the use of apomorphine, which is administered either as a sublingual film (Kynmobi) or via subcutaneous injection (Apokyn).

TABLE 18-1: Pharmacokinetics of Available Dopamine Receptor Agonists

Generic Name	Trade Name	Route of Administration	Tmax	Half-life	Metabolism	Excretion
Apomorphine	Apokyn, Kynmobi	Subcutaneous injection	10–60 minutes	0.5–1 hour	Hepatic, via auto-oxidation, O-glucuronidation, O-methylation, sulfation, and N-demethylation catabolized by CYP2B6, 2C8, and 3A4/5[b]	Primary urine, largely in bound form
Bromocriptine	Parlodel	Oral	1.5–3 hours	2–8 hours	Hepatic, CYP3A4[b]	Primarily feces
Cabergoline	Dostinex, Caberlin	Oral	2.5 hours	63–109 hours	Hepatic via hydrolysis	≈60% feces and ≈22% urine
Carbidopa-levodopa[a]	Numerous	Oral	60–120 minutes	90 minutes	decarboxylation, O-methylation, transamination, and oxidation	Primarily urine
Levodopa	Numerous	Oral	30–120 minutes	50 minutes	Decarboxylation, O-methylation, transamination, and oxidation	Almost exclusively urine
Pramipexole	Mirapex	Oral	2 hours	8–12 hours	Minimal metabolization	≈90% recovered in urine, almost all as unchanged drug
Ropinirole	Requip	Oral	1.5–3 hours	6 hours	Hepatic, CYP1A2[b]	Primarily urine
Rotigotine	Neupro	Transdermal patch	15–18 hours	5–7 hours[c]	Hepatic	≈71% urine and ≈23% feces

[a]CYP: Cytochrome P450 system.
[b]Figures represent data for levodopa, as carbidopa inhibits aromatic-L-amino-acid decarboxylase and enhance the effect of the coadministered levodopa.
[c]Following the removal of the patch.

Medication-Induced Movement Disorders

DAs are regularly used for the treatment of medication-induced parkinsonism, EPS, akinesia, and focal perioral tremors. However, their use has diminished sharply because the incidence of medication-induced movement disorders is much lower with the use of the newer, atypical antipsychotics (serotonin–dopamine antagonists [SDAs]). DAs are effective in treating idiopathic RLS and may also be helpful when this is a medication side effect.

For the treatment of medication-induced movement disorders, most clinicians rely on anticholinergics, amantadine, and antihistamines because they are equally effective and have few adverse effects.

DAs are also used to counteract the hyperprolactinemic effects of dopamine receptor antagonists (DRAs), which result in the side effects of amenorrhea and galactorrhea. Bromocriptine and cabergoline are indicated for the treatment of acromegaly and hyperprolactinemia.

Restless Leg Syndrome

Rotigotine, ropinirole, and pramipexole have been approved to treat RLS, while many of the other drugs covered in this chapter are often used off-label to treat RLS. Currently, only the short-acting version of ropinirole (Requip) is indicated for the treatment of RLS. The long-acting medication (Requip XL) is only indicated for use in the treatment of PD.

Type II Diabetes Mellitus

Bromocriptine received FDA approval in 2009 for use in the treatment of type II diabetes to assist with glycemic control.

Off-Label Uses

Mood Disorders

Bromocriptine has long been used to enhance response to antidepressant drugs in refractory patients. Ropinirole has been reported to be useful as augmentation to antidepressant therapy and as a treatment for treatment-resistant bipolar II depression. Ropinirole may also be helpful in the treatment of antidepressant-induced sexual dysfunction. Pramipexole is often used in the augmentation of antidepressants in treatment-resistant major depressive disorder and bipolar disorder. Some studies have found pramipexole to be superior to sertraline (Zoloft) in the treatment of depression in PD, as well as reducing anhedonia in Parkinson's patients.

Restless Leg Syndrome

Though several DAs are indicated for the treatment of RLS, levodopa, apomorphine, and bromocriptine may reduce symptoms of RLS.

Neuroleptic Malignant Syndrome

DAs have been used to treat NMS. Bromocriptine has been shown to be particularly effective, as has amantadine and the muscle relaxant dantrolene (Dantrium). However, the incidence of this disorder is diminishing with the decreasing use of DRAs.

Sexual Dysfunction

DAs improve sexual dysfunction, including erectile dysfunction, in some patients. However, they are rarely used because they frequently cause adverse effects even at therapeutic dosages. Phosphodiesterase-5 inhibitor agents are better tolerated and more effective (see Chapter 30).

Other Medical Conditions

Bromocriptine has been shown to be effective in treating hepatic encephalopathy.

Cabergoline may be effective at treating Cushing disease in some patients. A retrospective multicenter study found between 20% and 25% of patients are good responders to the therapy, though there is no single parameter that can allow clinicians to predict efficacy.

Pramipexole may improve the analgesic qualities of low-dose morphine when treating acute pain. Pramipexole may also reduce morphine tolerance and shorten withdrawal symptoms. A case report found that pramipexole, when used in conjunction with antidepressants and buprenorphine, may reduce pain and depressive symptoms in patients with opioid use disorder, chronic pain, and depression.

Precautions and Adverse Reactions

Adverse effects are common with DAs, thus limiting the usefulness of these drugs. Adverse effects are dosage dependent and include nausea, vomiting, orthostatic hypotension, headache, dizziness, and cardiac arrhythmias. To reduce the risk of orthostatic hypotension, the initial dosage of all DAs should be quite low, with incremental increases at intervals of at least 1 week. These drugs should be used with caution in persons with hypertension, cardiovascular disease, and hepatic disease. After long-term use, persons, particularly elderly persons, may experience choreiform and dystonic movements and psychiatric disturbances—including hallucinations, delusions, confusion, depression, and mania—and other behavioral changes.

Long-term use of bromocriptine can produce retroperitoneal and pulmonary fibrosis, pleural effusions, and pleural thickening.

In general, ropinirole and pramipexole have a similar but milder adverse-effect profile than levodopa and bromocriptine. Pramipexole and ropinirole may cause irresistible sleep attacks that occur suddenly without warning and have caused motor vehicle accidents.

The most common adverse effects of apomorphine are yawning, dizziness, nausea, vomiting, drowsiness, bradycardia, syncope, and perspiration. Hallucinations have also been reported. Apomorphine's sedative effects are exacerbated with concurrent use of alcohol or other CNS depressants.

Use in Pregnancy and Lactation

DAs are contraindicated during pregnancy, especially for nursing mothers because they inhibit lactation.

Drug Interactions

DRAs are capable of reversing the effects of DAs, but this is not usually clinically significant. The concurrent use of tricyclic drugs and DAs has been reported to cause symptoms of neurotoxicity, such as rigidity, agitation, and tremor. They may also potentiate the hypotensive effects of diuretics and other antihypertensive medications. DAs should not be used in conjunction with monoamine oxidase inhibitors (MAOIs), including selegiline (Eldepryl), and MAOIs should be discontinued at least 2 weeks before the initiation of DA therapy.

Benzodiazepines, phenytoin (Dilantin), and pyridoxine may interfere with the therapeutic effects of DAs. Ergot alkaloids and bromocriptine should not be used concurrently because they may cause hypertension and myocardial infarction. Progestins, estrogens, and oral contraceptives may interfere with the effects of bromocriptine and may raise plasma concentrations of ropinirole. Ciprofloxacin (Cipro) can raise plasma concentrations of ropinirole, and cimetidine (Tagamet) can raise plasma concentrations of pramipexole.

Laboratory Interferences

Levodopa administration has been associated with false reports of elevated serum and urinary uric acid concentrations, urinary glucose test results, urinary ketone test results, and urinary catecholamine concentrations. No laboratory interferences have been associated with the administration of the other DAs.

Dosage and Clinical Guidelines

Table 18-2 lists the various DAs and their formulations. For the treatment of antipsychotic-induced parkinsonism, the clinician should start with a 100-mg dose of levodopa three times a day, which may be increased until the person is functionally improved. The maximum dosage of levodopa is 2,000 mg a day, but most persons respond to dosages below 1,000 mg per day. The dosage of

TABLE 18-2: Available Preparations of Dopamine Receptor Agonists and Carbidopa

Generic Name	Trade Name	Preparations
Amantadine	Symmetrel	100-mg capsule, 50-mg/5-mL syrup (teaspoon)
Apomorphine	Apokyn	3-mL cartridges containing 10 mg active pharmaceutical ingredient (API)
Apomorphine	Kynmobi	10-, 15-, 20-, 25-, 30-mg sublingual films
Bromocriptine	Parlodel	2.5-, 5-mg tablets
Cabergoline	Dostinex, Caberlin	0.5-mg tablets
Carbidopa	Lodosyn	25 mg[a]
Levodopa (L-Dopa)	Larodopa	100-, 250-, 500-mg tablets
Levodopa-carbidopa (Co-careldopa)	Sinemet, Atamet	100/10-mg, 100/25-mg, 250/25-mg tablets; 100/25-, 200/50-mg extended-release tablets
Pramipexole	Mirapex	0.125-, 0.375-, 0.75-, 1.5-, 3-, 4-mg extended-release tablets
Ropinirole	Requip	0.25-, 0.5-, 1-, 2-, 5-mg tablets
Rotigotine	Neupro	1-, 2-, 3-, 4-, 6-, 8-mg transdermal patches

[a]Drug only available directly through the manufacturer.

the carbidopa component of the levodopa–carbidopa formulation should total at least 75 mg a day.

The dosage of bromocriptine for mental disorders is uncertain, although it seems prudent to begin with low dosages (1.25 mg twice daily) and to increase the dosage gradually. Bromocriptine is usually taken with meals to help reduce the likelihood of nausea.

The starting dosage of pramipexole is 0.125 mg three times daily, which is increased to 0.25 mg three times daily in the second week and is increased by 0.25 mg per dose each week until therapeutic benefit or adverse effects emerge. Persons with idiopathic PD usually experience benefits at total daily doses of 1.5 mg, and the maximum daily dose is 4.5 mg.

For ropinirole, the starting dosage is 0.25 mg three times daily and is increased by 0.25 mg per dose each week to a total daily dose of 3 mg, then by 0.5 mg per dose each week to a total daily dose of 9 mg, and then by 1 mg per dose each week to a maximum dosage of 24 mg a day until therapeutic benefit or adverse effects emerge. The average daily dose for persons with idiopathic PD is about 16 mg.

The recommended subcutaneous dose of apomorphine in PD is 0.2 to 0.6 mL subcutaneously during acute hypomobility episodes delivered via metered injector pen. Apomorphine can be administered three times daily, with a maximum dose of 0.6 mL five times daily. The 10-mg sublingual formulation of apomorphine is typically administered as needed by patients, with a maximum daily dose of 30 mg.

Rotigotine is a transdermal patch that should be applied once per day. To apply, the patch should be firmly placed on the skin for 30 seconds. The same site should not be used more than once in a 14-day period. The starting dosage should be 1 mg/24 hours, and then increase as needed by 1 mg/24 hours at weekly intervals when treating RLS or 2 mg/24 hours at weekly intervals when treating PD. Maximum dosage should not exceed 3 mg/24 hours for RDS or 8 mg/24 hours for PD.

AMANTADINE

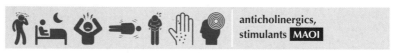

anticholinergics, stimulants MAOI

Amantadine (Symmetrel) is an antiviral drug that was initially used for the prophylaxis and treatment of influenza. It was found to have antiparkinsonian properties and is now used to treat the disorder as well as akinesias and other extrapyramidal signs, including focal perioral tremors (rabbit syndrome).

Pharmacologic Actions

Amantadine is well absorbed from the GI tract after oral administration, reaches peak plasma concentrations in approximately 2 to 3 hours, has a half-life of 12 to 18 hours, and attains steady-state concentrations after approximately 4 to 5 days of therapy. Amantadine is excreted largely unmetabolized (85% to 95%) in the urine. Amantadine plasma concentrations can be twice as high in elderly persons as in younger adults. Patients with renal failure accumulate amantadine in their bodies.

Amantadine augments dopaminergic neurotransmission in the CNS; however, the precise mechanism for the effect is unknown. The mechanism may involve dopamine release from presynaptic vesicles, blocking reuptake of dopamine into presynaptic nerve terminals, or an agonist effect on postsynaptic dopamine receptors.

Therapeutic Indications

The primary indication for amantadine's use in psychiatry is to treat extrapyramidal signs and symptoms, such as parkinsonism, akinesia, and the so-called rabbit syndrome (focal perioral tremor of the choreoathetoid type) caused by the administration of DRA or SDA drugs. Amantadine is as effective as the anticholinergics (e.g., benztropine [Cogentin]) for these indications and results in improvement in approximately half of all persons who take it. Amantadine, however, is not generally considered as effective as the anticholinergics for the treatment of acute dystonic reactions and is not effective in treating tardive dyskinesia and akathisia.

Amantadine is a reasonable compromise for persons with EPS who would be sensitive to additional anticholinergic effects, particularly those taking a low-potency DRA or the elderly. Elderly persons are susceptible to anticholinergic adverse effects, both in the CNS, such as anticholinergic delirium, and in the peripheral nervous system, such as urinary retention. Amantadine is associated with less memory impairment than are the anticholinergics.

Off-Label Uses

Amantadine is used in general medical practice for the treatment of parkinsonism of all causes, including idiopathic parkinsonism. In addition, amantadine has been reported to be of benefit in treating some selective serotonin reuptake inhibitor–associated side effects, such as lethargy, fatigue, anorgasmia, and ejaculatory inhibition. Limited evidence suggests that it may stabilize the weight of patients taking the antipsychotic olanzapine (Zyprexa) and enhance the effects of antidepressants in patients with acute bipolar depression.

Some studies have also suggested that amantadine may possess neuroprotective properties that can aid dementia patients and assist in the management of sequelae following cerebrovascular events, including traumatic brain injury. Research indicates that the drug may substantially improve executive functioning in patients with head injuries, particularly among individuals with frontal lobe syndrome.

Precautions and Adverse Effects

The most common CNS effects of amantadine are mild dizziness, insomnia, and impaired concentration (dosage related), which occur in 5% to 10% of all persons. Irritability, depression, anxiety, dysarthria, and ataxia occur in 1% to 5% of persons. More severe CNS adverse effects, including seizures and psychotic symptoms, have been reported. Nausea is the most common peripheral adverse effect of amantadine. Headache, loss of appetite, and blotchy spots on the skin have also been reported.

Livedo reticularis of the legs (a purple discoloration of the skin caused by dilation of blood vessels) has been reported in up to 5% of persons who take the drug for longer than 1 month. It usually diminishes with elevation of the legs and resolves in almost all cases when drug use is terminated.

Amantadine is relatively contraindicated in persons with renal disease or a seizure disorder. Amantadine should be used with caution in persons with edema or cardiovascular disease. Some evidence indicates that amantadine is teratogenic and therefore should not be taken by pregnant women. Because amantadine is excreted in breast milk, women who are breastfeeding should not take the drug.

Suicide attempts with amantadine overdosages are life-threatening. Symptoms can include toxic psychoses (confusion, hallucinations, aggressiveness) and cardiopulmonary arrest. Emergency treatment beginning with gastric lavage is indicated.

Use in Pregnancy and Lactation

Amantadine is classified as a pregnancy category C drug. Consequently, pregnant or nursing individuals should only be prescribed the drug in instances where potential risks are outweighed by its benefits.

Drug Interactions

Coadministration of amantadine with phenelzine (Nardil) or other MAOIs can result in a significant increase in resting blood pressure. The coadministration of amantadine with CNS stimulants can result in insomnia, irritability, nervousness, and possibly seizures or irregular heartbeat. Amantadine should not be coadministered with anticholinergics because unwanted side effects—such as confusion, hallucinations, nightmares, dry mouth, and blurred vision—may be exacerbated.

Dosage and Clinical Guidelines

Amantadine is available in 100-mg capsules and as a 50-mg per 5-mL syrup. The usual starting dosage of amantadine is 100 mg given orally twice a day, although the dosage can be cautiously increased up to 200 mg given orally twice a day if indicated. Amantadine should be used in persons with renal impairment *only* in consultation with the physician treating the renal condition.

If amantadine is beneficial for the treatment of the drug-induced EPS, it should be continued for 4 to 6 weeks and then discontinued to see whether the person has become tolerant to the neurologic adverse effects of the antipsychotic medication. Amantadine should be tapered over 1 to 2 weeks after a decision has been made to discontinue the drug.

Persons taking amantadine should not drink alcoholic beverages.

Dopamine Receptor Antagonists (First-Generation Antipsychotics)

19

Generic Name	Trade Name	Adverse Effects	Drug Interactions	CYP Interactions
Chlorpromazine	Thorazine	EPS, sedation, anticholinergic, hypotension, sexual dysfunction	See Table 19-4	2D6, 1A2, 3A4, 2E1
Prochlorperazine	Compazine	EPS, sedation, sexual dysfunction	See Table 19-4	2D6
Perphenazine	Trilafon	EPS, sedation, sexual dysfunction	See Table 19-4	2D6
Trifluoperazine	Stelazine	EPS, sedation, anticholinergic, sexual dysfunction	See Table 19-4	1A2
Fluphenazine	Prolixin	EPS, sexual dysfunction	See Table 19-4	2D6, 2E1
Thioridazine	Mellaril	Sedation, anticholinergic, sexual dysfunction	See Table 19-4	2D6, 2E1, 2C19
Haloperidol	Haldol	EPS, sexual dysfunction	See Table 19-4	2D6, 2C19, 2C9, 1A1, 1A2, 3A4, 3A5, 3A7
Thiothixene	Navane	EPS, hypotension, sexual dysfunction	See Table 19-4	2D6, 1A2
Loxapine	Loxitane	EPS, sedation, anticholinergic, sexual dysfunction	See Table 19-4	N/A
Molindone	Moban	Sedation, sexual dysfunction	See Table 19-4	N/A
Pimozide	Orap	EPS, sexual dysfunction	See Table 19-4	3A4, 3A5, 3A7, 1A2, 2D6

Introduction

The first group of agents proven to be effective in the treatment of schizophrenia and virtually all disorders with psychotic symptoms were dopamine receptor antagonists (DRAs). Historically known as neuroleptics or major tranquilizers, they are also commonly referred to as first-generation antipsychotics (FGAs) or typical antipsychotics. The first of these drugs, phenothiazine chlorpromazine (Thorazine) was introduced in the early 1950s. Other DRAs include all the antipsychotics in the following groups: phenothiazines, butyrophenones, thioxanthenes, dibenzoxazepines, dihydroindoles, and diphenylbutylpiperidines. Because these agents are associated with extrapyramidal syndromes (EPSs) at clinically effective dosages, newer antipsychotic drugs—the serotonin–dopamine antagonists (SDAs)—have gradually replaced them. The SDAs are differentiated from earlier drugs by their lower liability to cause extrapyramidal side effects. However, these newer drugs have other liabilities, most notably a propensity to cause weight gain, lipid elevations, and diabetes. Consequently, clinicians should still consider use of DRAs in patients with high risk of metabolic abnormalities that could lead to diabetes, cardiovascular disease, or other chronic ailments.

Intermediate-potency DRAs, such as perphenazine (Trilafon), have been shown to be as effective and well tolerated as the SDAs. Manufacturing of molindone (Moban), the DRA with the lowest risk of weight gain and metabolic side effects, was discontinued in the United States, but manufacturing resumed in 2018.

Pharmacologic Actions

All of the DRAs are well absorbed after oral administration, with liquid preparations being absorbed more efficiently than tablets or capsules. Peak plasma concentrations are usually reached 1 to 4 hours after oral administration and 30 to 60 minutes after parenteral administration. Smoking, coffee, antacids, and food interfere with absorption of these drugs. Steady-state levels are reached in approximately 3 to 5 days. The half-lives of these drugs are approximately 24 hours. All can be given in one daily oral dose, if tolerated, after the person is in a stable condition. Most DRAs are highly protein bound. Parenteral formulation of the DRAs results in a more rapid and more reliable onset of action. Bioavailability is also up to 10-fold higher with parenteral administration. Most DRAs are metabolized by CYP2D6 and 3A isozymes. However, there are differences among the specific agents.

Long-acting depot parenteral formulations of haloperidol (Haldol, Decanoate) and fluphenazine are available in the United States. They are usually administered once every 1 to 4 weeks, depending on the dose and the person. It can take up to 6 months of treatment with depot formulations to reach steady-state plasma levels, indicating that oral therapy should be continued during the first month or so of depot antipsychotic treatment.

Antipsychotic activity derives from inhibition of dopaminergic neurotransmission. The DRAs are effective when approximately 72% of D_2 receptors in the brain are occupied. The DRAs also block noradrenergic, cholinergic, and histaminergic receptors, with different drugs having different effects on these receptor systems.

There are some generalizations that can be made about the DRAs based on their potency. Potency refers to the amount of drug that is required to achieve therapeutic effects. Low-potency drugs such as chlorpromazine (Thorazine) and thioridazine (Mellaril), given in doses of several 100 mg/day, typically produce more weight gain and sedation than high-potency agents such as haloperidol and fluphenazine, usually given in doses of less than 10 mg/day. High-potency agents are also more likely to cause EPS. Some factors influencing the pharmacologic actions of DRAs are listed in Table 19-1.

Therapeutic Indications

DRAs are useful in numerous psychiatric and neurologic disorders. Some of these indications and off-label uses are shown in Table 19-2.

Schizophrenia and Schizoaffective Disorder

DRAs are effective in both the short- and long-term management of schizophrenia and schizoaffective disorder. They reduce both acute symptoms and prevent

TABLE 19-1: Factors Influencing the Pharmacokinetics of Antipsychotics

Age	Elderly patients may demonstrate reduced clearance rates
Medical condition	Decreased hepatic blood flow can reduce clearance
	Hepatic disease can decrease clearance
Enzyme inducers	Carbamazepine, phenytoin, ethambutol, barbiturates
Clearance inhibitors	Include SSRIs, TCAs, cimetidine, β-blockers, isoniazid, methylphenidate, erythromycin, triazolobenzodiazepines, ciprofloxacin, and ketoconazole
Changes in binding protein	Hypoalbuminemia can occur with malnutrition or hepatic failure

SSRI, selective serotonin reuptake inhibitor; TCA, tricyclic antidepressant.
Ereshefsky L. Pharmacokinetics and drug interactions: Update for new antipsychotics. *J Clin Psychiatry.* 1996;57(Suppl 11):12–25. Copyright 1996, Physicians Postgraduate Press. Adapted by permission.

TABLE 19-2: Approved Indications and Off-Label Uses of Dopamine Receptor Antagonists

Drug	FDA-Approved Indication	Off-Label Uses
Chlorpromazine	• Management of manifestations of psychotic disorders • Nausea and vomiting • Relief of restlessness before surgery • Acute intermittent porphyria • Management of manifestations of bipolar disorder • Relief of intractable hiccups	• Migraine treatment
Droperidol	• Prevention of postoperative vomiting	• Migraine treatment • Rapid tranquilization
Fluphenazine	• Management of manifestations of psychotic disorders	• Tic disorders • Chorea associated with Huntington disease • Dementia-related psychosis and agitation
Haloperidol	• Treatment of positive symptoms of schizophrenia • Management and control of tics and coprolalia associated with Tourette syndrome • Second-line treatment for severe behavior problems in children • Second-line and short-term treatment for hyperactive children with excessive motor activity and conduct disorders	• Acute mania • Agitation associated with psychiatric disorders • Chemotherapy-induced nausea and vomiting • Intractable hiccups
Loxapine	• Acute treatment of agitation associated with schizophrenia or bipolar I disorder	• Dementia-related psychosis and agitation • Irritability and aggression in ASD
Molindone	• Management of schizophrenia	• Dementia-related psychosis and agitation
Perphenazine	• Management of schizophrenia • Nausea and vomiting	• Acute mania

TABLE 19-2: Approved Indications and Off-Label Uses of Dopamine Receptor Antagonists (*continued*)

Drug	FDA-Approved Indication	Off-Label Uses
Pimozide	• Second-line treatment of motor tics and coprolalia associated with severe Tourette syndrome	• Delusional parasitosis
Prochlorperazine	• Treatment of schizophrenia • Nausea and vomiting • Second-line and short-term treatment of generalized, nonpsychotic anxiety	• Adult migraine • Pediatric migraine
Thioridazine	• Refractory schizophrenia	• Depression with psychotic features • Pediatric behavioral disorders • Geriatric psychoneurotic manifestations
Thiothixene	• Management of schizophrenia	• Dementia-related psychosis and agitation
Trifluoperazine	• Management of schizophrenia • Second-line and short-term treatment of generalized, nonpsychotic anxiety	
ASD, autism spectrum disorder.		

future exacerbations. DRAs produce their most dramatic effects against the positive symptoms of schizophrenia (e.g., hallucinations, delusions, and agitation). Negative symptoms (e.g., emotional withdrawal and ambivalence) are less likely to improve significantly, and they may appear to worsen because these drugs produce constriction of facial expression and akinesia, side effects that mimic negative symptoms. Consequently, adjunctive therapies are often necessary.

Schizophrenia and schizoaffective disorder are characterized by remission and relapse. DRAs decrease the risk of reemergence of psychosis in patients who have recovered while on medication. After a first episode of psychosis, patients should be maintained on medication for 1 to 2 years; after multiple episodes, for 2 to 5 years. However, patients with schizophrenia may require lifelong treatment and length of antipsychotic therapy should be tailored individually.

Acute Mania

DRAs are effective to treat psychotic symptoms of acute mania. Because antimanic agents (e.g., lithium) generally have a slower onset of action than do antipsychotics in the treatment of acute symptoms, it is standard practice to initially combine either a DRA or an SDA with lithium (Eskalith), divalproex (Depakote), lamotrigine (Lamictal), or carbamazepine (Tegretol), and to then gradually withdraw the antipsychotic.

Tourette Syndrome

DRAs are used to treat Tourette syndrome, a neurobehavioral disorder marked by motor and vocal tics. Haloperidol and pimozide (Orap) are the drugs most frequently used, but other DRAs are also effective. Use of pimozide should be avoided unless other treatment options have been unsuccessful and the patient's motor or verbal tics adversely affect quality of life. Some clinicians prefer to use clonidine (Catapres) for this disorder because of its lower risk of neurologic side effects.

Severe Agitation and Violent Behavior

Severely agitated and violent patients, regardless of diagnosis, may be treated with DRAs, though loxapine is specifically indicated for the treatment of agitation associated with schizophrenia or bipolar I disorder. Symptoms such as extreme irritability, lack of impulse control, severe hostility, gross hyperactivity, and agitation respond to short-term treatment with these drugs. Haloperidol is routinely used for treatment of acute agitation associated with schizophrenia, bipolar disorder, and numerous other conditions as monotherapy or in combination with lorazepam.

Bipolar Disorder

Chlorpromazine may help manage manic symptoms of bipolar disorder (e.g., increased excitability, impulsivity, and energy; decreased need for sleep; grandiose ideation), and some evidence suggest that it could serve as a prophylactic treatment for bipolar disorder.

Generalized Anxiety Disorder

Both prochlorperazine and trifluoperazine have been used as second-line and short-term treatments for generalized, nonpsychotic anxiety.

Behavioral Problems in Children

Haloperidol is an effective treatment for combative and explosive hyperexcitability in children. It is also an effective treatment for extreme hyperactivity that includes difficulty sustaining attention, impulsivity, aggression, poor frustration tolerance, and mood lability. This medication should be reserved for children who have not responded to psychotherapy and/or other medications.

Miscellaneous Medical Conditions

Other miscellaneous indications for the use of DRAs include the treatment of nausea, emesis, intractable hiccups, and preoperative apprehension.

Off-Label Uses

Depression with Psychotic Symptoms

Combination treatment with an antipsychotic and an antidepressant is one of the treatments of choice for major depressive disorder with psychotic features; the other is electroconvulsive therapy (ECT).

Delusional Disorder

Patients with delusional disorder often respond favorably to treatment with these drugs. Some persons with borderline personality disorder who may develop paranoid thinking in the course of their disorder may respond to antipsychotic drugs.

Chronic Pruritus and Delusional Parasitosis

Literature dating back to the 1950s has shown that DRAs can treat chronic pruritus, possibly via blockade of histamine H_1 receptors. A case series noted pimozide was effective at treating delusional parasitosis.

Dementia and Delirium

About two-thirds of agitated, elderly patients with various forms of dementia improve when given a DRA. Low doses of high-potency drugs (e.g., 0.5 to 1 mg a day of haloperidol) are recommended. DRAs are also used to treat psychotic symptoms and agitation associated with delirium. The cause of the delirium needs to be determined because toxic deliriums caused by anticholinergic agents can be exacerbated by low-potency DRAs, which often have significant antimuscarinic activity. Orthostasis, parkinsonism, and worsened cognition are the most problematic side effects in this elderly population.

Substance-Induced Psychotic Disorder

Intoxication with cocaine, amphetamines, alcohol, phencyclidine (PCP), or other drugs can cause psychotic symptoms. Because these symptoms tend to be time limited, it is preferable to avoid use of a DRA unless the patient is severely agitated and aggressive. Usually, benzodiazepines can be used to calm the patient. Benzodiazepines should be used instead of DRAs in cases of PCP intoxication, since PCP is highly anticholinergic. When a patient is experiencing hallucinations or delusions as a result of alcohol withdrawal, DRAs, especially low-potency antipsychotics, may increase the risk of seizure.

Childhood Schizophrenia

Children with schizophrenia benefit from treatment with antipsychotic medication, although considerably less research has been devoted to this population. Studies are currently underway to determine if intervention with medication at the very earliest signs of disturbance in children genetically at risk for schizophrenia can prevent the emergence of more florid symptoms. Careful consideration needs to be given to side effects, especially those involving cognition and alertness.

Irritability or Aggression Associated with Autism Spectrum Disorder

Adults and children with mental disabilities, especially those with autism spectrum disorder (ASD) level 2 or level 3, often have associated episodes of violence, aggression, and agitation that respond to treatment with antipsychotic drugs; however, the repeated administration of antipsychotics to control disruptive behavior in children is controversial.

Borderline Personality Disorder

Patients with borderline personality disorder who experience transient psychotic symptoms, such as perceptual disturbances, suspiciousness, ideas of reference, and aggression, may need to be treated with a DRA. This disorder is also associated with mood instability, so patients should be evaluated for possible treatment with mood-stabilizing agents.

Other Psychiatric and Nonpsychiatric Indications

The DRAs reduce the chorea in the early stages of Huntington disease. Patients with this disease may develop hallucinations, delusions, mania, or hypomania. These and other psychiatric symptoms respond to DRAs, especially high-potency DRAs. However, clinicians should be aware that patients with the rigid form of this disorder may experience acute EPS.

The use of DRAs to treat impulse control disorders should be reserved for patients in whom other interventions have failed. Patients with pervasive developmental disorder may exhibit hyperactivity, screaming, and agitation with combativeness. Some of these symptoms respond to high-potency DRAs, but there is little research evidence supporting benefits in these patients.

The rare neurologic disorders ballismus and hemiballismus (which affect only one side of the body), characterized by propulsive movements of the limbs away from the body, also respond to treatment with antipsychotic agents. Endocrine disorders and temporal lobe epilepsy may be associated with psychosis that responds to antipsychotic treatment. Numerous case reports suggest that DRAs are effective in treating adult and pediatric migraines based on the theoretical model that overactivity of dopaminergic systems is at least partially responsible for migraines.

The most common side effects of DRAs are neurologic. As a rule, low-potency drugs cause most nonneurologic adverse effects, and the high-potency drugs cause most neurologic adverse effects.

Precautions and Adverse Reactions

Table 19-3 summarizes the most common adverse events associated with the use of DRAs.

Neuroleptic Malignant Syndrome

A potentially fatal side effect of DRA treatment, neuroleptic malignant syndrome, can occur at any time during the course of treatment. Symptoms include extreme hyperthermia, severe muscular rigidity and dystonia, akinesia, mutism, confusion, agitation, and increased pulse rate and blood pressure (BP). Laboratory findings include increased white blood cell (WBC) count, creatinine phosphokinase, liver enzymes, plasma myoglobin, and myoglobinuria, occasionally associated with renal failure. The symptoms usually evolve over 24 to 72 hours, and the untreated syndrome lasts 10 to 14 days. The diagnosis is often missed in the early stages, and the withdrawal or agitation may mistakenly be considered to reflect increased psychosis. Men are affected more frequently than are women, and young persons are affected more commonly than are elderly persons. The mortality rate can reach 20% to 30% or even higher when depot medications are involved. Rates are also increased when high doses of high-potency agents are used.

If neuroleptic malignant syndrome is suspected, causative agent should be stopped immediately and supportive care started without delay: Request medical support and patient may need care in an intensive care unit; use cooling blankets to lower fever; monitor vital signs, electrolytes, fluid balance, and renal output; and maintain cardiorespiratory stability. Antiparkinsonian medications may

TABLE 19-3: Dopamine Receptor Antagonists: Potency and Adverse Effects

Drug Name	Chlorpromazine Therapeutic Equivalent (Oral Dose mg/d)	Adverse Effect Potential			
		Sedation	Anticholinergic Effects	Extrapyramidal Symptoms	Hypotensive Effects
Pimozide	2	Low	Low	High	Very low
Fluphenazine	2–3	Low	Low	Very high	Low
Haloperidol	2–3	Very low	Very low	Very high	Very low
Trifluoperazine	2–5	Low	Low	High	Low
Thiothixene	4	Low	Low	High	Low
Perphenazine	8–10	Low	Low	High	Low
Molindone	10	Very low	Low	Moderate	Low
Loxapine	10	Moderate	Low	Moderate	Moderate
Prochlorperazine	15	High	Low	High	Moderate
Chlorpromazine	100	High	High	Low	Moderate[a]
Thioridazine	100	High	High	Low	High

[a]Moderate when taken orally. The risk of adverse hypotensive effects increases to high with intermuscular administration.
Data from https://psychopharmacologyinstitute.com/publication/first-generation-antipsychotics-an-introduction-2110; https://aapp.org/guideline/essentials/antipsychotic-dose-equivalents; https://www.ncbi.nlm.nih.gov/pmc/articles/PMC4960429/

reduce muscle rigidity. Dantrolene (Dantrium), a skeletal muscle relaxant (0.8 to 2.5 mg/kg every 6 hours, up to a total dosage of 10 mg a day) may also be useful in the treatment of this disorder. When the person can take oral medications, dantrolene can be given in doses of 100 to 200 mg a day. Bromocriptine (20 to 30 mg a day in four divided doses) or amantadine can be added to the regimen. Treatment will typically need to be continued for 5 to 10 days. When drug treatment is restarted, the clinician should consider switching to a low-potency drug or an SDA, although these agents—including clozapine—may also cause neuroleptic malignant syndrome.

Seizure Threshold

DRAs may lower seizure threshold. Chlorpromazine, thioridazine, and other low-potency drugs are thought to be more epileptogenic than are high-potency drugs. The risk of inducing a seizure by drug administration warrants consideration when the person already has a seizure disorder or brain lesion.

Sedation

Blockade of histamine H_1 receptors is the usual cause of sedation associated with DRAs. Chlorpromazine is the most sedating of the drugs covered in this chapter. The relative sedative properties of the drugs are summarized in Table 19-3. Giving the entire daily dose at bedtime usually eliminates any problems of sedation, and tolerance for this adverse effect often develops.

Central Anticholinergic Effects

The symptoms of central anticholinergic activity include sedation, cognitive slowing, confusion, restlessness, severe agitation; disorientation to time, person, and place; hallucinations; seizures; high fever; and dilated pupils. Stupor and coma may ensue. The treatment of anticholinergic toxicity consists of discontinuing the causal agent or agents; close medical supervision; and administration of physostigmine (Antilirium, Eserine), 2 mg by slow intravenous (IV) infusion, repeated within 1 hour as necessary. Too much physostigmine is dangerous, and symptoms of physostigmine toxicity include hypersalivation and sweating. Atropine sulfate (0.5 mg) can reverse the effects of physostigmine toxicity.

Cardiac Effects

The DRAs decrease cardiac contractility, disrupt enzyme contractility in cardiac cells, increase circulating levels of catecholamines, and prolong atrial and ventricular conduction time and refractory periods. Low-potency DRAs, particularly the phenothiazines (chlorpromazine, prochlorperazine, and thioridazine), are usually more cardiotoxic than are high-potency drugs (haloperidol and fluphenazine). One exception is haloperidol, which has been linked to abnormal heart rhythm, ventricular arrhythmias, torsades de pointes, and sudden death when injected IV. Pimozide and droperidol (a butyrophenone) also prolong the QTc interval and have clearly been associated with torsades de pointes and sudden death, as does sulpiride, a selective antagonist at D_2, D_3, and $5\text{-}HT_{1A}$ that is not currently approved for use in the United States. In one study, thioridazine was responsible for 28 (61%) of the 46 sudden antipsychotic deaths. In 15 of these cases, it was the only drug ingested. Chlorpromazine also causes prolongation of the QT and PR intervals, blunting of the T waves, and depression of the ST segment. Clinicians should carefully assess cardiac status of the patient prior to prescribing these drugs.

Sudden Death

Occasional reports of sudden cardiac death during treatment with DRAs may be the result of cardiac arrhythmias. Other causes may include seizure, asphyxiation, malignant hyperthermia, heat stroke, and neuroleptic malignant syndrome. However, there does not appear to be an overall increase in the incidence of sudden death linked to the use of antipsychotics.

Orthostatic (Postural) Hypotension

Orthostatic (postural) hypotension is most common with low-potency drugs, particularly chlorpromazine, thioridazine, and chlorprothixene. When using intramuscular (IM) low-potency DRAs, the clinician should assess for orthostasis and measure the person's BP (lying and standing) before and after the first dose and during the first few days of treatment.

Orthostatic hypotension is mediated by adrenergic blockade and occurs most frequently during the first few days of treatment. Tolerance often develops for this side effect, which is why initial dosing of these drugs is lower than the usual therapeutic dose. Fainting or falls, although uncommon, may lead to injury. Patients should be warned of this side effect and instructed to rise slowly after sitting and reclining. Patients should avoid all caffeine and alcohol; should drink at least 2 L of fluid a day; and if not under treatment for hypertension, should add liberal amounts of salt to their diet. Support hose may help some persons.

Hypotension can usually be managed by having patients lie down with their feet higher than their heads and pump their legs as if bicycling. Volume expansion or vasopressor agents, such as norepinephrine (Levophed), may be indicated in severe cases. Because hypotension is produced by α-adrenergic blockade, the drugs also block the α-adrenergic–stimulating properties of epinephrine, leaving the β-adrenergic–stimulating effects untouched. Therefore, the administration of epinephrine results in a paradoxical worsening of hypotension and is contraindicated in cases of antipsychotic-induced hypotension. Pure α-adrenergic pressor agents, such as metaraminol (Aramine) and norepinephrine, are the drugs of choice in the treatment of the disorder.

Hematologic Effects

A temporary leukopenia with a WBC count of about 3,500 is a common but not serious problem. Agranulocytosis, a life-threatening hematologic problem, occurs in about 1 in 10,000 persons treated with DRAs. Thrombocytopenic or nonthrombocytopenic purpura, hemolytic anemias, and pancytopenia may occur rarely in persons treated with DRAs. Although routine complete blood counts (CBCs) are not indicated, if a person reports a sore throat and fever, a CBC should be done immediately to check for the possibility. If the blood indexes are low, administration of DRAs should be stopped, and the person should be transferred to a medical facility. The mortality rate for the complication may be as high as 30%.

Tardive Dyskinesia

As discussed in Chapter 42, medication-induced movement disorders can be one of the more concerning effects of long-term treatment with DRAs. It is an important reason to monitor patients being treated with these drugs. Clinical trials showed that patients who received 80 mg/day of the active treatment with valbenazine (Ingrezza) had a significant decrease in tardive dyskinesia (TD) symptoms on the Abnormal Involuntary Movement Scale (AIMS) at 6 weeks compared with those who received matching placebo. The group receiving the treatment at 40 mg/day also had a reduction on the AIMS measures.

Treatment with valbenazine may cause sleepiness and QT prolongation and its use should be avoided in patients with congenital long QT syndrome or with abnormal heartbeats associated with a prolonged QT interval. Valbenazine reduced involuntary movements without reducing the therapeutic effects of the DRA.

Peripheral Anticholinergic Effects

Peripheral anticholinergic effects, consisting of dry mouth and nose, blurred vision, constipation, urinary retention, and mydriasis are common, especially with low-potency DRAs such as chlorpromazine and thioridazine. Some persons may also experience nausea and vomiting.

Constipation should be treated with the usual laxative preparations, but severe constipation can progress to paralytic ileus. A decrease in the DRA dosage or a change to a less anticholinergic drug is warranted in such cases. Pilocarpine (Salagen) may be used to treat paralytic ileus, although the relief is only transitory. Bethanechol (Urecholine) (20 to 40 mg a day) may be useful in some persons with urinary retention.

Low-potency DRAs may cause significant weight gain but not as much as is seen with the SDAs like olanzapine (Zyprexa) and clozapine (Clozaril). Molindone and perhaps loxapine appear to be least likely to cause weight gain. Weight gain is associated with cardiometabolic complications that may lead to increase in morbidity and mortality as well as medication noncompliance. For relevant information about obesity, see Chapter 40.

Endocrine Effects

Blockade of the dopamine receptors in the tuberoinfundibular tract results in the increased secretion of prolactin, which can result in breast enlargement, galactorrhea, amenorrhea, and inhibited orgasm in women and impotence in men. The SDAs, with the exception of risperidone (Risperdal), are not particularly associated with an increase in prolactin levels and may be the drugs of choice for persons experiencing disturbing side effects from increased prolactin release.

Sexual Adverse Effects

Both men and women taking DRAs can experience anorgasmia and decreased libido. As many as 50% of men taking antipsychotics report ejaculatory and erectile disturbances. Sildenafil (Viagra), vardenafil (Levitra), and tadalafil (Cialis) are often used to treat psychotropic-induced orgasmic dysfunction, but they have not been studied in combination with the DRAs. Thioridazine is particularly associated with decreased libido and retrograde ejaculation in men. Priapism and reports of painful orgasms have also been described, both possibly resulting from α_1-adrenergic antagonist activity.

Skin and Eye Effects

Allergic dermatitis and photosensitivity may occur with use of DRAs, especially with low-potency agents. Urticarial, maculopapular, petechial, and edematous eruptions may occur early in treatment, generally in the first few weeks, and remit spontaneously. A photosensitivity reaction that resembles a severe sunburn also occurs in some persons taking chlorpromazine. Patients should be warned of this adverse effect, should spend no more than 30 to 60 minutes in the sun, and use sunscreens. Long-term chlorpromazine use is associated with blue-gray discoloration of skin areas exposed to sunlight. The skin changes often begin with a tan or golden-brown color and progress to such colors as slate gray, metallic blue, and purple. These discolorations resolve when the patient is switched to another medication.

Irreversible retinal pigmentation is associated with the use of thioridazine at dosages above 1,000 mg a day. An early symptom of the side effect can sometimes be nocturnal confusion related to difficulty with night vision. The pigmentation can progress even after thioridazine administration is stopped, finally resulting in blindness. It is for this reason that the maximum recommended dosage of thioridazine is 800 mg/day.

Patients taking chlorpromazine may develop a relatively benign pigmentation of the eyes, characterized by whitish brown granular deposits concentrated in the anterior lens and posterior cornea and visible only by slit-lens examination. The deposits can progress to opaque white and yellow-brown granules, often stellate. Occasionally, the conjunctiva is discolored by a brown pigment. No retinal damage is seen, and vision is almost never impaired. This condition gradually resolves when chlorpromazine is discontinued.

Jaundice

Elevations of liver enzymes during treatment with a DRA tend to be transient and not clinically significant. When chlorpromazine first came into use, cases of obstructive or cholestatic jaundice were reported. It usually occurred in the first month of treatment and was portended by symptoms of upper abdominal pain, nausea, and vomiting. This was followed by fever; rash; eosinophilia; bilirubin in the urine; and increases in serum bilirubin, alkaline phosphatase, and hepatic transaminases. Reported cases are now extremely rare, but if jaundice occurs, the medication should be discontinued.

Overdoses

Overdoses typically consist of exaggerated DRA side effects. Symptoms and signs include CNS depression, extrapyramidal side effects, mydriasis, rigidity, restlessness, decreased deep tendon reflexes, tachycardia, and hypotension. The severe symptoms of overdose include delirium, coma, respiratory depression, and seizures. Haloperidol may be among the safest typical antipsychotics in overdose. After an overdose, the electroencephalogram (EEG) shows diffuse slowing and low voltage. Extreme overdose may lead to delirium and coma, with respiratory depression and hypotension. Life-threatening overdose usually involves concomitant ingestion of other CNS depressants, such as alcohol or benzodiazepines.

Activated charcoal, if possible, and gastric lavage should be administered if the overdose is recent. Emetics are not indicated because the antiemetic actions of the DRAs inhibit their efficacy. Seizures can be treated with IV diazepam (Valium) or phenytoin (Dilantin). Hypotension can be treated with either norepinephrine or dopamine but not epinephrine.

Use in Pregnancy and Lactation

There is a low correlation between the use of antipsychotics during pregnancy and congenital malformations. Nevertheless, antipsychotics should be avoided during pregnancy, particularly in the first trimester unless the benefit outweighs the risk. High-potency drugs are preferable to low-potency drugs because the low-potency drugs are associated with hypotension.

DRAs are secreted in the breast milk, although concentrations are low. Women taking these agents should be advised against breastfeeding.

Drug Interactions

Many pharmacokinetic and pharmacodynamic drug interactions are associated with these drugs (Table 19-4). CYP2D6 is the most common hepatic isozyme involved in DRA pharmacokinetic interactions. Other common drug interactions affect the absorption of the DRAs.

TABLE 19-4: Antipsychotic Drug Interactions

Interacting Medication	Mechanism	Clinical Effect
Drug Interactions Assessed to Have Major Severity		
β-Adrenergic receptor antagonists	Synergistic pharmacologic effect; antipsychotic inhibits metabolism of propranolol; antipsychotic increases plasma concentrations	Severe hypotension
Anticholinergics	Pharmacodynamic effects	Decreased antipsychotic effect
	Additive anticholinergic effect	Anticholinergic toxicity
Barbiturates	Phenobarbital induces antipsychotic metabolism	Decreased antipsychotic concentrations
Carbamazepine	Induces antipsychotic metabolism	Up to 50% reduction in antipsychotic concentrations
Charcoal	Reduces GI absorption of antipsychotic and adsorbs drug during enterohepatic circulation	May reduce antipsychotic effect or cause toxicity when used to treat overdose or for GI disturbances
Cigarette smoking	Induction of microsomal enzymes	Reduced plasma concentrations of antipsychotic agents
Epinephrine, norepinephrine	Antipsychotic antagonizes pressor effect	Hypotension
Ethanol	Additive CNS depression	Impaired psychomotor status
Fluvoxamine	Fluvoxamine inhibits metabolism of haloperidol and clozapine	Increased concentrations of haloperidol and clozapine
Guanethidine	Antipsychotic antagonizes guanethidine reuptake	Impaired antihypertensive effect
Lithium	Unknown	Rare reports of neurotoxicity
Meperidine	Additive CNS depression	Hypotension and sedation
Drug Interactions Assessed to Have Minor or Moderate Severity		
Amphetamines anorexiants	Decreased pharmacologic effect of amphetamine	Diminished weight loss effect; amphetamines may exacerbate psychosis
ACEIs	Additive hypotensive crisis	Hypotension, postural intolerance
Antacids containing aluminum	Insoluble complex formed in GI tract	Possible reduced antipsychotic effect
AD nonspecific	Decreased metabolism of AD through competitive inhibition	Increased AD concentration
Benzodiazepines	Increased pharmacologic effect of the benzodiazepine	Respiratory depression, stupor, hypotension

(continued)

TABLE 19-4: Antipsychotic Drug Interactions (*continued*)

Interacting Medication	Mechanism	Clinical Effect
Bromocriptine	Antipsychotic antagonizes dopamine receptor stimulation	Increased prolactin
Caffeinated beverages	Form precipitate with antipsychotic solutions	Possible diminished antipsychotic effect
Cimetidine	Reduced antipsychotic absorption and clearance	Decreased antipsychotic effect
Clonidine	Antipsychotic potentiates α-adrenergic hypotensive effect	Hypotension or hypertension
Disulfiram	Impairs antipsychotic metabolism	Increased antipsychotic concentrations
Methyldopa	Unknown	BP elevations
Phenytoin	Induction of antipsychotic metabolism; decreased phenytoin metabolism	Decreased antipsychotic concentrations: increased phenytoin levels
SSRIs	Impair antipsychotic metabolism; pharmacodynamic interaction	Sudden onset of extrapyramidal symptoms
Valproic acid	Antipsychotic inhibits valproic acid metabolism	Increased valproic acid half-life and levels

ACEI, angiotensin-converting enzyme inhibitor; AD, antidepressant; BP, blood pressure; CNS, central nervous system; GI, gastrointestinal; SSRIs, selective serotonin reuptake inhibitors.
Data from Ereshosky L, Overman GP, Karp JK. Current psychotropic dosing and monitoring guidelines. *Prim Psychiatry*. 1996;3:21.

Antacids, activated charcoal, cholestyramine (Questran), kaolin, pectin, and cimetidine (Tagamet) taken within 2 hours of antipsychotic administration can reduce the absorption of these drugs. Anticholinergics may decrease the absorption of the DRAs. The additive anticholinergic activity of the DRAs, anticholinergics, and tricyclic drugs may result in anticholinergic toxicity. Digoxin (Lanoxin) and steroids, both of which decrease gastric motility, can increase DRA absorption.

Phenothiazines, especially thioridazine, may decrease the metabolism of and cause toxic concentrations of phenytoin. Barbiturates may increase the metabolism of DRAs.

Tricyclic drugs and selective serotonin reuptake inhibitors (SSRIs) that inhibit CYP2D6—paroxetine (Paxil), fluoxetine (Prozac), and fluvoxamine (Luvox)—interact with DRAs, resulting in increased plasma concentrations of both drugs. The anticholinergic, sedative, and hypotensive effects of the drugs may also be addictive.

Typical antipsychotics may inhibit the hypotensive effects of α-methyldopa (Aldomet). Conversely, typical antipsychotics may have an additive effect on some hypotensive drugs. Antipsychotic drugs have a variable effect on the hypotensive effects of clonidine. Propranolol (Inderal) coadministration increases the blood concentrations of both drugs.

The DRAs potentiate the CNS-depressant effects of the sedatives, antihistamines, opiates, opioids, and alcohol, particularly in persons with impaired respiratory status. When these agents are taken with alcohol, the risk for heat stroke may be increased.

Cigarette smoking may decrease the plasma levels of the typical antipsychotic drugs. Epinephrine has a paradoxical hypotensive effect in persons taking typical antipsychotics. These drugs may decrease the blood concentration of warfarin (Coumadin), resulting in decreased bleeding time. The phenothiazines, thioridazine, and pimozide should not be coadministered with other agents that prolong the QT interval.

Thioridazine is contraindicated in patients taking drugs that inhibit the CYP2D6 isoenzyme or in patients with reduced levels of CYP2D6.

Laboratory Interferences

Chlorpromazine and perphenazine may cause both false-positive and false-negative results in immunologic pregnancy tests and falsely elevated bilirubin (with reagent test strips) and urobilinogen (with Ehrlich's reagent test) values. These drugs have also been associated with an abnormal shift in results of the glucose tolerance test, although that shift may reflect the effects of the drugs on the glucose-regulating system. Phenothiazines have been reported to interfere with the measurement of 17-ketosteroids and 17-hydroxycorticosteroids and produce false-positive results in tests for phenylketonuria.

Dosage and Clinical Guidelines

Contraindications to the use of DRAs include the following:

1. A history of a serious allergic response
2. The possible ingestion of a substance that will interact with the antipsychotic to induce CNS depression (e.g., alcohol, opioids, barbiturates, and benzodiazepines) or anticholinergic delirium (e.g., scopolamine and possibly PCP)
3. The presence of a severe cardiac abnormality
4. A high risk for seizures
5. The presence of narrow-angle glaucoma or prostatic hypertrophy if a drug with high anticholinergic activity is to be used
6. The presence or a history of TD

Antipsychotics should be administered with caution in persons with hepatic disease because impaired hepatic metabolism may result in elevated plasma concentrations. The usual assessment should include a CBC with WBC indexes, liver function tests, and electrocardiography (EKG), especially in women older than 40 years of age and men older than 30 years of age. Elderly persons and children are more sensitive to side effects than are young adults, so the dosage of the drug should be adjusted accordingly.

Various patients may respond to widely different dosages of antipsychotics; therefore, there is no set dosage for any given antipsychotic drug. Because of side effects, it is reasonable clinical practice to begin at a low dosage and increase it as necessary. It is important to remember that the maximal effects of a particular dosage may not be evident for 4 to 6 weeks. Available preparations and dosages of the DRAs are given in Table 19-5.

208

TABLE 19-5: Dopamine Receptor Antagonists

Name		Trade (mg)	Capsules (mg)	Solution	Parenteral	Rectal Suppositories (mg)	Adult Dose Range (mg/day)	
Generic or Chemical	Trade						Acute	Maintenance
Chlorpromazine	Thorazine	10, 25, 50, 100, 200	30, 75, 150, 200, 300	10 mg/5 mL, 30 mg/mL, 100 mg/mL	25 mg/mL	25, 100	100–1,600 PO 25–400 IM	50–400 PO
Prochlorperazine	Compazine	5, 10, 25	10, 15, 30	5 mg/5 mL	5 mg/mL	2.5, 5, 25	15–200 PO 40–80 IM	15–60 PO
Perphenazine	Trilafon	2, 4, 8, 16	—	16 mg/5 mL	5 mg/mL	—	12–64 PO 15–30 IM	8–24 PO
Trifluoperazine	Stelazine	1, 2, 5, 10	—	10 mg/mL	2 mg/mL	—	4–40 PO 4–10 IM	5–20 PO
Fluphenazine	Prolixin	1, 2.5, 5, 10	—	2.5 mg/5 mL, 5 mg/mL	2.5 mg/mL (IM only)	—	2.5–40.0 PO 5–20 IM	1.0–15.0 PO 12.5–50.0 IM (decanoate or enanthate, weekly or biweekly)
Fluphenazine decanoate	—	—	—	—	2.5 mg/mL	—	—	—
Fluphenazine enanthate	—	—	—	2.5 mg/mL	—	—	—	—
Thioridazine	Mellaril	10, 15, 25, 50, 100, 150, 200	—	25 mg/5 mL, 100 mg/5 mL, 30 mg/mL, 100 mg/mL	—	—	200–800 PO	100–300 PO
Haloperidol	Haldol	0.5, 1, 2, 5, 10, 20	—	2 mg/5 mL	5 mg/mL (IM only)	—	5–20 PO 12.5–25 IM	1–10 PO
Haloperidol decancate	—	—	—	—	50 mg/mL, 100 mg/mL (IM only)	—	—	25–200 IM (decanoate, monthly)
Thiothixene	Navane	—	1, 2, 5, 10, 20	5 mg/mL	5 mg/mL (IM only), 20 mg/mL (IM only)	—	6–100 PO 8–30 IM	6–30
Loxapine	Loxitane	—	5, 10, 25, 50	25 mg/5 mL	50 mg/mL	—	20–250 20–75 IM	20–100
Molindone	Moban	5, 10, 25, 50, 100	—	20 mg/mL	—	—	50–225	5–150
Pimozide	Orap	2	—	—	—	—	0.5–20	0.5–5.0

IM, intramuscular; PO, oral.

Short-Term Treatment

The equivalent of 5 to 20 mg of haloperidol is a reasonable dose for an adult in an acute state. A geriatric person may benefit from as little as 1 mg of haloperidol. The administration of more than 25 mg of chlorpromazine in one injection may result in serious hypotension. IM administration results in peak plasma levels in about 30 minutes versus 90 minutes using the oral route. Doses of drugs for IM administration are about half those given by the oral route. In a short-term treatment setting, the person should be observed for 1 hour after the first dose of medication. After that time, most clinicians administer a second dose or a sedative agent (e.g., a benzodiazepine) to achieve effective behavioral control. Possible sedatives include lorazepam (Ativan) (2 mg IM) or diphenhydramine (Benadryl) (50 mg IM), though clinicians should carefully assess its anticholinergic effects, especially in older patients.

Rapid Neuroleptization

Rapid neuroleptization (also called psychotolysis) is the practice of administering hourly IM doses of antipsychotic medications until marked sedation of the person is achieved. However, several research studies have shown that merely waiting several more hours after one dose yields the same clinical improvement as is seen with repeated doses. Nevertheless, clinicians must be careful to keep persons from becoming violent while they are psychotic. Clinicians can help prevent violent episodes by using adjuvant sedatives or by temporarily using physical restraints until the persons can control their behavior.

Early Treatment

A full 6 weeks may be necessary to evaluate the extent of the improvement in psychotic symptoms. However, agitation and excitement usually improve quickly with antipsychotic treatment. About 75% of persons with a short history of illness show significant improvement in their psychosis. Psychotic symptoms, both positive and negative, usually continue to improve 3 to 12 months after the initiation of treatment.

About 5 mg of haloperidol or 300 mg of chlorpromazine is a usual starting effective daily dose. In the past, much higher doses were used, but evidence suggests that it resulted in more side effects without additional benefits. A single daily dose is usually given at bedtime to help induce sleep and to reduce the incidence of adverse effects. However, bedtime dosing for elderly persons may increase their risk of falling if they get out of bed during the night. The sedative effects of typical antipsychotics last only a few hours in contrast to the antipsychotic effects, which last for 1 to 3 days.

Intermittent Medications

It is common clinical practice to order medications to be given intermittently as needed (PRN). Although this practice may be reasonable during the first few days that a person is hospitalized, the amount of time the person takes antipsychotic drugs, rather than an increase in dosage, is what produces therapeutic improvement. Clinicians on inpatient services may feel pressured by staff members to write PRN antipsychotic orders; such orders should include specific symptoms, how often the drugs should be given, and how many doses can be given each day. Clinicians may choose to use small doses for the PRN doses (e.g., 2 mg of haloperidol) or use a benzodiazepine instead (e.g., 2 mg of lorazepam IM). If PRN doses of an antipsychotic are necessary after the first week of treatment, the clinician may want to consider increasing the standing daily dose of the drug.

Maintenance Treatment

The first 3 to 6 months after a psychotic episode is usually considered a period of stabilization. After that time, the dosage of the antipsychotic can be decreased about 20% every 6 months until the minimum effective dosage is found. A person is usually maintained on antipsychotic medications for 1 to 2 years after the first psychotic episode. Antipsychotic treatment is often continued for 5 years after a second psychotic episode, and lifetime maintenance is considered after the third psychotic episode, although attempts to reduce the daily dosage can be made every 6 to 12 months.

Antipsychotic drugs are effective in controlling psychotic symptoms, but persons may report that they prefer being off the drugs because they feel better without them. The clinician must discuss maintenance medication with patients and take into account their wishes, the severity of their illnesses, and the quality of their support systems. It is essential for the clinician to know enough about the patient's life to try to predict upcoming stressors that might require increasing the dosage or closely monitoring compliance.

Long-Acting Depot Medications

Long-acting depot preparations may be needed to overcome problems with compliance. IM preparations are typically given once every 1 to 4 weeks.

Two depot preparations, a decanoate and an enanthate, of fluphenazine and a decanoate preparation of haloperidol are available in the United States. The preparations are injected IM into an area of large muscle tissue, from which they are absorbed slowly into the blood. Decanoate preparations can be given less frequently than enanthate preparations because they are absorbed more slowly. Although stabilizing a person on the oral preparation of the specific drugs is not necessary before initiating the depot form, it is good practice to give at least one oral dose of the drug to assess the possibility of an adverse effect, such as severe EPS or an allergic reaction.

It is reasonable to begin with either 12.5 mg (0.5 mL) of fluphenazine preparation or 25 mg (0.5 mL) of haloperidol decanoate. If symptoms emerge in the next 2 to 4 weeks, the person can be treated temporarily with additional oral medications or with additional small depot injections. After 3 to 4 weeks, the depot injection can be increased to a single dose equal to the total of the doses given during the initial period.

A good reason to initiate depot treatment with low doses is that the absorption of the preparations may be faster than usual at the onset of treatment, resulting in frightening episodes of dystonia that eventually discourage compliance with the medication. Some clinicians keep persons drug free for 3 to 7 days before initiating depot treatment and give small doses of the depot preparations (3.125 mg of fluphenazine or 6.25 mg of haloperidol) every few days to avoid those initial problems.

Plasma Concentrations

Genetic differences among persons and pharmacokinetic interactions with other drugs influence the metabolism of the antipsychotics. If a person has not improved after 4 to 6 weeks of treatment, the plasma concentration of the drug should be determined if feasible. After a patient has been on a particular dosage for at least five times the half-life of the drug and thus approaches steady-state concentrations, blood levels may be helpful. It is standard practice to obtain plasma samples at trough levels—just before the daily dose is given, usually at least 12 hours after the previous dose and most commonly 20 to 24 hours after the previous dose. In fact, most antipsychotics have no well-defined dose–response curve. The best-studied drug is haloperidol, which may have a therapeutic window ranging from 2 to 15 ng/mL. Other therapeutic ranges that have been reasonably well documented are 30 to 100 ng/mL for chlorpromazine and 0.8 to 2.4 ng/mL for perphenazine.

Treatment-Resistant Persons

Unfortunately, 10% to 35% of persons with schizophrenia do not obtain significant benefit from antipsychotic drugs. Treatment resistance is a failure on at least two adequate trials of antipsychotics from two pharmacologic classes. It is useful to determine plasma concentrations for such persons because it is possible that they are slow or rapid metabolizers or are not taking their medication. Clozapine has been conclusively shown to be effective when given to patients who have failed multiple trials of DRAs.

Adjunctive Medications

It is common practice to use DRAs in conjunction with other psychotropic agents, either to treat side effects or further improve symptoms. Most commonly, this involves the use of lithium or other mood-stabilizing agents, SSRIs, or benzodiazepines. In the past, it was thought that antidepressant drugs exacerbated psychosis in schizophrenic patients. In all likelihood, this observation involved patients with bipolar disorder who were misdiagnosed as being schizophrenic. Abundant evidence suggests that antidepressants in fact improve symptoms of depression in schizophrenic patients. In some cases, amphetamines, such as dextroamphetamine, can be added to DRAs if patients remain withdrawn and apathetic.

Choice of Drug

Given their proven efficacy in managing acute psychotic symptoms and the fact that prophylactic administration of antiparkinsonian medication prevents or minimizes acute motor abnormalities, DRAs are still valuable, especially for short-term therapy. There is a considerable cost advantage to a DRA antiparkinsonian regimen compared with monotherapy with a newer antipsychotic agent. Concern about the development of DRA-induced TD is the major deterrent to long-term use of these drugs, yet it is not clear that SDAs are completely free of this complication. Thus, DRAs still occupy an important role in psychiatric treatment.

DRAs are not predictably interchangeable. For reasons that cannot be explained, some patients do better on one drug than another. Choice of a particular DRA should be based on the known adverse effect profile of the drugs. Other than a significant advantage in terms of medication cost, the choice currently would be an SDA. If a DRA is thought to be preferable, a high-potency antipsychotic is favored even though it may be associated with more neurologic adverse effects, mainly because there is a higher incidence of other adverse effects (e.g., cardiac, hypotensive, epileptogenic, sexual, and allergic) with the low-potency drugs. If sedation is a desired goal, either a low-potency antipsychotic in divided doses or a benzodiazepine can be coadministered.

An unpleasant or dysphoric reaction (a subjective sense of restlessness, oversedation, and acute dystonia) to the first dose of an antipsychotic predicts future poor response and noncompliance. Prophylactic use of antiparkinsonian medications may prevent this reaction. In general, clinicians should be vigilant about serious side effects and adverse events (described above) regardless of which drug is used.

Lamotrigine

20

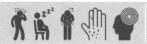

anticonvulsants, valproate, sertraline,
carbamazepine, phenytoin, phenobarbital

Introduction

Lamotrigine (Lamictal) is an antiepileptic drug that was first approved by the
Food and Drug Administration (FDA) in 1994 as an adjunctive treatment in
patients 2 years of age and older for partial seizures, primary generalized tonic–
clonic seizures, and generalized seizures of Lennox–Gestaut syndrome. It is still
considered a first-line treatment for these conditions. It has also been approved as
a monotherapy in patients with partial-onset seizures in patients 16 years of age
and older, who are switching treatment to lamotrigine from carbamazepine, phenytoin, phenobarbital, primidone, or valproate. Lamotrigine later demonstrated
efficacy and was approved for maintenance treatment of bipolar I disorder in
2003. However, lamotrigine has not received approval for the treatment of acute
bipolar depression or rapid cycling bipolar disorder, nor has lamotrigine been
shown to be effective as a main intervention in acute mania.

Pharmacologic Actions

Lamotrigine is completely absorbed, has a bioavailability of 98%, and has a
steady-state plasma half-life of 25 hours. However, the rate of lamotrigine's
metabolism varies over a sixfold range, depending on which other drugs are
administered concomitantly. Dosing is escalated slowly to twice-a-day maintenance dosing. Food does not affect its absorption, and it is 55% protein bound
in the plasma. Lamotrigine is metabolized primarily by glucuronic acid conjugation, and 94% of lamotrigine and its inactive metabolites are excreted in
the urine.

Among the better-delineated biochemical actions of lamotrigine are blockade
of voltage-sensitive sodium channels, which in turn modulate release of glutamate and aspartate as well as have slight effect on calcium channels. Lamotrigine
modestly increases plasma serotonin concentrations, possibly through inhibition
of serotonin reuptake, and is a weak inhibitor of serotonin 5-HT$_3$ receptors.

Psychiatric Indications

Bipolar Disorder

Lamotrigine is indicated in the treatment of bipolar disorder and may prolong the
time between episodes of depression and mania. It is more effective in lengthening the intervals between depressive episodes than manic episodes. It is also
effective as treatment for rapid cycling bipolar disorder.

Lamotrigine

213

Off-Label Indications

There have been reports of therapeutic benefit in the treatment of borderline personality disorder, binge-eating disorder, and in the treatment for various pain syndromes, though a 2013 review concluded that there is currently no convincing evidence that lamotrigine is an effective treatment for neuropathic pain or fibromyalgia. Some evidence suggests that lamotrigine may be effective at reducing the frequency and severity of migraine aura.

Reports have suggested that lamotrigine may be an effective monotherapy for the treatment of panic disorder with and without agoraphobia, while a case report describes efficacy of lamotrigine in reducing chronic anxiety and stress related to the COVID-19 pandemic. Research data suggest that lamotrigine, in conjunction with atypical antipsychotic drugs (particularly augmentation of clozapine), may improve outcomes in schizophrenia, especially in those with treatment resistance. Similarly, lamotrigine augmentation may assist in the treatment of unipolar depression.

Precautions and Adverse Reactions

Lamotrigine is remarkably well tolerated. The absence of sedation, weight gain, and other metabolic effects is noteworthy. The most common adverse effects— dizziness, ataxia, somnolence, headache, diplopia, blurred vision, and nausea— are typically mild. Anecdotal reports of cognitive impairment and joint or back pain are common.

The appearance of a rash, which is common and occasionally very severe, is a source of concern. About 8% of patients started on lamotrigine develop this benign maculopapular rash during the first 4 months of treatment, and the drug should be discontinued if a rash develops. Even though these rashes are benign, there is concern that in some cases, they may represent early manifestations of Stevens–Johnson syndrome or toxic epidermal necrolysis. Nevertheless, even if lamotrigine is discontinued immediately upon development of rash or other signs of hypersensitivity reaction, such as fever and lymphadenopathy, this may not prevent subsequent development of a life-threatening rash or permanent disfiguration.

Estimates of the rate of serious rash vary, depending on the source of the data. In some studies, the incidence of serious rashes was 0.08% in adult patients receiving lamotrigine as initial monotherapy and 0.13% in adult patients receiving lamotrigine as adjunctive therapy. German registry data, based on clinical practice, suggest that the risk of severe rash is significantly lower, and may only affect 1 in 5,000 patients. If a rash occurs the patient should be told to hold the next dose and contact their physician or go to an emergency room to be evaluated. Ideally, the patient should be evaluated by a dermatologist to determine if the rash is coincidental, drug related, or potentially serious. Characteristics of potentially serious rashes typically include confluent and widespread purpuric and tender lesions, with involvement of the neck or upper trunk. In addition, there may be possible involvement of the ears and mouth with redness, inflammation, and swelling around the eyes. There may also be peeling skin, and painful blisters. Concomitant fever, pharyngitis, anorexia, and lymphadenopathy may occur. Given that this is a systemic reaction, there is likely to be abnormal lab values. Patients who develop serious rashes should not be rechallenged. If on the other hand the rash is felt to be nondrug related or benign, it should be treated with a dose reduction, delay of any planned dose increases, or treatment with antihistamines and/or corticosteroids. Any rechallenge should be considered after a careful risk–benefit analysis. Patients who develop a serious rash should not be restarted on lamotrigine.

It is known that the likelihood of a rash increases if the recommended starting dose and titration of dose exceeds what is recommended. Concomitant administration of valproic acid also increases risk and should be avoided if possible. If valproate is used, a more conservative dosing regimen is followed. Children and adolescents younger than age 16 years appear to be more susceptible to rash with lamotrigine. If patients miss more than 4 consecutive days of lamotrigine treatment, they need to restart therapy at the initial starting dose and titrate upward as if they had not already been on the medication.

Use in Pregnancy and Lactation

Lamotrigine has a large pregnancy registry, which supports research data that lamotrigine is not associated with congenital malformations in humans. Still, it is classified as a pregnancy category C drug.

Breastfeeding during lamotrigine treatment does not appear to adversely affect neonatal development, though some mothers who have taken lamotrigine and breastfed have reported breathing problems and anemia in infants. People who are nursing while taking lamotrigine should watch for potential side effects, including rash, sleepiness, and poor suckling.

Drug Interactions

Lamotrigine has significant, well-characterized drug interactions involving other anticonvulsants. The most potentially serious lamotrigine drug interaction involves concurrent use of valproic acid, which doubles serum lamotrigine concentrations. Lamotrigine decreases the plasma concentration of valproic acid by 25%. Sertraline (Zoloft) also increases plasma lamotrigine concentrations but to a lesser extent than does valproic acid. Lamotrigine concentrations are decreased by 40% to 50% with concomitant administration of carbamazepine, phenytoin, or phenobarbital. Combinations of lamotrigine and other anticonvulsants have complex effects on the time of peak plasma concentration and the plasma half-life of lamotrigine.

Laboratory Testing

There is no proven correlation between lamotrigine blood concentrations and either antiseizure effects or efficacy in bipolar disorders. Laboratory tests are not useful in predicting the occurrence of adverse events.

Laboratory Interferences

Lamotrigine and topiramate do not interfere with any laboratory tests.

Dosage and Administration

In the clinical trials leading to the approval of lamotrigine as a treatment for bipolar disorder, no consistent increase in efficacy was associated with doses above 200 mg per day. Most patients should take between 100 and 200 mg a day.

TABLE 20-1: Lamotrigine Dosing (mg/day)			
Treatment	Weeks 1–2	Weeks 3–4	Weeks 4–5
Lamotrigine monotherapy	25	50	100–200 (500 maximum)
Lamotrigine + carbamazepine	50	100	200–500 (700 maximum)
Lamotrigine + valproate	25 every other day	25	50–200 (200 maximum)

In epilepsy, the drug is administered twice daily, but in bipolar disorder the total dose can be taken once a day, either in the morning or night, depending on whether the patient finds the drug activating or sedating.

Lamotrigine is available as unscored 25-, 100-, 150-, and 200-mg tablets. The major determinant of lamotrigine dosing is minimization of the risk of rash. Lamotrigine should not be taken by anyone younger than the age of 16 years for the treatment of bipolar disorder. Because valproic acid markedly slows the elimination of lamotrigine, concomitant administration of these two drugs necessitates a much slower titration (Table 20-1). People with renal insufficiency should aim for a lower maintenance dosage. Appearance of any type of rash necessitates immediate discontinuation of lamotrigine administration. Lamotrigine should usually be discontinued gradually over 2 weeks unless a rash emerges, in which case it should be discontinued over 1 to 2 days.

Lamotrigine orally disintegrating tablets (Lamictal ODT) are available for patients who have difficulty swallowing. It is the only antiepileptic treatment that is available in an orally disintegrating formulation. It is available in 25-, 50-, 100-, and 200-mg strengths and matches the dose of lamotrigine tablets. Chewable dispersible tablets of 2, 5, and 25 mg are also available.

Ketamine

 hypertension tachycardia opioids

Introduction

Ketamine hydrochloride (hereafter "ketamine") is a racemic mixture consisting of (S)- and (R)-ketamine that was initially developed as an anesthetic agent in the 1960s with the first clinical studies being published in 1965. The Food and Drug Administration (FDA) approved the use of ketamine as a rapid-acting intravenous (IV) anesthetic in 1970. At high doses, ketamine induces dissociative anesthesia, while at lower doses it exerts analgesic, anti-inflammatory, and rapid antidepressant actions. In 2019, esketamine (Spravato), a nasal spray consisting of only the (S)-ketamine isomer, received FDA approval for the treatment of treatment-resistant depression for individuals who failed prior trials or are suicidal. As of now, it is the only form of ketamine approved for treatment of depression along with an oral antidepressant, while IV ketamine infusions are not FDA approved, but remain an off-label treatment option for depression.

Esketamine is only available through a restricted distribution system and may only be administered under the supervision of a healthcare provider in a Risk Evaluation and Mitigation Strategy (REMS)–certified medical facility. These extra precautions have been deemed necessary because ketamine is a widely used street drug that can induce a state of intoxication that makes users feel as though they are in a dream-like state, euphoric, and numb.

Pharmacology

Ketamine is a racemic mixture of (S)- and (R)-ketamine isomers and is Schedule III controlled substance. It is a hydrosoluble aryl-cyclo-alkylamine with a molecular mass of 238 g/mol and a pKa 7.5.

Esketamine consists solely of the (S)-ketamine isomer and is an intranasal spray that is administered in two doses, 56 mg and 84 mg.

Pharmacokinetics

Absorption. Ketamine may be administered intravenously, intranasally, intrarectally, orally, sublingually, or via intramuscular or subcutaneous injection, with IV infusion being the most common prior to the FDA approval of esketamine. Ketamine reaches peak plasma concentrations rapidly except when taken orally, in which case peak concentration levels may not be achieved for 20 to 120 minutes.

TABLE 21-1: Ketamine Bioavailability by Route of Administration	
Route of Administration	Bioavailability (%)
Intravenous	100
Intramuscular	93
Intranasal	45–50
Intrarectal	25–30
Oral	16–29

Bioavailability. Depending on route of administration, ketamine may have a bioavailability ranging from as low as 16% (oral administration) to as high as 100% (IV infusion). See Table 21-1.

Distribution. Ketamine has a plasma protein binding between 10% and 50%, so it is rapidly distributed into highly perfused tissues like the brain.

Metabolism. Ketamine undergoes significant first-pass metabolism. Approximately 80% of ketamine is metabolized into norketamine primarily by cytochrome P450 liver enzymes CYP2B6 and CYP3A4. Norketamine is an active metabolite that retains the anesthetic qualities of the parent compound at approximately one-third the potency. It is then hydroxylated into 6-hydroxy-ketamine by CYP2A6. Less common metabolites of the original compound include 4-hydroxy-ketamine and 5-hydroxy-ketamine. In addition, ketamine is metabolized by the kidneys, the intestine, and the lungs.

Elimination and Excretion. Ketamine has a high rate of clearance ($\approx$95 L/h/ 70 kg) and a short elimination half-life (2 to 4 hours) and is primarily excreted in bile and urine. Clearance may be 20% higher in women than men. Repeated administration may prolong elimination time.

Pharmacodynamics

Ketamine is primarily an N-methyl-D-aspartate (NMDA) receptor antagonist. At high doses (1 to 2 mg/kg of an IV infusion), ketamine produces dissociative anesthetic effects that are characterized by catatonia, catalepsy, and amnesia.

Ketamine is also an analgesic. At lower doses (0.5 to 1 mg/kg), it may be used to treat acute pain and shares many similar properties with opioids but with notably less respiratory depressive effects. Similar doses have been shown to have antidepressant effects, as well as anti-inflammatory effects. While ketamine's role as an NMDA antagonist is believed to be the primary reason for the observed antidepressant effects, its anti-inflammatory properties and activity at glutamate-independent sites could also play a role in its psychiatric applications.

Peak ketamine plasma concentrations of 1,200 to 2,400 ng/mL are required to induce dissociative anesthesia, while awakening occurs when ranges drop to 640 to 1,100 ng/mL. Ketamine's analgesic effects can be felt when plasma concentrations range from 70 to 160 ng/mL, while the most common initial subanesthetic antidepressant dose (0.5 mg/kg; 40-minute infusion) results in a maximal plasma concentration (Cmax) of approximately 185 ng /mL, though even lower doses that result in a Cmax of 75 ng/mL may be enough to produce an antidepressant response. Improvements in mood are often immediate and may last 3 to 7 days initially. Repeated infusions may lead to improvements lasting for significantly longer.

The (S)-ketamine isomer is a more potent anesthetic when compared to the (R)-ketamine isomer.

Mechanism of Action.   Ketamine's antagonistic activity at NMDA receptors results in a reduction of γ-aminobutyric acid (GABA) inhibition and increases extracellular glutamate levels. The resultant surge in glutamate is believed to lead to synaptogenesis and elevated brain-derived neurotrophic factor (BDNF). Ketamine also acts as an inhibitor on HCN1-HCN2 heteromeric channels, which may account for ketamine's anesthetic and antidepressant properties, since HCN1 activity in the hippocampus is associated with antidepressant effects in rodents. Additional targets that may play a role in ketamine's antidepressant properties include muscarinic and nicotinic acetylcholine receptors, dopamine receptors (D2), serotonin receptors (5-HT1, 5-HT2, and 5-HT3), opioid receptors (delta, kappa, and mu), sigma receptors (σ-1 and σ-2), and L-type voltage-dependent calcium channels (see Table 21-2).

Therapeutic Index.   Ketamine has a wide therapeutic index, with an average lethal dose (LD50) of approximately 600 mg/kg in rodents.

TABLE 21-2: Ketamine Targets	
Target	Action
N-methyl-D-aspartate (NDMA)	Antagonist
Muscarinic acetylcholine	Antagonist
Alpha-7 nicotinic acetylcholine	Antagonist
Delta-type opioid	Binder
Kappa-type opioid	Agonist
Mu-type opioid	Binder
Dopamine (D2)	Partial agonist
5-hyrdoxytrytamine (5-HT₁, 5-HT₂)	Antagonist
5-hydroxytrytamine (5-HT3A)	Potentiator
Sigma-1 (σ-1)	Agonist
Sigma-2 (σ-2)	Agonist
Neurokinin 1	Antagonist
Hyperpolarization-activated cyclic nucleotide-gated channels (HCN-1 and HCN-2)	Inhibitor
Cholinesterase	Inhibitor
Nitric oxide synthase	Inhibitor
Sodium-dependent noradrenaline transporter	Inhibitor

Tolerance, Dependence, and Withdrawal.   Repeated use of ketamine can lead to the development of a tolerance and withdrawal. Though extremely rare in a clinical setting, frequent recreational users may still experience these issues. Withdrawal is characterized by cravings for the drug, lack of appetite, tiredness, difficulty sleeping, chills, irritability, restlessness, and irregular heartbeat.

Therapeutic Indications

There are three indications for ketamine that have been approved by the FDA:

1. As an anesthetic agent, oftentimes in conjunction with other anesthetic agents.
2. For depressive symptoms in adults diagnosed with major depressive disorder with acute suicidal ideation. (Esketamine only.)
3. For treatment-resistant depression in adults. (Esketamine only.)

Most patients seeking ketamine for depression have had treatment with four or more antidepressants, and a myriad of nonpharmacologic interventions with no success.

Off-Label Uses

Ketamine has been used to treat chronic pain, anxiety, bipolar disorder, postpartum depression, substance use disorder, obsessive compulsive disorder, and posttraumatic stress disorder (PTSD). Many research studies suggest that ketamine may also induce stress resilience in the aftermath of a traumatic event, thereby preventing the development of PTSD or other trauma- and stressor-related disorders. Clinical trials also suggest that subanesthetic infusions of ketamine may support abstinence among patients with alcohol use disorder.

Precautions and Adverse Effects

Acute ketamine intoxication can lead to psychedelic experiences, as well as euphoric, anxiolytic, and dissociative effects. In some cases, this experience can be unpleasant or too intense, but the effect can be mitigated by dose reductions or administration of lorazepam. Patients may also experience dizziness and gait instability following ketamine infusion. Consequently, patients should be monitored until they have recovered, while older patients should not attempt to walk for at least 1 hour after the infusion.

Precautions

Ketamine increases heart rate and blood pressure, so caution is warranted when considering treatment for patients with comorbid cardiovascular disease. Patients with kidney disease and other genitourinary disorders may not be ideal candidates for ketamine treatment, as excessive ketamine use is associated with some urinary tract pathologies.

Adverse Effects

Most adverse effects of ketamine resolve on their accord after the acute effects have dissipated. These include amnesia, anxiety, confusion, disorientation, dizziness, heart palpitations, hypersalivation, hyperreflexia, hypertension, nausea, spasms, tachycardia, and vomiting. Patients may also find the psychedelic experience induced by ketamine disturbing or unpleasant.

Frequent and long-term ketamine users may develop cognitive impairment, memory deficits, and genitourinary pathologies, including cystitis and detrusor overactivity. In extreme cases, habitual users may develop ketamine bladder syndrome, which is characterized by a painful bladder, incontinence, hematuria, and papillary necrosis.

Risk of Overdose or Abuse

Risk of overdose is extremely low, especially when used in a clinical setting. The risk of patients abusing ketamine is also quite low. However, ketamine's dissociative effects have made it a popular recreational drug, particularly in clubs where ketamine intoxication may be referred to as a "trip." It is known by names such as "Vitamin K," "Super K," "Special K," or just the letter "K," and may be snorted, added to drinks, added to cigarettes, or injected. Frequent use may lead to abuse or dependency or potentially even psychosis in some individuals who may be prone to psychotic events, though the risk of fatal overdose is low.

Pregnant and Nursing Women

Pregnant and nursing women should not use ketamine.

Drug Interactions

Ketamine is metabolized by cytochrome P450 enzymes CYP3A4 and CYP2B6, while the active ketamine metabolite norketamine is hydroxylated to 6-hydroxy-ketamine by CYP2A6. Inhibitors of CYP3A4 include clarithromycin, diltiazem, erythromycin, itraconazole, ketoconazole, ritonavir, verapamil, goldenseal, and grapefruit. Strong inhibitors of CYP2A6 include clotrimazole, letrozole, miconazole, pilocarpine, and tranylcypromine.

Ketamine also inhibits many human UDP-glucuronosyltransferase (UGT) enzymes, particularly UGT2B4, UGT2B7, and UGT2B15. UGT2B7 metabolizes morphine and codeine. Higher doses of ketamine may result in UGT2B7 inhibition that is clinically significant for metabolism of these two opioids, while analgesic (subanesthetic) doses of ketamine are only clinically significant for the metabolism of codeine.

Dosage and Clinical Guidelines

A typical dose of an IV ketamine infusion is usually 0.5 mg/kg infused over 40 minutes for the initial 2 to 3 weeks of treatment with 1-week intervals between infusions. Dosage can be gradually increased by 0.1 mg/kg to 1.0 mg/kg during subsequent sessions. Most patients receive treatment for 6 weeks but may need booster infusions depending on clinical need or may receive them periodically every few weeks or months. Intranasal esketamine can be administered two times per week for the first 2 to 4 weeks, once per week for weeks 5 to 9, and then once every week or every other week thereafter. Patients should begin with the 56-mg dose and if tolerated well may increase to the 84-mg dose. There is no standard guideline for maintenance treatment. A 4-week course of ketamine treatment with no response is considered a failed trial.

As a matter of practical protocol, patients should fast for 3 hours prior to ketamine infusion to limit nausea. Clinicians should then obtain patient's weight and baseline vitals, conduct a brief psychiatric interview, determine dose, and then begin the 40-minute infusion. Vital signs should be taken 20 minutes after starting the infusion and upon completion of the treatment. In addition, the patient's vital signs should be checked again after the treatment at 20 and 40 minutes to monitor downtrends in heart rate and blood pressure. Thereafter, it is recommended to offer and assist the patient to the restroom and assess gait and any signs of dizziness.

Special Populations

Children.   Ketamine is regularly used for procedural sedation and analgesia for neonates, infants, and young children in emergency departments due to its ease of administration and safety profile. However, esketamine is not indicated for use in individuals under the age of 18. While studies have found that ketamine infusions may potentially help children and adolescents with treatment-resistant depression or mood disorders, more studies are needed to determine its long-term safety.

Persons with Hepatic Insufficiency.   Patients with moderate hepatic impairment may need to be monitored for adverse reactions for longer than those with no such impairment. Use of ketamine in patients with severe hepatic impairment is not recommended.

Risk Evaluation and Mitigation Strategy

REMS is required by the FDA to manage potential risks associated with esketamine, including dissociation and sedation. All inpatient and outpatient healthcare settings should be certified to receive or dispense esketamine. In addition, pharmacies must also be certified, and all patients need to be enrolled with their prescriber to receive treatment.

Esketamine should be administered under the direct supervision of a healthcare provider and should be monitored for 2 hours post treatment. All patients should have a monitoring form completed by the healthcare provider that includes:

- Patients' demographic information
- Concomitant medications
- Healthcare provider and setting information
- Treatment session information, including:
  - Treatment date
  - Dose administered
  - Treatment duration
  - Vital signs monitoring
  - Adverse events
  - A report of all serious adverse events

Approved REMS for esketamine can be explored in greater detail on the esketamine and FDA's website.

Lithium

22

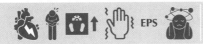 EPS 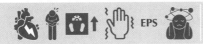   **see Table 22-6 for drug interactions**

Introduction

In 1948, Australian psychiatrist John Cade became the first clinician to treat a patient with lithium and observe its unequivocal benefits in patients who had been diagnosed with bipolar disorder (or manic depression, as it was known at the time). It proved to be the first effective medicine to treat a mental illness. Clinical observations, and associated and systematic clinical trials, subsequently led to its approval by most regulatory agencies for the treatment of acute mania. In the United States, it was not approved by the Food and Drug Administration until 1970, largely due to concerns about toxicity. The only other approved indication came in 1974, for maintenance therapy in bipolar patients with a history of mania.

For several decades, lithium was the only drug approved for both acute and maintenance treatment in bipolar I disorder. It is also used as an adjunctive medication in the treatment of major depressive disorder, though it has never been approved for this use by the FDA.

Lithium has neurotropic and neuroprotective activity that may extend its spectrum of use beyond bipolar disorder and as an off-label medication for conditions like major depressive disorder. For example, it has been shown to stimulate neurogenesis in adult rat hippocampus.

Studies have also shown an increase in total brain gray matter volume (by 3%) in 8 of 10 bipolar patients after 4 weeks of treatment.

Lithium (Li), a monovalent ion, is a member of the group IA alkali metals on the periodic table, a group that also includes sodium, potassium, rubidium, cesium, and francium. Lithium exists in nature as both ^{6}Li (7.42%) and ^{7}Li (92.58%). The latter isotope allows the imaging of lithium by magnetic resonance spectroscopy. Some 300 mg of lithium is contained in 1,597 mg of lithium carbonate (Li_2CO_3). Most lithium used in the United States is obtained from dry lake mining in Chile and Argentina.

Pharmacologic Actions

Lithium is rapidly and completely absorbed after oral administration, with peak serum concentrations occurring in 1 to 1.5 hours with standard preparations and in 4 to 4.5 hours with slow- and controlled-release preparations. Lithium does not bind to plasma proteins, is not metabolized, and is excreted through the kidneys. The plasma half-life is initially 1.3 days and is 2.4 days after administration for more than 1 year. The blood–brain barrier permits only slow passage of lithium,

223

which is why a single overdose does not necessarily cause toxicity and why long-term lithium intoxication is slow to resolve. The elimination half-life of lithium is 18 to 24 hours in young adults but is shorter in children and longer in elderly persons. Renal clearance of lithium is decreased with renal insufficiency. Equilibrium is reached after 5 to 7 days of regular intake. Obesity is associated with higher rates of lithium clearance. The excretion of lithium is complex during pregnancy; excretion increases during pregnancy but decreases after delivery. Lithium is excreted in breast milk and in insignificant amounts in the feces and sweat. Thyroid and renal concentrations of lithium are higher than serum levels.

An explanation for the mood-stabilizing effects of lithium remains elusive. Theories include alterations of ion transport and effects on neurotransmitters and neuropeptides, signal transduction pathways, and second messenger systems.

Therapeutic Indications

Lithium is currently approved for maintenance treatment of bipolar I disorder and to treat acute mania in patients 7 years of age and older.

Bipolar I Disorder

Manic Episodes.   Lithium controls acute mania and prevents relapse in about 80% of persons with bipolar I disorder and in a somewhat smaller percentage of persons with mixed (mania and depression) episodes, rapid cycling bipolar disorder, or mood changes in encephalopathy. Lithium has a relatively slow onset of action when used and exerts its antimanic effects over 1 to 3 weeks. Thus, a benzodiazepine, dopamine receptor antagonist (DRA), serotonin-dopamine antagonist (SDA), or valproic acid is usually administered for the first few weeks. Patients with mixed or dysphoric mania, rapid cycling, comorbid substance abuse, or organicity respond less well to lithium than those with classic mania.

Maintenance.   Maintenance treatment with lithium markedly decreases the frequency, severity, and duration of manic and depressive episodes in persons with bipolar I disorder. Lithium provides relatively more effective prophylaxis for mania than for depression, and supplemental antidepressant strategies may be necessary either intermittently or continuously. Lithium maintenance is almost always indicated after the first episode of bipolar I disorder, depression or mania, and should be considered after the first episode for adolescents or for persons who have a family history of bipolar I disorder. Others who benefit from lithium maintenance are those who have poor support systems, had no precipitating factors for the first episode, have a high suicide risk, had a sudden onset of the first episode, or had a first episode of mania. Clinical studies have shown that lithium reduces the incidence of suicide in bipolar I disorder patients six- or sevenfold. Lithium is also an effective treatment for persons with severe cyclothymic disorder.

Initiating maintenance therapy after the first manic episode is considered a wise approach based on several observations. First, each episode of mania increases the risk of subsequent episodes. Second, among people responsive to lithium, relapses are 28 times more likely after lithium use is discontinued. Third, case reports describe persons who initially responded to lithium, discontinued taking it, and then had a relapse but no longer responded to lithium in subsequent episodes. Continued maintenance treatment with lithium is often associated with increasing efficacy and reducing mortality. Therefore, an episode of depression or mania that occurs after a relatively short time of lithium maintenance does not necessarily represent treatment failure. However, lithium treatment alone may begin to lose its effectiveness after several years of successful use. If this occurs, then supplemental treatment with carbamazepine (Tegretol) or valproate may be useful.

Maintenance lithium dosages can often be adjusted to achieve plasma concentration somewhat lower than that needed for treatment of acute mania. If lithium use is to be discontinued, then the dosage should be slowly tapered. Abrupt discontinuation of lithium therapy is associated with an increased risk of recurrence of manic and depressive episodes.

Off-Label Uses

Bipolar Depression

Lithium has been shown to be effective in the treatment of depression associated with bipolar I disorder, as well as in the role of add-on therapy for patients with severe major depressive disorder. Augmentation of lithium therapy with valproic acid (Depakene) or carbamazepine is usually well tolerated, with little risk of precipitation of mania.

When a depressive episode occurs in a person taking maintenance lithium, the differential diagnosis should include lithium-induced hypothyroidism, substance abuse, and lack of compliance with the lithium therapy. Possible treatment approaches include increasing the lithium concentration (up to 1 to 1.2 mEq/L), adding supplemental thyroid hormone (e.g., 25 µg a day of liothyronine [Cytomel]) even in the presence of normal findings on thyroid function tests, augmentation with valproate or carbamazepine, the judicious use of antidepressants, or electroconvulsive therapy (ECT). After the acute depressive episode resolves, other therapies should be tapered off in favor of lithium monotherapy, if clinically tolerated.

Major Depressive Disorder

Lithium is effective in the long-term treatment of major depression but is not more effective than antidepressant drugs. The most common role for lithium in major depressive disorder is as an adjuvant to antidepressant use in persons who have failed to respond to the antidepressants alone. About 50% to 60% of antidepressant nonresponders do respond when lithium, 300 mg three times daily, is added to the antidepressant regimen. In some cases, a response may be seen within days, but most often, several weeks are required to see the efficacy of the regimen.

Lithium alone may effectively treat depressed persons who have bipolar I disorder but have not yet had their first manic episode. Lithium has been reported to be effective in persons with major depressive disorder whose disorder has a particularly marked cyclicity.

Schizoaffective Disorder and Schizophrenia

Persons with prominent mood symptoms—either bipolar type or depressive type—with schizoaffective disorder are more likely to respond to lithium than those with predominant psychotic symptoms. Although SDAs and DRAs are the treatments of choice for persons with schizoaffective disorder, lithium is a useful augmentation agent. This is particularly true for persons whose symptoms are resistant to treatment with SDAs and DRAs. Lithium augmentation of an SDA or DRA treatment may be an effective treatment for persons with schizoaffective disorder even in the absence of a prominent mood disorder component. Some persons with schizophrenia who cannot take antipsychotic drugs may benefit from lithium treatment alone.

Suicide Prevention

Though lithium reduces the incidence of suicide in bipolar I disorder patients and observational evidence suggests lithium may reduce suicidality in patients with a variety of psychiatric disorders, these benefits do not necessarily extend to suicidal patients with other mood disorders. A randomized clinical trial published in 2021 found that augmenting an existing treatment regimen with lithium does not appear to be an effective strategy in the prevention of suicide-related events.

Neuroprotective Agent

There is a growing body of evidence about the neurobiologic benefits of lithium, particularly its neuroprotective properties and effects on several mechanisms associated with neuronal homeostasis. These processes include the modulation of inflammatory cascades and oxidative stress; the inhibition of tryptophan catabolism via the kynurenine pathway; the upregulation of mitochondrial function; and the activation of neurotrophic responses. Given these properties, pre-clinical and clinical studies are underway to determine the therapeutic utility of lithium in a host of neuropsychiatric disorders and multiple neurodegenerative and dementing conditions.

Other Off-Label Uses

Over the years, reports have appeared about the use of lithium to treat a wide range of other psychiatric and nonpsychiatric conditions (Tables 22-1 and 22-2). The effectiveness and safety of lithium for most of these disorders have not been confirmed. Lithium is used to target aggressive behavior that is separate from its effects on mood. Aggressive outbursts in persons with schizophrenia, violent prison inmates, and children with conduct disorder and aggression, or

TABLE 22-1: Psychiatric Uses of Lithium
Historical
Gouty mania
Well established (FDA approved)
Acute mania
Maintenance therapy for bipolar disorder
Reasonably well established
Acute depressive episodes
Bipolar disorder—depressive episodes
Bipolar disorder—rapid cycling
Maintenance in major depressive disorder
Schizoaffective disorder

TABLE 22-1: Psychiatric Uses of Lithium (*continued*)

Evidence of benefit in particular groups
    Children and adolescents
    Conduct disorders
    Individuals with cognitive disorders
    Patients with autism spectrum disorder
    Schizophrenics
        Aggression (episodic)
        Explosive behavior
        Self-mutilation

Anecdotal, controversial, unresolved, or doubtful
    Alcohol use disorder
    Attention deficit hyperactivity disorder (ADHD)
    Eating disorders
        Anorexia nervosa
        Bulimia nervosa
    Impulse-control disorders
    Kleine–Levine syndrome
    Obsessive-compulsive disorder
    Pathologic hypersexuality
    Periodic catatonia
    Periodic hypersomnia
    Personality disorders
        Antisocial
        Borderline
        Schizotypal
    Posttraumatic stress disorder (PTSD)
    Premenstrual dysphoric disorder
    Specific phobias
    Substance use disorders
    Substance-induced mood disorders with manic features

self-mutilation in persons with level 2 or level 3 autism spectrum disorder can sometimes be pacified with lithium.

Preclinical evidence has found that lithium may augment ketamine treatment for major depressive disorder.

TABLE 22-2: Nonpsychiatric Uses of Lithium[a]

Cardiovascular
    Antiarrhythmic agent

Dermatologic
    Genital herpes
    Eczematoid dermatitis
    Seborrheic dermatitis

Endocrine
    Thyroid cancer as an adjunct to radioactive iodine
    Thyrotoxicosis
    Syndrome of inappropriate antidiuretic hormone secretion

Gastrointestinal
    Cyclic vomiting
    Gastric ulcers
    Pancreatic cholera
    Ulcerative colitis

Lithium

(*continued*)

TABLE 22-2: Nonpsychiatric Uses of Lithium[a] (continued)

Hematologic
    Aplastic anemia
    Cancer (chemotherapy-induced, radiotherapy-induced)
    Felty syndrome
    Leukemia
    Neutropenia
    Drug-induced neutropenia (e.g., from carbamazepine, antipsychotics, immunosuppressives, and
    zidovudine)

Historical   Gout
Miscellaneous medical conditions   Bovine spastic paresis

Neurologic
    Anticonvulsant
    Epilepsy
    Headache (chronic cluster, hypnic, migraine, particularly cyclic)
    Huntington disease
    Levodopa-induced hyperkinesias
    Ménière disease
    Movement disorders
    On–off phenomenon in Parkinson disease
    Spasmodic torticollis
    Tardive dyskinesia
    Tourette disorder
    Pain (facial pain syndrome, painful shoulder syndrome, fibromyalgia)
    Periodic paralysis (hypokalemic and hypermagnesic but not hyperkalemic)

Respiratory
    Asthma
    Cystic fibrosis

[a]All the uses listed here are experimental and do not have Food and Drug Administration (FDA)-approved labeling. There are conflicting reports about many of these uses—some have negative findings in controlled studies, and a few involve reports of possible adverse effects.

Precautions and Adverse Effects

More than 80% of patients taking lithium experience side effects. It is important to minimize the risk of adverse events through monitoring of lithium blood levels and to use appropriate pharmacologic interventions to counteract unwanted effects when they occur. The most common adverse effects are summarized in Table 22-3. Patient education can play an important role in reducing the incidence and severity of side effects. Patients taking lithium should be advised that changes in the body's water and salt content can affect the amount of lithium excreted, resulting in either increases or decreases in lithium concentrations. Excessive sodium intake (e.g., a dramatic dietary change) lowers lithium concentrations. Conversely, too little sodium (e.g., fad diets) can lead to potentially toxic concentrations of lithium. Decreases in body fluid (e.g., excessive perspiration) can lead to dehydration and lithium intoxication. Patients should report whenever medications are prescribed by another clinician because many commonly used agents can affect lithium concentrations.

TABLE 22-3: Adverse Effects of Lithium

Cardiovascular
    Benign T-wave changes
    Sinus node dysfunction

Dermatologic
    Acne
    Hair loss
    Psoriasis
    Rash

Endocrine

Parathyroid
    Hyperparathyroidism
    Adenoma
Thyroid
    Exophthalmos
    Goiter
    Hyperthyroidism (rare)
    Hypothyroidism

Gastrointestinal
    Appetite loss
    Diarrhea
    Nausea
    Vomiting

Miscellaneous
    Altered carbohydrate metabolism
    Weight gain

Neurologic
    Benign, nontoxic
    Altered creativity
    Benign intracranial hypertension
    Dysphoria
    Lack of spontaneity
    Lowered seizure threshold
    Memory difficulties
    Myasthenia gravis–like syndrome
    Peripheral neuropathy
    Slowed reaction time
    Tremor (postural, occasional extrapyramidal)

Toxic
    Ataxia
    Coarse tremor
    Coma
    Dysarthria
    Neuromuscular irritability
    Seizures

Renal
    Concentrating defect
    Fluid retention
    Morphologic changes
    Nephrotic syndrome
    Polyuria (nephrogenic diabetes insipidus)
    Reduced GFR
    Renal tubular acidosis

GFR, glomerular filtration rate.

Lithium

Cardiac Effects

Lithium can cause diffuse slowing, widening of frequency spectrum, potentiation, and disorganization of background rhythm on electrocardiograms (EKGs/ECGs). Bradycardia and cardiac arrhythmias may occur, especially in people with cardiovascular disease. Lithium infrequently reveals Brugada syndrome—an inherited, life-threatening heart problem that some people may have without knowing it. It can cause a serious abnormal heartbeat and other symptoms (such as severe dizziness, fainting, shortness of breath) that need medical attention right away. *Before starting lithium treatment, clinicians should ask about known heart conditions, unexplained fainting, and family history of problems or sudden unexplained death before age 45.* Obtaining a baseline EKG/ECG is recommended.

Gastrointestinal Effects

Gastrointestinal (GI) symptoms—which include nausea, decreased appetite, vomiting, and diarrhea—can be diminished by dividing the dosage, administering the lithium with food, or switching to another lithium preparation. The lithium preparation least likely to cause diarrhea is lithium citrate. Some lithium preparations contain lactose, which can cause diarrhea in lactose-intolerant persons. Persons taking slow-release formulations of lithium who experience diarrhea caused by unabsorbed medication in the lower part of the GI tract may experience less diarrhea than with standard-release preparations. Diarrhea may also respond to antidiarrheal preparations such as loperamide (Imodium, Kaopectate), bismuth subsalicylate (Pepto-Bismol), or diphenoxylate with atropine (Lomotil).

Weight Gain

Weight gain results from a poorly understood effect of lithium on carbohydrate metabolism. Weight gain can also result from lithium-induced hypothyroidism, lithium-induced edema, or excessive consumption of soft drinks and juices to quench lithium-induced thirst.

Neurologic Effects

Tremor. A lithium-induced postural tremor may occur that is usually 8 to 12 Hz and is most notable in outstretched hands, especially in the fingers, and during tasks involving fine manipulations. The tremor can be reduced by dividing the daily dosage, using a sustained-release formulation, reducing caffeine intake, reassessing the concomitant use of other medicines, and treating comorbid anxiety. β-Adrenergic receptor antagonists, such as propranolol, 30 to 120 mg a day in divided doses, and primidone (Mysoline), 50 to 250 mg a day, are usually effective in reducing the tremor. In persons with hypokalemia, potassium supplementation may improve the tremor. When a person taking lithium has a severe tremor, the possibility of lithium toxicity should be suspected and evaluated.

Cognitive Effects. Lithium use has been associated with dysphoria, lack of spontaneity, slowed reaction times, and impaired memory. The presence of these symptoms should be noted carefully because they are a frequent cause of non-compliance. The differential diagnosis for such symptoms should include depressive disorders, hypothyroidism, hypercalcemia, other illnesses. Other drugs may also be implicated in these symptoms. Some, but not all, persons have reported that fatigue and mild cognitive impairment decrease with time.

Other Neurologic Effects. Uncommon neurologic adverse effects include symptoms of mild parkinsonism, ataxia, and dysarthria, although the last two symptoms may also be attributable to lithium intoxication. Lithium is rarely associated with the development of peripheral neuropathy, benign intracranial hypertension (pseudotumor cerebri), findings resembling myasthenia gravis, and increased risk of seizures.

Renal Effect

The most common adverse renal effect of lithium is polyuria with secondary polydipsia. The symptom is particularly a problem in 25% to 35% of persons taking lithium who may have a urine output of more than 3 L a day (reference range: 1 to 2 L a day). The polyuria primarily results from lithium antagonism to the effects of antidiuretic hormone, which thus causes diuresis. When polyuria is a significant problem, the person's renal function should be evaluated and followed-up with 24-hour urine collections for creatinine clearance determinations. Treatment consists of fluid replacement, the use of the lowest effective dosage of lithium, and single daily dosing of lithium. Treatment can also involve the use of a thiazide or potassium-sparing diuretic—for example, amiloride (Midamor), spironolactone (Aldactone), triamterene (Dyrenium), or amiloride–hydrochlorothiazide (Moduretic). If treatment with a diuretic is initiated, the lithium dosage should be halved, and the diuretic should not be started for 5 days because the diuretic is likely to increase lithium retention.

The most serious renal adverse effects, which are rare and associated with continuous lithium administration for 10 years or more, involve appearance of nonspecific interstitial fibrosis, associated with gradual decreases in glomerular filtration rate and increases in serum creatinine concentrations, and rarely with renal failure. Lithium is occasionally associated with nephrotic syndrome and features of distal renal tubular acidosis. Another pathologic finding in patients with lithium nephropathy is the presence of microcysts. Magnetic resonance imaging (MRI) can be used to demonstrate renal microcysts secondary to chronic lithium nephropathy and therefore avoid renal biopsy. It is prudent for persons taking lithium to check their serum creatinine concentration, urine chemistries, and 24-hour urine volume at 6-month intervals. If creatinine levels do rise, then more frequent monitoring and MRI might be considered.

Thyroid Effects

Lithium causes a generally benign and often transient diminution in the concentrations of circulating thyroid hormones. Reports have attributed goiter (5% of persons), benign reversible exophthalmos, hyperthyroidism, and hypothyroidism (7% to 10% of persons) to lithium treatment. Lithium-induced hypothyroidism is more common in women (14%) than in men (4.5%). Women are at highest risk during the first 2 years of treatment. Persons taking lithium to treat bipolar disorder are twice as likely to develop hypothyroidism if they develop rapid cycling. About 50% of persons receiving long-term lithium treatment have laboratory abnormalities, such as an abnormal thyrotropin-releasing hormone response, and about 30% have elevated concentrations of thyroid-stimulating hormone (TSH). If symptoms of hypothyroidism are present, replacement with levothyroxine (Synthroid) is indicated. Even in the absence of hypothyroid symptoms, some clinicians treat persons with significantly elevated TSH concentrations with levothyroxine. In lithium-treated persons, TSH concentrations should be measured every 6 to 12 months. Lithium-induced hypothyroidism should be considered when evaluating depressive episodes that emerge during lithium therapy.

Cardiac Effects

The cardiac effects of lithium resemble those of hypokalemia on the EKG. They are caused by the displacement of intracellular potassium by the lithium ion. The most common changes on the EKG are T-wave flattening or inversion. The changes are benign and disappear after lithium is excreted from the body.

Lithium depresses the pacemaking activity of the sinus node, sometimes resulting in sinus dysrhythmias, heart block, and episodes of syncope. Lithium treatment, therefore, is contraindicated in persons with sick sinus syndrome. In rare cases, ventricular arrhythmias and congestive heart failure have been associated with lithium therapy. Lithium cardiotoxicity is more prevalent in persons on a low-salt diet, those taking certain diuretics or angiotensin-converting enzyme inhibitors (ACEIs), and those with fluid–electrolyte imbalances or any renal insufficiency.

Dermatologic Effects

Dermatologic effects may be dose dependent. They include acneiform, follicular, and maculopapular eruptions; pretibial ulcerations; and worsening of psoriasis. Occasionally, aggravated psoriasis or acneiform eruptions may force the discontinuation of lithium treatment. Alopecia has also been reported. Persons with many of those conditions respond favorably to changing to another lithium preparation and the usual dermatologic measures. Lithium concentrations should be monitored if tetracycline is used for the treatment of acne because it can increase the retention of lithium.

Lithium Toxicity and Overdoses

The early signs and symptoms of lithium toxicity include neurologic symptoms, such as coarse tremor, dysarthria, and ataxia; GI symptoms; cardiovascular changes; and renal dysfunction. The later signs and symptoms include impaired consciousness, muscular fasciculations, myoclonus, seizures, and coma. Signs and symptoms of lithium toxicity are outlined in Table 22-4.

Risk factors of overdose include exceeding the recommended dosage, renal impairment, low sodium diet, drug interaction (see Table 22-6), and dehydration. Elderly persons are more vulnerable to the effects of increased serum lithium concentrations. The greater the degree and duration of elevated lithium concentrations, the worse are the symptoms of lithium toxicity.

TABLE 22-4: Signs and Symptoms of Lithium Toxicity

1. Mild to moderate intoxication (lithium level, 1.5–2.0 mEq/L)

GI	Vomiting
	Abdominal pain
	Dryness of mouth
Neurologic	Ataxia
	Dizziness
	Slurred speech
	Nystagmus
	Lethargy or excitement
	Muscle weakness

2. Moderate to severe intoxication (lithium level: 2.0–2.5 mEq/L)

GI	Anorexia
	Persistent nausea and vomiting
Neurologic	Blurred vision
	Muscle fasciculations
	Clonic limb movements
	Hyperactive deep tendon reflexes
	Choreoathetoid movements
	Convulsions
	Delirium
	Syncope
	Electroencephalographic changes
	Stupor
	Coma
	Circulatory failure (lowered BP, cardiac arrhythmias, and conduction abnormalities)

3. Severe lithium intoxication (lithium level >2.5 mEq/L)
Generalized convulsions
Oliguria and renal failure
Death

Lithium toxicity is a medical emergency, potentially causing permanent neuronal damage and death. In cases of toxicity (see Table 22-5), lithium should be stopped and treatment for dehydration should be initiated. Unabsorbed lithium can be removed from the GI tract by ingestion of sodium polystyrene sulfonate (Kayexalate) or polyethylene glycol solution (GoLYTELY), but not activated charcoal. Ingestion of a single large dose may create clumps of medication in the stomach, which can be removed by gastric lavage with a wide-bore tube. The value of forced diuresis is still debated. In severe cases, hemodialysis rapidly

TABLE 22-5: Management of Lithium Toxicity

1. Contact personal physician or go to a hospital emergency department
2. Lithium should be discontinued
3. Vital signs and a neurologic examination with complete formal mental status examination
4. Lithium level, serum electrolytes, renal function tests, and EKG
5. Emesis, gastric lavage, and absorption with activated charcoal
6. For any patient with a serum lithium level greater than 4.0 mEq/L, hemodialysis

removes excessive amounts of serum lithium. Postdialysis serum lithium concentrations may increase as lithium is redistributed from tissues to blood, so repeat dialysis may be needed. Neurologic improvement may lag behind clearance of serum lithium by several days because lithium crosses the blood–brain barrier slowly.

Adolescents

The serum lithium concentrations for adolescents are similar to those for adults. Weight gain and acne associated with lithium use can be particularly troublesome to adolescents.

Elderly Persons

Lithium is a safe and effective drug for elderly persons. However, the treatment of elderly persons taking lithium may be complicated by the presence of other medical illnesses, decreased renal function, special diets that affect lithium clearance, and generally increased sensitivity to lithium. Elderly persons should initially be given low dosages, their dosages should be switched less frequently than those of younger persons, and a longer time must be allowed for renal excretion to equilibrate with absorption before lithium can be assumed to have reached its steady-state concentrations.

Use in Pregnancy and Lactation

Lithium should not be administered to pregnant women in the first trimester because of the risk of birth defects. The most common malformations involve the cardiovascular system, most commonly Ebstein's anomaly of the tricuspid valves. The risk of Ebstein's malformation in lithium-exposed fetuses is 1 in 1,000, which is 20 times the risk in the general population. The possibility of fetal cardiac anomalies can be evaluated with fetal echocardiography preferably at 20-week gestation. The teratogenic risk of lithium (4% to 12%) is higher than that for the general population (2% to 3%) but appears to be lower than that associated with the use of valproate or carbamazepine.

A woman who continues to take lithium during pregnancy should use the lowest effective dosage. The maternal lithium concentration must be monitored closely during pregnancy and especially after pregnancy because of the significant decrease in renal lithium excretion as renal function returns to normal in the first few days after delivery. It is recommended to evaluate fetal growth and monitor for signs of preterm labor. Adequate hydration can reduce the risk of lithium toxicity during labor. Lithium prophylaxis is recommended for all women with bipolar disorder as they enter the postpartum period.

Lithium is excreted into breast milk and should be taken by a nursing mother only after careful evaluation of potential risks and benefits. Signs of lithium toxicity in infants include lethargy, cyanosis, abnormal reflexes, and sometimes hepatomegaly.

Lithium is classified as a pregnancy category D drug.

Miscellaneous Effects

Lithium should be used with caution in diabetic patients, and they should monitor their blood glucose concentrations carefully to avoid diabetic ketoacidosis. Benign, reversible leukocytosis is commonly associated with lithium treatment, which may be a helpful intervention when used in conjunction with clozapine, as the latter carries risk of leukopenia. Dehydrated, debilitated, and medically ill persons are most susceptible to adverse effects and toxicity.

Drug Interactions

Lithium drug interactions are summarized in Table 22-6.

Lithium is commonly used in conjunction with DRAs. This combination is typically effective and safe. However, coadministration of higher dosages of a DRA and lithium may result in a synergistic increase in the symptoms of lithium-induced neurologic side effects and neuroleptic extrapyramidal symptoms. In rare instances, encephalopathy has been reported with this combination.

The coadministration of lithium and carbamazepine, lamotrigine, valproate, and clonazepam may increase lithium concentrations and aggravate lithium-induced neurologic adverse effects. Treatment with the combination should be initiated at slightly lower dosages than usual, and the dosages should be increased gradually. Changes from one to another treatment for mania should be made carefully, with as little temporal overlap between the drugs as possible.

Most diuretics (e.g., thiazide and potassium sparing) can increase lithium concentrations; when treatment with such diuretics is stopped, the clinician may need to increase the person's daily lithium dosage. Osmotic and loop diuretics, carbonic anhydrase inhibitors, and xanthines (including caffeine) may reduce lithium concentrations to below therapeutic concentrations. Whereas ACEIs may cause an increase in lithium concentrations, the AT_1 angiotensin II receptor inhibitors losartan (Cozaar) and irbesartan (Avapro) do not alter lithium concentrations. A wide range of nonsteroidal anti-inflammatory drugs (NSAIDs) can decrease lithium clearance, thereby increasing lithium concentrations. These drugs include indomethacin (Indocin), phenylbutazone (Azolid), diclofenac (Voltaren), ketoprofen (Orudis), oxyphenbutazone (Oxalid), ibuprofen (Motrin, Advil), piroxicam (Feldene), and naproxen (Naprosyn). *Patient should be clearly warned of this interaction since many of these medicines are available over the counter and commonly used by patients.* Aspirin and sulindac (Clinoril) do not affect lithium concentrations.

The coadministration of lithium and quetiapine (Seroquel) may cause somnolence but is otherwise well tolerated. The coadministration of lithium and ziprasidone (Geodon) may modestly increase the incidence of tremor. The coadministration of lithium and calcium channel inhibitors should be avoided because of potentially fatal neurotoxicity.

TABLE 22-6: Drug Interactions with Lithium	
Drug Class	**Reaction**
Antipsychotics	Case reports of encephalopathy, worsening of extrapyramidal adverse effects, and neuroleptic malignant syndrome; inconsistent reports of altered red blood cell and plasma concentrations of lithium, antipsychotic drug, or both
Antidepressants	Occasional reports of a serotonin-like syndrome with potent serotonin reuptake inhibitors
Anticonvulsants	No significant pharmacokinetic interactions with carbamazepine or valproate; reports of neurotoxicity with carbamazepine; combinations helpful for treatment resistance
NSAIDs	May reduce renal lithium clearance and increase serum concentration; toxicity reported (exception is aspirin)
Diuretics	
Thiazides	Well-documented reduced renal lithium clearance and increased serum concentration; toxicity reported
Potassium sparing	Limited data; may increase lithium concentration
Loop	Lithium clearance unchanged (some case reports of increased lithium concentration)
Osmotic (mannitol, urea)	Increase renal lithium clearance and decrease lithium concentration
Xanthine (aminophylline, caffeine, theophylline)	Increase renal lithium clearance and decrease lithium concentration
Carbonic anhydrase inhibitors (acetazolamide)	Increase renal lithium clearance
ACEIs	Reports of reduced lithium clearance, increased concentrations, and toxicity
Calcium channel inhibitors	Case reports of neurotoxicity; no consistent pharmacokinetic interactions
Miscellaneous	
Succinylcholine, pancuronium	Reports of prolonged neuromuscular blockade
Metronidazole	Increased lithium concentration
Methyldopa	Few reports of neurotoxicity
Sodium bicarbonate	Increased renal lithium clearance
Iodides	Additive antithyroid effects
Propranolol	Used for lithium tremor; possible slight increase in lithium concentration

ACEI, angiotensin-converting enzyme inhibitor; NSAID, nonsteroidal anti-inflammatory drug.

   A person taking lithium who is about to undergo ECT should discontinue taking lithium 2 days before beginning ECT to reduce the risk of delirium.

Laboratory Interferences

Lithium does not interfere with any laboratory tests, but lithium-induced alterations include an increased white blood cell count, decreased serum thyroxine, and increased serum calcium. Blood collected in a lithium–heparin anticoagulant tube will produce falsely elevated lithium concentrations.

Dosage and Clinical Guidelines

Initial Medical Workup

All patients should have a routine laboratory workup and physical examination before being started on lithium. The laboratory tests should include serum creatinine concentration (or a 24-hour urine creatinine if the clinician has any reason to be concerned about renal function), electrolytes, thyroid function (TSH, T_3 [triiodothyronine], and T_4 [thyroxine]), a complete blood count (CBC), EKG, and a pregnancy test in women of childbearing age.

Dosage Recommendations

Lithium formulations include immediate-release 150-, 300-, and 600-mg lithium carbonate capsules (Eskalith and generic), 300-mg lithium carbonate tablets (Lithotabs), 450-mg controlled-release lithium carbonate capsules (Eskalith CR and Lithonate), and 8 mEq/5 mL of lithium citrate syrup.

The starting dosage for most adults is 300 mg of the regular-release formulation three times daily. The starting dosage for elderly persons or persons with renal impairment should be 300 mg once or twice daily. After stabilization, dosages between 900 and 1,200 mg a day usually produce a therapeutic plasma concentration of 0.6 to 1 mEq/L, and a daily dose of 1,200 to 1,800 mg usually produces a therapeutic concentration of 0.8 to 1.2 mEq/L.

Maintenance dosing can be given either in two or three divided doses of the regular-release formulation or in a single dosage of the sustained-release formulation equivalent to the combined daily dosage of the regular-release formulation. The use of divided doses reduces gastric upset and avoids single high-peak lithium concentrations.

Discontinuation of lithium should be gradual to minimize the risk of early recurrence of mania and to permit recognition of early signs of recurrence.

Laboratory Monitoring

The periodic measurement of serum lithium concentration is an essential aspect of patient care, but it should always be combined with sound clinical judgment. A laboratory report listing the therapeutic range as 0.5 to 1.5 mEq/L may lull a clinician into disregarding early signs of lithium intoxication in patients whose levels are less than 1.5 mEq/L. Clinical toxicity, especially in elderly persons, has been well documented within this so-called therapeutic range.

Regular monitoring of serum lithium concentrations is essential. Lithium levels should be obtained every 2 to 6 months except when there are signs of toxicity, during dosage adjustments, and in persons suspected to be noncompliant with the prescribed dosages. Under these circumstances, levels may be done weekly. Baseline EKGs are essential and should be repeated annually.

When obtaining blood for lithium levels, patients should be at steady-state lithium dosing (usually after 5 days of constant dosing), preferably using a twice- or thrice-daily dosing regimen, and the blood sample must be drawn 12 hours

(±30 minutes) after a given dose. Lithium concentrations 12 hours postdose in persons treated with sustained-release preparations are generally about 30% higher than the corresponding concentrations obtained from those taking the regular-release preparations. Because available data are based on a sample population following a multiple-dosage regimen, regular-release formulations given at least twice daily should be used for initial determination of the appropriate dosages. Factors that may cause fluctuations in lithium measurements include dietary sodium intake, mood state, activity level, body position, and use of an improper blood sample tube.

Laboratory values that do not seem to correspond to clinical status may result from the collection of blood in a tube with a lithium–heparin anticoagulant (which can give results falsely elevated by as much as 1 mEq/L) or aging of the lithium ion–selective electrode (which can cause inaccuracies of up to 0.5 mEq/L). After the daily dose has been set, it is reasonable to change to the sustained-release formulation given once daily.

Effective serum concentrations for mania are 1.0 to 1.5 mEq/L, a level associated with 1,800 mg a day. The recommended range for maintenance treatment is 0.4 to 0.8 mEq/L, which is usually achieved with a daily dose of 900 to 1,200 mg. A small number of persons will not achieve therapeutic benefit with a lithium concentration of 1.5 mEq/L, but will have no signs of toxicity. For such persons, titration of the lithium dosage to achieve a concentration above 1.5 mEq/L may be warranted. Some patients can be maintained at concentrations below 0.4 mEq/L. There may be considerable variation from patient to patient, so it is best to follow the maxim, "Treat the patient, not the laboratory results." The only way to establish an optimal dose for a patient may be through trial and error.

US package inserts for lithium products list effective serum concentrations for mania between 1.0 and 1.5 mEq/L (usually achieved with 1,800 mg of lithium carbonate daily) and for long-term maintenance between 0.6 and 1.2 mEq/L (usually achieved with 900 to 1,200 mg of lithium carbonate daily). The dose–blood level relationship may vary considerably from patient to patient. The likelihood of achieving a response at levels above 1.5 mEq/L is usually outweighed greatly by the increased risk of toxicity, although rarely a patient may both require and tolerate a higher-than-usual blood concentration.

What constitutes the lower end of the therapeutic range remains a matter of debate. A prospective 3-year study found patients who maintained a concentration between 0.4 and 0.6 mEq/L (mean: 0.54) were 2.6 times more likely to relapse than those who maintained between 0.8 and 1.0 mEq/L (mean: 0.83). However, the higher blood concentrations produced more adverse effects and were less well tolerated.

If there is no response after 2 weeks at a concentration that is beginning to cause adverse effects, then the person should taper off lithium over 1 to 2 weeks and other mood-stabilizing drugs should be tried.

Patient Education

Lithium has a narrow therapeutic index, and many factors can upset the balance between lithium concentrations that are well tolerated and therapeutic, and those that produce side effects or toxicity. It is thus imperative that persons taking

TABLE 22-7: Instructions to Patients Taking Lithium

Lithium can be remarkably effective in treating your disorder. If not used appropriately and not monitored closely, it can be ineffective and potentially harmful. It is important to keep the following instructions in mind.

Dosing

Take lithium exactly as directed by your doctor—never take more or less than the prescribed dose.

Do not stop taking without speaking to your doctor.

If you miss a dose, take it as soon as possible. If it is within 4 hours of the next dose, skip the missed dose (about 6 hours in the case of extended- or slow-release preparations). Never double up doses.

Blood Tests

Comply with the schedule of recommended regular blood tests.

Despite their inconvenience and discomfort, your lithium blood levels, thyroid function, and kidney status need to be monitored as long as you take lithium.

When going to have lithium levels checked, you should have taken your last lithium dose 12 hours earlier.

Use of Other Medications

Do not start any prescription or over-the-counter medications without telling your doctor.

Even drugs such as ibuprofen (Advil, Motrin) and naproxen (Aleve) can significantly increase lithium levels.

Diet and Fluid Intake

Avoid sudden changes in your diet or fluid intake. If you do go on a diet, your doctor may need to increase the frequency of blood tests.

Caffeine and alcohol act as diuretics and can lower your lithium concentrations.

During treatment with lithium, it is recommended that you drink about 2 or 3 quarts of fluid daily and use normal amounts of salt.

Inform your doctor if you start or stop a low-salt diet.

Recognizing Potential Problems

If you engage in vigorous exercise or have an illness that causes sweating, vomiting, or diarrhea, consult your doctor because these might affect lithium levels.

Nausea, constipation, shakiness, increased thirst, frequency of urination, weight gain, or swelling of the extremities should be reported to your doctor.

Blurred vision, confusion, loss of appetite, diarrhea, vomiting, muscle weakness, lethargy, shakiness, slurred speech, dizziness, loss of balance, inability to urinate, or seizures could indicate severe toxicity and should prompt immediate medical attention.

lithium be educated about signs and symptoms of toxicity, factors that affect lithium levels, how and when to obtain laboratory testing, and the importance of regular communication with the prescribing physician. Lithium concentrations can be disrupted by common factors such as excessive sweating from ambient heat or exercise or use of widely prescribed agents such as ACEIs or NSAIDs. Patients may stop taking their lithium because they are feeling well or because they are experiencing side effects. They should be advised against discontinuing or modifying their lithium regimen. Table 18-7 lists some important instructions for patients.

23 Agents for Insomnia and Excessive Daytime Sleepiness

Generic Name	Trade Name	Adverse Effects	Drug Interactions	CYP Interactions
Melatonin	N/A	Sedation, dizziness, fatigue, headache	N/A	1A1, 1A2, 1B1, 2C19, 2C9
Ramelteon	Rozerem	Sedation, dizziness, fatigue	Fluvoxamine	1A2, 2C19, 3A4, 2C9
Tasimelteon	Hetlioz	Sedation, increases in alanine aminotransferase, headache	Alcohol, fluvoxamine	1A2, 3A4
Agomelatine	Valdoxan	Sedation, GI symptoms, dizziness	N/A	1A2, 2C9
Suvorexant	Belsomra	Sedation, dizziness, headache	CNS	3A4, 2C19
Lemborexant	Dayvigo	Sedation, dizziness, headache	CNS	3A4, 3A5, 2B6
Daridorexant	Quviviq	Sedation, dizziness, headache	CNS	3A4
Modafinil	Provigil	Sedation, skin rash, confusion, headache	CNS	3A4, 3A5, 2C19, 1A2, 2B6, 2C9, 2D6
Armodafinil	Nuvigil	Sedation, rash, confusion, headache	CNS	3A4, 3A5, 2C19, 1A2, 2B6, 2C9
Pitolisant	Wakix	Cardiac arrhythmia, headache	Antihistamines, QT	2D6, 3A4, 1A2, 2B6
Solriamfetol	Sunosi	Cardiac arrhythmia, hypertension, agitation, insomnia, GI symptoms, headache	MAOIs, DRAs	N/A
Calcium, magnesium, potassium, and sodium oxybates	Xywav	Respiratory suicidality, confusion, memory impairment, dizziness, GI symptoms, headache	CNS, valproate	N/A

Introduction

While several agents can be prescribed as hypnotics, this chapter will focus on drugs for insomnia that specifically target melatonin and orexin receptors, as well as medications used for excessive daytime sleepiness.

Melatonin is a hormone that plays a key role in the regulation of sleep–wake cycle and its dysfunction is linked not only to insomnia but to depression and other disorders. It is a natural ligand at melatonin receptors, which are G protein-coupled receptors. Two subtypes of receptors (MT_1 and MT_2) are found in humans and other mammals. MT_1 receptors are found in various locations within the central nervous system (CNS)—particularly the suprachiasmatic nuclei (SCN) of the hypothalamus—and play a role in sleep promotion; MT_2 receptors are located primarily in the retina and are linked to phase-shifting activity.

As the link between poor sleep architecture or insomnia and numerous psychiatric conditions has been galvanized in recent years, interest in how melatonin dysfunction impacts sleep, and potentially contributes to psychiatric pathologies, has also grown. Consequently, melatonergic ligands that have recently been introduced as pharmacologic agents to promote sleep and normalize circadian rhythm may also mitigate the symptoms of certain psychiatric and neurodegenerative disorders.

Melatonin, ramelteon (Rozerem), and Tasimeleteon (Hetlioz) are the only melatonin receptor agonists commercially available in the United States. Melatonin is available as a dietary supplement in various preparations in health food stores and is not covered under Food and Drug Administration (FDA) regulations. Ramelteon is an FDA-approved drug for the treatment of insomnia characterized by difficulties with sleep onset. Tasimeleteon was approved to treat sleep disturbances experienced by Smith–Magenis patients and blind individuals with non-24-hour sleep–wake disorder.

Also included in this chapter are orexin antagonists. Orexin is a neuropeptide that promotes wakefulness. Antagonistic activity at orexin receptors (OX_1 and OX_2) has been shown to promote somnolence and has led to the development of several dual orexin receptor antagonists (DORAs). Suvorexant (Belsomra), lemborexant (Dayvigo), and daridorexant (Quviviq) are all highly selective antagonists for orexin receptors.

Finally, this chapter includes five drugs that are FDA indicated to improve wakefulness in patients with excessive daytime sleepiness (including narcolepsy), obstructive sleep apnea (OSA), and shift-work disorder. These include: modafinil (Provigil); armodafinil (Nuvigil); pitolisant (Wakix); solriamfetol (Sunosi); and calcium, magnesium, potassium, and sodium oxybates (Xywav).

Agents for Insomnia

MELATONIN

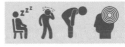 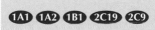

Melatonin (*N*-acetyl-5-methoxytryptamine) is a hormone mainly produced at night in the pineal gland. Ingested melatonin has been shown to be capable of reaching and binding to melatonin-binding sites in the brains of mammals and to produce somnolence when used at high doses. Melatonin is available as a dietary supplement and is not a medication. Few well-controlled clinical trials have been conducted to determine its effectiveness in treating such conditions as insomnia, jet lag, and sleep disturbances related to shift work, though preliminary evidence suggests that it is a safe supplement to improve sleep quality and total sleep time.

Pharmacologic Actions

Melatonin's secretion is stimulated by the dark and inhibited by the light. It is naturally synthesized from the amino acid tryptophan. Tryptophan is converted to serotonin and finally converted to melatonin. Melatonin may have a direct action on the SCN to influence circadian rhythms, which include jet lag and sleep disturbances. In addition to the pineal gland, melatonin is also produced in the retina (where M_2 receptors are located) and gastrointestinal tract.

Melatonin has a very short half-life of 0.5 to 6 minutes. Plasma concentrations are a function of the dose administered and the endogenous rhythm. Approximately 90% of melatonin is cleared through first-pass metabolism via the CYP1A1 and CYP1A2 pathways. Elimination occurs principally in urine.

Exogenous melatonin interacts with the melatonin receptors that suppress neuronal firing and promote sleep. There does not appear to be a dose–response relationship between exogenous melatonin administrations and sleep effects.

Therapeutic Indications

Melatonin is not regulated by the FDA. Individuals have used exogenous melatonin to address sleep difficulties (insomnia, circadian rhythm disorders), cancer (breast, prostate, colorectal), seizures, depression, anxiety, and seasonal affective disorder. Some studies suggest that exogenous melatonin may have some antioxidant effects, as well as neuroprotective, and antiaging properties.

None of these claims have been substantiated by the FDA.

Precautions and Adverse Reactions

Adverse events associated with melatonin include fatigue, dizziness, headache, irritability, and somnolence. Disorientation, confusion, sleepwalking, vivid dreams, and nightmares have also been observed, often with effects resolving after melatonin administration was discontinued.

Melatonin may reduce fertility in both men and women. In men, exogenous melatonin reduces sperm motility and long-term administration has been shown to inhibit testicular aromatase levels. In women, exogenous melatonin may inhibit ovarian function; and for that reason, it has been evaluated as a contraceptive, but with inconclusive results.

Use in Pregnancy and Lactation

Melatonin occurs naturally in the body, so it is considered safe to take during pregnancy. However, there is no good scientific evidence of either its safety or risks. Doses above 3 mg/day should not be used.

Drug Interactions

As a dietary supplement preparation, exogenous melatonin is not regulated by the FDA and has not been subjected to the same type of drug interaction studies that were performed for other melatonin agonists (ramelteon, tasimelteon). Caution is suggested in coadministering melatonin with blood thinners (e.g., warfarin [Coumadin], aspirin, and heparin), antiseizure medications, and medications that lower blood pressure.

Laboratory Interference

Melatonin is not known to interfere with any commonly used clinical laboratory tests.

Dosage and Administration

Over-the-counter melatonin is available in myriad formulations, strengths, and routes of administration. Since it is considered a supplement and has not been approved by the FDA, individual formulations are not regulated and may vary in quality (see Chapter 39).

Standard recommendations are to take the desired melatonin dose at bedtime, but some evidence from clinical trials suggests that dosing up to 2 hours before habitual bedtime may produce greater improvement in sleep onset.

RAMELTEON

 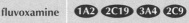

Ramelteon (Rozerem) is a melatonin receptor agonist used to treat sleep-onset insomnia. Unlike the benzodiazepines, ramelteon has no appreciable affinity for the γ-aminobutyric acid (GABA) receptor complex.

Pharmacologic Actions

Ramelteon is rapidly absorbed and eliminated over a dose range of 4 to 64 mg. Maximum plasma concentration (C_{max}) is reached approximately 45 minutes after administration, and the elimination half-life is 1 to 2.6 hours. The total absorption of ramelteon is at least 84%, but extensive first-pass metabolism results in a bioavailability of just 2%. Ramelteon is primarily metabolized via the cytochrome P450 isoenzyme CYP1A2 and principally eliminated in urine. Repeated once-daily dosing does not appear to result in accumulation, likely because of the compound's short half-life.

Ramelteon essentially mimics melatonin's sleep-promoting properties and has high affinity for melatonin MT_1 and MT_2 receptors.

Therapeutic Indications

Ramelteon was approved by the FDA in 2005 for the treatment of insomnia characterized by difficulty with sleep onset. Clinical trials and animal studies failed to find evidence of rebound insomnia or withdrawal effects.

Off-Label Uses

Potential off-label usage is centered on use in circadian rhythm disorders, predominantly jet lag, delayed sleep phase syndrome, and shift-work sleep disorder.

Precautions and Adverse Events

Headache is the most common side effect of ramelteon. Other adverse effects may include somnolence, fatigue, dizziness, worsening insomnia, depression, nausea, and diarrhea. The drug should not be used in patients with severe hepatic impairment. It is also not recommended in patients with severe sleep apnea or severe chronic obstructive pulmonary disease. Prolactin levels may be increased in women.

Ramelteon has been found to sometimes decrease blood cortisol and testosterone and to increase prolactin. Female patients should be monitored for cessation of menses and galactorrhea, as well as decreased libido, and fertility problems. The safety and effectiveness of ramelteon in children has not been established.

Use in Pregnancy and Lactation

This drug should only be used in pregnancy if the potential benefit justifies the possible risk to the fetus. It is not known if ramelteon is excreted in human breast milk. Ramelteon is classified as a pregnancy category C drug.

Drug Interactions

CYP1A2 is the major isozyme involved in the hepatic metabolism of ramelteon. Accordingly, fluvoxamine (Luvox) and other CYP1A2 inhibitors may increase side effects of ramelteon.

Ramelteon should be administered with caution in patients taking CYP1A2 inhibitors, strong CYP3A4 inhibitors such as ketoconazole, and strong CYP2C inhibitors such as fluconazole (Diflucan). No clinically meaningful interactions were found when ramelteon was coadministered with omeprazole, theophylline, dextromethorphan, midazolam, digoxin, and warfarin.

Dosing and Clinical Guidelines

The usual dose of ramelteon is 8 mg within 30 minutes of going to bed. It should not be taken with or immediately after high-fat meals. See Table 23-1 for dosing guidelines.

TABLE 23-1: Agents for Insomnia

Generic Name	Trade Name	Preparations	Initial Daily Dose	Usual Daily Dosage Range	Maximum Daily Dose
Melatonin	N/A	Myriad	N/A[a]	N/A[a]	N/A[a]
Ramelteon	Rozerem	8-mg tablet	8 mg	8 mg	8 mg
Tasimelteon	Hetlioz[b]	20-mg capsules	20 mg	20 mg	20 mg
Tasimelteon	Hetlioz LQ[c]	4 mg/mL oral suspension	0.7 mg for patients ≤28 kg; 20 mg for patients >28 kg	0.7 mg for patients ≤28 kg; 20 mg for patients >28 kg	0.7 mg for patients ≤28 kg; 20 mg for patients >28 kg
Suvorexant	Belsomra	5-, 10-, 15-, and 20-mg tablets	10 mg	10–20 mg	20 mg
Lemborexant	Dayvigo	5- and 10-mg tablets	5 mg	5–10 mg	10 mg
Daridorexant	Quviviq	25- and 50-mg tablets	25 mg	25–50 mg	50 mg

[a]Melatonin has not been approved for use by the FDA and is widely available as an over-the-counter medication. Patients should follow dosing instructions on the label of the OTC container.
[b]Hetlioz is indicated for patients 16 years of age and older.
[c]Hetlioz is indicated for patients 3 years to 15 years of age.

TASIMELTEON

 alcohol, fluvoxamine

Tasimelteon (Hetlioz) was approved by the FDA in 2014 for use in non-24-hour sleep–wake disorder, a disorder in which one's circadian rhythm fails to synchronize to a 24-hour day. The approval was limited to individuals who are blind and have no perception of light. In 2020, tasimelteon was approved for use in Smith–Magenis syndrome in patients 3 years of age and older for the treatment of nighttime sleep disturbances.

Pharmacologic Action

Tasimelteon is rapidly absorbed upon oral administration and reaches a peak concentration in 0.5 to 3 hours when taken in a fasting state. The absorption time is delayed by 1.75 hours after a high-fat meal, suggesting that the drug should be taken without food for maximum effect. Tasimelteon is 90% bound to proteins and extensively metabolized by cytochrome P450 isoenzymes CYP1A2 and CYP3A4, with only 1% of the parent compound being excreted in urine unchanged. Approximately 80% of radiolabeled tasimelteon is excreted in urine, while only 4% is excreted in feces. The mean elimination half-life of tasimelteon is 1.3 ± 0.4 hours. Repeated once-daily dosing does not appear to result in accumulation.

Tasimelteon's sleep-promoting effect is believed to be mediated by its interaction with melatonin receptors. It is an agonist at both MT_1 and MT_2 receptors and has a greater affinity for MT_2 receptors than MT_1 receptors. Tasimelteon's metabolites have less than one-tenth the binding affinity of the parent compound at either receptor.

Therapeutic Indications

Tasimelteon capsule formulation is approved for use in adult blind patients with non-24-hour sleep–wake disorder and nighttime sleep disturbances in Smith–Magenis syndrome in patients 16 years of age and older. The oral suspension is approved for use in pediatric patients with Smith–Magenis syndrome who are between the ages of 3 and 15 years of age.

Off-Label Uses

Tasimelteon may help patients with primary insomnia and other sleep-related disorders (e.g., jet lag disorder, advanced sleep phase disorder, shift-work disorder).

Precautions and Adverse Events

Patients should limit activity after taking tasimelteon, as it causes somnolence and can impair the performance of activities requiring an individual's full attention.

The most common side effects reported during clinical trials are headache, increases in alanine aminotransferase (twice as high as placebo group), and abnormal dreams.

Use in Pregnancy and Lactation

In animal studies, tasimelteon administration at higher than recommended doses resulted in developmental toxicity. However, no controlled studies have been conducted in pregnant humans, so the drug is classified as pregnancy category C.

It is not known if tasimelteon is excreted in human milk. Administration of the drug in nursing patients is warranted only if the benefits outweigh the potential risks.

Drug Interactions

As CYP1A2 and CYP3A4 are the major isozyme involved in the hepatic metabolism of tasimelteon, it should be administered with caution in patients taking CYP1A2 or CYP3A4 inhibitors or inducers. Coadministration with fluvoxamine (a strong CYP1A2 inhibitor) increases tasimeleteon C_{max} two-fold, while coadministration with ketoconazole (a strong CYP3A4 inhibitor) increases tasimelteon exposure by 50%. Exposure of tasimelteon declines by 90% when coadministered with rifampin (a strong CYP3A4 inducer), indicating the efficacy of tasimelteon may be limited if used in conjunction with a strong CYP3A4 inducer.

No clinically meaningful interactions were found when tasimelteon was coadministered with midazolam or rosiglitazone.

Clinical studies found a trend for additive effect with alcohol consumption.

Laboratory Interference

Tasimelteon is not known to interfere with any commonly used clinical laboratory tests.

Dosage and Administration

Tasimelteon is available as a 20-mg hard gelatin capsule and in an oral suspension. An oral suspension (Hetlioz LQ) is supplied in 4 mg/mL of yellow-white opaque suspension in 48 mL or 158 mL bottles.

The capsule is indicated for use in adults 16 years of age or older. The oral solution is indicated for pediatric patients aged 3 to 15 years of age. Prior to every administration, the oral solution should be shaken for at least 30 seconds and stored refrigerated when not in use. Tasimelteon has a short shelf life and depending on the packaging should be discarded within 5 to 8 weeks after opening.

The recommended dosage of tasimelteon for adults is one 20-mg capsule taken 1 hour before bedtime without food. Similarly, administration of tasimelteon in pediatric patients should occur 1 hour before bedtime without food. For children weighing more than 28 kg, the dose should be 20 mg. In pediatric patients weighting 28 kg or less, the dose should be 0.7 mg/kg. See Table 23-1 for dosing guidelines.

The drug's full effect may not be experienced for weeks or months.

No dose adjustments are necessary in patients with mild or moderate hepatic or renal impairment.

AGOMELATINE

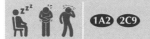

Agomelatine (Valdoxan) is structurally related to melatonin and is used in Europe for the treatment of major depressive disorder. It acts as an agonist at melatonin (MT_1 and MT_2) receptors. It also acts as a serotonin antagonist. It is primarily indicated for use in treating major depressive disorder. Analysis of agomelatine clinical trial data raised serious questions about the efficacy and safety of the drug and currently is not being marketed in the United States.

DUAL OREXIN RECEPTOR ANTAGONISTS

As of this writing, the FDA has approved three DORAs for the treatment of insomnia in adults. They include suvorexant (approved August 2014), lemborexant (approved December 2019), and daridorexant (approved January 2022).

Pharmacologic Actions

Suvorexant typically reaches maximum concentrations in 2 hours under fasted conditions. A high-fat meal can delay the time to peak concentrations by approximately 1.5 hours but does not result in meaningful change to exposure. It is extensively bound to plasma proteins and has an estimated bioavailability of 82% for a 10-mg dosage. Suvorexant is primarily metabolized by cytochrome P450 CYP3A isoenzymes with a minor contribution from CYP2C19 isoenzymes; it is primarily eliminated through feces (66%) and to a lesser extent urine (23%). The systemic pharmacokinetics of suvorexant are linear with an accumulation of one to two-fold with once-daily dosing, a mean half-life of 12 hours and steady state is achieved in 3 days. Although the FDA has determined that suvorexant is effective, it cautions that it may not be safe at the higher doses.

Lemborexant reaches maximum concentration in 1 to 3 hours in fasting state and food can affect absorption. A high-fat, high-calorie meal decreases C_{max} by 23%, delays T_{max} by 2 hours, and increases AUC_{0-inf} by 18%. Protein binding is approximately 94%. Lemborexant is metabolized by cytochrome P450 CYP3A4 isoenzymes and to a lesser extent CYP3A5 isoenzymes and is primarily eliminated through feces (57.4%) and 29.1% through urine. Mean half-life for 5-mg and 10-mg doses are 17 and 19 hours, respectively. Following single doses of lemborexant 2.5 to 75 mg (10 mg being the maximum recommended dose), exposure increases slightly less than in proportion to dose. The extent of accumulation of lemborexant at steady-state is 1.5- to 3-fold across this dose range.

Daridorexant reaches maximum concentration in 1 to 2 hours in a fasting state. A high-fat, high-calorie meal decreases C_{max} and delays T_{max} by 1.3 hours but does not affect total exposure. Daridorexant has an absolute bioavailability of 62% and protein binding is 99.7%. The drug is extensively metabolized, primarily by cytochrome P450 CYP3A4 isoenzymes (89%), and is excreted in feces (57%) and urine (28%) with only trace amounts of the parent drug found in either. Terminal half-life is 8 hours. Plasma exposure is dose proportional with no accumulation. As noted above, the three DORAs described in this chapter block orexin receptors, thereby preventing the binding of orexin A and orexin B neuropeptides to reduce wakefulness. They have no effects on the GABAergic system.

Therapeutic Indications

All three drugs are indicated for the treatment of insomnia in adults. Clinical trials and animal studies failed to find evidence of rebound insomnia or withdrawal effects.

Precautions and Adverse Events

DORAs are CNS depressants and can impair daytime wakefulness, especially in patients who do not get a full night's sleep while taking these drugs. Consequently, patients should not operate heavy machinery or drive while experiencing the acute effects of the drug.

More common side effects include drowsiness, dizziness, headache, unusual dreams, dry mouth, cough, and diarrhea. Some serious side effects include temporary inability to move or speak for up to several minutes while going to sleep or waking up, and temporary leg weakness during the day or at night. Symptoms of overdose typically include extreme drowsiness.

Older patients may be at higher risk of somnolence and drowsiness after taking DORAs. This may put them at a greater risk for falls. Exercise caution when prescribing doses of more than 5 mg daily in older patients (≥65 years old). The effects of DORAs on patients with compromised respiratory function should be considered. Unfortunately, no clinical studies on individuals with respiratory conditions have been conducted at this time.

Blood levels of suvorexant are increased in obese compared with nonobese patients, and in women compared with men. Particularly in obese women, the increased risk of exposure-related adverse effects should be considered before increasing the dose.

Unlike melatonin agonists, DORAs are classified as Schedule IV controlled substances.

Use in Pregnancy and Lactation

The safety and effectiveness of DORAs during pregnancy has not been established.

No information has been published about the use of DORAs during nursing, but their high protein binding suggests that small amounts are excreted in breast milk.

Drug Interactions

There are no serious interactions, but coadministration with strong CYP3A4 inhibitors, including grapefruit juice, is not recommended. Coadministration with other CNS depressants, including alcohol, can cause additive effects and may lead to increased drowsiness and more severe side effects.

Laboratory Interference

DORAs are not known to interfere with any commonly used clinical laboratory tests.

Dosage and Clinical Guidelines

See Table 23-1 for an outline of dosing guidelines.

Suvorexant

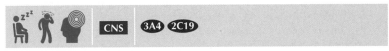

The recommended starting dose of suvorexant is 10 mg at night within 30 minutes of going to bed, with at least 7 hours of planned sleep time before awakening. If the 10-mg dose is well tolerated but not effective, the dose can be increased to 20 mg but should not exceed 20 mg a day. No dosage adjustment is required in patients with renal impairment or in patients with mild to moderate hepatic impairment. The drug is not recommended if hepatic impairment is severe. Suvorexant is available as 5-, 10-, 15- and 20-mg tablets.

Lemborexant

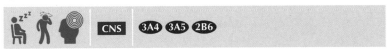

Lemborexant is available in 5- and 10-mg tablets. Patients are advised to start with 5 mg at night immediately before going to bed with at least 7 hours of planned sleep time before awakening. The dose may be increased to 10 mg based on patient tolerability. The maximum dose of lemborexant in patients with moderate hepatic impairment is 5 mg per night. Patients with severe hepatic impairment should not take lemborexant.

Daridorexant

Daridorexant is available in 25- and 50-mg tablets. The recommended dosage range of daridorexant is 25 to 50 mg taken within 30 minutes of going to bed with at least 7 hours of planned sleep time before waking. The maximum dose of daridorexant in patients with moderate hepatic impairment is 25 mg per night. Patients with severe hepatic impairment should not take daridorexant.

Agents for Excessive Daytime Sleepiness

Modafinil (Provigil) is a racemic compound. Both modafinil and its R-enantiomer, armodafinil (Nuvigil), exert clinical effects by enhancing catecholamine neurotransmission. Modafinil has been found to activate lateral hypothalamus orexin (hypocretin) neurons. In addition to the wake-promoting effects, modafinil increases motor activity, euphoria, and alterations in perception, emotions, and cognition typical of CNS stimulants. Both drugs have similar clinical effects and side effects.

Pitolisant (Wakix) is a first-in-class histamine 3 receptor (H_3) antagonist/ inverse agonist. H_3 receptors are expressed primarily in the CNS and may play an inhibitory role in the release of other neurotransmitters such as dopamine, GABA, acetylcholine, noradrenaline, serotonin, and histamine.

Solriamfetol (Sunosi) is a norepinephrine-dopamine reuptake inhibitor (NDRI) that is believed to induce wakefulness by increasing levels of norepinephrine and dopamine in the CNS.

A combination of calcium, magnesium, potassium, and sodium oxybates marketed under the trade name Xywav has been approved for the treatment of excessive daytime sleepiness in patients 7 years of age and older with narcolepsy. The therapeutic effects of the oxybate salts are believed to be mediated through $GABA_B$ actions during sleep at noradrenergic and dopaminergic neurons. Thalamocortical neurons may also be involved.

MODAFINIL AND ARMODAFINIL

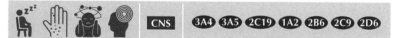

Pharmacologic Actions

The enantiomers of modafinil (a 1:1 ratio of R-modafinil and S-modafinil) have different pharmacokinetics and do not interconvert. Peak plasma levels of modafinil and armodafinil occur 2 to 4 hours after dosing. Food intake does not affect bioavailability, but the time to reach peak concentrations may be delayed by up to 1 hours if taken with food. Both drugs are moderately bound to plasma protein (approximately 60%), mainly albumin, and both drugs are extensively metabolized by the liver, with cytochrome P450 isoenzymes CYP3A4 and CYP3A5 both playing significant roles in metabolism. Approximately 80% of both drugs are excreted in urine within 11 days, compared to only 1% in feces. Only 10% of the parent compound is excreted in urine.

After multiple doses, the elimination half-life of modafinil is 15 hours and the half-life of R-modafinil is approximately 3 times that of S-modafinil. Apparent steady states of total modafinil and R-modafinil are achieved after 2 to 4 days of dosing, while steady states for armodafinil are achieved in 7 days.

Narcolepsy–cataplexy results from deficiency of hypocretin, a hypothalamic neuropeptide. Modafinil and armodafinil activate hypocretin-producing neurons and do not work through dopaminergic mechanism. They both have α_1-adrenergic agonist properties, which may account for their alerting effects and consequent wakefulness can be attenuated by prazosin, an α_1-adrenergic antagonist. Some evidence suggests that modafinil and armodafinil have some norepinephrine reuptake blocking effects.

Therapeutic Indications

Modafinil and armodafinil are indicated to improve wakefulness in adults who have excessive sleepiness associated with OSA, narcolepsy, or shift-work disorder. In direct comparison with amphetamine-like drugs, modafinil and armodafinil are equally effective at maintaining wakefulness but with a lower risk of excessive activation.

Off-Label Uses

Attention Deficit Hyperactivity Disorder

Though there is some conflicting evidence about the efficacy of modafinil and armodafinil in treating symptoms associated with attention deficit hyperactivity disorder (ADHD) in adults and children, multiple trials have demonstrated the clinical effectiveness of modafinil on the core symptoms of inattention, hyperactivity, and impulsivity, both at school and at home. Additionally, use of modafinil or armodafinil may be preferred over stimulants because the risk of abuse is low and properly regimented use of the drugs does not affect sleep architecture.

Acute Unipolar and Bipolar Depressive Episodes

Modafinil and armodafinil can reduce the severity of depressive episodes when taken in conjunction with antidepressants.

Cocaine Dependence

Limited data suggests that modafinil, when used in conjunction with individual behavioral therapy, may decrease cocaine cravings and increase cocaine nonuse days in patients with cocaine use disorder without comorbid alcohol dependence.

Fatigue

Some evidence suggests that a low-dose regimen of modafinil may treat some fatigue symptoms associated with cancer or multiple sclerosis (MS) though some double-blind trials show that modafinil was not superior to placebo in treating MS-related fatigue and caused more frequent adverse events than placebo.

Precautions and Adverse Events

Modafinil or armodafinil may cause a serious rash and lead to Stevens–Johnson syndrome or multiorgan hypersensitivity reaction, at which point the drug should be discontinued immediately. Angioedema has also been observed with use of the medications and should be discontinued at the first sign of angioedema or anaphylaxis. Excessive sleepiness may persist following use of modafinil or armodafinil, so clinicians should ask patients about their degree of sleepiness to reassess treatment and advise about the risks of certain behaviors or actions. Depending on the level of excessive sleepiness, it may be advisable to encourage patients to avoid driving or other potentially dangerous activities.

Caution should be advised in patients with a history of psychosis, depression, or mania, as treatment with modafinil or armodafinil may exacerbate these

Agents for Insomnia and Excessive Daytime Sleepiness

conditions. More common psychiatric adverse effects include anxiety, nervousness, insomnia, confusion, agitation, and depression. Other adverse events include headache, nausea, diarrhea, anorexia, and dry mouth.

Cardiovascular events, including chest pain, palpitations, dyspnea, and transient ischemic T-wave changes on ECG, were reported in subjects with mitral valve prolapse or left ventricular hypertrophy. Consequently, patients with either cardiovascular condition should not be treated with modafinil or armodafinil if already receiving CNS stimulants.

The pharmacokinetics of modafinil may be altered in older males and in patients with chronic hepatic impairment.

As both modafinil and armodafinil are Schedule IV drugs, there is a mild risk of abuse, particularly in patients with a history of substance abuse.

Use in Pregnancy and Lactation

Modafinil and armodafinil should only be used in pregnancy if the potential benefit justifies the possible risk to the fetus. It is not known if ramelteon is excreted in human breast milk. Both drugs are classified as pregnancy category C drugs.

Drug Interactions

In vitro, modafinil has been shown to inhibit the cytochrome P450 (CYP) isoenzyme CYP2C19 (moderately potent, reversible inhibition); modestly induce CYP1A2, CYP3A4/5, and CYP2B6; and suppress CYP2C9. More frequent monitoring of prothrombin times/INR should be considered if patients are taking both warfarin and modafinil.

Laboratory Interference

Modafinil and armodafinil are not known to interfere with any commonly used clinical laboratory tests.

Dosage and Clinical Guidelines

The starting dosage of modafinil is 200 mg in the morning in medically healthy individuals and 100 mg in the morning in persons with hepatic impairment. Some persons take a second 100- or 200-mg dose in the afternoon. The maximum recommended daily dosage is 400 mg, although dosages of 600 to 1,200 mg a day have been used safely. Adverse effects become prominent at dosages above 400 mg a day. Compared with amphetamine like drugs, modafinil promotes wakefulness but produces less attentiveness and less irritability. Modafinil and armodafinil are generally well tolerated.

Some persons with excessive daytime sleepiness extend the activity of the morning modafinil dose with an afternoon dose of methylphenidate. Armodafinil is virtually identical to modafinil, but is dosed differently, with the range being 50 to 250 mg daily.

For patients with severe hepatic impairment, dosing of both drugs should be reduced by 50% to that of patients with normal hepatic function.

See Table 23-2 for an outline of dosing guidelines.

TABLE 23-2: Agents for Excessive Daytime Sleepiness

Generic Name	Trade Name	Preparations	Initial Daily Dose	Usual Daily Dosage Range	Maximum Daily Dose
Modafinil	Provigil	100- and 200-mg tablets	100 mg	100–200 mg	400 mg
Armodafinil	Nuvigil	50-, 150-, and 250-mg tablets	50 mg	150–250 mg	250 mg
Pitolisant	Wakix	4.45- and 17.8-mg tablets	8.9 mg	17.8–35.6 mg	35.6 mg
Solriamfetol	Sunosi	75- and 150-mg tablets	37.5 mg or 75 mg[a]	37.5–150 mg	150 mg

[a]The initial dosage for treating obstructive sleep apnea with solriamfetol is 37.5 mg once daily. For treating narcolepsy, it is 75 mg once daily.

PITOLISANT

  antihistamines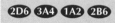

Pharmacologic Actions

Oral absorption of pitolisant is 90% and mean time to maximum plasma concentration is 3.5 hours. Pharmacokinetics is not affected by concomitant consumption of a high-fat meal and the plasma protein binding is 91% to 96%. Pitolisant is extensively metabolized primarily by cytochrome P450 isoenzymes CYP2D6 and to a lesser extent by CYP3A4 and does not produce active metabolites. It has a half-life of 20 hours and is excreted primarily in urine (90%) and only a small amount in feces (2.3%). Less than 2% of the parent compound is excreted in urine unchanged. Exposure increases proportionally with dose. With regular dosing, steady state is achieved in 7 days.

Pitolisant is an antagonist/inverse agonist at histamine 3 (H$_3$) receptors and has virtually no binding affinity to other histamine receptors. A full understanding of the role that H$_3$ receptors play in regulating the sleep–wake cycle has yet to be elucidated.

Therapeutic Indications

Pitolisant is indicated for the treatment of daytime sleepiness in adult patients with narcolepsy.

Off-Label Uses

Cataplexy

A randomized, double-blind, placebo-controlled trial involving patients with narcolepsy found that pitolisant was well-tolerated and efficacious for the treatment of cataplexy in patients with narcolepsy.

Pediatric Uses

Preliminary studies suggest that pitolisant may be safe for use in pediatric patients with narcolepsy, but more pharmacokinetic analyses need to be conducted in pediatric patients. There is limited evidence that pitolisant may relieve disease burden of pediatric patients with Prader–Willi syndrome, including excessive daytime sleepiness, poor-quality nighttime sleep, and cognitive difficulties.

Precautions and Adverse Events

Pitolisant prolongs the QT interval and should be avoided in patients with established QT prolongation or in patients who are using other drugs known to prolong QT interval. Patients with cardiac arrhythmias may be at a heightened risk of torsade de pointes and severe adverse events. Patients with hepatic or renal impairment may be at a higher risk of adverse events due to increased serum drug concentrations.

Pitolisant is contraindicated in patients with severe hepatic impairment and not recommended for patients with end-stage renal disease.

Some of the most common side effects associated with pitolisant include headache, insomnia, nausea, abdominal discomfort, anxiety, and loss of appetite.

Use in Pregnancy and Lactation

Though no definitive studies have shown that pitolisant can adversely affect developing fetus, the drug should not be used during pregnancy unless the benefits outweigh any clear risks. Though tests have not concluded if pitolisant is present in the milk of nursing mothers, it has been determined that pitolisant is present in the milk of lactating rats and likely present in human breast milk.

Drug Interactions

Strong CYP2D6 inhibitors increase pitolisant exposure by 2.2-fold and strong CYP3A4 inducers decrease exposure of pitolisant by 50%. H_1 receptor antagonists that cross the blood–brain barrier may inhibit the efficacy of pitolisant and should not be coadministered.

Pitolisant is a borderline/weak inducer of CYP3A4 and if coadministered with some medications, including contraceptives, may reduce efficacy

Laboratory Interference

Pitolisant is not known to interfere with any commonly used clinical laboratory tests.

Dosage and Clinical Guidelines

The recommended dosage range of pitolisant is 17.8 to 35.6 mg administered once daily upon waking. Doses are available in 4.45- and 17.8-mg oral tablets and should be administered according to the following schedule:

- Week 1: Initiate with a dose of 8.9 mg (two 4.45-mg tablets) once daily.
- Week 2: Increase dose to 17.8 mg (one 17.8-mg tablet) once daily.
- Week 3: If tolerated, increase dose to 35.6 mg (two 17.8-mg tablets) once daily.

If well-tolerated, double dose if coadministered with CYP3A4 inducers, and then return to normal dose if inducer is discontinued. Reduce dose by half if coadministered with CYP2D6 inhibitors. Dosage reductions are recommended in patients who are poor CYP2D6 metabolizers.

In patients with moderate hepatic impairment, initiate at the normal, 8.9 mg daily dose, but wait 2 weeks before increasing the dosage to 17.8 mg once daily. Pitolisant is contraindicated in patients with severe hepatic impairment.

In patients with renal impairment, initiate at the normal, 8.9 mg daily dose and increase the dosage to 17.8 mg once daily after 7 days, but do not exceed the 17.8-mg dosage.

SOLRIAMFETOL

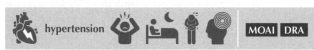

Solriamfetol was approved to treat excessive daytime sleepiness associated with narcolepsy and OSA by the FDA in 2019.

Pharmacologic Actions

Oral bioavailability of solriamfetol is 95%. The mean time to maximum plasma concentration is 2 hours, which can be delayed when consumed with a high-fat meal, though food does not appear to affect exposure. It has low plasma protein binding ranging from 13.3% to 19.4%. Solriamfetol is minimally metabolized, with 95% of the parent compound being excreted unchanged in urine. The apparent mean half-life of solriamfetol is 7.1 hours and steady state is achieved in 3 days.

Solriamfetol inhibits the reuptake of norepinephrine and dopamine by binding to transporters with low affinities though it is unclear why this improves wakefulness in patients.

Therapeutic Indications

Solriamfetol is indicated to treat excessive daytime sleepiness associated with narcolepsy and OSA.

Off-Label Uses

Solriamfetol has been used to treat excessive daytime sleepiness in people with idiopathic hypersomnia.

Precautions and Adverse Events

Solriamfetol is contraindicated in patients taking monoamine oxidase inhibitors (MAOIs) or patients who have discontinued the use of MAOIs within 14 days. Patients with cardiovascular disease should be cautioned before using solriamfetol, as it increases heart rate and both systolic and diastolic blood pressure in a dose-dependent fashion. Of note, this can increase the risk of stroke, heart attack, and cardiovascular death.

Some patients have experienced anxiety, irritability, and insomnia, and individuals with moderate or severe renal impairment may experience an increased risk of psychiatric symptoms due to the drug's prolonged half-life. Clinicians should use caution when prescribing solriamfetol to patients with a history of psychosis or bipolar disorder. Additionally, solriamfetol is a Schedule IV drug with some risk of abuse.

The most commonly adverse reactions include headache, decreased appetite, nausea, anxiety, insomnia, irritability, dry mouth, constipation, palpitations, abdominal pain, feelings of jitteriness, chest discomfort, and hyperhidrosis.

Agents for Insomnia and Excessive Daytime Sleepiness

Use in Pregnancy and Lactation

Though no definitive studies have shown that solriamfetol can adversely affect developing fetuses, the drug should not be used during pregnancy unless the benefits outweigh any clear risks. Though tests have not concluded if solriamfetol is present in the milk of nursing mothers, it has been determined that it is present in the milk of lactating rats and likely present in human breast milk.

Drug Interactions

Solriamfetol is contraindicated in patients who are receiving concomitant MAOIs or who have discontinued use of MAOIs within the last 14 days before beginning solriamfetol use. Caution should be used when administering solriamfetol with other drugs that increase blood pressure. Dopaminergic drugs may result in pharmacodynamic interactions when coadministered with solriamfetol.

Laboratory Interference

Solriamfetol is not known to interfere with any commonly used clinical laboratory tests.

Dosage and Clinical Guidelines

Solriamfetol is administered as a tablet available in two strengths: 75 mg and 150 mg. The 75-mg tablets are functionally scored that can be split in half to administer dose of 37.5 mg. It should be administered once daily upon waking, without food, and at least 9 hours before planned bedtime.

For narcolepsy, the initial dosage is 75 mg once daily. Based on efficacy and tolerability, the dosage may be increased to 150 mg after 3 days though the dosage should not exceed 150 mg per day. For OSA, the initial dosage should be 37.5 mg once daily. Based on efficacy and tolerability, the dosage may double every 3 days, but should not exceed 150 mg per day (see Table 23-2).

For patients with moderate or severe renal impairment, initiate dosing at 37.5 mg once daily. For patients with severe renal impairment, the maximum dosage is 37.5 mg once daily. For patients with moderate renal impairment, the dosage may be increased to 75 mg once daily after 7 days at the 37.5 mg dose, provided it is well-tolerated; but the dosage for this population should not exceed 75 mg.

CALCIUM, MAGNESIUM, POTASSIUM, AND SODIUM OXYBATES

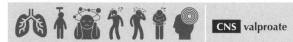

CNS valproate

A combination of calcium, magnesium, potassium, and sodium oxybate (the oxybate salts) marketed under the trade name Xywav received FDA approval in July 2020 for the treatment of cataplexy or excessive daytime sleepiness in patients 7 years of age and older. The active moiety of Xywav is oxybate or gamma-hydroxybutyrate (GHB), which is known colloquially as "the date rape drug," as it can result in decreased levels of consciousness, respiratory depression, coma, and even death. *Consequently, Xywav is available only through a restricted program under Risk Evaluation and Mitigation Strategy (REMS) called the XYWAV and XYREM REMS.*

Pharmacologic Actions

Following oral administration, the oxybate salts reach peak plasma concentration within 1.3 hours, and the plasma levels of GHB increase more than dose-proportionately. Coadministration with a high-fat meal reduces total exposure of GHB by 16%. Less than 1% of GHB is bound to plasma proteins and less than 5% of the drug is excreted unchanged (in urine) within 6 to 8 hours. Primary metabolism occurs via the tricarboxylic acid (Krebs) cycle, as well as via beta-oxidation, and clearance of GHB is almost entirely via expiration as carbon dioxide. No active metabolites have been identified.

It is believed that the therapeutic effects of the oxybate salts are mediated through $GABA_B$ actions during sleep at noradrenergic, dopaminergic, and thalamocortical neurons.

Therapeutic Indications

The oxybate salts marketed under the trade name Xywav are indicated for cataplexy or excessive daytime sleepiness in patients 7 years of age and older.

Precautions and Adverse Events

There is a black box warning for Xywav since it is a CNS depressant and may lead to clinically significant respiratory depression and obtundation. Consequently, Xywav is only available through a restricted program called the XYWAV and XYREM REMS. Xywav is a Schedule III controlled substance and may be misused or abused.

Additional precautions to consider include adverse effects that include sleepwalking, depression, suicidality, anxiety, and confusion. Less serious side effects include headache, nausea, dizziness, decreased appetite, diarrhea, hyperhidrosis, vomiting, fatigue, and dry mouth.

In pediatric studies, suicidal ideation, tactile hallucinations, weight loss, affect lability, and sleep apnea syndrome may lead to treatment discontinuation. Other common side effects include bedwetting, nausea, headache, vomiting, decrease appetite, and dizziness. In geriatric studies, frequency of headache is significantly higher than in nonelderly individuals.

Use in Pregnancy and Lactation

Xywav has not been assigned a pregnancy category, but GHB is classified as a pregnancy category B drug. Consequently, use of this drug among pregnant women is not recommended. As GHB is excreted in human milk following oral administration, women who are nursing should not use Xywav.

Drug Interactions

Coadministration of GHB with divalproex sodium (valproic acid) increases the mean systemic exposure of GHB by approximately 25%, though coadministration

TABLE 23-3: Adult Dosage of Xywav		
Total Nightly Dosage	Dosage at Bedtime	Dosage 2.5–4 Hours Later
4.5 g per night	2.25 g	2.25 g
6 g per night	3 g	3 g
7.5 g per night	3.75 g	3.75 g
9 g per night	4.5 g	4.5 g

does not appear to affect the pharmacokinetics of valproic acid. Tests on attention and working memory appear to be more impaired following coadministration than with either drug alone.

Laboratory Interference

Xywav is not known to interfere with any commonly used clinical laboratory tests.

Dosing and Clinical Guidelines

Xywav is administered as an oral solution at a total salt concentration of 0.5 g per mL. The salts are broken down into 0.234 g calcium oxybate, 0.096 g magnesium oxybate, 0.13 g potassium oxybate, and 0.04 g sodium oxybate.

Dosages should be diluted in ¼ cup of water in the empty pharmacy container provided. Dilutions should be consumed within 24 hours. Nightly dosages should be divided into two doses, the first taken at least 2 hours after eating dinner, the second dose 2.5 to 4 hours after the first. Patients should prepare both doses prior to bedtime and immediately lie down after dosing and remain in bed following ingestion of each dose, as one may fall asleep suddenly without feeling drowsy within 5 to 15 minutes. Patients will likely need to set an alarm to wake up for their second dose. If the second dose is missed, that dose should be skipped, and the next dose taken the next night.

The recommended starting dosage is 4.5 g split evenly as 2.25 g for the first and second dose (see Table 23-3). Dosages can be increased 1.5 g per night per week to the recommended range of 6 to 9 g per night. Dosages should not exceed 9 g per night. Some patients may experience better results with unequal doses. The starting dosage should be reduced in half for patients with hepatic impairment.

Depending on weight, dosages for pediatric patients may need to be significantly lower (see Table 23-4).

TABLE 23-4: Xywav Dosing Guidance for Patients 7 Years of Age and Older						
	Initial Dosage		Maximum Weekly Increase		Maximum Recommended Dosage	
Patient Weight	Bedtime Dose	Dosage 2.5–4 Hours Later	Bedtime Dose	Dosage 2.5–4 Hours Later	Bedtime Dose	Dosage 2.5–4 Hours Later
20 kg to <30 kg	≤1 g	≤1 g	0.5 g	0.5 g	3 g	3 g
30 kg to <45 kg	≤1.5 g	≤1.5 g	0.5 g	0.5 g	3.75 g	3.75 g
≥45 kg	≤2.25 g	≤2.25 g	0.75 g	0.75 g	4.5 g	4.5 g

Insufficient evidence exists to provide dosing recommendations for pediatric patients 7 years of age and older who weigh less than 20 kg.

Methylenedioxymetham-phetamine

24

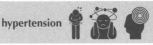 hypertension **SERO** antidepressants **2D6** **1A2** **3A4**

Introduction

MDMA (3,4-methylenedioxymethamphetamine) is a psychoactive substance that promotes the release of neurotransmitters like dopamine, serotonin, and norepinephrine, as well as neurohormones, most notably oxytocin. The subjective effects of MDMA include euphoria and increased levels of empathy or connectivity to others and for that reason it is often referred to as an empathogen or entactogen. MDMA also attenuates fear or anxiety, even when one is exposed to frightening or stressful stimuli. This includes stressful or negative memories.

During the 1970s and early 1980s, a small number of psychotherapists began using MDMA as an adjunctive during individual and group therapy. They reported that its use could allow patients struggling with poor emotional regulation to process painful or negative memories more effectively and to gain greater emotional insight into their conditions, relationships, or situations. Concurrently, news of the prosocial effects of the drug became more widely known and MDMA became a recreational drug, particularly within the context of dance clubs, which led to its familiar name outside of clinical settings: ecstasy.

Despite its association with dance clubs, particularly the underground "rave" scenes of the late 1980s and 1990s and subsequent stigma in the field of medicine, interest in MDMA's clinical utility never faded entirely. After years of lobbying, research in MDMA resumed in the early 2000s and has continued ever since. The primary focus has been how MDMA can be used to reduce symptoms of posttraumatic stress disorder (PTSD) when used in conjunction with psychotherapy. The underlying premise behind this course of treatment is that MDMA allows the patient to revisit the traumatic memory without triggering negative emotional symptoms characteristic of PTSD, and to then work with the therapist to mitigate the fear or anxiety associated with the trauma. This model relies on fear extinction and memory reconsolidation, and shares many of the same theoretical foundations of one of the most conventional treatment modalities for PTSD, prolonged exposure.

While most of the research into MDMA-assisted psychotherapy has focused on its potential to treat symptoms associated with PTSD, some believe that it could be useful for the treatment of anxiety, substance use, eating, and obsessive-compulsive disorders as well as suicidality.

259

Description and Route of Administration

MDMA was first synthesized in 1912. It quickly lapsed into obscurity but was rediscovered in the 1970s by a small group of psychotherapists who believed it could be used to help patients gain emotional insight while in individual or group therapy. Before the efficacy of MDMA-assisted psychotherapy could be studied, the drug became popular among recreational users, who referred to it as ecstasy, E, X, XTC, or molly. The Drug Enforcement Agency criminalized its use in 1985 and classified it as a Schedule I drug in 1986.

The base of MDMA is a colorless oil. Its more common form is a hydrochloride salt, which is a white or off-white powder or crystal that is soluble in water. Bromide and phosphate salts may also be encountered. Outside of clinical settings, it may be snorted if in powder form, but the more common route of administration is by mouth as a capsule or tablet. Tablets are often branded with symbols or logos. Within drug culture, tablets of E or ecstasy may contain MDMA in conjunction with a cornucopia of other illicit substances, while the appellation molly is supposed to be reserved for pure MDMA. In a clinical setting, MDMA is administered orally as a capsule or tablet.

Pharmacokinetics

Absorption and Distribution

Following oral administration, MDMA is absorbed in the intestinal tract within 30 minutes and reaches peak plasma concentration in approximately 2 hours. Peak blood concentrations of 106, 131, and 236 ng/mL are reached in healthy volunteers following oral doses of 50, 75, and 125 mg, respectively.

Metabolism

MDMA is primarily metabolized in the liver by cytochrome P450 CYP2D6 into 3,4-dihydroxymethamphetamine (HHMA), an unstable compound that is converted into 4-hydroxy-3-methoxymethamphetamine (HMMA) before being metabolized into 4-hydroxy-3-methoxyamphetamine (HMA) by CYP1A2. In a secondary metabolic pathway, MDMA is N-demethylated by CYP3A4 to form 3,4-methylenedioxyamphetamine (MDA), which then undergoes further demethylation via CYP2D6 to form 3,4-dihydroxyamphetamine (HHA).

Many of these metabolites are psychoactive members of the methamphetamine family, but only MDA appears to be used as a recreational drug with any degree of regularity. Derived from the oil of the sassafras plant, MDA is commonly referred to as sass or sally.

Elimination and Excretion

The elimination half-life of MDA is 7.7 ± 0.4 hours, though it may take upwards of five half-lives (approximately 40 hours) for 95% of the drug to be cleared following administration. MDMA and its metabolites are excreted in urine, primarily as sulfate and glucuronide conjugates, though 20% of MDMA may be excreted unchanged in urine. After a single dose of MDMA the maximum concentration in urine is highly variable (3.3 to 30.4 hours) and metabolites may be detected for more than 7 days following administration.

Pharmacodynamics

The subjective and psychological effects of MDMA are typically felt 30 to 75 minutes following oral administration. Patients are likely to become more appreciative of sensory stimuli or may observe alterations in perceptions (e.g., colors are more vivid, time appears to move slower, sounds possess unusual qualities), while thoughts and memories may be given new or heighted significance. Peak subjective effects typically occur 70 to 90 minutes following administration and may persist for 1 to 3 hours. Throughout this time, patients may experience increasingly intense visual or auditory hallucinations, euphoria, anxiety, enhanced connectivity to others, and a wide range of emotional states. Adverse effects are noted below.

Mechanism of Action

MDMA acts by increasing the net release of monoamine neurotransmitters from their axon terminals by binding to transporters and preventing reuptake. These effects are most pronounced in serotonin, as well as norepinephrine and to a lesser extent dopamine. The increase in net release of serotonin (and to some degree dopamine) is the major mechanism of action for MDMA, whereas the net increase of norepinephrine results in effects akin to other amphetamines. On a dose-dependent basis, MDMA also increases plasma levels of the neurohormone oxytocin.

Therapeutic Index

An effective dose of MDMA for a 70 kg (154 lbs) person is 125 mg, while a lethal dose is 2 g (therapeutic index = 16), which is considered relatively safe.

Tolerance, Dependence, and Withdrawal

Chronic users of MDMA appear to develop a tolerance to the psychoactive effects of the drug and cross-tolerance with methamphetamines has been evidenced in rodent models. Real-world data about tolerance to MDMA in humans is difficult to establish, since illicit MDMA tends to contain myriad impurities and other drugs.

Withdrawal symptoms are typically felt after first-time use and appear to be mediated by depletions in serotonin. Following use, one may feel depressed, anxious, fatigued, and exhausted, though these negative effects tend to dissipate within a few days. Chronic use of MDMA may result in more severe depletions of serotonin, more severe withdrawal symptoms, and persistent emotional and cognitive impairments.

Therapeutic Indications

As of this writing, MDMA is considered a Schedule I drug and is not indicated for any condition. However, clinical trials are investigating the possibility that MDMA-assisted psychotherapy may be effective at treating PTSD, existential crisis in terminally ill patients, as well as anxiety and depressive disorders. Phase 3 trials are currently underway to assess the value of MDMA-assisted psychotherapy in treating PTSD.

Precautions and Adverse Effects

MDMA-assisted psychotherapy in general is typically contraindicated for people with a personal or family history of severe and persistent mental illnesses or existing psychiatric comorbidities that make them more susceptible to psychosis. Even those who are not predisposed to mental illness or psychosis may experience adverse psychological effects during the acute phase of the treatment, including confusion, fear, paranoia, depersonalization, and unpleasant hallucinations. These effects typically wear off within a few hours.

Common adverse effects include hyperthermia, dehydration, hyponatremia, headache, increased blood pressure, pupil dilation, nausea, involuntary jaw clenching or teeth grinding, restlessness, and excessive sweating. If used in a recreational setting, particularly in a dance club, the combination of hyperthermia, excessive sweating, hyponatremia, and dehydration can become life-threatening. MDMA may also cause tachycardia, posing a risk to patients with cardiovascular diseases.

In rare instances, MDMA may cause liver injury or acute liver failure.

Long-term use of MDMA can lead to impairments in executive functioning, memory, and visual processing, as well as sleep disturbances. Additionally, long-term use is associated with depleted serotonin, which can lead to depression, anxiety, irritability, and fatigue.

Risk of Overdose

The risk of overdose or abuse in a clinical setting is very low. MDMA overdose is possible in a recreational setting, but still relatively rare unless used in conjunction with alcohol or other drugs.

Drug Interactions

In a recreational setting, MDMA is often ingested with alcohol or illicit drugs (e.g., cannabis, cocaine, opioids), which may lead to severe adverse events or even death. Clinical studies on drug interactions between common pharmaceuticals and MDMA are currently lacking, though it is known that MDMA is primarily metabolized by cytochrome P450 CYP2D6 and that coadministration with other pharmaceuticals that are metabolized by this enzyme may lead to adverse events. Similarly, patients who have been prescribed antidepressant drugs that inhibit serotonin reuptake (see Table 24-1) should taper and discontinue use at least 2 weeks prior to administration of MDMA. In the case of fluoxetine, patients should taper and discontinue use at least 6 weeks prior to administration of MDMA. Patients run a higher risk of developing serotonin syndrome if MDMA is taken in conjunction with other drugs that elevate serotonin levels (see Table 24-2).

Dosage and Clinical Guidelines

While there are no set guidelines for administering MDMA at this time, the protocol for MDMA-assisted psychotherapy established by the Multidisciplinary Association of Psychedelic Studies (MAPS) recommends two to three sessions prior to the administration of MDMA to create a rapport between the patient and

TABLE 24-1: Drug–Drug Interactions Between Antidepressants and Classic Psychedelics

Drug Type	Examples
Monoamine oxidase inhibitors	Isocarboxazid, moclobemide, phenelzine, selegiline, tranylcypromine
Noradrenergic and specific serotonergic antidepressants	Mianserin, mirtazapine, setiptiline
Select serotonin reuptake inhibitors	Citalopram, escitalopram, fluvoxamine, fluoxetine[a], paroxetine, sertraline
Serotonin modulators	Nefazodone, trazodone, vilazodone, vortioxetine
Serotonin norepinephrine reuptake inhibitors	Desvenlafaxine, duloxetine, levomilnacipran, venlafaxine
Serotonin partial agonist reuptake inhibitors	Vilazodone, vortioxetine
Tricyclic antidepressants	Amitriptyline, chlorpheniramine, clomipramine, desipramine, imipramine, nortriptyline
Other	Buspirone

Listed drugs should be tapered and discontinued at least 2 weeks prior to acute MDMA-assisted psychotherapy.

[a]Fluoxetine should be tapered and discontinued at least 6 weeks prior to acute MDMA-assisted psychotherapy.

the therapist and to introduce the patient to the drug. This is followed by a session where the drug is administered, oftentimes with a 125-mg dose and a smaller, supplemental dose midway through the session. Following the session where the drug is administered, the patient will be expected to attend several follow-up sessions, often over the course of several weeks, to talk about the experience and to take steps to incorporate it into a larger psychotherapeutic framework. This may be repeated two to three times in total.

TABLE 24-2: Drugs Associated with Elevated Serotonin Levels and Serotonin Syndrome

Drug Type	Examples
Analgesics	Fentanyl, meperidine, pentazocine, tramadol
Antibiotics	Linezolide, ritonavir
Anticonvulsants	Valproate
Antidepressants	Buspirone, clomipramine, nefazodone, trazodone, venlafaxine
Antiemetics	Granisetron, metoclopramide, ondansetron
Antimigraine medications	Sumatriptan
Bariatric drugs	Sibutramine
Monoamine oxidase inhibitors	Clorgiline, isocarboxazid, moclobemide, phenelzine
Over-the-counter drugs	Dextromethorphan
Selective serotonin reuptake inhibitors	Citalopram, fluoxetine, fluvoxamine, paroxetine, sertraline

No clinical programs that utilize MDMA-assisted psychotherapy currently support the perpetual administration of MDMA.

Conclusion

MDMA holds tremendous promise as an adjunctive to traditional treatment modalities for conditions that are notoriously difficult to treat, particularly trauma- and stressor-related disorders like PTSD. Preliminary and anecdotal evidence suggests that patients who have struggled with these disorders for years or even decades are experiencing breakthroughs or progressing on an accelerated timeline following the treatment. However, as much optimism as there is around the use of MDMA to help patients with these conditions, it remains an experimental treatment as of this writing and more research is still needed to determine if it should be rescheduled or if its potential risks are too high.

Mirtazapine

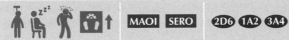

25

Introduction

First introduced in 1996, mirtazapine (Remeron) is an atypical antidepressant currently indicated to treat major depression. It is a tetracyclic drug that belongs to the piperazino-azepine group of compounds and increases both norepinephrine and serotonin without having a significant effect on monoamine oxidase inhibition (as is the case with phenelzine or tranylcypromine) or monoamine uptake (as in the case of tricyclic agents or selective serotonin reuptake inhibitors [SSRIs]). Its effects are the result of inhibition of α_2-adrenergic receptors and blockade of postsynaptic serotonin type 2 (5-HT$_2$) and type 3 (5-HT$_3$) receptors.

Mirtazapine is more likely to reduce rather than induce nausea and diarrhea due to its effects on serotonin 5-HT$_3$ receptors. Characteristic side effects include increased appetite and sedation. Its potent antagonistic activity at histamine H$_1$ receptors accounts for its sedative and appetite-enhancing properties. Weight gain is also a common unwanted side effect of mirtazapine therapy and affects approximately 15% to 25% of patients.

Pharmacologic Actions

Mirtazapine is administered orally and is rapidly, completely absorbed, and has a bioavailability of approximately 50%. It has a half-life of about 30 hours. Peak concentration is achieved within 2 hours of ingestion, and steady state is reached after 6 days. Plasma clearance may be slowed up to 30% in persons with impaired hepatic function, up to 50% in those with impaired renal function, up to 40% slower in elderly men, and up to 10% slower in elderly women. Mirtazapine is extensively metabolized, with major pathways of biotransformation being demethylation and hydroxylation, followed by glucuronide conjunction. Cytochrome P450 isoenzymes CYP2D6, CYP1A2, and the CYP3A subfamily are involved in metabolism. Mirtazapine is primarily eliminated via urine (75%), with 15% in feces.

The mechanism of action of mirtazapine is antagonism of central presynaptic α_2-adrenergic receptors and blockade of postsynaptic serotonin 5-HT$_2$ and 5-HT$_3$ receptors. The α_2-adrenergic receptor antagonism causes increased firing of norepinephrine and serotonin neurons. The potent antagonist of serotonin 5-HT$_2$ and 5-HT$_3$ receptors serves to decrease anxiety, relieve insomnia, and stimulate appetite. Mirtazapine is a potent antagonist of histamine H$_1$ receptors and is a moderately potent antagonist at α_1-adrenergic and muscarinic–cholinergic receptors.

Therapeutic Indications

Mirtazapine is effective for the treatment of depression. It is highly sedating, making it a reasonable choice for use in depressed patients with severe or long-standing insomnia. Some patients find the residual daytime sedation associated with initiation of treatment to be quite pronounced and even overwhelming. However, the more extreme sedating properties of the drug generally lessen over the first week of treatment. Combined with the tendency to cause sometimes a ravenous appetite, mirtazapine is well suited for depressed patients with melancholic features such as insomnia, weight loss, and agitation. Elderly depressed patients in particular are good candidates for mirtazapine; young adults are more likely to object to this side-effect profile.

Off-Label Uses

Chemotherapy (as Appetite Stimulant and Sedative)

Mirtazapine's blockade of 5-HT$_3$ receptors, a mechanism associated with medications used to combat the severe gastrointestinal side effects of cancer chemotherapy agents, has led to the use of the drug in a similar role. In this population, sedation and stimulation of appetite clearly could be seen as being beneficial instead of unwelcome side effects.

Anti–Depressant-Induced Side Effects

Mirtazapine is often combined with SSRIs or venlafaxine to augment antidepressant response or counteract serotonergic side effects of those drugs, particularly nausea, agitation, and insomnia. Mirtazapine has no significant pharmacokinetic interactions with other antidepressants.

Posttraumatic Stress Disorder

Mirtazapine has been used as adjunctive treatment with SSRIs in the treatment of posttraumatic stress disorder (PTSD). It can also help treat comorbid depression and sleep difficulties.

Insomnia

Mirtazapine has been shown to increase deep sleep and REM sleep in patients, but may lead to rebound insomnia upon discontinuation of the medicine.

Anxiety Disorders

Though there are very few clinical trials assessing mirtazapine for anxiety disorders, limited evidence shows efficacy in treating panic disorder and, to a lesser extent, social anxiety disorder.

Other Off-Label Uses

Some studies have found that mirtazapine can be used to treat pain, sleep problems, and various quality of life issues for patients with fibromyalgia. It may also be used in the prophylactic treatment of tension-type headaches.

TABLE 25-1: Adverse Reactions Reported with Mirtazapine Clinical Trials

Event	Percentage (%)
Somnolence	54
Dry mouth	25
Increased appetite	17
Constipation	13
Weight gain	12
Dizziness	7
Myalgias	5
Disturbing dreams	4

Precautions and Adverse Reactions

Suicide Warning

Like all antidepressants, mirtazapine has a black box warning because it may cause an increase in suicidal ideation or actions in children, teenagers, and young adults. Suicidality is also more pronounced during the initial months of treatment and following changes to dosage.

Side Effects

Somnolence, the most common adverse effect of mirtazapine, occurs in more than 50% of patients (see Table 25-1). Individuals starting mirtazapine should thus exercise caution when driving or operating dangerous machinery and even when getting out of bed at night. This is one reason why mirtazapine is almost always given before sleep. Mirtazapine potentiates the sedative effects of other central nervous system depressants, so potentially sedating prescription or over-the-counter drugs and alcohol should be avoided during use of mirtazapine. Mirtazapine also causes dizziness in 7% of persons. It does not appear to increase the risk for seizures. Mania or hypomania occurred in clinical trials at a rate similar to that of other antidepressant drugs.

Mirtazapine increases appetite and may also increase serum cholesterol concentration to 20% or more above the upper limit of normal in 15% of persons and increase triglycerides to 500 mg/dL or more in 6% of persons. Elevations of alanine transaminase levels to more than three times the upper limit of normal were seen in 2% of mirtazapine-treated persons, as opposed to 0.3% of placebo-controlled subjects.

In limited premarketing experience, the absolute neutrophil count dropped to 500/mm^3 or less within 2 months of the onset of use in 0.3% of persons, some of whom developed symptomatic infections. This hematologic condition was reversible in all cases and was more likely to occur when other risk factors for neutropenia were present. Increases in the frequency of neutropenia have not, however, been reported during the extensive postmarketing period. Persons who develop fever, chills, sore throat, mucous membrane ulceration, or other signs of

Mirtazapine

infection should nevertheless be evaluated medically. If a low white blood cell count is found, mirtazapine should be immediately discontinued, and the infectious disease status should be followed closely.

A small number of persons experience orthostatic hypotension while taking mirtazapine.

Use in Pregnancy and Lactation

Mirtazapine use by pregnant women has not been studied, so no data exist regarding the effects on fetal development and mirtazapine should be used with caution during pregnancy. Since the drug may be excreted in breast milk, it should not be taken by nursing mothers.

Because of the risk of agranulocytosis associated with mirtazapine use, persons should be attuned to signs of infection.

Mirtazapine is classified as a pregnancy category C drug.

Drug Interactions

Mirtazapine can potentiate the sedation of alcohol and benzodiazepines. Mirtazapine should not be used within 14 days of use of a monoamine oxidase inhibitor.

Mirtazapine can induce serotonin syndrome. While rare when used in monotherapy, it becomes more common when taken in conjunction with other serotonergic agents, particularly methadone, sertraline, linezolid, and methylene blue. Symptoms of serotonin syndrome include confusion, agitation, difficulty thinking, coordination problems, hallucinations, twitching, and coma. Patients may also experience significant blood pressure changes (increases or decreases), stiffened muscles, tachycardia, fever, sweating, nausea, vomiting, and diarrhea.

Laboratory Interferences

No laboratory interferences have yet been described for mirtazapine.

Dosage and Administration

Mirtazapine is available in 15-, 30-, and 45-mg scored tablets. Mirtazapine is also available in 15-, 30- and 45-mg orally disintegrating tablets for persons who have difficulty swallowing pills. If persons fail to respond to the initial dose of 15 mg of mirtazapine before sleep, the dose may be increased in 15-mg increments every 5 days to a maximum of 45 mg before sleep. Lower dosages may be necessary in elderly persons or persons with renal or hepatic insufficiency.

Monoamine Oxidase Inhibitors

26

Generic Name	Trade Name	Adverse Effects	Drug Interactions	CYP Interactions
Isocarboxazid	Marplan	Suicidality, hypotension, weight gain, insomnia, sexual dysfunction, dizziness, confusion	See Table 26-2	N/A
Moclobemide	Manerix	Suicidality, hypotension, weight gain, insomnia, dizziness, confusion	See Table 26-2	2D6, 2C19, 1A2, 2C9
Phenelzine	Nardil	Suicidality, hypotension, weight gain, insomnia, sexual dysfunction, dizziness, confusion	See Table 26-2	2C19, 2C8, 3A4, 3A5, 3A7, 2D6, 2E1
Rasagiline	Azilect	Suicidality, hypotension, weight gain, insomnia, sexual dysfunction, dizziness, confusion	See Table 26-2	1A2
Selegiline	Eldepryl, Emsam	Suicidality, hypotension, weight gain, insomnia, sexual dysfunction, dizziness, confusion	See Table 26-2	2B6, 2C9, 3A4, 3A5
Tranylcypromine	Parnate	Suicidality, hypotension, weight gain, insomnia, sexual dysfunction, dizziness, confusion	See Table 26-2	2D6, 2C9, 2C19, 1A2, 2A6, 3A4

Introduction

First discovered in the 1950s, monoamine oxidase inhibitors (MAOIs) were the first class of approved antidepressant drugs. Their antidepressant properties were discovered by chance while the drug isoniazid (Marsilid) was being investigated as a treatment for tuberculosis in 1952. Some patients treated for tuberculosis experienced elevation of mood during treatment. A subsequent study of psychotically depressed patients showed substantial improvement of symptoms in 70% of those taking the drug. In 1961, isoniazid was withdrawn from the US market because it caused jaundice and hepatotoxicity. Other MAOIs without these side effects have continued to be commercially available.

The currently available MAOIs include phenelzine (Nardil), isocarboxazid (Marplan), and tranylcypromine (Parnate). These drugs are irreversible inhibitors of MAO, and are nonselective, inactivating the MAO-A and MAO-B isoforms. Another MAOI, selegiline (Eldepryl), is an irreversible and selective inhibitor of the MAO-B isoform. In its oral form, it is used for the treatment of Parkinson disease; while in a transdermal delivery form (Emsam), it is approved as an antidepressant.

Two other MAOIs should be mentioned. Rasagiline (Azilect), an irreversible MAO-B inhibitor, is used in Parkinson disease. It has no approved psychiatric indications. Moclobemide (Manerix), a selective reversible inhibitor of MAO-A (RIMA), is approved as an antidepressant in many countries, but not the United States.

Despite the proven effectiveness of phenelzine, isocarboxazid, and tranyl-cypromine, prescription of these drugs as first-line agents has always been limited by concern about the development of potentially lethal hypertension and the consequent need for a restrictive diet. Use of MAOIs declined further after the introduction of the selective serotonin reuptake inhibitors (SSRIs) and other new agents. They are now mainly relegated to use in treatment-resistant cases. Thus, the second-line status of MAOIs has less to do with considerations of efficacy than with concerns for safety.

Pharmacologic Actions

Phenelzine, tranylcypromine, and isocarboxazid are readily absorbed after oral administration and reach peak plasma concentrations within 2 hours. Whereas their plasma half-lives are in the range of 2 to 3 hours, their tissue half-lives are considerably longer. Because they irreversibly inactivate MAOs, the therapeutic effect of a single dose of irreversible MAOIs may persist for as long as 2 weeks.

The RIMA moclobemide is rapidly absorbed and has a half-life of 0.5 to 3.5 hours. Because it is a reversible inhibitor, moclobemide has a much briefer clinical effect after a single dose than do irreversible MAOIs.

A transdermal patch containing selegiline that is marketed under the trade name Emsam is delivered systematically over 24 hours and results in significantly higher exposure with lower exposure to metabolites when compared to selegiline when administered orally. Drug absorption may be 33% higher than in this formulation. The mean half-lives of selegiline and its three metabolites range from 18 to 25 hours, and it's extensively metabolized by cytochrome P450 isoenzymes CYP2B6, CYP2C9, CYP3A4, and CYP3A5.

The MAO enzymes are found on the outer membranes of mitochondria, where they degrade cytoplasmic and extraneuronal monoamine neurotransmitters such as norepinephrine, serotonin, dopamine, epinephrine, and tyramine. MAOIs act in the central nervous system (CNS), the sympathetic nervous system, the liver, and the gastrointestinal (GI) tract. There are two types of MAOs, MAO_A and MAO_B. MAO_A primarily metabolizes norepinephrine, serotonin, and epinephrine; dopamine and tyramine are metabolized by both MAO_A and MAO_B.

The structures of phenelzine and tranylcypromine are like those of amphetamine and have similar pharmacologic effects in that they increase the release of dopamine and norepinephrine with attendant-stimulant effects on the brain.

Therapeutic Indications

MAOIs are used for treatment of depression. Due to their side effect profiles, MAOIs are typically only used in treatment-resistant patients. Some research indicates that phenelzine is more effective than tricyclic antidepressants (TCAs) in depressed patients with mood reactivity, extreme sensitivity to interpersonal loss or rejection, prominent anergia, hyperphagia, and hypersomnia—a constellation of symptoms conceptualized as atypical depression. Evidence also suggests that MAOIs are more effective than TCAs as a treatment for bipolar depression.

Off-Label Uses

Due to safety concerns, MAOIs are not commonly used off-label and should only be considered when all other treatment options have been exhausted. Patients with panic disorder and social phobia respond well to MAOIs. MAOIs have also been used to treat bulimia nervosa, posttraumatic stress disorder, anginal pain, atypical facial pain, migraine, attention-deficit hyperactivity disorder, idiopathic orthostatic hypotension, and depression associated with traumatic brain injury.

Precautions and Adverse Reactions

The most frequent adverse effects of MAOIs are orthostatic hypotension, insomnia, weight gain, edema, and sexual dysfunction. Orthostatic hypotension can lead to dizziness and falls. Thus, cautious upward tapering of the dosage should be used to determine the maximum tolerable dosage. Treatment for orthostatic hypotension includes avoidance of caffeine; intake of 2 L of fluid per day; addition of dietary salt or adjustment of antihypertensive drugs (if applicable); support stockings; and in severe cases, treatment with fludrocortisone (Florinef), a mineralocorticoid, 0.1 to 0.2 mg a day. Orthostatic hypotension associated with tranylcypromine use can usually be relieved by dividing the daily dosage.

Insomnia can be treated by dividing the dose, not giving the medication after dinner, and using trazodone (Desyrel) or a benzodiazepine hypnotic if necessary. Weight gain, edema, and sexual dysfunction often do not respond to any treatment and may warrant switching to another agent. When switching from one MAOI to another, the clinician should taper and stop use of the first drug for 10 to 14 days before beginning use of the second drug.

Paresthesias, myoclonus, and muscle pains are occasionally seen in persons treated with MAOIs. Paresthesias may be secondary to MAOI-induced pyridoxine deficiency, which may respond to supplementation with pyridoxine, 50 to 150 mg orally each day. Occasionally, persons complain of feeling drunk or confused, perhaps indicating that the dosage should be reduced and then increased gradually. Reports that the hydrazine MAOIs are associated with hepatotoxic effects are relatively uncommon. MAOIs are less cardiotoxic and less epileptogenic than are the tricyclic and tetracyclic drugs.

The most common adverse effects of the RIMA moclobemide are dizziness, nausea, and insomnia or sleep disturbance. RIMAs cause fewer GI adverse effects than do SSRIs. Moclobemide does not have adverse anticholinergic or cardiovascular effects, and it has not been reported to interfere with sexual function.

MAOIs should be used with caution by persons with renal disease, cardiovascular disease, or hyperthyroidism. MAOIs may alter the dosage of a hypoglycemic agent required by diabetic persons. MAOIs have been particularly associated with induction of mania in persons in the depressed phase of bipolar I disorder and triggering of a psychotic decompensation in persons with schizophrenia.

Suicide Warning

As with all antidepressants, MAOIs have a black box warning, as they may cause an increase in suicidal ideation or actions in children, teenagers, and young adults even though they are not usually prescribed in this population. Suicidality is also more pronounced during the initial months of treatment and following changes in dosage.

Use in Pregnancy and Lactation

Little is known about the MAOIs during pregnancy. Data on their teratogenic risk are minimal. MAOIs should not be taken by nursing women because the drugs can pass into the breast milk. MAOIs are classified as pregnancy category C drugs.

Tyramine-Induced Hypertensive Crisis

The most worrisome side effect of MAOIs is the tyramine-induced hypertensive crisis. The amino acid tyramine is normally transformed via GI metabolism. However, MAOIs inactivate GI metabolism of dietary tyramine, thus allowing intact tyramine to enter circulation. A hypertensive crisis may subsequently occur as a result of a powerful pressor effect of the amino acid. Tyramine-containing foods should be avoided for 2 weeks after the last dose of an irreversible MAOI to allow resynthesis of adequate concentrations of MAO enzymes.

Accordingly, foods rich in tyramine (Table 26-1) or other sympathomimetic amines, such as ephedrine, pseudoephedrine (Sudafed), or dextromethorphan (Trocal), should be avoided by persons who are taking irreversible MAOIs. Patients should be advised to continue the dietary restrictions for 2 weeks after they stop MAOI treatment to allow the body to resynthesize the enzyme. Bee stings may also cause a hypertensive crisis. In addition to severe hypertension, other symptoms may include headache, stiff neck, diaphoresis, nausea, and vomiting. A patient with these symptoms should seek immediate medical treatment.

An MAOI-induced hypertensive crisis should be treated with α-adrenergic antagonists, such as phentolamine (Regitine) or chlorpromazine (Thorazine). These drugs lower blood pressure within 5 minutes. Intravenous furosemide (Lasix) can be used to reduce fluid load, and a β-adrenergic receptor antagonist can control tachycardia. A sublingual 10-mg dose of nifedipine (Procardia) can be given and repeated after 20 minutes. MAOIs should not be used by persons with thyrotoxicosis or pheochromocytoma.

The risk of tyramine-induced hypertensive crises is relatively low for persons who are taking RIMAs, such as moclobemide. These drugs have relatively little inhibitory activity for MAO_B, and because they are reversible, normal activity of existing MAO_A returns within 16 to 48 hours of the last dose of an RIMA. Therefore, the dietary restrictions are less stringent for RIMAs, applying only to foods containing high concentrations of tyramine, which need be avoided for 3 days after the last dose of an RIMA. A reasonable dietary recommendation for persons taking RIMAs is to avoid eating tyramine-containing foods 1 hour before and 2 hours after taking an RIMA.

Spontaneous, nontyramine-induced hypertensive crisis is a rare occurrence, usually shortly after the first exposure of an MAOI. Persons experiencing such a crisis should avoid MAOIs altogether.

TABLE 26-1: Tyramine-Rich Foods to Be Avoided in Planning MAOI Diets
High tyramine content[a] (≥2 mg of tyramine a serving)
Cheese: English Stilton, blue cheese, white (3 years old), extra old, old cheddar, Danish blue, mozzarella, cheese snack spreads
Fish, cured meats, sausage, and pâtés
Alcoholic beverages[b]: liqueurs and concentrated after-dinner drinks
Marmite (concentrated yeast extract)
Sauerkraut
Moderate tyramine content[a] (0.5–1.99 mg of tyramine a serving)
Cheese: Swiss Gruyere, muenster, feta, parmesan, gorgonzola, blue cheese dressing, Black Diamond
Fish, cured meats, sausage, and pâtés: chicken liver (5 days old), bologna, aged sausage, smoked meat, salmon mousse
Alcoholic beverages: beer and ale (12 oz per bottle) or Rioja red wine (4-oz glass)
Low tyramine content[a] (>0.5 mg of tyramine a serving)
Cheese: Brie, Camembert, Cambozola with or without rind
Fish, cured meat, sausage, and pâtés; pickled herring, smoked fish, kielbasa sausage, chicken liver (fresh), liverwurst (<2 days old)
Alcoholic beverages: most red wines (4-oz glass), sherry, scotch[c]
Others: banana or avocado (ripe or not), banana peel
[a]Any food left out to age or spoil can spontaneously develop tyramine through fermentation.
[b]Alcohol can produce profound orthostasis interacting with MAOIs but cannot produce direct hypotensive reactions.
[c]White wines, gin, and vodka have no tyramine content.
Table by Jonathan M. Himmelhoch, MD.
MAOI, monoamine oxidase inhibitor.

Withdrawal

Abrupt cessation of regular doses of MAOIs may cause a self-limited discontinuation syndrome consisting of arousal, mood disturbances, and somatic symptoms. To avoid these symptoms when discontinuing use of an MAOI, dosages should be gradually tapered over several weeks.

Overdose

There is often an asymptomatic period of 1 to 6 hours after an MAOI overdose before the occurrence of the symptoms of toxicity. MAOI overdose is characterized by agitation that can progress to coma with hyperthermia, hypertension, tachypnea, tachycardia, dilated pupils, and hyperactive deep tendon reflexes. Involuntary movements may be present, particularly in the face and the jaw. Acidification of the urine markedly hastens the excretion of MAOIs, and dialysis can be of some use. Phentolamine or chlorpromazine may be useful if hypertension is a problem. Moclobemide alone in overdosage causes relatively mild and reversible symptoms.

Drug Interactions

The major drug–drug and food–drug interactions involving MAOIs are listed in Table 26-2. Most antidepressants as well as precursor agents should be avoided. Persons should be instructed to tell any other physicians or dentists who are

TABLE 26-2: Drugs to Be Avoided During Monoamine Oxidase Inhibitor Treatment (Part of Listing)

Never Use

Antiasthmatics

Antihypertensives (methyldopa, guanethidine, reserpine)

Buspirone

Levodopa

Opioids (especially meperidine, dextromethorphan, propoxyphene, tramadol; morphine or codeine may be less dangerous.)

Cold, allergy, or sinus medications containing dextromethorphan or sympathomimetics

SSRIs, clomipramine, venlafaxine, sibutramine

Sympathomimetics (amphetamines, cocaine, methylphenidate, dopamine, epinephrine, norepinephrine, isoproterenol, ephedrine, pseudoephedrine, phenylpropanolamine)

L-Tryptophan

Use Carefully

Anticholinergics

Antihistamines

Disulfiram

Bromocriptine

Hydralazine

Sedative-hypnotics

Terpin hydrate with codeine

Tricyclics and tetracyclics (avoid clomipramine)

SSRI, selective serotonin reuptake inhibitor.

treating them that they are taking an MAOI. MAOIs may potentiate the action of CNS depressants, including alcohol and barbiturates. MAOIs should not be coadministered with serotonergic drugs, such as SSRIs and clomipramine (Anafranil), because this combination can trigger a serotonin syndrome. Use of lithium or tryptophan with an irreversible MAOI may also induce a serotonin syndrome. Initial symptoms of a serotonin syndrome can include tremor, hypertonicity, myoclonus, and autonomic signs, which can then progress to hallucinosis, hyperthermia, and even death. Fatal reactions have occurred when MAOIs were combined with meperidine (Demerol), methadone, or fentanyl (Sublimaze).

When switching from an irreversible MAOI to any other type of antidepressant drug, persons should wait at least 14 days after the last dose of the MAOI before beginning use of the next drug to allow replenishment of the body's MAOs. When switching from an antidepressant to an irreversible MAOI, persons should wait 10 to 14 days (or 5 weeks for fluoxetine [Prozac]) before starting use of the MAOI to avoid drug–drug interactions. In contrast, MAO activity recovers completely 24 to 48 hours after the last dose of an RIMA.

Considering the recent interest in psychedelic drugs and their potential use in psychiatric conditions, it is important to note that they should not be taken by patients being treated with MAOIs. Patients should taper MAOI use, and then wait for 14 days after their final dose before administration of any psychedelic drug. This topic is explored in greater depth in Chapter 31.

The effects of the MAOIs on hepatic enzymes are poorly studied. Tranyl-cypromine inhibits CYP2C19. Moclobemide inhibits CYP2D6, CYP2C19, and CYP1A2 and is a substrate for 2C19.

Cimetidine (Tagamet) and fluoxetine significantly reduce the elimination of moclobemide. Modest doses of fluoxetine and moclobemide administered concurrently may be well tolerated, with no significant pharmacodynamic or pharmacokinetic interactions.

Laboratory Interferences

MAOIs may lower blood glucose concentrations. MAOIs artificially raise urinary metanephrine concentrations and may cause a false-positive test result for pheochromocytoma or neuroblastoma. MAOIs have been reported to be associated with a minimal false elevation in thyroid function test results.

Dosage and Clinical Guidelines

There is no definitive rationale for choosing one irreversible MAOI over another. Table 26-3 lists MAOI preparations and typical dosages. Phenelzine use should begin with a test dose of 15 mg on the first day. The dosage can be increased to 15 mg three times daily during the first week and increased by 15 mg a day each week thereafter until the dosage of 90 mg a day, in divided doses, is reached by the end of the fourth week. Tranylcypromine and isocarboxazid use should begin with a test dosage of 10 mg and may be increased to 10 mg three times daily by the end of the first week. Many clinicians and researchers have recommended upper limits of 50 mg a day for isocarboxazid and 40 mg a day for

TABLE 26-3: Selectivity, Reversibility, Typical Dosage Forms, and Recommended Dosages for Currently Available Monoamine Oxidase Inhibitors

Drug	Selectivity/ Reversibility	Usual Dose (mg/day)	Maximum Dose (mg/day)	Dosage Formulation
Isocarboxazid (Marplan)	MAO-A and MAO-B/irreversible	20–40	60	10-mg tablets (oral)
Phenelzine (Nardil)	MAO-A and MAO-B/irreversible	30–60	90	15-mg tablets (oral)
Tranylcypromine (Parnate)	MAO-A and MAO-B/irreversible	20–60	60	10-mg tablets (oral)
Rasagiline (Azilect)[a]	MAO-B/irreversible	0.5–1.0	1.0	0.5- or 1.0-mg tablets (oral)
Selegiline (Eldepryl)	MAO-B/irreversible	10	30	5-mg tablets (oral)
Selegiline (Emsam)	MAO-B/irreversible	6–12	12	6-, 9-, and 12-mg patches (transdermal)
Moclobemide (Manerix)[b]	MAO-A/reversible	300–600	600	100- or 150-mg tablets (oral)

[a]Indicated for Parkinson disease.
[b]Not available in the United States but indicated for depression in countries where it is available.

tranylcypromine. Administration of tranylcypromine in multiple small daily doses may reduce its hypotensive effects.

A transdermal patch containing selegiline is available in dosages of 6, 9, and 12 mg per patch and sold under the trade name Emsam. Patches should be applied to dry, intact skin. Patients should only apply one patch per day, preferably at the same time each day. The starting dose of the patch is usually 6 mg that can be increased by 3 mg/24 hours after 2 weeks at one treatment but should not exceed 12 mg/24 hours.

Even though coadministration of MAOIs with TCAs, SSRIs, or lithium is generally contraindicated, these combinations have been used successfully and safely to treat patients with refractory depression. However, they should be used with extreme caution.

Hepatic transaminase serum concentrations should be monitored periodically because of the potential for hepatotoxicity, especially with phenelzine and isocarboxazid. Elderly persons may be more sensitive to MAOI adverse effects than are younger adults. MAO activity increases with age, so MAOI dosages for elderly persons are the same as those required for younger adults. The use of MAOIs in children has not been extensively studied.

There have been studies that suggest transdermal selegiline has antidepressant properties. Although selegiline is a type B inhibitor at low doses, as the dose is increased, it becomes less selective.

Table 26-4 summarizes the reversibility, selectivity, and indications for MAOIs.

TABLE 26-4: Classification of Monoamine Oxidase Inhibitors

Drug	Reversibility	Selectivity	Indication
Iproniazid[a] (Marsilid)	Irreversible	MAO-A MAO-B	Depression
Isocarboxazid (Marplan)	Irreversible	MAO-A MAO-B	Depression
Phenelzine (Nardil)	Irreversible	MAO-A MAO-B	Depression
Tranylcypromine (Parnate)	Irreversible	MAO-A MAO-B	Depression
Isoniazid (Nydrazid)	Irreversible	MAO-A MAO-B	Antituberculosis
Nialamide[a] (Niamid)	Irreversible	MAO-A MAO-B	Depression
Procarbazine (Matulane)	Weak irreversible	MAO-A MAO-B	Antineoplastic
Clorgyline[b]	Irreversible	MAO-A only	Depression
Selegiline (Eldepryl, Emsam)	Irreversible	MAO-B only	Depression, Parkinson disease
Rasagiline (Azilect)	Irreversible	MAO-B only	Parkinson disease
Pargyline[a] (Eutonyl)	Irreversible	MAO-B only	Antihypertensive
Linezolid	Reversible	MAO-A MAO-B	Antibiotic

TABLE 26-4: Classification of Monoamine Oxidase Inhibitors *(continued)*			
Drug	Reversibility	Selectivity	Indication
Lazabemide[c] (Pakio)	Reversible	MAO-B only	Parkinson disease
Moclobemide[c] (Aurorix/Manerix)	Reversible	MAO-A only	Depression
Brofaromine[a] (Consonar)	Reversible	MAO-A only	Depression
Befloxatone[a] (Synthelabo)	Reversible	MAO-A only	Depression
Pirlindole[c] (Pirazidol)	Reversible	MAO-A only	Depression
Toloxatone[a] (Humoryl)	Reversible	MAO-A only	Depression

[a]Discontinued.
[b]Used in research only.
[c]Available outside the United States only.
Borrowed from Sadock BJ, Sadock VA, Kaplan HI, eds. *Kaplan & Sadock's Comprehensive Textbook of Psychiatry*. 10th ed. Philadelphia, PA: Lippincott Williams & Wilkins; 2017.

27 Nefazodone and Trazodone

Generic Name	Trade Name	Adverse Effects	Drug Interactions	CYP Interactions
Nefazodone	Serzone	Suicidality, tachycardia, confusion, dizziness, sedation, fatigue, headache	CNS, SERO, MAOI, LITH, haloperidol, digoxin	3A4, 2D6
Trazodone	Desyrel, Oleptro	Suicidality, sedation, GI symptoms, agitation, hypotension, insomnia, confusion, tachycardia, headache	CNS, SERO, TRI, MAOI, digoxin, phenytoin	3A4, 3A5, 3A7, 2D6

Introduction

The drugs nefazodone (Serzone) and trazodone (Desyrel, Oleptro) are approved as treatments for depression with similar mechanisms of action and are structurally similar, as nefazodone is a structural analogue of trazodone. Though the two drugs have differing pharmacologic properties, they both have demonstrated antagonistic activity at serotonin type 2A (5-HT$_{2A}$) receptors. This is believed to account for their antidepressant effects.

Trazodone was the first of these drugs to be introduced, in 1981. Because of its generally benign side-effect profile, there were high expectations that it would replace older drugs as a mainstay of treatment for depression. However, the extreme sedation associated with trazodone, even at subtherapeutic doses, limited the clinical effectiveness of the drug, though it did make trazodone a favorite off-label alternative to standard hypnotics as a sleep-inducing agent. It is also used off-label for bulimia, anxiety, substance abuse, Alzheimer disease, and fibromyalgia. Unlike conventional sleeping pills, trazodone is not a controlled substance. In 2010, the Food and Drug Administration (FDA) approved an extended-release, once-daily formulation (Oleptro) as a treatment for major depressive disorder (MDD) in adults. In the trial leading to the approval of the extended-release formulation, the most common adverse events were somnolence or sedation, dizziness, constipation, and blurred vision.

Nefazodone is an analog of trazodone. When nefazodone was introduced in 1995, there were expectations that it would become widely used because it did not cause the sexual side effects and sleep disruption associated with the selective serotonin reuptake inhibitors (SSRIs). Although it was devoid of these side effects, it was nevertheless found to produce problematic sedation, nausea, dizziness, and visual disturbances. Consequently, nefazodone was never extensively adopted in clinical practice. This fact, as well as reports of rare cases of sometimes fatal hepatotoxicity, led the original manufacturer to discontinue production of branded nefazodone in 2004. Generic nefazodone remains available in the US market though its clinical utilization continues to decline. Sales of nefazodone in Canada were discontinued in 2003.

NEFAZODONE

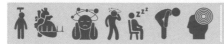

| CNS | SERO | MAOI | LITH | | 3A4 |
| haloperidol, digoxin | | | | | 2D6 |

Pharmacologic Actions

Nefazodone is rapidly and completely absorbed. The drug is extensively metabolized in the liver primarily by cytochrome P450 isoenzyme CYP3A4 so that the bioavailability of active compounds is only about 20% of the oral dose. Approximately 1% is excreted in urine unchanged. Its half-life is 2 to 4 hours. Steady-state concentrations of nefazodone and its principal active metabolite, hydroxynefazodone, are achieved within 4 to 5 days. Metabolism of nefazodone in elderly persons, especially women, is about half of that seen in younger persons, so lowered doses are recommended for this population. An important metabolite of nefazodone is meta-chlorophenylpiperazine (mCPP), which has some serotonergic effects and may cause migraine, anxiety, and weight loss.

Although nefazodone is an inhibitor of serotonin uptake and, to a lesser extent, of norepinephrine reuptake, its antagonism of serotonin 5-HT$_{2A}$ receptors is thought to produce its antianxiety and antidepressant effects. Nefazodone is also a mild antagonist of the α_1-adrenergic receptors, which predisposes some persons to orthostatic hypotension but is not sufficiently potent to produce priapism.

Therapeutic Indications

Nefazodone is effective for the treatment of major depression. The usual effective dosage is 300 to 600 mg a day. In direct comparison with SSRIs, nefazodone is less likely to cause inhibition of orgasm or decreased sexual desire.

Off-Label Uses

There is some evidence that nefazodone can be effective for the treatment of panic disorder and panic with comorbid depression or depressive symptoms, generalized anxiety disorder, and premenstrual dysphoric disorder. At this time, no controlled studies have been conducted to properly assess the efficacy of nefazodone in treating these conditions. Nefazodone is also of use in patients with posttraumatic stress disorder (PTSD) and chronic fatigue syndrome. It may also be effective in patients who have been treatment-resistant to other antidepressant drugs or those who have depression with comorbid insomnia because nefazodone increases rapid eye movement (REM) sleep and increases sleep continuity.

There is also evidence that chronic administration of nefazodone can induce antinociceptive effects and that it may be effective in the prophylaxis of chronic headaches.

Nefazodone is not effective for the treatment of obsessive-compulsive disorder.

Precautions and Adverse Reactions

The most common reasons for discontinuing nefazodone use are sedation, nausea, dizziness, insomnia, weakness, and agitation (see Table 27-1). Many patients

TABLE 27-1: Adverse Reactions Reported with Nefazodone (300 to 600 mg a Day)

Reaction	Patients (%)
Headache	36
Dry mouth	25
Somnolence	25
Nausea	22
Dizziness	17
Constipation	14
Insomnia	11
Weakness	11
Lightheadedness	10
Blurred vision	9
Dyspepsia	9
Infection	8
Confusion	7
Scotomata	7

report no specific side effect but describe a vague sense of feeling medicated. Nefazodone also causes visual trails, in which patients see an afterimage when looking at moving objects or when moving their heads quickly.

Some patients taking nefazodone may experience a decrease in blood pressure that can cause episodes of postural hypotension. Nefazodone should therefore be used with caution by persons with underlying cardiac conditions or history of stroke or heart attack, dehydration, or hypovolemia or by persons being treated with antihypertensive medications. Patients switched from SSRIs to nefazodone may experience an increase in side effects, possibly because nefazodone does not protect against SSRI withdrawal symptoms. One of its metabolites, mCPP, may actually intensify these discontinuation symptoms.

Patients have survived nefazodone overdoses in excess of 10 g, but deaths have been reported when it has been combined with alcohol. Nausea, vomiting, and somnolence are the most common signs of toxicity. The nefazodone dosage should be lowered in persons with severe hepatic disease, but no adjustment is necessary in persons with renal disease.

Liver Failure

A major safety concern with the use of nefazodone is severe elevation of hepatic enzymes, and, in some instances, liver failure. Accordingly, serial hepatic function tests need to be done when patients are treated with nefazodone. Hepatic effects can be seen early in treatment and are more likely to develop when nefazodone is combined with other drugs metabolized in the liver.

Suicide Warning

As with all antidepressants, nefazodone has a black box warning because it may cause an increase in suicidal ideation or actions in children, teenagers, and young adults. Suicidality is also more pronounced during the initial months of treatment and following changes in dosage.

Use in Pregnancy and Lactation

The effects of nefazodone in human mothers are not as well understood as those of the SSRIs, mainly due to the paucity of its clinical use. Nefazodone should therefore be used during pregnancy only if the potential benefit to the mother outweighs the potential risks to the fetus. It is not known whether nefazodone is excreted in human breast milk and should be used with caution by lactating mothers.

Nefazodone is classified as a pregnancy category C drug.

Drug Interactions

Nefazodone should not be given concomitantly with monoamine oxidase inhibitors (MAOIs). In addition, nefazodone has particular drug–drug interactions with the triazolobenzodiazepines, triazolam (Halcion), and alprazolam (Xanax) because of the inhibition of CYP3A4 by nefazodone. Potentially elevated levels of each of these drugs can develop after administration of nefazodone, but the levels of nefazodone are generally not affected. The dose of triazolam should be lowered by 75% and the dose of alprazolam should be lowered by 50% when given concomitantly with nefazodone.

Nefazodone may slow the metabolism of digoxin; therefore, digoxin levels should be monitored carefully in persons taking both medications. Nefazodone also slows the metabolism of haloperidol (Haldol) so that the dosage of haloperidol should be reduced in persons taking both medications. Addition of nefazodone may also exacerbate the adverse effects of lithium carbonate (Eskalith).

Patients can develop serotonin syndrome when nefazodone is taken in conjunction with other serotonergic agents. Symptoms of serotonin syndrome include confusion, agitation, difficulty thinking, coordination problems, hallucinations, twitching, and coma. Patients may also experience significant blood pressure changes (increases or decreases), stiffened muscles, tachycardia, fever, sweating, nausea, vomiting, and diarrhea.

Laboratory Interferences

There are no known laboratory interferences associated with nefazodone.

Dosage and Clinical Guidelines

Nefazodone is available in 50-, 200-, and 250-mg unscored tablets and 100- and 150-mg scored tablets. Dosage guidelines are outlined in Table 27-2. The recommended starting dosage of nefazodone is 100 mg twice a day, but 50 mg twice a day may be better tolerated, especially by elderly persons. To limit the development of adverse effects, the dosage should be slowly raised in increments of 100 to 200 mg a day at intervals of no less than 1 week per increase.

TABLE 27-2: Dosing Guidelines for Nefazodone

	Adults	Older Adults
Initial dosage	200 mg per day in two divided doses	100 mg per day in two divided doses
Titration rate	100–200 mg per day; changes should occur at intervals of no less than 1 week	50–100 mg per day; changes should occur at intervals of no less than 1 week
Maintenance dosage	300–600 mg per day	200–400 mg per day

The optimal dosage is 300 to 600 mg daily in two divided doses. However, some studies report that nefazodone is effective when taken once a day, especially at bedtime. Geriatric persons should receive dosages about two-thirds of the usual nongeriatric dosages, with a maximum of 400 mg a day.

Similar to other antidepressants, clinical benefit of nefazodone usually appears after 2 to 4 weeks of treatment. Patients with premenstrual syndrome are treated with a flexible dosage that averages about 250 mg a day.

TRAZODONE

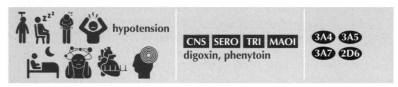

hypotension

CNS SERO TRI MAOI
digoxin, phenytoin

3A4 3A5 3A7 2D6

Pharmacologic Actions

Trazodone is readily absorbed from the gastrointestinal tract and reaches peak plasma levels in about 1 hour. It has a half-life of 5 to 9 hours. Trazodone is metabolized in the liver primarily by cytochrome P450 isoenzyme CYP3A4, and 75% of its metabolites are excreted in the urine.

Trazodone is a weak inhibitor of serotonin reuptake and a potent antagonist of serotonin 5-HT$_{2A}$ and 5-HT$_{2C}$ receptors. The active metabolite of trazodone is mCPP, which is an agonist at 5-HT$_{2C}$ receptors and has a half-life of 14 hours. mCPP has been associated with migraine, anxiety, and weight loss. The adverse effects of trazodone are partially mediated by α_1-adrenergic receptor antagonism.

Therapeutic Indications

The main indication for the use of trazodone is MDD. There is a clear dose–response relationship, with dosages of 250 to 600 mg a day necessary to have therapeutic benefit. Trazodone increases total sleep time, decreases the number and the duration of nighttime awakenings, and decreases the amount of REM sleep. Unlike tricyclic drugs, trazodone does not decrease stage 4 sleep. Therefore, it is useful for depressed persons with anxiety and insomnia.

Off-Label Uses

Insomnia

Trazodone is a first-line agent for the treatment of insomnia in patients with and without concurrent depression because of its marked sedative qualities and favorable effects on sleep architecture combined with its lack of anticholinergic effects but is not approved by the FDA for this indication. Trazodone is effective for insomnia caused by depression or use of drugs. When used as a hypnotic, the usual initial dosage is 25 to 100 mg at bedtime.

Erectile Disorder

Trazodone is associated with an increased risk of priapism and can potentiate erections resulting from sexual stimulation. It has thus been used to prolong erectile time and turgidity in some men with erectile disorder. The dosage for this indication is 150 to 200 mg a day. Trazodone-triggered priapism (an erection lasting more than 3 hours with pain) is a medical emergency. The use of trazodone for treatment of male erectile dysfunction has diminished considerably since the introduction of phosphodiesterase type 5 (PDE5) agents (see Chapter 30).

Other Indications

Trazodone may be useful in low dosages (50 mg a day) for controlling severe agitation in children with developmental disabilities and elderly persons with dementia. At dosages above 250 mg a day, trazodone reduces the tension and apprehension associated with generalized anxiety disorder. It has been used to treat depression in schizophrenic patients. Trazodone may have a beneficial effect on insomnia and nightmares in persons with PTSD. Some evidence suggests that trazodone may reduce the frequency of binge eating and vomiting episodes in individuals with bulimia nervosa. An open-label study showed that trazodone was effective at improving sleep quality and some quality-of-life issues in patients with fibromyalgia.

Precautions and Adverse Reactions

The most common adverse effects associated with trazodone are sedation, orthostatic hypotension, dizziness, headache, and nausea (see Table 27-3). Some persons experience dry mouth or gastric irritation. The drug is not associated with anticholinergic adverse effects, such as urinary retention, weight gain, and constipation. A few case reports have noted an association between trazodone and arrhythmias in persons with preexisting premature ventricular contractions or mitral valve prolapse. Neutropenia, usually not of clinical significance, may develop, which should be considered if persons have fever or sore throat.

Trazodone may cause significant orthostatic hypotension 4 to 6 hours after a dose is taken, especially if taken concurrently with antihypertensive agents or if a large dose is taken without food. Administration of trazodone with food slows absorption and reduces the peak plasma concentration, thus reducing the risk of orthostatic hypotension.

Trazodone causes priapism, prolonged erection in the absence of sexual stimuli, in 1 of every 10,000 men. Trazodone-induced priapism usually appears

TABLE 27-3: Adverse Reactions Reported with Trazodone
Blurred vision
Constipation
Dry mouth
Tachycardia/Palpitations
Confusion
Dizziness
Drowsiness
Fatigue
Headache
Insomnia
Nervousness
Nausea/Vomiting
Nasal/Sinus congestion
Nightmares/Vivid dreams

in the first 4 weeks of treatment but may occur as late as 18 months into treatment and can occur at any dose. Use of trazodone should be discontinued, and the patient should be switched to another antidepressant. Painful erections or erections lasting more than 1 hour are warning signs that warrant immediate discontinuation of the drug and medical evaluation. The first step in the emergency management of priapism is intracavernosal injection of an α_1-adrenergic agonist pressor agent, such as metaraminol (Aramine) or epinephrine. In about one-third of reported cases, surgical intervention is required, and sometimes permanent impairment of erectile function or impotence may result.

Trazodone should be used with caution in persons with hepatic and renal diseases.

Trazodone Intoxication

Because suicide attempts often involve ingestion of sleeping pills, it is important to be familiar with the symptoms and treatment of trazodone overdose. Patients have survived trazodone overdoses of more than 9 g. Symptoms of overdose include lethargy, vomiting, drowsiness, headache, orthostasis, dizziness, dyspnea, tinnitus, myalgias, tachycardia, incontinence, shivering, and coma. Treatment consists of emesis or lavage and supportive care. Forced diuresis may enhance elimination. In addition, hypotension and sedation should be managed appropriately.

Suicide Warning

As with all antidepressants, trazodone has a black box warning because it may cause an increase in suicidal ideation or actions in children, teenagers, and young adults. Suicidality is also more pronounced during the initial months of treatment and following changes in dosage.

Use in Pregnancy and Lactation

This drug should only be used in pregnancy if the potential benefit justifies the possible risk to the fetus. Very small amounts of trazodone are excreted in human breast milk. Trazodone is a pregnancy category C drug.

Drug Interactions

Trazodone potentiates the central nervous system depressant effects of other centrally acting drugs and alcohol. Concurrent use of trazodone and antihypertensives may cause hypotension. No cases of hypertensive crisis have been reported when trazodone has been used to treat MAOI-associated insomnia. Trazodone can increase levels of digoxin and phenytoin. Trazodone should be used with caution in combination with warfarin. Drugs that inhibit CYP3A4 can increase levels of trazodone's major metabolite, mCPP, leading to an increase in side effects.

Some patients may develop serotonin syndrome or neuroleptic malignant syndrome (NMS)-like reactions with trazodone treatment, particularly if used in conjunction with other serotoninergic drugs (including SSRIs, SNRIs, and triptans) and with drugs that impair metabolism of serotonin (including MAOIs), or with antipsychotics or other dopamine antagonists. Symptoms of serotonin syndrome include confusion, agitation, difficulty thinking, coordination problems, hallucinations, twitching, and coma. Patients may also experience significant blood pressure changes (increases or decreases), stiffened muscles, tachycardia, fever, sweating, nausea, vomiting, and diarrhea.

Laboratory Interferences

No known laboratory interferences are associated with the administration of trazodone.

Dosage and Clinical Guidelines

Trazodone is available in 50-, 100-, 150-, and 300-mg tablets. An outline of the dosing guidelines can be found in Table 27-4. Once-a-day dosing is as effective as divided doses and reduces daytime sedation. The usual starting dose is 150 mg in divided doses, with first dose at bedtime. The dosage can be increased in increments of 50 mg every 3 to 4 days unless patient experiences excessive sedation or orthostatic hypotension. The therapeutic range for trazodone is 200 to 600 mg a day in divided doses. Some reports indicate that dosages of 400 to 600 mg a day are required for maximal therapeutic effects, particularly in inpatient settings;

TABLE 27-4: Dosing Guidelines for Trazodone		
	Tablets	Extended Release
Initial dosage	150 mg/day, given in divided doses	150 mg per day once daily
Titration rate	50 mg per day every 3–4 days	75 mg per day every 3–4 days
Maintenance dosage	250–600 mg per day, given in divided doses	150–375 mg per day
Maximum dosage	600 mg per day	375 mg per day

other reports indicate that a more modest range of 250 to 400 mg a day is sufficient, particularly in outpatient settings. The dosage may be titrated up to 300 mg a day; thereafter the person can be evaluated for further dosage increases based on clinical improvement.

Once-daily trazodone marketed under the name Oleptro is available as bisectable tablets of 150 mg or 300 mg. The starting dosage of the extended-release formulation is 150 mg once daily. It may be increased by 75 mg per day every 3 days. The maximum dosage is 375 mg per day. Dosing should be at the same time every day in the late evening, preferably at bedtime, on an empty stomach. Tablets should be swallowed whole or broken in half along the score line.

Opioid Receptor Agonists: Methadone, Buprenorphine, and Tramadol

28

Generic Name	Trade Name	Adverse Effects	Drug Interactions	CYP Interactions
Methadone	N/A	Sedation, dizziness, insomnia, GI symptoms, weight gain, sexual dysfunction, agitation, seizures, respiratory depression	CNS, DRA, TRI/ TET, MAOI, Anticholinergics, muscle relaxants	3A4, 2B6, 2C19, 2C9, 2C8, 2D6, 3A7, 2C18
Buprenorphine	Buprenex	Sedation, dizziness, insomnia, GI symptoms, weight gain, sexual dysfunction, agitation, seizures, respiratory depression	CNS, DRA, TRI/ TET, MAOI, Anticholinergics, muscle relaxants	3A4, 3A5, 2C9, 2C8, 3A7, 2D6, 2C18, 2C19
Tramadol	Ultram	Sedation, dizziness, insomnia, GI symptoms, weight gain, sexual dysfunction, agitation, seizures, respiratory depression	CNS, DRA, SERO, TRI/TET, MAOI, Anticholinergics, muscle relaxants	2D6, 3A4, 2B6

Introduction

Opioid receptor agonists have been used for millennia to provide pain management. While highly effective as analgesics, they often cause dependence and are frequently diverted for recreational use and rates of death from overdose of opioids has reached epidemic proportions throughout the United States. The number of synthetic opioid receptor agonist overdoses in the United States in 2021 was estimated to be 71,238—up from 57,834 just a year earlier.

Commonly used opioid agonists for pain relief include morphine, hydromorphone (Dilaudid), codeine, meperidine (Demerol), oxycodone (OxyContin), buprenorphine (Buprenex), hydrocodone (Robidone), tramadol (Ultram), and fentanyl (Duragesic). Though heroin was introduced as a pharmaceutical by Bayer in 1898, it is now solely used as an illicit drug. Methadone is used both for pain management and for treatment of opiate addiction. The efficacy of opioid agonist medications, such as methadone and buprenorphine, has been clearly established in the treatment of opioid dependence.

There are multiple types of opioid receptors, with μ- and κ-opioid receptors representing functionally opposing endogenous systems (Table 28-1). All the compounds noted above, which represent the most extensively used opioid analgesics, are agonists at μ-opioid receptors. However, analgesic and antidepressant effects also result from antagonist effects on the κ-opioid receptor. This chapter focuses on the μ-opioid receptor agonists, drugs that are most likely to be used in the treatment of pain management, but κ-opioid receptor antagonism has been shown to have antidepressant activity.

TABLE 28-1: Agonist and Antagonist Effects at Opiate Receptors		
Receptor	Agonist Effects	Antagonist Effects
Mu (μ)	Analgesia	Anxiety
	Euphoria	Hostility
	Antidepressant	
	Anxiety	
Kappa (κ)	Analgesia	Antidepressant
	Dysphoria	
	Depression	
	Stress-induced anxiety	

While there is growing interest in the use of some drugs that act on opioid receptors as alternative treatments for a subpopulation of patients with refractory depression, as well as treatment for cutting behavior in patients with borderline personality disorder, no medications have been indicated for these purposes at this time. A drug that combines buprenorphine and samidorphan, which is also an opioid receptor ligand, has been proposed as a potential add-on to antidepressants in treatment-resistant depression, but a panel from the Food and Drug Administration (FDA) voted against approval in 2018.

Before using opioid receptor agonists with patients who have failed on multiple conventional therapeutic agents, clinicians should carefully screen for history of drug abuse, document the rationale for off-label use, establish treatment ground rules, obtain written consent, consult with primary care physician, and monitor closely. Consideration of off-label use should always consider that ongoing, regular use of opioids produces dependence and tolerance and may lead to maladaptive use, functional impairment, withdrawal symptoms, and death. Avoid replacing "lost" prescriptions and providing early prescription renewals.

Pharmacologic Actions

Methadone and buprenorphine are absorbed rapidly from the gastrointestinal (GI) tract. Hepatic first-pass metabolism significantly affects the bioavailability of each of the drugs but in markedly different ways. For methadone, hepatic enzymes reduce the bioavailability of an oral dosage by about half, an effect that is easily managed with dosage adjustments.

For buprenorphine, first-pass intestinal and hepatic metabolism eliminates oral bioavailability almost completely. When used in opioid detoxification, buprenorphine is given sublingually in either a liquid or a tablet formulation.

The peak plasma concentrations of oral methadone are reached within 2 to 6 hours, and the plasma half-life is 4 to 6 hours initially in opioid-naive persons and 24 to 36 hours after steady dosing of any type of opioid. Methadone is highly protein bound and equilibrates widely throughout the body, which ensures little postdosage variation in steady-state plasma concentrations. In opioid-naïve patients, methadone can be lethal in relatively small doses.

Elimination of a sublingual dosage of buprenorphine occurs in two phases: an initial phase with a half-life of 3 to 5 hours and a terminal phase with a half-life of more than 24 hours. Buprenorphine dissociates from its receptor binding site slowly, which permits an every-other-day dosing schedule.

Methadone acts as pure agonists at μ-opioid receptors and has negligible agonist or antagonist activity at κ- or δ-opioid receptors. Buprenorphine is a partial agonist at μ-receptors, a potent antagonist at κ-receptors, and neither an agonist nor an antagonist at δ-receptors.

Tramadol has a more complex pharmacology. It is a weak μ-opioid receptor agonist, a 5-HT–releasing agent, a DA-releasing agent, a 5-HT_{2C} receptor antagonist, an NE reuptake inhibitor, an NMDA receptor antagonist, a nicotinic acetylcholine receptor antagonist, a TRPV1 receptor agonist, and M_1 and M_3 muscarinic acetylcholine receptor antagonist.

Other relevant properties of tramadol are its relatively long half-life, which reduces the potential for misuse. Its habituating effects are found to be much less than other opiate agonists, but abuse, withdrawal, and dependence are risks. Tramadol requires the patient metabolized the drug to exhibit analgesic properties: individuals who are CYP2D6 "poor metabolizers," or use drugs that are CYP2D6 inhibitors reduce the efficacy of tramadol (the same is true of codeine).

Therapeutic Indications

At this time, the only psychiatric indication for any opioid agonist is for the treatment of opioid addiction.

METHADONE

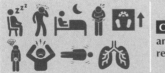

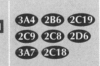

CNS | DRA | TRI/TET | MAOI
anticholinergics, muscle relaxants

3A4 | 2B6 | 2C19
2C9 | 2C8 | 2D6
3A7 | 2C18

Methadone is used for short-term detoxification (7 to 30 days), long-term detoxification (up to 180 days), and maintenance (treatment beyond 180 days) of opioid-dependent individuals. For these purposes, it is only available through designated clinics called methadone maintenance treatment programs (MMTPs) and in hospitals and prisons. Methadone is a schedule II drug, which means that its administration is tightly governed by specific federal laws and regulations.

Prior to the ascendency of fentanyl, studies showed that enrollment in a methadone program had numerous benefits for individuals with opioid use disorder and reduced the risk of death by 70%. It is unclear if this figure is still accurate, but studies indicate that many of the same benefits from before the fentanyl era still apply. Enrollment in methadone programs reduces illicit use of opioids and other substances of abuse; reduces criminal activity; reduces the risk of infectious diseases of all types, most importantly HIV and hepatitis B and C infection; and in pregnant women, reduces the risk of fetal and neonatal morbidity and mortality. However, it should be noted that the use of methadone maintenance frequently requires lifelong treatment.

Some opioid-dependence treatment programs use a stepwise detoxification protocol in which a person addicted to heroin switches first to the strong agonist methadone, then to the weaker agonist buprenorphine, and then finally to maintenance on an opioid receptor antagonist, such as naltrexone (ReVia). This approach minimizes the appearance of opioid withdrawal effects, which, if they occur, are mitigated with clonidine (Catapres). However, compliance with opioid receptor antagonist treatment is poor in the absence of intensive cognitive-behavioral techniques. In contrast, noncompliance with methadone maintenance precipitates opioid withdrawal symptoms, which serve to reinforce the use of methadone and make cognitive-behavioral therapy less than essential. Thus, some well-motivated, socially integrated former heroin addicts are able to use methadone for years without participation in a psychosocial support program.

Data pooled from many reports indicate that methadone is more effective when taken at dosages in excess of 60 mg a day.

The analgesic effects of methadone are sometimes used in the management of chronic pain when less addictive agents are ineffective.

BUPRENORPHINE

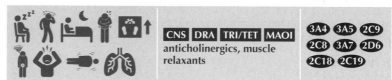

CNS | DRA | TRI/TET | MAOI
anticholinergics, muscle relaxants

3A4 3A5 2C9
2C8 3A7 2D6
2C18 2C19

The analgesic effects of buprenorphine are sometimes used in the management of chronic pain when less addictive agents are ineffective. Since buprenorphine is a partial agonist rather than a full agonist at the μ-receptor and is a weak antagonist at the κ-receptor, this agent produces a milder withdrawal syndrome and has a wider margin of safety than the full μ-agonist compounds generally used in treatment. Buprenorphine has a ceiling effect beyond which dose increases prolong the duration of action of the drug without further increasing the agonist effects. Because of this, buprenorphine has a high clinical safety profile, with limited respiratory depression, therefore decreasing the likelihood of lethal overdose. Buprenorphine does have the capacity to cause typical side effects associated with opioids, including sedation, nausea and vomiting, constipation, dizziness, headache, and sweating. A relevant pharmacokinetic consideration when using buprenorphine is the fact that it requires hepatic conversion to produce analgesia (*N*-dealkylation catalyzed by CYP3A4). This may explain why some patients do not benefit from buprenorphine. Genetics, grapefruit juice, and many medications (including fluoxetine and fluvoxamine) can reduce a person's ability to metabolize buprenorphine into its bioactive form.

To reduce the likelihood of abusing buprenorphine via the intravenous route, buprenorphine has been combined with the narcotic antagonist naloxone for sublingual administration. Because naloxone is poorly absorbed by the sublingual route, when the combination drug is taken sublingually, there is no effect of the naloxone on the efficacy of buprenorphine. If an opioid-dependent individual injects the combination medication, the naloxone precipitates a withdrawal reaction, therefore reducing the likelihood of illicit injection use of the sublingual preparation.

Inducting and stabilizing a patient on buprenorphine is analogous to inducting and stabilizing a patient on methadone except that, as a partial agonist, buprenorphine has the potential to cause precipitated withdrawal in patients who have recently taken full agonist opioids. Thus, a patient must abstain from the use of short-acting opioids for 12 to 24 hours before starting buprenorphine and from longer-acting opioids such as methadone for 24 to 48 hours or longer. The physician must assess the patient clinically and determine that the patient is in mild to moderate opioid withdrawal with objectively observable withdrawal signs before initiating buprenorphine.

In most instances, a relatively low dose of buprenorphine (2 to 4 mg) can then be administered with additional doses given in 1 to 2 hours if withdrawal signs persist. The goal for the first 24 hour is to suppress withdrawal signs and symptoms, and the total 24-hour dose to do so can range from 2 to 16 mg on the first day. In subsequent days, the dose can be adjusted upward or downward to resolve withdrawal fully and, as with methadone, to achieve an absence of craving, adequate tolerance to prevent reinforcement from the use of other opioids, and ultimately abstinence from other opioids while minimizing side effects. Dose-ranging studies have demonstrated that dosages of 6 to 16 mg per day are associated with improved treatment outcomes compared with lower doses of buprenorphine (1 to 4 mg). In some cases, patients seem to need dosages higher than 16 mg per day, but there is no evidence for any benefit of dosages beyond 32 mg per day.

For the treatment of opioid dependence, a dose of approximately 4 mg of sublingual buprenorphine is the equivalent of a daily dose of 40 mg of oral methadone. It has also been demonstrated that daily, alternate-day, or three-times-per-week administration have equivalent effects in suppressing the symptoms of opioid withdrawal in dependent individuals. The combination tablet is recommended for most clinical purposes, including induction and maintenance. The buprenorphine mono should be used only for pregnant patients or for patients who have a documented anaphylactic reaction to naloxone.

Newer forms of buprenorphine delivery, including a transdermal skin patch and a subcutaneous buprenorphine implant that may provide therapeutic plasma levels for 6 months, are being investigated. The latter delivery system could obviate the need for taking medications daily while virtually eliminating the risk of medication nonadherence.

A long-acting depot intramuscular injection of buprenorphine that provides therapeutic plasma levels is being marketed under the name Sublocade. It is a once-monthly injection that was approved for the treatment of moderate-to-severe opioid use disorder by the FDA in 2017.

Buprenorphine is a Schedule III drug.

TRAMADOL

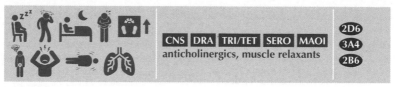

CNS	DRA	TRI/TET	SERO	MAOI	2D6
anticholinergics, muscle relaxants					3A4
					2B6

Tramadol is currently indicated to treat mild to severe pain, both acute and chronic. It is a Schedule IV drug.

Off-Label Use

There are multiple reports of tramadol's antidepressant effects, both as monotherapy and augmentation agent in treatment-resistant depression. Clinical and experimental data suggest that tramadol has an inherent antidepressant-like activity. Consistent with the evidence of its antidepressant effects is the fact that tramadol has a close structural similarity to the antidepressant venlafaxine.

Both venlafaxine and tramadol inhibit norepinephrine/serotonin reuptake and inhibit the reserpine-induced syndrome completely. Both compounds also have an analgesic effect on chronic pain. Venlafaxine may have an opioid component and naloxone reverses the antipain effect of venlafaxine. Nonopioid activity is demonstrated by the fact that its analgesic effect is not fully antagonized by the μ-opioid receptor antagonist naloxone. Indicative of their structural similarities, venlafaxine may cause false-positive results on liquid chromatography tests to detect urinary tramadol levels.

Precautions and Adverse Reactions

The most common adverse effects of opioid receptor agonists are lightheadedness, dizziness, sedation, nausea, constipation, vomiting, perspiration, weight gain, decreased libido, inhibition of orgasm, and insomnia or sleep irregularities. Opioid receptor agonists are capable of inducing tolerance as well as producing physiologic and psychological dependence. Other central nervous system (CNS) adverse effects include depression, sedation, euphoria, dysphoria, agitation, and seizures. Delirium has been reported in rare cases. Occasional non-CNS adverse effects include peripheral edema, urinary retention, rash, arthralgia, dry mouth, anorexia, biliary tract spasm, bradycardia, hypotension, hypoventilation, syncope, antidiuretic hormone–like activity, pruritus, urticaria, and visual disturbances. Menstrual irregularities are common in women, especially in the first 6 months of use. Various abnormal endocrine laboratory indexes of little clinical significance may also be seen.

Most persons develop tolerance to the pharmacologic adverse effects of opioid agonists during long-term maintenance, and relatively few adverse effects are experienced after the induction period.

Overdosage

The acute effects of opioid receptor agonist overdosage include sedation, hypotension, bradycardia, hypothermia, respiratory suppression, miosis, and decreased GI motility. Severe effects include coma, cardiac arrest, shock, and death. The risk of overdosage is greatest in the induction stage of treatment and in persons with slow drug metabolism caused by preexisting hepatic insufficiency. Deaths have been caused during the first week of induction by methadone dosages of only 50 to 60 mg a day.

The risk of overdosage with buprenorphine appears to be lower than with methadone, and the risk of overdose with tramadol appears to be ever lower but is still possible. In addition, deaths have occurred by use of buprenorphine in combination with benzodiazepines.

Withdrawal Symptoms

Abrupt cessation of opioid receptor agonists can induce severe withdrawal symptoms. Methadone cessation triggers withdrawal symptoms within 3 to 4 days, which usually reach peak intensity on day 6. Withdrawal symptoms include weakness, anxiety, anorexia, insomnia, gastric distress, headache, sweating, and hot and cold flashes. The withdrawal symptoms usually resolve after 2 weeks. However, a protracted methadone abstinence syndrome is possible that may include restlessness and insomnia.

The withdrawal symptoms associated with buprenorphine are similar to, but less marked than, those caused by methadone. In particular, buprenorphine is sometimes used to ease the transition from methadone to opioid receptor antagonists or abstinence because of the relatively mild withdrawal reaction associated with discontinuation of buprenorphine.

The withdrawal symptoms of tramadol are milder than either buprenorphine or methadone.

Use in Pregnancy and Lactation

Methadone maintenance, combined with effective psychosocial interventions and regular obstetric monitoring, significantly improves obstetric and neonatal outcomes for women addicted to heroin. Enrollment of a heroin-addicted pregnant woman in such a maintenance program reduces the risk of malnutrition, infection, preterm labor, spontaneous abortion, preeclampsia, eclampsia, abruptio placenta, and septic thrombophlebitis.

The dosage of methadone during pregnancy should be the lowest effective dosage, and no withdrawal to abstinence should be attempted during pregnancy. Methadone is metabolized more rapidly in the third trimester, which may necessitate higher dosages. To avoid potentially sedating postdose peak plasma concentrations, the daily dose can be administered in two divided doses during the third trimester. Methadone treatment has no known teratogenic effects.

Methadone, buprenorphine, and tramadol are all classified as a pregnancy category C drugs. Clinicians should be advised to avoid their use in pregnant or nursing women whenever possible.

Neonatal Opioid Withdrawal Symptoms

Withdrawal symptoms in newborns frequently include tremor, a high-pitched cry, increased muscle tone and activity, poor sleep and appetite, mottling, yawning, perspiration, and skin excoriation. Convulsions that require aggressive anticonvulsant therapy may also occur. Withdrawal symptoms may be delayed in onset and prolonged in neonates because of their immature hepatic metabolism.

Women taking methadone are sometimes counseled to initiate breastfeeding as a means of gently weaning their infants from methadone dependence, but they should not breastfeed their babies while still taking methadone.

Drug–Drug Interactions

Opioid receptor agonists can potentiate the CNS-depressant effects of alcohol, barbiturates, benzodiazepines, other opioids, low-potency dopamine receptor antagonists, tricyclic and tetracyclic drugs, and monoamine oxidase inhibitors (MAOIs). Carbamazepine (Tegretol), phenytoin (Dilantin), barbiturates, rifampin (Rimactane, Rifadin), and heavy long-term consumption of alcohol may induce hepatic enzymes, which may lower the plasma concentration of methadone, buprenorphine, or tramadol and thereby precipitate withdrawal symptoms. In contrast, hepatic enzyme induction may increase the plasma concentration of active levomethadyl metabolites and cause toxicity.

Acute opioid withdrawal symptoms may be precipitated in persons on methadone maintenance therapy who take pure opioid receptor antagonists such as naltrexone, nalmefene (Revex), and naloxone (Narcan); partial agonists such as buprenorphine; or mixed agonist–antagonists such as pentazocine (Talwin). These symptoms may be mitigated by use of clonidine, a benzodiazepine, or both.

Competitive inhibition of methadone or buprenorphine metabolism after short-term use of alcohol or administration of cimetidine (Tagamet), erythromycin, ketoconazole (Nizoral), fluoxetine (Prozac), fluvoxamine (Luvox), loratadine (Claritin), quinidine (Quinidex), and alprazolam (Xanax) may lead to higher plasma concentrations or a prolonged duration of action of methadone or buprenorphine. Medications that alkalinize the urine may reduce methadone excretion. Additional drug interactions are outlined in Table 28-2.

Methadone maintenance may also increase plasma concentrations of desipramine (Norpramin, Pertofrane) and fluvoxamine. Use of methadone may increase zidovudine (Retrovir) concentrations, which increases the possibility of zidovudine toxicity at otherwise standard dosages. Moreover, in vitro human liver microsome studies demonstrate competitive inhibition of methadone demethylation by several protease inhibitors, including ritonavir (Norvir), indinavir (Crixivan), and saquinavir (Invirase). The clinical relevance of this finding is unknown.

Fatal drug–drug interactions with the MAOIs are associated with use of the opioids fentanyl (Sublimaze) and meperidine (Demerol), but not with use of methadone, levomethadyl, or buprenorphine.

Tramadol may interact with drugs that inhibit serotonin reuptake. Such combinations can trigger seizures and serotonin syndrome. These events may also develop during tramadol monotherapy, either at routine or excessive doses. Risk of interactions is increased when tramadol is combined with virtually all classes of antidepressants and with drugs that lower the seizure threshold, especially the antidepressant bupropion.

TABLE 28-2: Potential Interactions Involving Buprenorphine and Other Classes of Drugs

Class of Drugs	Potential Interactions
Anticholinergics (e.g., benztropine, ipratropium bromide, tiotropium, trihexyphenidyl)	Urinary retention and/or severe constipation. In severe cases, patient may develop paralytic ileus.
Benzodiazepines (e.g., diazepam, alprazolam, clonazepam)	Misuse of buprenorphine (particularly via injection) in combination with benzodiazepines can result in coma or death due to decreased ceiling effects on buprenorphine-induced respiratory depression, as coadministration can mimic the respiratory effects of full mu opioid agonists. Dose reductions of one or both medications may be necessary.
Central nervous system depressants (e.g., alcohol, hypnotics, general anesthetics, other opioids, sedatives, tranquilizers)	Hypotension, severe sedation, respiratory depression, coma, and death.
CYP3A4 inducers (e.g., carbamazepine, phenobarbital, phenytoin, rifampicin)	May cause enhanced clearance of buprenorphine, resulting in decreased plasma concentrations, lack of efficacy, or even symptoms of withdrawal. Dose adjustments may be necessary.
CYP3A4 inhibitors (e.g., amitriptyline, azole, erythromycin, fluoxetine, fluvoxamine, ketoconazole)	May cause decreased clearance of buprenorphine, resulting in elevated plasma concentrations and prolonged or enhanced opioid effects. Monitor patients for excessive sedation or respiratory depression. Dose reduction of either buprenorphine or the CYP3A4 inhibitor may be required.
Nonbenzodiazepine muscle relaxants (e.g., carisoprodol, cyclobenzaprine)	Excessive respiratory depression.
Psychostimulants (e.g., cocaine)	Increased metabolism, resulting in diminished plasma concentrations of buprenorphine.

Opioid Receptor Agonists: Methadone, Buprenorphine, and Tramadol

Laboratory Interferences

Methadone and buprenorphine can be tested for separately in urine toxicology to distinguish them from other opioids. No known laboratory interferences are associated with the use of methadone or buprenorphine.

Dosage and Clinical Guidelines

Methadone

Methadone is supplied in 5-, 10-, and 40-mg dispersible scored tablets; 40-mg scored wafers; 5-mg/5-mL, 10-mg/5-mL, and 10-mg/mL solutions; and a 10-mg/mL parenteral form. In maintenance programs, methadone is usually dissolved in water or juice, and dose administration is directly observed to ensure compliance. For induction of opioid detoxification, an initial methadone dose of 15 to 20 mg will usually suppress craving and withdrawal symptoms. However, some individuals may require up to 40 mg a day in single or divided doses. Higher dosages should be avoided during induction of treatment to reduce the risk of acute toxicity from overdosage.

Over several weeks, the dosage should be raised to at least 70 mg a day. The maximum dosage is usually 120 mg a day, and higher dosages require prior approval from regulatory agencies. Dosages above 60 mg a day are associated with much more complete abstinence from use of illicit opioids than are dosages less than 60 mg a day.

The duration of treatment should not be predetermined but should be based on response to treatment and assessment of psychosocial factors. All studies of methadone maintenance programs endorse long-term treatment (i.e., several years) as more effective than short-term programs (i.e., less than 1 year) for prevention of relapse into opioid abuse. In actual practice, however, a minority of programs are permitted by policy or approved by insurers to provide even 6 months of continuous maintenance treatment. Moreover, some programs actually encourage withdrawal from methadone in less than 6 months after induction. This is quite ill conceived because more than 80% of persons who terminate methadone maintenance treatment eventually return to illicit drug use within 2 years. In programs that offer both maintenance and withdrawal treatments, the overwhelming majority of participants enroll in the maintenance treatment.

Buprenorphine

Buprenorphine is supplied as a 0.3-mg/mL solution in 1-mL ampules. Sublingual tablet formulations of buprenorphine containing buprenorphine only or buprenorphine combined with naloxone in a 4:1 ratio is used for opioid maintenance treatment. Other formulations are explored in Table 28-3. Buprenorphine is not used for short-term opioid detoxification. Maintenance dosages of 8 to 16 mg thrice weekly have effectively reduced heroin use.

Sublocade is prepared and injected into the abdomen of the patient by a health care provider once per month with a minimum of 26 days between doses. There are two dosages available, 100 mg/0.5 mL and 300 mg/1.5 mL. In both cases, the solution is provided in a prefilled syringe with a 19-gauge 5/8-inch needle.

Physicians must be trained and certified to carry out this therapy in their private offices. There are a number of approved training programs in the United States.

Tramadol

There are no controlled trials establishing the appropriate dosing schedule for tramadol when used for conditions other than pain. Tramadol is available in many formulations. These range from capsules (regular and extended release) to tablets (regular, extended release, chewable tablets) that can be taken sublingually, as suppositories, or injectable ampules. It also comes as tablets and capsules containing acetaminophen or aspirin. Doses reported in case reports of treatment for depression or obsessive-compulsive disorder range from 50 to 200 mg/day and involve short-term use. The long-term use of tramadol in the treatment of psychiatric disorders has not been studied.

TABLE 28-3: Buprenorphine Formulations

Product Name	Active Ingredients	Recommended Once-Daily Target Maintenance Dosage (mg)	Dosage Range (mg)	Available Strengths (mg)	Route of Administration
Bunavail	• Buprenorphine hydrochloride • Naloxone hydrochloride	8.4/1.4	2.1/0.3–12.6/2.1	2.1/0.3 4.2/0.7 6.3/1.0	Buccal film
Suboxone	• Buprenorphine hydrochloride • Naloxone hydrochloride	16/4	4/1–24/6	2.0/0.5 4/1 8/2 12/3	Sublingual film
Zubsolv	• Buprenorphine hydrochloride • Naloxone hydrochloride	11.4/2.9	2.9/0.71–17.2/4.2	1.4/0.36 2.9/0.71 5.7/1.4 8.6/2.1 11.4/2.9	Sublingual tablet
Generic	• Buprenorphine hydrochloride • Naloxone hydrochloride	16/4	4/1–24/6	2.0/0.5 8.0/2.0	Sublingual tablet
Generic	• Buprenorphine hydrochloride	16	4–24	2 8	Sublingual tablet

All ratios are listed as buprenorphine hydrochloride/naloxone hydrochloride and all units of measurement are in milligrams (mg). For example, "1.4/0.36" in the above chart translates into 1.4 mg of buprenorphine hydrochloride and 0.36 mg of naloxone hydrochloride.

Opioid Receptor Agonists: Methadone, Buprenorphine, and Tramadol

29 Opioid Receptor Antagonists: Naltrexone, Nalmefene, and Naloxone

Generic Name	Trade Name	Adverse Effects	Drug Interactions	CYP Interactions
Naltrexone	ReVia, Depade	GI symptoms, insomnia, dizziness, fatigue, skin rash, headache	Opioids, DRA, disulfiram	N/A
Nalmefene	Revex	Dizziness, GI symptoms, headache	Opioids, flumazenil	3A4, 3A5
Naloxone	Narcan	Dizziness, hypotension, hypertension, tachycardia, GI symptoms, headache	Opioids	3A4, 2C18, 2C19

Introduction

Unlike opioid agonists (covered in Chapter 28), competitive opioid antagonists bind to opioid receptors without causing their activation and induces opioid withdrawal in people using full opioid agonists. Naltrexone and naloxone are the most widely used of these drugs. Naltrexone is more widely used for preventing relapse of opioid use disorder in detoxified opioid addicts because it has a relatively long half-life, is orally effective, is not associated with dysphoria, and is administered once daily.

Since its introduction, naltrexone (ReVia, Depade) has been tried for the treatment of a wide range of psychiatric disorders, but only has been approved by the Food and Drug Administration (FDA) for two indications. Naltrexone is approved for the treatment of opiate dependence and alcohol dependence. An extended-release, once-a-month injectable suspension (Vivitrol) is also available. Some individuals may lose a considerable amount of weight from naltrexone treatment. In 2014, the FDA-approved Contrave, which is the trade name for the combination of naltrexone hydrochloride and bupropion hydrochloride in an extended-release formulation, for the treatment of obesity. This combination drug is covered in more detail in Chapter 41.

Naloxone (Narcan), an opiate antagonist, has been FDA approved for reversal of opioid overdose. It is an effective medication in reversing respiratory depression and preventing fatalities secondary to opioid overdose, particularly in an emergency setting.

Nalmefene is indicated for the complete or partial reversal of opioid drug effects and in the management of known or suspected opioid overdose. It is administered as an immediate-release injection. An oral formulation of nalmefene is available in some countries but not in the United States.

Samidorphan, a more recently developed naltrexone analogue and opioid antagonist in combination with the atypical antipsychotic olanzapine—under the trade name Lybalvi—is indicated for the treatment of schizophrenia and bipolar I disorder A combination of opioid agonist buprenorphine and samidorphan was proposed as a potential add-on to antidepressants in treatment-resistant depression, but a panel from the Food and Drug Administration (FDA) voted against approval in 2018. Samidorphan has not been approved for any use as a standalone treatment.

Pharmacologic Actions

Oral opioid receptor antagonists are rapidly absorbed from the gastrointestinal (GI) tract. Due to first-pass hepatic metabolism, only 60% of a dose of naltrexone and between 40% to 50% of a dose of nalmefene or intranasal naloxone reach the systemic circulation unchanged. Peak concentrations of naltrexone and its active metabolite, 6β-naltrexol, are achieved within 1 hour of ingestion. The half-life of naltrexone is 1 to 3 hours and the half-life of 6β-naltrexol is 13 hours. Peak concentrations of intranasal naloxone are achieved in 15 to 30 minutes, while peak concentrations of intramuscular and intravenous naloxone are achieved in 10 and 2 minutes, respectively. The half-life of naloxone is approximately 60 minutes. Peak concentrations of nalmefene are achieved in about 1 to 2 hours, and the half-life is 8 to 10 hours.

Clinically, a single dose of naltrexone effectively blocks the rewarding effects of opioids for 72 hours. Traces of 6β-naltrexol may linger for up to 125 hours after a single dose.

Naltrexone, naloxone, and nalmefene are competitive antagonists of opioid receptors. Understanding the pharmacology of opioid receptors can explain the difference in adverse effects caused by the three drugs. Opioid receptors in the body are typed pharmacologically as μ, κ, or δ. Whereas activation of the κ- and δ-receptors is thought to reinforce opioid and alcohol consumption centrally, activation of μ-receptors is more closely associated with central and peripheral antiemetic effects. Because naltrexone is a relatively weak antagonist of κ- and δ-receptors and a potent μ-receptor antagonist, dosages of naltrexone that effectively reduce opioid and alcohol consumption also strongly block μ-receptors and therefore may cause nausea. Nalmefene, in contrast, is an equally potent antagonist of all three opioid receptor types, and dosages of nalmefene that effectively reduce opioid and alcohol consumption have no particularly increased effect on μ-receptors. Thus, nalmefene is associated clinically with few GI adverse effects.

Naloxone has the highest affinity for the μ-receptor but is a competitive antagonist at the κ- and δ-receptors.

Whereas the effects of opioid receptor antagonists on opioid use are easily understood in terms of competitive inhibition of opioid receptors, the effects of opioid receptor antagonists on alcohol dependence are less straightforward and probably relate to the fact that the desire for and the effects of alcohol consumption appear to be regulated by several neurotransmitter systems, both opioid and nonopioid.

Samidorphan is an antagonist or weak partial agonist at μ-receptors and a partial agonist at κ- and δ-receptors.

Therapeutic Indications

The combination of a cognitive-behavioral program plus use of opioid receptor antagonists is more successful than either the cognitive-behavioral program or use of opioid receptor antagonists alone. Naltrexone is used as a screening test to ensure that the patient is opioid-free before the induction of therapy with naltrexone (see Table 29-1).

TABLE 29-1: Common and Less Common Side Effects of Opioid Receptor Antagonists

	Naltrexone	Nalmefene	Naloxone
Common side effects	• Abdominal pain • Alanine aminotransferase increased • Anxiety • Aspartate aminotransferase increased • Decreased appetite • Diarrhea • Difficulty concentrating • Dizziness • Fatigue • Headache • Injection site tenderness • Insomnia • Joint stiffness • Nausea/Vomiting • Pharyngitis/Nasopharyngitis • Rash	• Chills • Dizziness • Fever • Headache • Nausea/Vomiting	• Dizziness • Headache • Hypertension • Hypotension • Joint or muscle pain • Nausea/Vomiting • Tachycardia
Less common side effects	• Back pain • Chest pain • Gamma-glutamyl transferase increased • Depression • Dry mouth • Muscle cramps • Somnolence	• Agitation • Arrhythmia • Bradycardia • Confusion • Depression • Diarrhea • Dry mouth • Hypertension • Hypotension • Myoclonus • Nervousness • Pharyngitis • Somnolence • Tachycardia • Tremor • Vasodilation	• Arrhythmia • Bradycardia • Diarrhea • Dry mouth • Tremor

Opioid Dependence

Patients in detoxification programs are usually weaned from potent opioid agonists such as heroin or fentanyl over a period of days to weeks, during which emergent adrenergic withdrawal effects are treated as needed with clonidine (Catapres). A serial protocol is sometimes used in which potent agonists are gradually replaced by weaker agonists followed by mixed agonist–antagonists and then finally by pure antagonists. For example, an abuser of the potent agonist heroin would switch first to the weaker agonist methadone (Dolophine), then to the partial agonist buprenorphine (Buprenex) or levomethadyl acetate (OrLAAM)—commonly called LAAM—and finally, after a 7- to 10-day washout period, to a pure antagonist, such as naltrexone or nalmefene. However, even with gradual detoxification, some persons continue to experience mild adverse effects or opioid withdrawal symptoms for the first several weeks of treatment with naltrexone.

As the opioid receptor agonist potency diminishes, so do the adverse consequences of discontinuing the drug. Since there are no pharmacologic barriers to discontinuation of pure opioid receptor antagonists, the social environment and frequent cognitive-behavioral intervention become extremely important factors in supporting continued opioid abstinence. Because of withdrawal symptoms, most persons not simultaneously enrolled in a cognitive-behavioral program stop taking opioid receptor antagonists within 3 months. Compliance with the administration of an opioid receptor antagonist regimen can also be increased with participation in a well-conceived voucher program.

Issues of medication compliance should be a central focus of treatment. If a person with a history of opioid addiction stops taking a pure opioid receptor antagonist, the person's risk of relapse into opioid abuse is exceedingly high because reintroduction of a potent opioid agonist would yield an extremely rewarding subjective "high." Additionally, this may lead to hazardous and unpredictable levels of receptor activation (see Precautions and Adverse Reactions). In contrast, compliant persons do not develop tolerance to the therapeutic benefits of naltrexone even if it is administered continuously for 1 year or longer. Individuals may undergo several relapses and remissions before achieving long-term abstinence.

Rapid Detoxification

To avoid the 7- to 10-day period of opioid abstinence generally recommended before use of opioid receptor antagonists, rapid detoxification protocols have been developed. Continuous administration of adjunct clonidine—to reduce the adrenergic withdrawal symptoms—and adjunct benzodiazepines, such as oxazepam (Serax)—to reduce muscle spasms and insomnia—can permit use of oral opioid receptor antagonists on the first day of opioid cessation. Detoxification can thus be completed within 48 to 72 hours, at which point opioid receptor antagonist maintenance is initiated. Moderately severe withdrawal symptoms may be experienced on the first day, but they tail off rapidly thereafter.

Because of the potential hypotensive effects of clonidine, the blood pressure (BP) of persons undergoing rapid detoxification must be closely monitored for the first 8 hours. Outpatient rapid detoxification settings must therefore be adequately prepared to administer emergency care.

The main advantage of rapid detoxification is that the transition from opioid abuse to maintenance treatment occurs over just 2 or 3 days. The completion of detoxification in as little time as possible minimizes the risk that the person will relapse into opioid abuse during the detoxification protocol.

Alcohol Dependence

Opioid receptor antagonists are also used as adjuncts to cognitive-behavioral programs for treatment of alcohol dependence, though only naltrexone has received formal approval from the FDA for this indication. Opioid receptor antagonists reduce alcohol craving and alcohol consumption, and they ameliorate the severity of relapses. The risk of relapse into heavy consumption of alcohol attributable to an effective cognitive-behavioral program alone may be halved with concomitant use of opioid receptor antagonists.

Nalmefene has a number of potential pharmacologic and clinical advantages over its predecessor naltrexone for treatment of alcohol dependence. Whereas naltrexone may cause reversible transaminase elevations in persons who take dosages of 300 mg a day (which is six times the recommended dosage for treatment of alcohol and opioid dependence [50 mg a day]), nalmefene has not been associated with any hepatotoxicity. Clinically effective dosages of naltrexone are discontinued by 10% to 15% of persons because of adverse effects, most commonly nausea. In contrast, discontinuation of nalmefene because of an adverse event is rare at the clinically effective dosage of 20 mg a day and in the range of 10% at excessive dosages—that is, 80 mg a day. Because of its pharmacokinetic profile, a given dosage of nalmefene may also produce a more sustained opioid antagonist effect than does naltrexone.

The efficacy of opioid receptor antagonists in reducing alcohol craving may be augmented with a selective serotonin reuptake inhibitor, although data from large trials are needed to assess this potential synergistic effect more fully.

Off-Label Uses

Studies have found that opioid antagonists may have multiple uses beyond treating opioid use disorder, opioid overdoses, or alcohol use disorder. Due to their anti-inflammatory effects, opioid antagonists may treat several dermatologic conditions (e.g., pruritus, psoriasis, systemic sclerosis), autoimmune disorders (e.g., interstitial cystitis, rheumatoid arthritis, Crohn disease), and chronic disorders like fibromyalgia and chronic fatigue syndrome. Although no clinical studies have evaluated the use of naltrexone to treat chronic fatigue syndrome, multiple case studies and anecdotal evidence suggest that it can significantly improve quality of life.

Substance Use Disorders

Opioid antagonists may treat other substance use disorders besides alcohol use disorder and opioid use disorder. Some evidence has shown that naltrexone is effective at reducing cravings in individuals with either cocaine or cannabis use disorders.

Smoking Cessation

Naltrexone is found to be effective at helping individuals quit smoking. Limited studies have shown that naltrexone treatment can improve quit rates, decrease cravings, reduce the number of cigarettes smoked, and lessen the amount of weight gained while in the process of quitting.

Compulsive Behaviors

Opioid antagonists may reduce the urge to engage in compulsive behaviors, such as pathologic gambling and self-injurious behavior in individuals with and without autism spectrum disorder.

Chronic Pain

Perhaps the most promising off-label use for opioid antagonists is in the treatment of chronic pain. Some evidence suggests that very low doses of naltrexone (<5 mg a day) may provide relief to patients.

Precautions and Adverse Reactions

Because opioid receptor antagonists are used to maintain a drug-free state after opioid detoxification, great care must be taken to ensure that an adequate wash-out period elapses—at least 5 days for a short-acting opioid such as heroin and at least 10 days for longer-acting opioids such as methadone—after the last dose of opioids and before the first dose of an opioid receptor antagonist is taken. The opioid-free state should be determined by self-report and urine toxicology screens.

If there are any doubts about the presence of opioids in the body despite a negative urine screen result, a *naloxone challenge test* should be performed. Naloxone challenge is used because its opioid antagonism lasts less than 1 hour, but those of naltrexone and nalmefene may persist for more than 24 hours. Thus, any withdrawal effects elicited by naloxone will be relatively short-lived (see Dosage and Clinical Guidelines). Symptoms of acute opioid withdrawal include drug craving, feeling of temperature change, musculoskeletal pain, and GI distress. In addition, other signs of opioid withdrawal include confusion, drowsiness, vomiting, and diarrhea. Naltrexone and nalmefene should not be taken if naloxone infusion causes any signs of opioid withdrawal except as part of a supervised rapid detoxification protocol.

A set of adverse effects resembling a vestigial withdrawal syndrome tends to affect up to 10% of persons who take opioid receptor antagonists. Up to 15% of persons taking naltrexone may experience abdominal pain, cramps, nausea, and vomiting, which may be limited by transiently halving the dosage or altering the time of administration. Adverse central nervous system effects of naltrexone, experienced by up to 10% of persons, include headache, low energy, insomnia, anxiety, and nervousness. Rash, joint and muscle pains may occur in up to 10% of persons taking naltrexone.

Naltrexone may cause dosage-related hepatic toxicity at dosages well in excess of 50 mg a day; 20% of persons taking 300 mg a day of naltrexone may experience serum aminotransferase concentrations 3 to 19 times the upper limit of normal. The hepatocellular injury of naltrexone appears to be a dose-related toxic effect rather than an idiosyncratic reaction. At the lowest dosages of naltrexone required for effective opioid antagonism, hepatocellular injury is not typically observed. However, naltrexone dosages as low as 50 mg a day may be hepatotoxic in persons with underlying liver disease, such as persons with cirrhosis of the liver caused by chronic alcohol abuse. *Serum aminotransferase concentrations should be monitored monthly for the first 6 months of naltrexone therapy and thereafter on the basis of clinical suspicion.* Hepatic enzyme concentrations usually return to normal after discontinuation of naltrexone therapy.

If analgesia is required while a dose of an opioid receptor antagonist is pharmacologically active, opioid agonists should be avoided in favor of benzodiazepines or other nonopioid analgesics. Persons taking opioid receptor antagonists should be instructed that low dosages of opioids will have no effect, but larger dosages could overcome the receptor blockade and suddenly produce symptoms of profound opioid overdosage, with sedation possibly progressing to coma or death. Use of any opioid receptor antagonist is contraindicated in persons who

TABLE 29-2: Naloxone (Narcan) Challenge Test
The naloxone challenge test should not be performed in a patient showing clinical signs or symptoms of opioid withdrawal or in a patient whose urine contains opioids. The naloxone challenge test may be administered by either the intravenous (IV) or the subcutaneous route.
IV challenge: After appropriate screening of the patient, 0.8 mg of naloxone should be drawn into a sterile syringe. If the IV route of administration is selected, 0.2 mg of naloxone should be injected, and while the needle is still in the patient's vein, the patient should be observed for 30 seconds for evidence of withdrawal signs or symptoms. If there is no evidence of withdrawal, the remaining 0.6 mg of naloxone should be injected, and the patient observed for an additional 20 minutes for signs and symptoms of withdrawal.
Subcutaneous challenge: If the subcutaneous route is selected, 0.8 mg should be administered subcutaneously, and the patient observed for signs and symptoms of withdrawal for 20 minutes.
Conditions and technique for observation of patient: During the appropriate period of observation, the patient's vital signs should be monitored, and the patient should be monitored for signs of withdrawal. It is also important to question the patient carefully. The signs and symptoms of opioid withdrawal include, but are not limited to, the following:
Withdrawal signs: Stuffiness or running nose, tearing, yawning, sweating, tremor, vomiting, or piloerection
Withdrawal symptoms: Feeling of temperature change, joint or bone and muscle pain, abdominal cramps, and formication (feeling of bugs crawling under skin)
Interpretation of the challenge: Warning—the elicitation of the enumerated signs or symptoms indicates a potential risk for the subject, and naltrexone should not be administered. If no signs or symptoms of withdrawal are observed, elicited, or reported, naltrexone may be administered. If there is any doubt in the observer's mind that the patient is not in an opioid-free state or is in continuing withdrawal, naltrexone should be withheld for 24 hours and the challenge repeated.

are taking opioid agonists, small amounts of which may be present in over-the-counter antiemetic and antitussive preparations; in persons with acute hepatitis or hepatic failure; and in persons who are hypersensitive to the drugs.

A list of the side effects of naltrexone, nalmefene, and naloxone can be found in Table 29-2.

Use in Pregnancy and Lactation

Because naltrexone is transported across the placenta, it should only be taken by pregnant women if a compelling need outweighs the potential risks to the fetus. A minimal amount of naltrexone is passed in maternal milk. It is a pregnancy category C drug, as is naloxone. The safety of nalmefene in pregnancy and breastfeeding has not been confirmed, but it is classified as a pregnancy category B drug.

Overdose

Opioid receptor antagonists are relatively safe drugs, and ingestion of high doses of opioid receptor antagonists should be treated with supportive measures combined with efforts to decrease GI absorption.

Drug Interactions

Many drug interactions involving opioid receptor antagonists have been discussed, including those with opioid agonists associated with drug abuse as well as those involving antiemetics and antitussives. Because of its extensive hepatic metabolism, naltrexone may affect or be affected by other drugs that influence hepatic enzyme levels. However, the clinical importance of these potential interactions is not known.

One potentially hepatotoxic drug that has been used in some cases with opioid receptor antagonists is disulfiram (Antabuse). Although no adverse effects were observed, frequent laboratory monitoring is indicated when such combination therapy is contemplated. Opioid receptor antagonists have been reported to potentiate the sedation associated with use of thioridazine (Mellaril), an interaction that probably applies equally to all low-potency dopamine receptor antagonists.

Intravenous nalmefene has been administered after benzodiazepines, inhalational anesthetics, muscle relaxants, and muscle relaxant antagonists administered in conjunction with general anesthetics without any adverse reactions. Care should be taken when using and nalmefene together because both of these agents have been shown to induce seizures in preclinical studies.

Because buprenorphine has a high affinity and slow displacement from the opioid receptors, nalmefene may not completely reverse buprenorphine-induced respiratory depression.

Laboratory Interferences

The potential for a false-positive urine for opiates using less specific urine screens such as enzyme multiplied immunoassay technique (EMIT) may exist, given that naltrexone and nalmefene are derivatives of oxymorphone. Thin-layer, gas–liquid, and high-pressure liquid chromatographic methods used for the detection of opiates in the urine are not interfered by naltrexone.

Dosage and Clinical Guidelines

To avoid the possibility of precipitating an acute opioid withdrawal syndrome, several steps should be taken to ensure that the person is opioid-free. Within a supervised detoxification setting, at least 5 days should elapse after the last dose of short-acting opioids, such as heroin, hydromorphone (Dilaudid), meperidine (Demerol), or morphine; and at least 10 days should elapse after the last dose of longer-acting opioids, such as methadone, before opioid antagonists are initiated. Briefer periods off opioids have been used in rapid detoxification protocols. To confirm that opioid detoxification is complete, urine toxicologic screens should demonstrate no opioid metabolites. However, an individual may have a negative urine opioid screen result, yet still be physically dependent on opioids and thus susceptible to antagonist-induced withdrawal effects. Therefore, after the urine screen result is negative, a naloxone challenge test is recommended unless an adequate period of opioid abstinence can be reliably confirmed by observers (Table 29-2).

The initial dosage of naltrexone for treatment of opioid or alcohol dependence is 50 mg a day, which should be achieved through gradual introduction, even when the naloxone challenge test result is negative. Various authorities begin with 5, 10, 12.5, or 25 mg and titrate up to the 50-mg dosage over a period ranging from 1 hour to 2 weeks while constantly monitoring for evidence of opioid withdrawal. When a daily dose of 50 mg is well tolerated, it may be averaged over a week by giving 100 mg on alternate days or 150 mg every third day. Such schedules may increase compliance. The corresponding therapeutic dosage of nalmefene is 20 mg a day divided into two equal doses. Gradual titration of nalmefene to this daily dose is probably a wise strategy, although clinical data on dosage strategies for nalmefene are not yet available.

For the extended-release injectable formulation of naltrexone (Vivitrol), a 380-mg dose delivered intramuscularly every 4 weeks or once a month is recommended. The needles provided in the carton are customized for the drug. Vivitrol should be stored in the refrigerator and requires 45 minutes for drug to reach room temperature prior to preparation and administration.

To maximize compliance, it is recommended that family members directly observe ingestion of each dose. Random urine tests for opioid receptor antagonists and their metabolites as well as for ethanol or opioid metabolites should also be taken. Opioid receptor antagonists should be continued until the person is no longer considered psychologically at risk for relapse into opioid or alcohol abuse. This generally requires at least 6 months but may take longer, particularly if there are external stresses.

Nalmefene is available as a sterile solution for intravenous, intramuscular, and subcutaneous administration in two concentrations, containing 100 µg or 1 mg of nalmefene free base per mL. The 100 µg/mL concentration contains 110.8 µg of nalmefene hydrochloride, and the 1.0 mg/mL concentration contains 1.108 mg of nalmefene hydrochloride per mL. Both concentrations contain 9.0 mg of sodium chloride per mL and the pH is adjusted to 3.9 with hydrochloric acid. Pharmacodynamic studies have shown that nalmefene has a longer duration of action than naloxone at fully reversing opiate activity.

Rapid Detoxification

Rapid detoxification has been standardized using naltrexone, although nalmefene would be expected to be equally effective with fewer adverse effects. In rapid detoxification protocols, the addicted person stops opioid use abruptly and begins the first opioid-free day by taking clonidine, 0.2 mg, orally every 2 hours for nine doses, to a maximum dose of 1.8 mg, during which time the BP is monitored every 30 to 60 minutes for the first 8 hours. Naltrexone, 12.5 mg, is administered 1 to 3 hours after the first dose of clonidine. To reduce muscle cramps and later insomnia, a short-acting benzodiazepine, such as oxazepam, 30 to 60 mg, is administered simultaneously with the first dose of clonidine, and half of the initial dose is readministered every 4 to 6 hours as needed. The maximum daily dosage of oxazepam should not exceed 180 mg. The person undergoing rapid detoxification should be accompanied home by a reliable escort. On the second day, similar doses of clonidine and the benzodiazepine are administered but with a single dose of naltrexone, 25 mg, taken in the morning. Relatively asymptomatic persons may return home after 3 to 4 hours. Administration of the daily maintenance dose of 50 mg of naltrexone is begun on the third day, and the dosages of clonidine and the benzodiazepine are gradually tapered off over 5 to 10 days.

Emergency Administration

Naloxone can be administered intravenously, intramuscularly, and intranasally. Intravenous administration is preferable in emergency situations when an opioid overdose is known or suspected, as it has the most rapid onset of action.

An initial dose of 0.4 to 2 mg should be administered intravenously. If there is insufficient improvement in respiratory function, this may be repeated at intervals of 2 to 3 minutes. If there is no response after 10 mg of naloxone, the diagnosis of opioid-induced toxicity should be questioned. Intramuscular or subcutaneous injection may be necessary when the intravenous route is not available.

In children suspected of overdosing on opioids, the initial dose should be 0.01 mg/kg body weight. When using intranasal naloxone, do not prime the nasal spray, as each container holds one dose of naloxone (4 mg for Narcan; 8 mg for Kloxxado). The intranasal spray requires specific instructions for administration and clinicians may need to familiarize themselves with the guidelines.

30 Medications for Sexual Dysfunction

Generic Name	Trade Name	Adverse Effects	Drug Interactions	CYP Interactions
Sildenafil	Viagra	Myocardial infarction, GI symptoms, skin rash, headache	Organic nitrates	3A4, 2C9, 3A5, 3A7, 2C19, 2D6, 2E1
Vardenafil	Levitra	Myocardial infarction, GI symptoms, skin rash, headache	Organic nitrates	3A4, 3C5
Tadalafil	Cialis	Myocardial infarction, GI symptoms, skin rash, headache	Organic nitrates	3A4
Avanafil	Stendra	Myocardial infarction, GI symptoms, skin rash, headache	Organic nitrates	3A4, 2C9

Introduction

Since the introduction of sildenafil (Viagra) in 1998, phosphodiesterase (PDE)-5 inhibitors have revolutionized the treatment of the major sexual dysfunction affecting men—erectile disorder. Sildenafil (Viagra) was the first drug of this class, with three congeners that subsequently came on the market—vardenafil (Levitra), tadalafil (Cialis), and avanafil (Stendra). All four cause vasodilation in the penis, thus prolonging penile erections.

Moreover, all four drugs work the same way. The development of sildenafil provided important information about the physiology of erection. Sexual stimulation causes the release of the neurotransmitter nitric oxide (NO), which increases the synthesis of cyclic guanosine monophosphate (cGMP), causing smooth muscle relaxation in the corpus cavernosum that allows blood to flow into the penis and that results in turgidity and tumescence. The concentration of cGMP is regulated by the enzyme PDE-5, which, when inhibited, allows cGMP to increase and enhance erectile function. Because sexual stimulation is required to cause the release of NO, PDE-5 inhibitors have no effect in the absence of such stimulation, an important point to understand when providing information to patients about their use. The congeners vardenafil, tadalafil, and avanafil work in the same way, by inhibiting PDE-5, thus allowing an increase in cGMP and enhancing the vasodilatory effects of NO. For this reason, these drugs are sometimes referred to as NO enhancers.

Although indicated only for the treatment of male erectile dysfunction (ED), there is anecdotal evidence that they can treat sexual dysfunction in women, as well. These drugs are also used recreationally by individuals without ED because they are believed to enhance sexual performance.

Pharmacologic Actions

Sildenafil, vardenafil, tadalafil, and avanafil are fairly rapidly absorbed from the gastrointestinal tract, with maximum plasma concentrations reached in 30 to

120 minutes (median, 60 minutes) in a fasting state. Because they are lipophilic, concomitant ingestion of a high-fat meal delays the rate of absorption by up to 60 minutes and reduces the peak concentration by one-quarter. These drugs are principally metabolized by cytochrome P450 CYP3A4 isoenzymes, which may lead to clinically significant drug–drug interactions, not all of which have been documented. Excretion of 80% of the dose is via feces, and another 13% is eliminated in the urine. Elimination is reduced in persons older than age 65 years, which results in plasma concentrations 40% higher than in persons aged 18 to 45 years. Elimination is also reduced in the presence of severe renal or hepatic insufficiency.

The mean half-lives of sildenafil and vardenafil are 3 to 4 hours, that of tadalafil 18 hours, and avanafil is 5 hours. Tadalafil can be detected in the bloodstream 5 days after ingestion; and because of its long half-life, it has been marketed as effective for up to 36 hours—the so-called weekend pill. The onset of sildenafil occurs about 30 minutes after ingestion on an empty stomach; avanafil takes 45 minutes, while tadalafil and vardenafil act somewhat more quickly.

Clinicians need to be aware of the important clinical observation that these drugs do not by themselves create an erection. Rather, the mental state of sexual arousal brought on by erotic stimulation must first lead to activity in the penile nerves, which then release NO into the cavernosum, triggering the erectile cascade. The resulting erection is prolonged by the NO enhancers. Thus, full advantage may be taken of a sexually exciting stimulus, but the drug is not a substitute for foreplay and emotional arousal.

Therapeutic Indications

Erectile Dysfunction

ED has traditionally been classified as organic, psychogenic, or mixed. Organic causes of ED include diabetes mellitus, hypertension, hypercholesterolemia, cigarette smoking, peripheral vascular disease, pelvic or spinal cord injury, pelvic or abdominal surgery (especially prostate surgery), multiple sclerosis, peripheral neuropathy, and Parkinson disease. The use of alcohol, nicotine, and other substances (including prescription drugs) can also cause organic ED. Psychogenic ED can arise for myriad reasons.

PDE-5 inhibitors are indicated for use in organic, psychogenic, and mixed instances of ED.

Moreover, these drugs are effective regardless of the baseline severity of ED, race, or age. Among those responding to them are men with coronary artery disease, hypertension, other cardiac disease, peripheral vascular disease, diabetes mellitus, depression, coronary artery bypass graft surgery, radical prostatectomy, transurethral resection of the prostate, spina bifida, and spinal cord injury, as well as persons taking antidepressants, antipsychotics, antihypertensives, and diuretics. However, the response rate is variable.

PDE-5 inhibitors may also manage concomitant premature ejaculation, but do not appear to benefit patients with premature ejaculation alone.

Benign Prostatic Hyperplasia

Tadalafil is indicated for the use of treating signs and symptoms associated with benign prostatic hyperplasia.

Off-Label Uses

Sildenafil has been reported to reverse selective serotonin reuptake inhibitor–induced anorgasmia in men.

There are anecdotal reports of PDE-5 inhibitors having a therapeutic effect on sexual inhibition in women, as well. It may benefit women who have a healthy sex drive but struggle with sexual arousal. PDE-5 inhibitors do not have any effect on libido.

Additionally, PDE-5 inhibitors have been used to treat pulmonary arterial hypertension (typically administered intravenously), altitude sickness, diabetic neuropathy, peripheral neuropathy, and peripheral arterial disease. They also have antianginal properties and may have some efficacy in the treatment of ischemic heart disease.

Precautions and Adverse Reactions

A major potential adverse effect associated with use of these drugs is myocardial infarction (MI). The Food and Drug Administration (FDA) distinguished the risk of MI caused directly by these drugs from that caused by underlying conditions such as hypertension, atherosclerotic heart disease, diabetes mellitus, and other atherogenic conditions. The FDA concluded that when used according to the approved labeling, the drugs do not by themselves confer an increased risk of death. However, there is increased oxygen demand and stress placed on the cardiac muscle by sexual intercourse. Thus, coronary perfusion may be severely compromised, and cardiac failure may occur as a result. For that reason, any person with a history of MI, stroke, renal failure, hypertension, or diabetes mellitus and any person older than the age of 70 years should discuss plans to use these drugs with an internist or a cardiologist. The cardiac evaluation should specifically address exercise tolerance and the use of nitrates.

Use of PDE-5 inhibitors is contraindicated in persons who are taking organic nitrates in any form. Also, amyl nitrate (poppers), a popular substance of abuse to enhance the intensity of orgasm, should not be used with any of the erection-enhancing drugs. *The combination of organic nitrates and PDE inhibitors can cause a precipitous lowering of blood pressure and can reduce coronary perfusion to the point of causing MI and death.*

Adverse effects are dose dependent, occurring at higher rates with higher dosages. The most common adverse effects are headache, flushing, and stomach pain. Other, less common adverse effects include nasal congestion, urinary tract infection, abnormal vision (colored tinge [usually blue], increased sensitivity to light, or blurred vision), diarrhea, dizziness, and rash. Supportive management is indicated in cases of overdosage. Tadalafil has been associated with back and muscle pain in about 10% of patients.

There have been numerous reports and verified cases of a serious condition in men taking PDE-5 inhibitors called nonarteritic anterior ischemic optic neuropathy (NAION). This is an eye ailment that causes restriction of blood flow to the optic nerve and can result in permanent vision loss. The first symptoms appear within 24 hours after use of PDE-5 inhibitors and include blurred vision and some degree of vision loss. The incidence of this effect is very rare—1 in

1 million. In the reported cases, many patients had preexisting eye problems that may have increased their risk, and many had a history of heart disease and diabetes, which may indicate vulnerability in these men to endothelial damage.

In addition to vision problems, in 2010, a warning of possible hearing loss was reported based on 29 incidents of the problem since introduction of these drugs. Hearing loss usually occurs within hours or days of using the drug and in some cases is both unilateral and temporary.

Use in Pregnancy and Lactation

No data are available on the effects on human fetal growth and development or testicular morphologic or functional changes. However, because these drugs are not considered an essential treatment, they should not be used during pregnancy.

Treatment of Priapism

Priapism occurs infrequently with the use of PDE-5 inhibitors. Phenylephrine is the drug of choice and first-line treatment of priapism because the drug has almost pure α-agonist effects and minimal β-activity. In short-term priapism (less than 6 hours), especially for drug-induced priapism, an intracavernosal injection of phenylephrine can be used to cause detumescence. A mixture of one ampule of phenylephrine (1 mL/1,000 μg) should be diluted with an additional 9 mL of normal saline. Using a 29-gauge needle, 0.3 to 0.5 mL should be injected into the corpora cavernosa, with 10 to 15 minutes between injections. Vital signs should be monitored, and compression should be applied to the area of injection to help prevent hematoma formation.

Phenylephrine can also be used orally, 10 to 20 mg every 4 hours as needed, but it may not be as effective or act as rapidly as the injectable route.

Drug Interactions

The major route of PDE-5 metabolism is through CYP3A4, and the minor route is through CYP2C9. Inducers or inhibitors of these enzymes will therefore affect the plasma concentration and half-life of sildenafil. For example, 800 mg of cimetidine (Tagamet), a nonspecific CYP inhibitor, increases plasma sildenafil concentrations by 56%, and erythromycin (E-Mycin) increases plasma sildenafil concentrations by 182%. Other, stronger inhibitors of CYP3A4 include ketoconazole (Nizoral), itraconazole (Sporanox), and mibefradil (Posicor). In contrast, rifampicin, a CYP3A4 inducer, decreases plasma concentrations of sildenafil.

Laboratory Interferences

No laboratory interferences have been described.

Dosage and Clinical Guidelines

Sildenafil is available as 25-, 50-, and 100-mg tablets. The recommended dose of sildenafil is 50 mg taken by mouth 1 hour before intercourse. However, sildenafil may take effect within 30 minutes. The duration of the effect is usually 4 hours. In healthy young men, the effect may persist for 8 to 12 hours. Based on effectiveness and adverse effects, the dose should be titrated between 25 and

100 mg. Sildenafil is recommended for use no more than once a day. The dosing guidelines for use by women, an off-label use, are the same as those for men.

Increased plasma concentrations of sildenafil may occur in persons older than 65 years of age and those with cirrhosis, severe renal impairment, or using CYP3A4 inhibitors. A starting dose of 25 mg should be used in these circumstances.

Vardenafil is supplied in 2.5-, 5-, 10-, and 20-mg tablets. The initial dose is usually 10 mg taken with or without food about 1 hour before sexual activity. The dose can be increased to a maximum of 20 mg or decreased to 5 mg based on efficacy and side effects. The maximum dosing frequency is once per day. As with sildenafil, dosages may have to be adjusted in patients with hepatic impairment or in patients using certain CYP3A4 inhibitors. A 10-mg orally disintegrating form of vardenafil (Staxyn) is available. It is placed on the tongue approximately 60 minutes before sexual activity and should not be used more than once a day.

Tadalafil is available in 2.5-, 5-, or 20-mg tablets for oral administration. The recommended dose of tadalafil is 10 mg before sexual activity, which may be increased to 20 mg or decreased to 5 mg depending on efficacy and side effects. Once-a-day use of the 2.5- or 5-mg pill is acceptable for most patients. Similar cautions apply as mentioned earlier in patients with hepatic impairment and in those taking concomitant potent inhibitors of CYP3A4. As with other PDE-5 inhibitors, concomitant use of nitrates in any form is contraindicated.

Avanafil is available in 50-, 100-, and 200-mg tablets for oral administration. The recommended starting dose is 100 mg. It can be taken as early as approximately 15 minutes before sexual activity and dosage can be adjusted to 200 mg or decreased to 50 mg depending on tolerability and any potential adverse effects. It should be taken once per day and sexual stimulation is required for a response to treatment. Similar cautions apply as mentioned earlier in patients with hepatic impairment and in those taking concomitant potent inhibitors of CYP3A4. As with other PDE-5 inhibitors, concomitant use of nitrates in any form is contraindicated.

Psychedelics

31

Generic Name	Trade Name	Adverse Effects	Drug Interactions	CYP Interactions
Psilocybin	N/A	Confusion, dizziness, tachycardia, hypertension, GI symptoms, headache, paranoia, temporary psychosis	SERO, antidepressants	N/A
Lysergic acid diethylamide (LSD)	N/A	Confusion, dizziness, tachycardia, hypertension, GI symptoms, headache, paranoia, temporary psychosis	SERO, antidepressants	1A2, 2C19, 2D6, 2E1, 3A4

Introduction

Psychedelic ("mind-manifesting") or entheogenic ("spiritually inspiring") drugs induce powerful alterations in consciousness, sensory hallucinations, and synesthesia, and have been used by cultures throughout the world for millennia for spiritual, ritualistic, and medicinal purposes. Despite widespread use by practitioners of traditional medicine from myriad cultures and significant clinical interest in the middle of the 20th century, only limited clinical research on these drugs has occurred since the 1960s. In addition to being stigmatized because of their popularity with various countercultural groups of the era, the Controlled Substances Act of 1970 classified the most well-known psychedelics of the time as Schedule I drugs and erected numerous barriers to research.

Within the last 20 years, these barriers have been increasingly torn down and significant clinical research is now being conducted on psychedelics. Evidence now suggests that these drugs may aid in the treatment of anxiety, substance use, mood, and affective disorders. They may also aid in palliative care for patients who have a terminal disease and are struggling with the emotional distress following their diagnosis. These effects appear to be sustained for months or even years following a single acute psychedelic experience with concomitant psychotherapy. These lasting effects are mediated by the mystical-like experiences induced by the drugs rather than a sustained physiologic change, though these drugs do typically produce autonomic effects, including mydriasis, tachycardia, tachypnea, hyperthermia, hypertonia, diaphoresis, and increases in blood pressure and salivation with occasional nausea.

While there are numerous types of compounds capable of producing mystical-like experiences, this chapter will focus on the two most well-understood "classic psychedelics," psilocybin and lysergic acid diethylamide (LSD). Both drugs share many similar pharmacologic properties including tolerance, dependence, withdrawal, drug interactions, therapeutic indications, as well as adverse effects, and will be discussed together at the end of this chapter. Other classic psychedelics include mescaline (the active ingredient in peyote) and *N,N*-dimethyltryptamine (the active ingredient in ayahuasca), and they appear to have similar properties and mechanisms of action (i.e., demonstrating agonistic

313

activity at 5-HT2A receptors). However, as of now, not enough clinical work has been done on mescaline or *N,N*-dimethyltryptamine (DMT) to warrant discussion in this book.

Finally, it should be noted that none of these drugs mentioned have yet been approved by the Food and Drug Administration for any indication though recent research and data suggests that this may be forthcoming. At this time, they are all still considered Schedule I drugs.

PSILOCYBIN

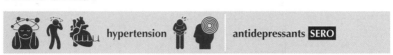

Psilocybin was isolated in 1957 from the Central American mushroom Psilocybe mexicana by Albert Hoffman. The compound has since been found in more than 100 species of mushrooms in varying concentrations.

Mushrooms containing psilocybin may be consumed raw, dried, or steeped in hot water to create a form of tea. Psilocybin can also be created synthetically and administered as a capsule. In its purified state, psilocybin is a white, needle-like crystalline powder. Of note, psilocybin is a prodrug and is converted into the pharmacologically active psilocin following dephosphorylation.

Pharmacokinetics

Absorption, Bioavailability, and Distribution

Following oral administration, psilocybin is rapidly converted to psilocin, of which approximately 50% is absorbed. The bioavailability of psilocin following oral administration is 52.7 ± 20%. The compound is uniformly distributed throughout the body and is detectable in significant concentrations in plasma within 20 to 40 minutes of administration. It reaches maximum concentrations within 80 to 100 minutes after administration.

Metabolism

Psilocybin is converted into psilocin in the stomach, intestines, kidney, and blood. Within 5 hours, up to 80% of psilocin undergoes glucuronidation via glucuronosyltransferase enzymes UGT1A9 and UGT1A10 to form psilocin O-glucuronide, which is then excreted through urine. Psilocin may also be metabolized into 4-hydroxyindole-3-acetaldehyde, 4-hydroxytryptophol, and 4-hydroxyindole-3-acetic acid by liver monoamine oxidase (MAO) or aldehyde dehydrogenase.

Elimination and Excretion

Psilocybin's elimination half-life is 160 minutes, while psilocin's is only 50 minutes. Psilocin is excreted within 8 hours primarily through urine (65%), as well as bile and feces (15% to 20%). Psilocin or one of its metabolites may be detectable in urine for up to 7 days after oral administration and approximately 25% of psilocybin will be excreted unaltered.

Pharmacodynamics

Onset of action is typically 40 minutes after ingestion. Intoxication may last 4 to 6 hours and can be characterized by a spectrum of psychological effects. In small doses, individuals are likely to experience euphoria and minor sensory distortions. In larger doses, psilocybin can induce mystical experiences and ego dissolution. A great deal of the therapeutic value of psilocybin and other psychedelics may be the experience of the latter, particularly for individuals facing existential duress due to a terminal illness.

The intensity of one's subjective experience is dose-dependent and can be influenced by experience with psychedelics, as well as mental outlook and environmental factors (i.e., "set and setting"). Research is ongoing to establish proper dosing guidelines and best practices for administering psychotherapy before, during, and after patients' psychedelic experiences.

Mechanism of Action

Psilocybin's active metabolite, psilocin, is a partial agonist at 5-HT2A receptor (<40% activation efficacy) and binds to 5-HT2C, 5-HT1A, and 5-HT1B receptors in the thalamus and prefrontal cortex. Of note, alterations in perception are primarily mediated by 5-HT2A receptors. This is evidenced by the fact that such alterations can be eliminated following the administration of the 5-HT2A antagonist ketanserin.

Evidence suggests that alterations in sensory perception stem from the activation of serotonin receptors in the thalamus and downstream effects on the cerebral cortex. The former is primarily responsible for relaying motor and sensory signals to the latter, which in turn plays an integral role in regulating mood, social behavior, personality expression, and executive functioning. Downstream effects on dopaminergic pathways and on the glutamate system may also be partially responsible for psilocybin's effects on mood, particularly as euphoria, and the commonly reported phenomenon of depersonalization.

Repeated doses of classic psychedelics have also been linked with the downregulation of 5-HT2A receptors in the cerebral cortex, which may contribute to the therapeutic effects of psychedelics like psilocybin. 5-HT2A density was found to be significantly higher in postmortem samples from patients with major depression. A strong correlation has been observed in rodent models linking increased 5-HT2A receptor density and anxiety-like behavior.

Therapeutic Index

Psilocybin has a wide therapeutic index, with an average lethal dose (LD50) of approximately 280 mg/kg in rodents.

LYSERGIC ACID DIETHYLAMIDE

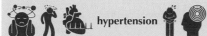   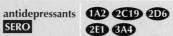

hypertension   antidepressants SERO   1A2 2C19 2D6 2E1 3A4

LSD was first synthesized from ergoline alkaloids in 1938 by Swiss chemist Albert Hoffman while working at Sandoz AG Pharmaceutical Company. Five years later,

Psychedelics

on April 16, 1943, a small amount of the substance was accidentally ingested by Hoffman, which produced a sensation he described as, "characterized by an extremely stimulated imagination." Three days later, on April 19, Hoffman dosed himself with 250 mg of the substance and became the first person to experience what has become colloquially known as an "acid trip."

By the 1950s and early 1960s, LSD-assisted psychotherapy had become immensely popular, particularly as a treatment for alcoholism. A few years later, it became a popular recreational drug among various countercultural movements due to its ability to alter consciousness and break familiar patterns of thought. As non-clinical use increased, clinical research declined as the drug became increasingly stigmatized amongst the medical community. Clinical research was effectively discontinued following the passage of the Controlled Substances Act of 1970.

Within the last 20 years, there has been resurgent interest in LSD-assisted psychotherapy coupled with reduced restrictions of use in clinical settings. There is now some evidence to suggest that LSD, when used in a clinical setting, may help alleviate anxiety, depression, substance use disorders, and existential distress among terminally ill patients.

LSD is a semisynthetic product of lysergic acid, which is produced by the rye fungus ergot (Claviceps purpurea). It is a white odorless crystalline substance in its pure state. More commonly, LSD is diluted in a solution, and then administered orally, sublingually, or buccally via dropper. Small amounts of the solution may also be placed on mediums such as a gelatin sheets, pieces of blotting paper, or sugar cubes, and then administered orally.

Pharmacokinetics

Absorption, Bioavailability, and Distribution

Following oral administration, LSD is completely absorbed in the digestive tract and has an estimated bioavailability of 71%. Absorption typically occurs within 1 hour but may be slowed if administration is preceded by a meal.

LSD is rapidly distributed throughout the body and crosses the blood–brain barrier, but a full understanding of how it is distributed across organ systems has yet to be quantified. Peak plasma concentrations are achieved 40 to 130 minutes after administration. There is some confusion as to whether the effects of LSD and concentrations of the drug are related in a linear fashion, a logarithmic fashion, or neither.

Metabolism

LSD undergoes extensive first-pass metabolism in humans and is almost fully metabolized into inactive metabolites. The major human metabolite of LSD is 2-oxo-3-hydroxy LSD. Other metabolites include lysergic acid ethylamide (LAE), lysergic acid ethyl-e-hydroxyethylamide (LEO), nor-LSD, 2-oxo-LSD, and 13 or 14-Hydroxy-LSD glucuronide. CYP1A2, CYP2C19, CYP2D6, CYP2E1, and CYP3A4 each play a role in the metabolism of LSD.

Elimination and Excretion

The half-life of LSD is estimated to be approximately 175 minutes in humans. It is excreted primarily through urine within 8 hours and may be detectable in urine for

96 hours following administration. The rate of excretion reaches a maximum rate 4 to 6 hours after administration and the elimination half-life for LSD is 3.6 hours. Less than 1% of LSD is excreted unchanged.

Pharmacodynamics

LSD's subjective effects can be felt 30 to 120 minutes following ingestion and typically last between 6 and 10 hours. Peak effects following a moderate dose (100 to 250 μg po) can occur 90 to 150 minutes following administration.

The intensity of one's subjective experience is dose-dependent and can be influenced by experience with psychedelics, as well as mental outlook and environmental factors (i.e., "set and setting"). LSD can produce a wide variety of effects ranging from euphoria and minor sensory distortions in small doses (<100 μg po) to mystical-like experiences in larger doses. A great deal of the therapeutic value of LSD comes from these experiences coupled with psychotherapy.

Research is ongoing to establish proper dosing guidelines.

Mechanism of Action

LSD is a partial agonist of 5-HT2A receptors, and its most acute effects can be eliminated via the administration of the 5-HT2A antagonist ketanserin. Repeated doses of psychedelics like LSD have also been linked with the downregulation of 5-HT2A receptors in the cerebral cortex.

As with psilocybin, LSD's activity at thalamic 5-HT2A receptors alters communication between the thalamus and the cerebral cortex, thereby disrupting the brain's ability to filter sensory stimuli and convert experienced reality into a familiar narrative, thereby accounting for patients' increasingly disorganized thoughts while experiencing the acute effects of the drug. Disruptions to typical cerebral cortex functioning via LSD's activity at 5-HT2A receptors may also contribute to its effects on mood, social behavior, personality expression, and executive functioning.

Additionally, LSD has been shown to have an affinity for several 5-HT subtypes and other receptors (see Table 31-1), though a full understanding of the relationship between the activation of these receptors and the subject effects of the drug are still poorly understood. Downstream effects on dopaminergic pathways and on the glutamate system may also be partially responsible for LSD's effects on mood and the phenomenon of ego dissolution.

Therapeutic Index

The average lethal dose (LD50) of LSD is 16.5 mg/kg (iv) for rats and 46 to 60 mg/kg (iv) for mice. There have been no documented human deaths attributed solely to LSD toxicity.

Shared Characteristics of Psilocybin and LSD
Therapeutic Indications and Off-Label Uses

As of this writing, psilocybin and LSD are considered Schedule I drugs and are not indicated for any condition. However, clinical trials are investigating their potential efficacy in treating anxiety, depression, posttraumatic stress disorder,

Psychedelics

TABLE 31-1: Lysergic Acid Diethylamide Affinity at Receptors		
Receptor	Ki (nM)	Species
5-HT$_{1A}$	1.1	Human
5-HT$_{1B}$	3.9	Rat
5-HT$_{1D}$	14	Human
5-HT$_{1E}$	93	Rat
5-HT$_{2A}$	2.7	Human
5-HT$_{2B}$	30	Rat
5-HT$_{2C}$	5.5	Rat
5-HT$_{4L}$	1,000	Rat
5-HT$_{5A}$	9	Rat
5-HT$_{5B}$	3.23	Rat
5-HT$_6$	2.3	Human
5-HT$_7$	6.6	Rat
5-HT$_{7L}$	10	Rat
Adrenergic Alpha	220	Rat
Adrenergic Beta$_1$	140	Rat
Adrenergic Beta$_2$	740	Rat
Dopamine D$_1$	180	Rat
Dopamine D$_2$	120	Rat
Dopamine D$_3$	27	Rat
Dopamine D$_4$	56	Rat
Dopamine D$_5$	340	Rat
Histamine H$_1$	1,540	Rat

and substance use disorders. Classic psychedelics may also be useful in end-of-life care as a means of reducing existential distress. Emerging evidence also suggests that those who have used psilocybin and LSD may be at a reduced risk of developing opioid use disorder.

Tolerance, Dependence, and Withdrawal

Tolerance to psilocybin and LSD is readily established but dissipates quickly, and cross-tolerance to other classical psychedelics has also been observed. Physical dependence and symptoms of withdrawal are extremely rare.

Precautions and Adverse Effects

Psilocybin, LSD, and psychedelic-assisted therapy in general are typically contraindicated for people with a personal or family history of severe and persistent mental illnesses or existing psychiatric comorbidities that make them more susceptible to psychosis. It is also not recommended for patients who express significant fear about psychedelics, because the wrong mindset can precipitate a distressing experience (a "bad trip") that can be deeply traumatic.

Even those who view psychedelics in a positive light may experience adverse psychological effects during the acute phase of the treatment, including confusion, fear, paranoia, and unpleasant hallucinations. Other common adverse effects include headache, pupil dilation, tachycardia, nausea, and increased blood pressure. Consequently, patients with cardiovascular disease may not be suitable candidates for psychedelic-assisted therapy.

There is minimal risk of abuse or overdose. Likewise, the risk of prolonged psychosis following use in a clinical setting is negligible in otherwise healthy adults.

Drug Interactions

Psilocybin and LSD target serotonin receptors, which are also the targets of many antidepressants as well as atypical antipsychotic medications. Acute administration of selective serotonin reuptake inhibitors (SSRIs) potentiates the effects of psilocybin and LSD whereas chronic administration downregulates serotonin receptors, thereby attenuating the effects of these drugs. Most medicines that alter the effects of psychedelics should be tapered and discontinued at least 2 weeks prior to initiating psychedelic therapy. Considering the long half-life of fluoxetine, it should be tapered and discontinued at least 6 weeks prior to beginning psychedelic therapy. For a more robust list of drug–drug interactions, see Table 31-2.

There is a mild to moderate risk of patients developing serotonin syndrome if psilocybin and LSD are taken concurrently with another drug that increases serotonin levels (see Table 31-3).

TABLE 31-2: Drug–Drug Interactions between Antidepressants and Classic Psychedelics

Drug Type	Examples
Monoamine oxidase inhibitors	Isocarboxazid, moclobemide, phenelzine, selegeline, tranylcypromine
Noradrenergic and specific serotonergic antidepressants	Mianserin, mirtazapine, setiptiline
Select serotonin reuptake inhibitors	Citalopram, escitalopram, fluvoxamine, fluoxetine[a], paroxetine, sertraline
Serotonin modulators	Nefazodone, trazodone, vilazodone, vortioxetine
Serotonin norepinephrine reuptake inhibitors	Desvenlafaxine, duloxetine, levomilnacipran, venlafaxine
Serotonin partial agonist reuptake inhibitors	Vilazodone, vortioxetine
Tricyclic antidepressants	Amitriptyline, chlorpheniramine, clomipramine, desipramine, imipramine, nortriptyline
Other	Buspirone

Listed drugs should be tapered and discontinued at least 2 weeks prior to acute psychedelic therapy.
[a]Fluoxetine should be tapered and discontinued at least 6 weeks prior to acute psychedelic therapy.

Psychedelics

TABLE 31-3: Drugs Associated with Elevated Serotonin Levels and Serotonin Syndrome

Drug Type	Examples
Analgesics	Fentanyl, meperidine, pentazocine, tramadol
Antibiotics	Linezolide, ritonavir
Anticonvulsants	Valproate
Antidepressants	Buspirone, clomipramine, nefazodone, trazodone, venlafaxine
Antiemetics	Granisetron, metoclopramide, ondansetron
Antimigraine medications	Sumatriptan
Bariatric drugs	Sibutramine
Monoamine oxidase inhibitors	Clorgiline, isocarboxazid, moclobemide, phenelzine
Over-the-counter drugs	Dextromethorphan
Selective serotonin reuptake inhibitors	Citalopram, fluoxetine, fluvoxamine, paroxetine, sertraline

Dosage and Clinical Guidelines

At this time, there are no dosage or clinical guidelines pertaining to the administration of these drugs.

Conclusion

Any optimism about the clinical utility of psychedelic-assisted therapy needs to be tempered by the reality that the current state of clinical research into classic psychedelics like LSD and psilocybin remains preliminary. While early phase studies suggest that psychedelic-assisted therapy holds a great deal of promise to bring relief to patients who are experiencing difficult to treat conditions like anxiety, substance use, mood, and affective disorders, strong clinical evidence is currently lacking to support their use for any indication. However, anecdotal evidence suggests that psychedelic-assisted therapy can help individuals figuratively open up and accelerate their ability to process difficult emotions or view traumatic memories with new and profound insights. Should these findings be supported by late phase clinical trials, there is no doubt that they will become integral tools to the field of psychiatry.

Selective Serotonin–Norepinephrine Reuptake Inhibitors

32

Generic Name	Trade Name	Adverse Effects	Drug Interactions	CYP Interactions
Venlafaxine	Effexor	Suicidality, GI symptoms, sexual dysfunction, sedation, insomnia, dizziness, hypertension, headache	MAOI, SERO	2D6, 3A4
Desvenlafaxine succinate	Pristiq, Aptryxol, Khedezla	Suicidality, GI symptoms, sexual dysfunction sedation, insomnia, dizziness, headache	MAOI, SERO	3A4, 2D6
Duloxetine	Cymbalta	Suicidality, GI symptoms, fatigue, sedation, hyperglycemia	MAOI, SERO	2D6, 1A2, 3A4, 2C9, 2B6, 2C19
Levomilnacipran	Fetzima	Suicidality, GI symptoms, tachycardia, sexual dysfunction	MAOI, SERO	3A4, 2C8, 2C19, 2D6, 2J2
Milnacipran	Savella	Suicidality, GI symptoms, tachycardia, sexual dysfunction	MAOI, SERO	3A4, 2C8, 2C19, 2D6, 2J2
Viloxazine	Qelbree	Suicidality, fatigue, GI symptoms, tachycardia, insomnia, headache	MAOI, SERO	1A2, 2D6, 3A4, 3A5, 2B6

Introduction

There are currently four serotonin–norepinephrine reuptake inhibitors (SNRIs) that have been approved for use as antidepressants in the United States: venlafaxine (Effexor and Effexor XR), desvenlafaxine succinate (Pristiq, Aptryxol, Khedezla), duloxetine (Cymbalta), and levomilnacipran (Fetzima). Milnacipran (Savella) is available in other countries as an antidepressant, but the Food and Drug Administration (FDA) has only approved its use as a treatment for fibromyalgia. More recently, viloxazine, which has been available in Europe as an antidepressant in immediate-release formulation for over two decades, was approved by the FDA for use in children and adolescents with attention-deficit hyperactivity disorder (ADHD). It is sold as an extended-release formulation under the trade name Qelbree.

As is the case with all antidepressant medications, there is an increased risk of suicidal thinking and behavior in children, adolescents, and young adults taking antidepressants for major depressive disorder.

Serotonin syndrome is a serious condition that usually occurs with coadministration of serotonin-based antidepressants and clinicians should be cautious if using SNRIs with drugs that have serotonergic effects.

Pharmacodynamics

Five of the drugs discussed in this chapter—venlafaxine, desvenlafaxine, duloxetine, levomilnacipran, and viloxazine—share similar pharmacodynamics and mechanisms of action. The pharmacodynamics of milnacipran are somewhat unique and will be covered below.

The term SNRI reflects the belief that the therapeutic effects of these medications are mediated by concomitant blockade of neuronal serotonin (5-HT) and norepinephrine uptake transporters. The SNRIs are also sometimes referred to as dual reuptake inhibitors, a broader functional class of antidepressant medications that includes tricyclic antidepressants (TCAs) such as clomipramine (Anafranil) and, to a lesser extent, imipramine (Tofranil) and amitriptyline. What distinguishes the SNRIs from TCAs is their relative lack of affinity for other receptors, especially muscarinic, histaminergic, and the families of α- and β-adrenergic receptors. This distinction is an important one because the SNRIs have a more favorable tolerability profile than the TCAs.

However, viloxazine has demonstrated a wider range of activity, including antagonistic activity at $5\text{-}HT_{2B}$ receptors and agonistic activity at $5\text{-}HT_{2C}$ receptors; weak activity at other sites including $5\text{-}HT_7$ (agonistic), adrenergic β_2-adrenoceptors (antagonistic), and α_{1B}-adrenoceptors (antagonistic); and very weak activity toward several other adrenoceptors (ADRs), including $ADR\alpha_{1A}$, $ADR\alpha_{2A}$, $ADR\alpha_{2B}$, $ADR\alpha_{2C}$, and $ADR_{\beta1}$.

VENLAFAXINE AND DESVENLAFAXINE

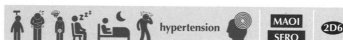

hypertension | MAOI SERO | 2D6 3A4

Pharmacokinetics

Venlafaxine is rapidly absorbed in the gastrointestinal tract, with a bioavailability of 45%. Immediate-release venlafaxine reaches maximum concentrations in an average of 2 hours, while extended-release formulations reach maximum concentrations in an average of 5.5 hours. Metabolism primarily occurs in the liver and involves the cytochrome P450 isoenzyme CYP2D6. Its major metabolite, O-desmethylvenlafaxine (ODV), reaches maximum concentrations within 3 hours after administration of immediate-release formulations and 9 hours after administration of extended-release formulations. Venlafaxine and ODV reach steady-state concentrations within 3 days of multiple oral dose therapy. Food does not affect the pharmacokinetics of venlafaxine.

Following oral administration, desvenlafaxine has a bioavailability of 80% and mean peak plasma concentrations are reached in 7.5 hours. Food may increase exposure, but the difference between fasting state and fed state is not clinically significant. Plasma protein binding is relatively low (30%) and independent of drug concentration. Desvenlafaxine undergoes first-pass metabolism involving multiple uridine 5′-diphospho-glucuronosyltransferase (UGT) isoforms and the cytochrome P450 isoenzyme CYP3A4, and as much as 45% of parent compound may be excreted in urine unchanged within 72 hours. The mean terminal half-life of desvenlafaxine is 11 hours. Steady-state plasma concentrations are reached within 4 to 5 days of consistent dosing.

Therapeutic Indications

Venlafaxine is approved for treatment of four psychiatric disorders: major depressive disorder, generalized anxiety disorder, social anxiety disorder, and panic disorder. Major depressive disorder is currently the only FDA-approved indication for desvenlafaxine.

Depression

The FDA does not recognize any class of antidepressant as being more effective than any other. This does not mean that differences do not exist, but no study to date has sufficiently demonstrated such superiority. It has been argued that direct modulation of serotonin and norepinephrine may convey greater antidepressant effects than are exerted by medications that selectively enhance only noradrenergic or serotoninergic neurotransmission alone. This greater therapeutic benefit could result from an acceleration of postsynaptic adaptation to increased neuronal signaling; simultaneous activation of two pathways for intracellular signal transduction; additive effects on the activity of relevant genes such as brain-derived neurotrophic factor; or, quite simply, broader coverage of depressive symptoms. Clinical evidence supporting this hypothesis first emerged in a pair of studies conducted by the Danish University Antidepressant Group, which found an advantage for the dual reuptake inhibitor clomipramine compared with the selective serotonin reuptake inhibitors (SSRIs) citalopram (Celexa) and paroxetine (Paxil). Another report, which compared the results of a group of patients prospectively treated with the combination of the TCA desipramine (Norpramin) and the SSRI fluoxetine (Prozac), with a historical comparison group treated with desipramine alone, provided additional support. A meta-analysis of 25 inpatient studies comparing the efficacy of TCAs and SSRIs yielded the strongest evidence. Specifically, although the TCAs were found to have a modest overall advantage, superiority versus SSRIs was almost entirely explained by the studies that used the TCAs that are considered to be dual reuptake inhibitors—clomipramine, amitriptyline, and imipramine. Meta-analyses of head-to-head studies suggest that venlafaxine has a potential to induce higher rates of remission in depressed patients than do the SSRIs. This difference of the venlafaxine advantage is about 6%. Desvenlafaxine has not been extensively compared with other classes of antidepressants with respect to efficacy.

Generalized Anxiety Disorder

The extended-release formulation of venlafaxine is approved for treatment of generalized anxiety disorder and the management of anxiety-related symptoms. In clinical trials lasting 6 months, dosages of 75 to 225 mg a day were effective in treating insomnia, poor concentration, restlessness, irritability, and excessive muscle tension related to generalized anxiety disorder.

Social Anxiety Disorder

The extended-release formulation of venlafaxine is approved for treatment of social anxiety disorder. Its efficacy was established in 12-week studies.

Panic Disorder

The extended-release formulation of venlafaxine is approved for treatment of panic disorder and its efficacy was established in two 12-week studies. The drug often takes upward of 2 weeks for adequate response to occur.

Off-Label Uses

Case reports and uncontrolled studies have indicated that venlafaxine may be beneficial in the treatment of obsessive-compulsive disorder, agoraphobia, social phobia, ADHD, and patients with a dual diagnosis of depression and cocaine dependence. It has also been used in chronic pain syndromes with good effect. Clinicians should be mindful of the fact that venlafaxine may trigger manic episodes in those with a predisposition for bipolar disorder. Therefore, addition of a mood-stabilizing agent may be necessary to avoid triggering a manic episode.

Desvenlafaxine has also been used as an alternative to estrogen to treat hot flashes during menopause.

Precautions and Adverse Reactions

Venlafaxine has a safety and tolerability profile similar to that of the more widely prescribed SSRI class. Nausea is the most frequently reported treatment-emergent adverse effect associated with therapies involving venlafaxine and desvenlafaxine. Initiating therapy at lower dosages and with food may attenuate nausea. When extremely problematic, treatment-induced nausea can be controlled by prescribing a selective $5-HT_3$ antagonist or mirtazapine (Remeron).

Venlafaxine and desvenlafaxine therapies are associated with sexual side effects, predominantly decreased libido and a delay to orgasm or ejaculation. The incidence of these side effects may range from 30% to 40% when there is direct, detailed assessment of sexual function.

Other common side effects include headache, insomnia, somnolence, dry mouth, dizziness, constipation, asthenia, sweating, and nervousness. Although several side effects are suggestive of anticholinergic effects, these drugs have no affinity for muscarinic or nicotinic receptors. Thus, noradrenergic agonism is likely to be the culprit.

Higher-dose venlafaxine therapy is associated with an increased risk of sustained elevations of blood pressure (BP). Experience with the instant-release (IR) formulation in studies of depressed patients indicated that sustained hypertension was dose related, increasing from 3% to 7% at doses of 100 to 300 mg per day and to 13% at doses greater than 300 mg per day. In this data set, venlafaxine therapy did not adversely affect BP control of patients taking antihypertensives and actually lowered mean values of patients with elevated BP readings before therapy. In controlled studies of the extended-release formulation, venlafaxine therapy resulted in only approximately a 1% greater risk of high BP when compared to placebo. Arbitrarily capping the upper dose of venlafaxine used in these studies thus greatly attenuated concerns about elevated BP. When higher doses of the extended-release formulation are used, however, monitoring of BP is recommended.

Venlafaxine and desvenlafaxine are commonly associated with a discontinuation syndrome. This syndrome is characterized by the appearance of a constellation of adverse effects during a rapid taper or abrupt cessation, including dizziness, dry mouth, insomnia, nausea, nervousness, sweating, anorexia, diarrhea, somnolence, and sensory disturbances. These may feel like tingling sensations, like getting an electric shock, or what some patients have described as "brain zaps." It is recommended that, whenever possible, a slow taper schedule should be used when longer-term treatment must be stopped. On occasion, substituting a few doses of the sustained-release formulation of fluoxetine may help to bridge this transition.

There were no overdose fatalities in premarketing trials of venlafaxine, although electrocardiographic changes (e.g., prolongation of QT interval, bundle branch block, QRS interval prolongation), tachycardia, bradycardia, hypotension, hypertension, coma, serotonin syndrome, and seizures were reported. Fatal overdoses have been documented subsequently, typically involving venlafaxine ingestion in combination with other drugs, alcohol, or both.

Use in Pregnancy and Lactation

Venlafaxine and desvenlafaxine are both classified as pregnancy category C drugs. Information concerning use of venlafaxine and desvenlafaxine by pregnant and nursing women is limited, but they appear to be relatively safe. Venlafaxine and desvenlafaxine are excreted in human milk.

Drug Interactions

Venlafaxine is metabolized in the liver primarily by the CYP2D6 isoenzyme. Because the parent drug and principal metabolite are essentially equipotent, medications that inhibit this isoenzyme usually do not adversely affect therapy. Venlafaxine is itself a relatively weak inhibitor of CYP2D6, although it can increase levels of substrates such as desipramine or risperidone (Risperdal). In vitro and in vivo studies have shown venlafaxine to cause little or no inhibition of CYP1A2, CYP2C9, CYP2C19, and CYP3A4.

Desvenlafaxine is metabolized in the liver primarily by the CYP3A4 isoenzyme. Potent inhibitors of CYP3A4 may result in higher concentrations of desvenlafaxine. Desvenlafaxine does not appear to inhibit cytochrome P450 isoenzymes CYP1A1, CYP1A2, CYP2A6, CYP2D6, CYP2C8, CYP2C9, CYP2C19, or CYP2E1.

Venlafaxine and desvenlafaxine are contraindicated in patients taking monoamine oxidase inhibitors (MAOIs) and serotonergic drugs because of the risk of a pharmacodynamic interaction (i.e., serotonin syndrome). An MAOI should not be started for at least 14 days after stopping venlafaxine or desvenlafaxine. Few data are available regarding the combination of venlafaxine or desvenlafaxine with atypical antipsychotics, benzodiazepines, lithium (Eskalith), and anticonvulsants; therefore, clinical judgment should be exercised when combining medications.

Laboratory Interferences

Data are not currently available on laboratory interferences with venlafaxine.

Dosage and Administration

Venlafaxine is available in 25-, 37.5-, 50-, 75-, and 100-mg tablets and 37.5-, 75-, and 150-mg extended-release capsules. The tablets and the extended-release capsules are equally potent, and persons stabilized with one can switch to an equivalent dosage of the other. Since the immediate-release tablets are rarely used because of their tendency to cause nausea and the need for multiple daily doses, the dosage recommendations that follow refer to the use of extended-release capsules.

In depressed persons, venlafaxine demonstrates a dose–response curve. The initial therapeutic dosage is 75 mg a day given once a day. However, most persons are started at a dosage of 37.5 mg for 4 to 7 days to minimize adverse effects, particularly nausea. A convenient starter kit for the drug contains a 1-week supply of both the 37.5- and 75-mg strengths. If a rapid titration is preferred, the dosage can be raised to 150 mg per day after day 4. As a rule, the dosage can be raised in increments of 75 mg a day every 4 or more days. Although the recommended upper dosage of the extended-release preparation (venlafaxine XR) is 225 mg per day, it is approved by the FDA for use at dosages up to 375 mg a day. The dosage of venlafaxine should be halved in persons with significantly diminished hepatic or renal function. If discontinued, venlafaxine use should be gradually tapered over 2 to 4 weeks to avoid withdrawal symptoms.

There are minor differences in the doses used for major depression, generalized anxiety disorder, and social anxiety disorder. In the treatment of these disorders, for example, a dose–response effect has not been found. In addition, lower mean dosages are typically used, with most patients taking 75 to 150 mg per day.

Desvenlafaxine is available as 50- and 100-mg extended-release tablets under the trade names Pristiq, Aptryxol, and Khedezla. The therapeutic dose for most patients is 50 mg a day. Although some patients may need higher doses, in clinical trials, no greater therapeutic benefit was noted when the dose was increased. At higher doses, adverse event and discontinuation rates were increased. Patients with severe renal impairment should reduce dosages to 50 mg every other day and should not take supplemental doses after dialysis.

DULOXETINE

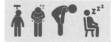 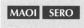

Pharmacologic Actions

Duloxetine is formulated as a delayed-release capsule to reduce the risk of severe nausea associated with the drug. It is well absorbed, but there is a 2-hour delay before absorption begins. Peak plasma concentrations occur 6 hours after ingestion. Food delays the time to achieve maximum concentrations from 6 to

10 hours and reduces the extent of absorption by about 10%. Duloxetine has an elimination half-life of about 12 hours (range: 8 to 17 hours) and steady-state plasma concentrations occur after 3 days. Elimination is mainly through the isozymes CYP2D6 and CYP1A2, and duloxetine undergoes extensive hepatic metabolism to numerous metabolites. About 70% of the drug appears in the urine as metabolites and about 20% is excreted in the feces. Duloxetine is 90% protein bound.

Therapeutic Indications

Depression

In contrast to venlafaxine, a small number of studies have compared duloxe-tine with the SSRIs. Although these studies are suggestive of some advantage in efficacy, their findings are limited by the use of fixed, low starting doses of paroxetine and fluoxetine, but dosages of duloxetine in some studies were as high as 120 mg per day. Any inferences on whether duloxetine is superior to SSRIs in any aspect of treatment for depression thus await more evidence from properly designed trials.

Generalized Anxiety Disorder

Duloxetine is approved for treatment of generalized anxiety disorder. Its efficacy was established in three randomized, double-blind, placebo-controlled trials.

Neuropathic Pain Associated with Diabetes and Stress Urinary Incontinence

Duloxetine was the first drug to be approved by the FDA as a treatment for neuro-pathic pain associated with diabetes. The drug has been studied for its effects on physical symptoms, including pain, in depressed patients, but these effects have not been compared with those seen with other widely used agents such as venlafaxine .and the TCAs. Duloxetine has been studied as a treatment for stress urinary incon-tinence, the inability to voluntarily control bladder voiding, which is the most fre-quent type of incontinence in women. The action of duloxetine in the treatment of stress urinary incontinence is associated with its effects in the sacral spinal cord, which in turn increase the activity of the striated urethral sphincter. Duloxetine is marketed under the name Yentreve in the United Kingdom.

Other Indications

Duloxetine is also FDA approved for use in treating fibromyalgia and chronic musculoskeletal pain.

Off-Label Uses

Duloxetine may be an effective treatment of panic disorder, schizophrenia, and borderline personality disorder.

Precautions and Adverse Reactions

The most common adverse reactions are nausea, dry mouth, dizziness, constipa-tion, fatigue, decreased appetite, anorexia, somnolence, and increased sweating.

Selective Serotonin–Norepinephrine Reuptake Inhibitors

Nausea was the most common side effect leading to treatment discontinuation in clinical trials. The true incidence of sexual dysfunction is unknown, though erectile dysfunction, difficulty orgasming, premature ejaculation, and decreased libido have all been anecdotally reported, particularly during the initial weeks of treatment. The long-term effects on body weight are also unknown. In clinical trials, treatment with duloxetine was associated with mean increases in BP averaging 2 mm Hg systolic and 0.5 mm Hg diastolic versus placebo. No studies have compared the BP effects of venlafaxine and duloxetine at equivalent therapeutic doses.

Close monitoring is suggested when using duloxetine in patients who have or are at risk for diabetes. Duloxetine has been shown to increase blood sugar and hemoglobin A1C levels during long-term treatment. Hepatic failure has been reported in patients taking duloxetine and the drug should be discontinued if they develop jaundice or show signs of liver dysfunction. Abnormal bleeding events have also been observed in patients taking duloxetine.

Patients with substantial alcohol use should not be treated with duloxetine because of possible hepatic effects. It also should not be prescribed for patients with hepatic insufficiency and end-stage renal disease or for patients with uncontrolled narrow-angle glaucoma.

Abrupt discontinuation of duloxetine should be avoided because it may produce a discontinuation syndrome similar to that of venlafaxine. A gradual dose reduction is recommended.

Use in Pregnancy and Lactation

Duloxetine is a pregnancy category C drug, which means that risk to fetal development cannot be ruled out. Though information concerning use of duloxetine by pregnant and nursing women is limited, fetal risk appears to be low. Levels of duloxetine excreted in human milk are low, but there still may be risks to infants if the mother takes duloxetine while nursing.

Drug Interactions

Duloxetine is a moderate inhibitor of cytochrome P450 isoenzymes CYP2D6 and CYP1A2. Duloxetine is contraindicated in patients taking MAOIs and patients should wait at least 14 days after stopping treatment with an MAOI before taking duloxetine.

Laboratory Interferences

Data are not currently available on laboratory interferences with duloxetine.

Dosage and Administration

Duloxetine is available in 20-, 30-, and 60-mg tablets. The recommended therapeutic, and maximum, dosage is 60 mg per day. The 20- and 30-mg doses are useful for either initial therapy or for twice-daily use as strategies to reduce side effects. In clinical trials, dosages of up to 120 mg per day were studied, but no consistent advantage in efficacy was noted at dosages higher than 60 mg per day. Duloxetine thus does not appear to demonstrate a dosage–response curve. However, there were difficulties in tolerability with single doses above 60 mg.

Accordingly, when dosages of 80 and 120 mg per day were used, they were administered as 40 or 60 mg twice daily.

MILNACIPRAN AND LEVOMILNACIPRAN

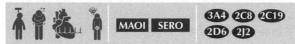

Milnacipran is approved by the FDA only for the treatment of fibromyalgia. Although some countries have approved milnacipran for general use as an antidepressant, efficacy is not as well established. Unlike milnacipran, levomilnacipran is not approved for the management of fibromyalgia. Compared with venlafaxine, milnacipran is approximately five times more potent for inhibition of norepinephrine uptake than for 5-HT reuptake inhibition. Milnacipran has a half-life of approximately 8 hours and shows linear pharmacokinetics between doses of 50 and 250 mg per day. Metabolized in the liver, milnacipran has no active metabolites and is primarily excreted by the kidneys.

Milnacipran is available as 12.5-, 25-, 50-, and 100-mg tablets. The standard recommended milnacipran dose is as follows: day 1, 12.5 mg once daily; days 2 and 3, 12.5 mg twice daily; days 4 to 7, 25 mg twice daily; and day 7 and beyond, 50 mg twice daily.

Levomilnacipran (Fetzima)

Levomilnacipran is an active enantiomer of the racemic drug milnacipran. In vitro studies have shown that it has greater potency for norepinephrine reuptake inhibition than for serotonin reuptake inhibition and does not directly affect the uptake of dopamine or other neurotransmitters.

Pharmacokinetics

Following oral administration, levomilnacipran reaches peak concentration in 6 to 8 hours and has a bioavailability of 92%. Food does not appear to affect levomilnacipran concentrations. Plasma protein binding is 22%. Levomilnacipran is primarily metabolized in the liver by cytochrome P450 isoenzyme CYP3A4 and excreted in urine. Isoenzymes CYP28C, CYP2C19, CYP2D6, and CYP2J2 play a less significant role. Approximately 58% of the parent compound is excreted in urine unchanged, and the terminal half-life is approximately 12 hours.

Therapeutic Indications

Levomilnacipran is indicated for the treatment of major depressive disorder. It is taken once daily as a sustained-release formulation. In clinical trials, doses of 40, 80, or 120 mg improved symptoms compared with placebo.

Precautions and Adverse Reactions

Adverse events associated with the use of levomilnacipran may include, but are not limited to, the following: nausea, constipation, hyperhidrosis, heart rate

Selective Serotonin–Norepinephrine Reuptake Inhibitors

increase, erectile dysfunction, tachycardia, vomiting, and palpitations. The only dose-related adverse events in clinical trials were urinary hesitation and erectile dysfunction.

As with all serotonergic drugs, a gradual dose reduction is recommended instead of an abrupt discontinuation. Levomilnacipran therapy is associated with increases in BP and caution is advised before beginning levomilnacipran treatment in patients with hypertension, cardiovascular disease, or cerebrovascular conditions that might be exacerbated by increases in BP. Abnormal bleeding events have also been observed in patients taking levomilnacipran.

Use in Pregnancy and Lactation

Levomilnacipran may pose some risk to fetal development, though information concerning its use by pregnant and nursing women is limited. Levels of levomilnacipran excreted in human milk are low, but there still may be risks to infants if the mother takes duloxetine while nursing.

Drug Interactions

The dose of levomilnacipran should not exceed 80 mg once daily when used with strong CYP3A4 inhibitors such as ketoconazole, clarithromycin, or ritonavir (Norvir). Levomilnacipran is contraindicated in patients taking MAOIs and patients should wait at least 14 days after stopping treatment with an MAOI before taking levomilnacipran.

Laboratory Interferences

Data are not currently available on laboratory interferences with levomilnacipran.

Dosage and Administration

Levomilnacipran is supplied as 20-, 40-, 80-, and 120-mg extended-release capsules for oral administration. The recommended dose range for levomilnacipran is 40 to 120 mg once daily, with or without food. Levomilnacipran should be initiated at 20 mg once daily for 2 days and then increased to 40 mg once daily. Based on efficacy and tolerability, the drug may then be increased in increments of 40 mg at intervals of 2 or more days. The maximum recommended dose is 120 mg once daily. Levomilnacipran should be taken at approximately the same time each day and should be swallowed whole. Capsules should not be opened, chewed, or crushed. As with most newly approved antidepressants, efficacy of levomilnacipran has not been established beyond 8 weeks.

Dose adjustment is not recommended in patients with mild renal impairment (creatinine clearance of 60 to 89 mL/min). For patients with moderate renal impairment (creatinine clearance of 30 to 59 mL/min), the maintenance dose should not exceed 80 mg once daily. For patients with severe renal impairment (creatinine clearance of 15 to 29 mL/min), the maintenance dose should not exceed 40 mg once daily. Levomilnacipran is not recommended for patients with end-stage renal disease.

VILOXAZINE

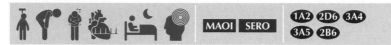

Pharmacokinetics

The relative bioavailability of viloxazine is 88%, while the mean peak plasma concentration following oral administration is 5 hours for extended-release viloxazine. Consumption of high-fat meals totaling 800 calories and 1,000 calories decrease exposure of viloxazine by 9% and 8%, respectively, and increase time to peak plasma concentrations by 2 hours. Viloxazine is 76% to 82% bound to plasma proteins and metabolized by the cytochrome P450 isoenzyme CYP2D6 and UGT isoforms UGT1A9 and UGT2B15. Ninety percent of radiolabeled viloxazine is recovered in urine within 24 hours, while only 1% is recovered in feces. The mean half-life for viloxazine is 7.02 hours.

Therapeutic Indications

Viloxazine is indicated for the treatment of ADHD in pediatric patients 6 to 17 years of age.

Off-Label Uses

The immediate-release formulation of viloxazine has long been used in Europe as an antidepressant. As viloxazine does not produce anticholinergic side effects, it may be an effective treatment for depression in geriatric populations.

Precautions and Adverse Reactions

Adverse events associated with the use of viloxazine may include, but are not limited to, the following: somnolence, nausea, headache, irritability, tachycardia, fatigue, decreased appetite, vomiting, and insomnia.

As with other antidepressants, patients with bipolar disorder may experience a manic episode during viloxazine treatment. As with all serotonergic drugs, a gradual dose reduction is recommended instead of an abrupt discontinuation. Viloxazine therapy is associated with increases in BP and caution is advised before beginning viloxazine treatment in patients with hypertension, cardiovascular disease, or cerebrovascular conditions that might be exacerbated by increases in BP. Abnormal bleeding events have also been observed in patients taking viloxazine.

Use in Pregnancy and Lactation

Viloxazine may pose some risk to fetal development, though information concerning its use by pregnant and nursing women is limited. Viloxazine is likely excreted in human milk, so there may be some risk associated with the use of viloxazine while nursing.

Drug Interactions

Viloxazine is contraindicated in patients taking MAOIs and patients should wait at least 14 days after stopping treatment with an MAOI before taking viloxazine.

Viloxazine is a strong inhibitor of CYP1A2. Some sensitive CYP1A2 substrates with a narrow therapeutic range such as alosetron (Lotronex), duloxetine (Cymbalta), ramelteon (Rozerem), tasimelteon (Hetlioz), tizanidine (Zanaflex), and theophylline (Theocron) are contraindicated with viloxazine, while dose adjustments may be necessary for sensitive CYP1A2 substrates without a narrow therapeutic range (e.g., clozapine, pirfenidone [Esbriet]).

Viloxazine is a weak inhibitor of CYP2D6 and CYP3A4. Other substrates of CYP2D6 (e.g., atomoxetine [Strattera], desipramine, dextromethorphan) and CYP3A4 (e.g., avanafil [Stendra], buspirone, conivaptan [Aquaretic]) isoenzymes may affect the pharmacology of viloxazine and vice versa, and dosage adjustments may be warranted.

Laboratory Interferences

Data are not currently available on laboratory interferences with viloxazine.

Dosage and Administration

Viloxazine is available in 100-, 150-, and 200-mg extended-release capsules and should be consumed whole with or without food. The recommended starting dosage for patients 6 to 11 years of age is 100 mg orally once daily. Dosages can be titrated in increments of 100 mg at weekly intervals if tolerated with the maximum dosage being 400 mg once daily. For patients 12 to 17 years of age, the recommended starting dosage is 200 mg orally once daily; and if well tolerated, the dosage can be titrated to 400 mg once daily after 1 week.

Dosage reduction is recommended in patients with severe renal impairment, though no such reductions are necessary in patients with mild or moderate renal impairment. The effect of hepatic impairment on viloxazine is unknown at this time.

Selective Serotonin Reuptake Inhibitors

33

Generic Name	Trade Name	Adverse Effects	Drug Interactions	CYP Interactions
Citalopram	Celexa	Suicidality, sexual dysfunction, GI symptoms, cardiac arrhythmia, EPS, insomnia, sedation, fatigue, increased prolactin levels, skin rash	QT, MAOI, SERO, NSAID, clozapine, zolpidem, cimetidine, metoprolol	3A4, 2C19, D26, 1A2
Escitalopram	Lexapro	Suicidality, sexual dysfunction, GI symptoms, cardiac arrhythmia, EPS, insomnia, sedation, fatigue, increased prolactin levels, skin rash	QT, MAOI, SERO, NSAID, warfarin, clozapine, zolpidem, metoprolol, desipramine	3A4, 2D6, 2C19
Fluoxetine	Prozac	Suicidality, sexual dysfunction, GI symptoms, cardiac arrhythmia, EPS, insomnia, sedation, fatigue, increased prolactin levels, headache, skin rash	QT, MAOI, SERO, TRI, BENZ, antipsychotics, LITH, NSAID, warfarin, clozapine, zolpidem, carbamazepine, antineoplastic agents, phenytoin	2D6, 2B6, 3A4, 3A5, 1A2, 2C19
Fluvoxamine	Luvox	Suicidality, sexual dysfunction, GI symptoms, cardiac arrhythmia, EPS, insomnia, sedation, fatigue, increased prolactin levels, skin rash	QT, MAOI, SERO, NSAID, BENZ, warfarin, clozapine, zolpidem, carbamazepine, methadone, propranolol, diltiazem	3A4, 2D6, 1A1, 1A2, 2C9, 2C19, 2B6
Paroxetine	Paxil	Suicidality, sexual dysfunction, GI symptoms, cardiac arrhythmia, EPS, insomnia, sedation, fatigue, increased prolactin levels, rash, anticholinergic effects	QT, MAOI, SERO, TRI, NSAID, cimetidine, warfarin, clozapine, zolpidem, phenytoin, phenobarbital	2D6, 2B6, 1A2, 3A4, 2C19, 2C9
Sertraline	Zoloft	Suicidality, sexual dysfunction, GI symptoms, cardiac arrhythmia, EPS, insomnia, sedation, fatigue, increased prolactin levels, skin rash	QT, MAOI, SERO, TRI, BENZ, LITH, NSAID, antipsychotics, warfarin, clozapine, zolpidem, carbamazepine, antineoplastic agents, phenytoin, cimetidine	2D6, 3A4, 2C19, 2C9, 2B6, 2E1
Vilazodone	Viibryd	Suicidality, sexual dysfunction, GI symptoms, cardiac arrhythmia, EPS, insomnia, sedation, fatigue, increased prolactin levels, skin rash	QT, MAOI, SERO, NSAID, warfarin, clozapine, zolpidem	3A4, 2C19, 2D6

Introduction

The selective serotonin reuptake inhibitors (SSRIs) have been the most widely used class of psychopharmacologic agents to treat depression and anxiety since they were introduced over 35 years ago. They are considered "selective" because they have little effect on reuptake of norepinephrine or dopamine and exert their therapeutic effects primarily through serotonin reuptake inhibition. From a historical perspective, the most significant impact of fluoxetine (Prozac), the first SSRI to be approved by the Food and Drug Administration (FDA) and to be marketed in the United States, was the positive attention it generated in the popular press and the consequent reduction in the longstanding stigma and fear of taking antidepressants. Patients also experienced the benefits of no longer having to experience side effects such as dry mouth, constipation, sedation, orthostatic hypotension, and tachycardia, which are more commonly associated with the earlier antidepressant drugs like the tricyclic antidepressants (TCAs) and monoamine oxidase inhibitors (MAOIs). Fluoxetine is also significantly safer when taken in overdose compared to older antidepressants.

Since the launch of fluoxetine, many other SSRIs have been approved. These include sertraline (Zoloft), paroxetine (Paxil), fluvoxamine (Luvox), citalopram (Celexa), escitalopram (Lexapro), and vilazodone (Viibryd). Vortioxetine (Trintellix) is unofficially considered to be an SSRI because its major pharmacologic effect is to inhibit the serotonin reuptake transporter. However, since the FDA has designated the drug a "serotonin modulator and stimulator," it is discussed separately at the end of this chapter.

Regardless of pharmacodynamic variations of these drugs, they are all equally effective in treating depression. Additionally, some have received FDA approval for other indications, such as obsessive-compulsive disorder (OCD), posttraumatic stress disorder (PTSD), premenstrual dysphoric disorder (PMDD), panic disorder, and social phobia (social anxiety disorder) (see Table 33-1). Of note, fluvoxamine is not FDA approved as an antidepressant, a fact that is due to a marketing decision though it is labeled an antidepressant in other countries.

While all SSRIs are equally effective, there are meaningful differences in pharmacodynamics, pharmacokinetics, and side effects, differences that might affect clinical responses among individual patients. This would explain why some patients have better clinical responses to a particular SSRI than another. The SSRIs have proven more problematic in terms of some side effects than the original clinical trials suggested. Quality-of-life–associated adverse effects such as nausea, sexual dysfunction, and weight gain sometimes mitigate the therapeutic benefits of the SSRIs. There can also be distressing withdrawal symptoms when SSRIs are stopped abruptly. This is especially true with paroxetine but also occurs when other SSRIs with short half-lives are stopped abruptly.

Pharmacologic Actions

Pharmacokinetics

A significant difference among the SSRIs is their broad range of serum half-lives. Fluoxetine has the longest half-life: 4 to 6 days; its active metabolite has a half-life of 7 to 9 days. The half-life of sertraline is 26 hours, and its less active

TABLE 33-1: Currently Approved Indications of the Selective Serotonin Reuptake Inhibitors in the United States for Adult and Pediatric Populations

	Citalopram (Celexa)	Escitalopram (Lexapro)	Fluoxetine (Prozac)	Fluvoxamine (Luvox)	Paroxetine (Paxil)	Sertraline (Zoloft)	Vilazodone (Viibryd)
Major depressive disorder	Adult	Adult and pediatric	Adult[a] and pediatric	—	Adult[c]	Adult	Adult
Generalized anxiety disorder	—	Adult	—	—	Adult	—	—
OCD	—	—	Adult and pediatric	Adult and pediatric	Adult	Adult and pediatric	—
Panic disorder	—	—	Adult	—	Adult[c]	Adult	—
PTSD	—	—	—	—	Adult	Adult	—
Social anxiety disorder	—	—	—	—	Adult[c]	Adult	—
Bulimia nervosa	—	—	Adult	—	—	—	—
Premenstrual dysphoric disorder	—	—	Adult[b]	—	Adult[d]	Adult	—
Menopausal vasomotor symptoms	—	—	—	—	Adult[e]	—	—
Body dysmorphic disorder	—	—	Pediatric[f]	—	—	—	—
Autism	—	—	Pediatric[f]	—	—	—	—

[a]Weekly fluoxetine is approved for continuation and maintenance therapy in adults.
[b]Marketed as Sarafem.
[c]Paroxetine- and paroxetine-controlled release.
[d]Paroxetine-controlled release is approved for premenstrual dysphoric disorder.
[e]Marketed as Brisdelle.
[f]Received orphan drug designation for this indication.
OCD, obsessive-compulsive disorder; PTSD, posttraumatic stress disorder.

metabolite has a half-life of 3 to 5 days. The half-lives of the other five SSRIs, which do not have metabolites with significant pharmacologic activity, are 35 hours for citalopram, 27 to 32 hours for escitalopram, 21 hours for paroxetine, 15 hours for fluvoxamine, and 25 hours for vilazodone. As a rule, the SSRIs are well absorbed after oral administration and have their peak effects in the range of 3 to 8 hours. Absorption of sertraline may be slightly enhanced by food, while vilazodone can lose approximately half of its bioavailability unless taken with food.

There are also differences in plasma protein–binding percentages among the SSRIs, with vilazodone, sertraline, fluoxetine, and paroxetine being the most highly bound and escitalopram being the least bound.

All SSRIs are metabolized in the liver by the CYP450 enzymes. Because the SSRIs have such a wide therapeutic index, it is rare that other drugs produce problematic increases in SSRI concentrations. The most important drug–drug interactions involving the SSRIs occur as a result of the SSRIs inhibiting the metabolism of coadministered medication. Each of the SSRIs possesses a potential for slowing or blocking the metabolism of many drugs (Table 33-2). Fluvoxamine is the most problematic of the drugs in this respect. It has a marked effect on several of the CYP enzymes. Examples of clinically significant interactions include fluvoxamine and theophylline (Theo-Dur) through CYP1A2 interaction; fluvoxamine and clozapine (Clozaril) through CYP1A2 inhibition; and fluvoxamine with alprazolam (Xanax) or clonazepam (Klonopin) through CYP3A4 inhibition. Fluoxetine and paroxetine also possess significant effects on the

TABLE 33-2: CYP450 Inhibitory Potential of Commonly Prescribed Antidepressants

Relative Rank	CYP1A2	CYP2C	CYP2D6	CYP3A
Higher	Fluvoxamine (Luvox)	Fluoxetine	Bupropion	Fluvoxamine
		Fluvoxamine	Fluoxetine	Nefazodone
			Paroxetine	Tricyclics
			Vortioxetine	Vilazodone
Moderate	Tertiary amine tricyclics	Sertraline	Secondary amine tricyclics	Fluoxetine
	Fluoxetine (Prozac)		Citalopram (Celexa)	Sertraline
			Escitalopram (Lexapro)	
			Sertraline	
Low or minimal	Bupropion (Wellbutrin)	Paroxetine	Fluvoxamine	Citalopram
	Mirtazapine (Remeron)	Venlafaxine (Effexor)	Mirtazapine	Escitalopram
	Nefazodone (Serzone)		Nefazodone	Mirtazapine
	Paroxetine (Paxil)		Venlafaxine	Paroxetine
	Sertraline (Zoloft)			Venlafaxine
	Venlafaxine			
CYP, cytochrome P450.				

CYP2D6 isozyme, which may interfere with the efficacy of opiate analogs, such as codeine and hydrocodone, by blocking the conversion of these agents to their active form. Thus, coadministration of fluoxetine and paroxetine with an opiate interferes with its analgesic effects. Sertraline, citalopram, and escitalopram are least likely to complicate treatment because of CYP450 interactions.

Pharmacodynamics

Often, adequate clinical activity and saturation of the 5-HT transporters are achieved at starting dosages. As a rule, higher dosages do not increase antidepressant efficacy but may increase the risk of adverse effects.

Citalopram and escitalopram are the most selective inhibitors of serotonin reuptake, with very little inhibition of norepinephrine or dopamine reuptake and very low affinities for histamine H_1, γ-aminobutyric acid (GABA), or benzodiazepine receptors. The other SSRIs have a similar profile except that fluoxetine weakly inhibits norepinephrine reuptake and binds to 5-HT_{2C} receptors, sertraline weakly inhibits norepinephrine and dopamine reuptake, vilazodone has 5-HT_{1A} receptor agonist properties, and paroxetine has significant anticholinergic activity at higher dosages and binds to nitric oxide synthase.

A pharmacodynamic interaction appears to underlie the antidepressant effects of combined fluoxetine–olanzapine. When taken together, these drugs increase brain concentrations of norepinephrine and can help treat symptoms associated with depressive episodes in bipolar I disorder and treatment-resistant depression (see Therapeutic Indications below). Concomitant use of SSRIs and drugs in the triptan class (sumatriptan [Imitrex], naratriptan [Amerge], rizatriptan [Maxalt], and zolmitriptan [Zomig]) may result in a serious pharmacodynamic interaction—the development of a serotonin syndrome (see Precautions and Adverse Reactions). However, many people use triptans while taking low doses of an SSRI for headache prophylaxis without adverse reaction. A similar reaction may occur when SSRIs are combined with tramadol (Ultram).

Therapeutic Indications

Depression

In the United States, all SSRIs other than fluvoxamine have been approved by the FDA for treatment of depression. Several studies have found that antidepressants with serotonin–norepinephrine activity—drugs such as the MAOIs, TCAs, venlafaxine, and mirtazapine—may produce higher rates of remission than SSRIs in head-to-head studies. The continued role of SSRIs as first line treatments thus reflects their simplicity of use, safety, and broad spectrum of action.

Direct comparisons of individual SSRIs have not revealed any one of them to be consistently superior over another. There nevertheless can be considerable diversity in response to the various SSRIs among individuals. For example, more than 50% of people who respond poorly to one SSRI will respond favorably to another. Thus, before shifting to non-SSRI antidepressants, it is most reasonable to try other agents in the SSRI class for persons who did not respond to the first SSRI.

Some clinicians have attempted to select a particular SSRI for a specific person on the basis of the drug's unique adverse effect profile. For example, thinking that fluoxetine is an activating and stimulating SSRI may lead them to assume that it is a better choice for an abulic person than paroxetine, which is presumed to be a sedating SSRI. These differences, however, usually vary from person to person. Analyses of clinical trial data show that the SSRIs are more effective in patients with more severe symptoms of major depression than those with milder symptoms.

Depression During Pregnancy and Breastfeeding.   Rates of relapse of major depression during pregnancy among women who discontinue, attempt to discontinue, or modify their antidepressant regimens are extremely high and may range from 68% to 100% of patients. Thus, many women need to continue taking their medication during pregnancy and postpartum period. The impact of maternal depression on infant development is unknown. Of note, there is no increased risk for major congenital malformations after exposure to SSRIs during pregnancy. Thus, the risk of relapse into depression when a newly pregnant mother is taken off SSRIs is severalfold higher than the risk to the fetus of exposure to SSRIs.

Postpartum depression (with or without psychotic features) affects a small percentage of mothers. Some clinicians start administering SSRIs if the postpartum blues extend beyond a few weeks or if a woman becomes depressed during pregnancy. If a woman is at risk for postpartum depression, it may be wise to begin SSRI administration during pregnancy to protect the newborn, as some women may have harmful thoughts toward their infant after parturition.

Depression in Elderly and Medically Ill Persons.   The SSRIs are safe and well tolerated when used to treat elderly and medically ill persons. As a class, they have little or no cardiotoxic, anticholinergic, antihistaminergic, or α-adrenergic adverse effects. The one exception is paroxetine, which has some anticholinergic activity and may lead to constipation and worsening of cognition. The SSRIs can produce subtle cognitive deficits, prolonged bleeding time, and hyponatremia, all of which may impact the health of this population. The SSRIs are effective in poststroke depression and dramatically reduce the symptom of crying.

Depression in Children and Adolescents.   The use of SSRI antidepressants in children and adolescents has been controversial. Few studies have shown clear-cut benefits from the use of these drugs, and studies show that there may be an increase in suicidal or aggressive impulses. However, some children and adolescents do exhibit dramatic responses to these drugs in terms of depression and anxiety. Both fluoxetine and escitalopram are indicated for acute and maintenance treatment of major depressive disorder in adolescents 12 to 17 years of age. Fluoxetine has most consistently demonstrated effectiveness in reducing symptoms of depressive disorder in both children and adolescents. This may be a function of the quality of the clinical trials involved. Sertraline has been shown to be effective in treating social anxiety disorder in this population, especially when combined with cognitive-behavioral therapy. Given the potential negative effect of untreated depression and anxiety in a young population and the uncertainty about many aspects of how children and adolescents might react to medication, any use of SSRIs should be undertaken only within the context of comprehensive management of the patient.

Anxiety Disorders

Obsessive-Compulsive Disorder.   Fluvoxamine, paroxetine, sertraline, and fluoxetine are indicated for treatment of OCD in persons older than the age of 18 years. Fluvoxamine and sertraline have also been approved for treatment of children with OCD (ages 6 to 17 years). About 50% of persons with OCD begin to show symptoms in childhood or adolescence, and more than half of these respond favorably to medication. Beneficial responses can be dramatic. Long-term data support the model of OCD as a genetically determined, lifelong condition that is best treated continuously with drugs and cognitive-behavioral therapy from the onset of symptoms in childhood throughout the lifespan.

SSRI dosages for OCD may need to be higher than those required to treat depression. Although some response can be seen in the first few weeks of treatment, it may take several months for the maximum effects to become evident. Patients who fail to obtain adequate relief of their OCD symptoms with an SSRI often benefit from the addition of a small dose of risperidone (Risperdal). Apart from the extrapyramidal side effects of risperidone, patients should be monitored for increases in prolactin levels when this combination is used. Clinically, hyperprolactinemia may manifest as gynecomastia and galactorrhea (in both men and women) and loss of menses.

A number of disorders are now considered to be within the OCD spectrum. This includes a number of conditions and symptoms characterized by nonsuicidal self-mutilation, such as trichotillomania, eyebrow picking, nose picking, nail biting, compulsive picking of skin blemishes, and cutting. Patients with these behaviors benefit from treatment with SSRIs. Other spectrum disorders include compulsive gambling, compulsive shopping, hypochondriasis, and body dysmorphic disorder.

Panic Disorder.   Paroxetine and sertraline are indicated for treatment of panic disorder, with or without agoraphobia. These agents work less rapidly than do the benzodiazepines alprazolam (Xanax) and clonazepam (Klonopin) but are far superior to the benzodiazepines for treatment of panic disorder with comorbid depression. Citalopram, fluvoxamine, and fluoxetine also may reduce spontaneous or induced panic attacks. Because fluoxetine can initially heighten anxiety symptoms, persons with panic disorder must begin taking small dosages (5 mg a day) and increase the dosage slowly. Low doses of benzodiazepines may be given to manage this side effect.

Social Anxiety Disorder.   SSRIs are effective agents in the treatment of social phobia. They reduce both symptoms and disability. The response rate is comparable to that seen with the MAOI phenelzine (Nardil), the previous standard treatment. The SSRIs are safer to use than MAOIs or benzodiazepines.

Generalized Anxiety Disorder.   The SSRIs may be useful for the treatment of specific phobias, generalized anxiety disorder, and separation anxiety disorder. A thorough, individualized evaluation is the first approach, with particular attention to identifying conditions amenable to drug therapy. In addition, cognitive-behavioral or other psychotherapies can be added for greater efficacy.

Posttraumatic Stress Disorder

Pharmacotherapy for PTSD must target specific symptoms in three clusters: Reexperiencing, avoidance, and hyperarousal. For long-term treatment, SSRIs appear to have a broader spectrum of therapeutic effects on specific PTSD symptom clusters than do TCAs and MAOIs. Benzodiazepine augmentation is useful in the acute symptomatic state. The SSRIs are associated with marked improvement of both intrusive and avoidant symptoms.

Bulimia Nervosa and Other Eating Disorders

Fluoxetine is indicated for treatment of bulimia, which is best done in the context of psychotherapy. Dosages of 60 mg a day are significantly more effective than 20 mg a day. In several well-controlled studies, fluoxetine in dosages of 60 mg a day was superior to placebo in reducing binge eating and induced vomiting. Some experts recommend an initial course of cognitive-behavioral therapy alone. If there is no response in 3 to 6 weeks, then fluoxetine administration is added. The appropriate duration of treatment with fluoxetine and psychotherapy has not been determined.

Fluvoxamine was not effective at a statistically significant level in one double-blind, placebo-controlled trial for inpatients with bulimia.

Anorexia Nervosa. Fluoxetine has been used in inpatient treatment of anorexia nervosa to attempt to control comorbid mood disturbances and obsessive-compulsive symptoms. However, at least two careful studies, one of 7 months and one of 24 months, failed to find that fluoxetine affected the overall outcome and the maintenance of weight. Effective treatments for anorexia include cognitive behavioral, interpersonal, psychodynamic, and family therapies in addition to a trial with SSRIs.

Obesity. Fluoxetine, in combination with a behavioral program, has been shown to be only modestly beneficial for weight loss. A significant percentage of all persons who take SSRIs, including fluoxetine, lose weight initially but later may gain weight. However, all SSRIs may cause initial weight gain.

Premenstrual Dysphoric Disorder

PMDD is characterized by debilitating mood and behavioral changes in the week preceding menstruation that interfere with normal functioning. Fluoxetine under a different brand name (Serafem) is approved to treat PMDD and is the only SSRI indicated for this condition, though sertraline, paroxetine, and fluvoxamine have been reported to reduce the symptoms of PMDD. Controlled trials of fluoxetine and sertraline administered either throughout the cycle or only during the luteal phase (the 2-week period between ovulation and menstruation) showed both schedules to be equally effective.

An additional observation of unclear significance was that fluoxetine was associated with changing the duration of the menstrual period by more than 4 days, either lengthening or shortening it. The effects of SSRIs on menstrual cycle length are mostly unknown and may warrant careful monitoring in women of reproductive age.

Acute Depressive Episodes in Bipolar I Disorder

Symbyax, the trade name of a combination of fluoxetine and olanzapine, is indicated for the treatment of acute depressive episodes in bipolar I disorder. Neither drug is indicated as monotherapy.

Treatment-Resistant Depression

Symbyax is also indicated for use in treating treatment resistant depression. Neither fluoxetine nor olanzapine is indicated as monotherapy for this indication.

Off-Label Uses

Premature Ejaculation

The antiorgasmic effects of SSRIs make them useful as a treatment for men with premature ejaculation. The SSRIs permit intercourse for a significantly longer period and are reported to improve sexual satisfaction in couples in which the man has premature ejaculation. Fluoxetine and sertraline have been shown to be effective for this purpose.

Paraphilias

The SSRIs may reduce obsessive-compulsive behavior in people with paraphilias. The SSRIs diminish the average time per day spent in unconventional sexual fantasies, urges, and activities. Evidence suggests a greater response for sexual obsessions than for paraphilic behavior.

Autism Spectrum Disorder

Obsessive-compulsive behavior, poor social relatedness, and aggression are prominent features of autism spectrum disorder (ASD) that may respond to serotonergic agents such as SSRIs and clomipramine. Sertraline and fluvoxamine have been shown in controlled and open-label trials to mitigate aggressiveness, self-injurious behavior, repetitive behaviors, some degree of language delay, and (rarely) lack of social relatedness in adults with autistic spectrum disorders. Fluoxetine has been reported to be effective for features of autism in children, adolescents, and adults.

Alcohol Use Disorder

Some studies have found limited evidence to suggest that SSRIs such as citalopram can reduce cue-induced alcohol cravings among people with alcohol use disorder.

Precautions and Adverse Reactions

SSRI side effects need to be considered in terms of their onset, duration, and severity. For example, nausea and jitteriness are early, generally mild, and time-limited side effects. Although SSRIs share common side-effect profiles, individual drugs in this class may cause a higher rate or carry a more severe risk of certain side effects depending on the patient.

Suicide

The FDA has issued a black box warning for antidepressants due to presumed increases in suicidal thoughts and behavior in children and young adults who begin treatment with antidepressants. This warning is based on a decade-old analysis of clinical trial data. More recent, comprehensive reanalysis of data has shown that suicidal thoughts and behavior decreased over time for adult and geriatric patients treated with antidepressants as compared with placebo. No differences were found for youths. In adults, reduction in suicide ideation and attempts occurred through a reduction in depressive symptoms. In all age groups, severity of depression improved with medication and was significantly related to suicide ideation or behavior. It appears that SSRIs, as well as SNRIs, have a protective effect against suicide that is mediated by decreases in depressive symptoms with treatment.

For youths, no significant effects of treatment on suicidal thoughts and behavior were found, although depression responded to treatment. No evidence of increased suicide risk was observed in youths receiving active medication. It is important to keep in mind that SSRIs, like all antidepressants, prevent potential suicides as a result of their primary action, the shortening and prevention of depressive episodes.

In clinical practice, a few patients become especially anxious and agitated when started on an SSRI. The appearance of these symptoms could conceivably provoke or aggravate suicidal ideation. Thus, all depressed patients should be closely monitored during the period of maximum risk, the first few days and weeks they are taking SSRIs.

Despite these analyses, clinicians should continue to monitor patients, especially younger patients, based on the FDA labeling, which states, "Antidepressants increase the risk of suicidal thinking and behavior (suicidality) in children and adolescents with MDD and other psychiatric disorders."

Sexual Dysfunction

All SSRIs cause sexual dysfunction, and it is the most common adverse effect of SSRIs associated with long-term treatment. It has an estimated incidence of between 50% and 80%. The most common complaints are anorgasmia, inhibited orgasm, and decreased libido. Some studies suggest that sexual dysfunction is dose-related, but this has not been clearly established. Unlike most of the other adverse effects of SSRIs, sexual inhibition rarely resolves in the first few weeks of use but usually continues as long as the drug is taken. In some cases, there may be improvement over time.

Strategies to counteract SSRI-induced sexual dysfunction are numerous, but none has been proven to be very effective. Some reports suggest decreasing the dosage or adding bupropion or amphetamine. Reports have described successful treatment of SSRI-induced sexual dysfunction with agents such as sildenafil (Viagra), which are used to treat erectile dysfunction (see Chapter 30). Ultimately, patients may need to be switched to antidepressants that do not interfere with sexual functioning, drugs such as mirtazapine or bupropion.

Gastrointestinal Adverse Effects

Gastrointestinal (GI) side effects are very common and are mediated largely through effects on the serotonin 5-HT$_3$ receptor. The most frequent GI complaints are nausea, diarrhea, anorexia, vomiting, flatulence, and dyspepsia. Sertraline and fluvoxamine produce the most intense GI symptoms. Delayed-release paroxetine, compared with the immediate-release preparation of paroxetine, has less intense GI side effects during the first week of treatment. However, paroxetine, because of its anticholinergic activity, frequently causes constipation. Nausea and loose stools are usually dose related and transient, usually resolving within a few weeks. Sometimes flatulence and diarrhea persist, especially during sertraline treatment.

Initial anorexia may also occur and is most common with fluoxetine. SSRI-induced appetite and weight loss begin as soon as the drug is taken and peaks at 20 weeks, after which weight often returns to baseline. Up to one-third of persons taking SSRIs will gain weight, sometimes more than 20 lb. This effect is mediated through a metabolic mechanism, increase in appetite, or both. It happens gradually and is usually resistant to diet and exercise regimens. Paroxetine is associated with more frequent, more rapid, and more pronounced weight gain than the other SSRIs, especially among young women.

Cardiovascular Effects

All SSRIs can lengthen the QT interval in otherwise healthy people and cause drug-induced long QT syndrome, especially when taken in overdose. The risk of QTc prolongation increases when an antidepressant and an antipsychotic are used in combination, an increasingly common practice. Citalopram stands out as the SSRI with the most pronounced effect on QT interval. A QT interval study in adults assessing the effects of 20- and 60-mg doses of citalopram compared with placebo found a maximum mean prolongation in the individually corrected QT interval of 8.5 ms for 20-mg citalopram and 18.5 ms for 60 mg. For 40 mg, prolongation of the corrected QT interval was estimated to be 12.6 ms. Based on these findings, the FDA has issued the following recommendation regarding citalopram use:

- 20 mg/day is the maximum recommended dose for patients with hepatic impairment, who are older than 60 years of age, who are CYP2C19 poor metabolizers, or who are taking concomitant cimetidine.
- Maximum daily dose should not be greater than 40 mg/day.
- Do not use in patients with congenital long QT syndrome.
- Correct hypokalemia and hypomagnesemia before administering citalopram.
- Monitor electrolytes monitored as clinically indicated.
- Consider more frequent EKGs in patients with CHF, bradyarrhythmias, or patients on concomitant medications that prolong the QT interval.

The fact that citalopram carries greater risk of causing fatal rhythm abnormalities seemed to be confirmed in a review of 469 SSRI poisoning admissions. Conversely, a study done at the Ann Arbor Veterans Affairs Medical Center (VAMC) and the University of Michigan failed to confirm an increased risk for arrhythmias or death associated with daily doses of more than 40 mg. These findings do raise questions about the continued legitimacy of the FDA warning. Nevertheless, patients should be advised to contact their prescriber immediately if they experience signs and symptoms of an abnormal heart rate or rhythm while taking citalopram.

The effect of vilazodone (20, 40, 60, and 80 mg) on the QTc interval was evaluated and a small effect was observed. The upper bound of the 90% confidence interval for the largest placebo-adjusted, baseline-corrected QTc interval was below 10 ms, based on the individual correction method (QTcI). This is below the threshold for clinical concern. However, it is unknown whether 80 mg is adequate to represent a high clinical exposure condition.

Physicians should consider whether the benefits of androgen deprivation therapy outweigh the potential risks in SSRI-treated patients with prostate cancer, as reductions in androgen levels can cause QTc interval prolongation.

Dextromethorphan/quinidine (Nuedexta) is available as a treatment for pseudobulbar affect, which is defined by involuntary, sudden, and frequent episodes of laughing and/or crying that are generally out of proportion or inappropriate to the situation. Quinidine, a potent inhibitor of CYP2D6 prolongs the QT interval, and therefore should not be used with medications that also prolong the QT interval and are metabolized by CYP2D6. This drug should be used with caution with any medications that can prolong the QT interval and inhibit CYP3A4, particularly in patients with cardiac disease.

Antepartum use of SSRIs is sometimes associated with QTc interval prolongation in exposed neonates. In a review of 52 newborns exposed to SSRIs in the immediate antepartum period and 52 matched control subjects, the mean QTc was significantly longer in the group of newborns exposed to antidepressants as compared with control subjects. Five (10%) newborns exposed to SSRIs had a markedly prolonged QTc interval (>460 ms) compared with none of the unexposed newborns. The longest QTc interval observed among exposed newborns was 543 ms. All of the drug-associated repolarization abnormalities normalized in subsequent electrocardiographic tracings.

Headaches

The incidence of headache in SSRI trials was 18% to 20%, only 1% point higher than the placebo rate. Fluoxetine is the most likely to cause headache. On the other hand, all SSRIs offer effective prophylaxis against both migraine and tension-type headaches in many individuals.

Central Nervous System or Psychiatric Adverse Effects

Anxiety.   Fluoxetine may cause anxiety, particularly in the first few weeks of treatment. However, these initial effects usually give way to an overall reduction in anxiety after a few weeks. Increased anxiety is caused considerably less frequently by paroxetine and escitalopram, which may be better choices if sedation is desired, as in mixed anxiety and depressive disorders.

Insomnia and Sedation.   The major effect SSRIs exert in the area of insomnia and sedation is improved sleep resulting from treatment of depression and anxiety. However, as many as 25% of persons taking SSRIs note trouble sleeping, excessive somnolence, or overwhelming fatigue. Fluoxetine is most likely to cause insomnia; and for this reason, it is often taken in the morning. Sertraline and fluvoxamine are about equally likely to cause insomnia or somnolence, and citalopram and especially paroxetine often cause somnolence. Escitalopram is more likely to interfere with sleep than its isomer, citalopram. Some patients benefit from taking their SSRI dose before going to bed, but others prefer to take it in the morning. SSRI-induced insomnia can be treated with benzodiazepines, trazodone (Desyrel) (though clinicians must explain the risk of priapism), or other sedating medicines. Significant SSRI-induced somnolence often requires switching to use of another SSRI or bupropion.

Other Sleep Effects.   Many patients taking SSRIs report recalling extremely vivid dreams or nightmares. They describe sleep as "busy." Other sleep effects of the SSRIs include bruxism, restless legs, nocturnal myoclonus, and sweating.

Emotional Blunting.   Emotional blunting is a largely overlooked but frequent side effect associated with chronic SSRI use. Patients report an inability to cry in response to emotional situations, a feeling of apathy or indifference, or a restriction in the intensity of emotional experiences. This side effect often leads to treatment discontinuation even when the drugs provide relief from depression or anxiety.

Yawning.   Close clinical observation of patients taking SSRIs reveals an increase in yawning. This side effect is not a reflection of fatigue or poor nocturnal sleep but is the result of SSRI's effect on the hypothalamus.

Seizures.   Seizures have been reported in 0.1% to 0.2% of all patients treated with SSRIs, an incidence comparable to that reported with other antidepressants and not significantly different from that with placebo. Seizures are more frequent at the highest doses of SSRIs (e.g., fluoxetine 100 mg a day or higher).

Extrapyramidal Symptoms.   The SSRIs may rarely cause akathisia, dystonia, tremor, cogwheel rigidity, torticollis, opisthotonos, gait disorders, and bradykinesia. Rare cases of tardive dyskinesia have been reported. Some people with well-controlled Parkinson disease may experience acute worsening of their motor symptoms when they take SSRIs.

Anticholinergic Effects

Paroxetine has mild anticholinergic activity that causes dry mouth, constipation, and sedation in a dose-dependent fashion. Nevertheless, most persons taking paroxetine do not experience cholinergic adverse effects. Other SSRIs are associated with dry mouth, but this effect is not mediated by muscarinic activity.

Hematologic Adverse Effects

The SSRIs can cause functional impairment of platelet aggregation but not a reduction in platelet number. Easy bruising and excessive or prolonged bleeding manifest this pharmacologic effect. When patients exhibit these signs, a test for bleeding time should be performed. Special monitoring is suggested when patients use SSRIs in conjunction with anticoagulants or aspirin. *Concurrent use of SSRIs and nonsteroidal anti-inflammatory drugs (NSAIDs) is associated with a significantly increased risk of gastric bleeding. In cases where this combination is necessary, use of proton pump inhibitors should be considered.*

Electrolyte and Glucose Disturbances

The SSRIs may acutely decrease glucose concentrations; therefore, diabetic patients should be carefully monitored. Long-term use may be associated with increased glucose levels, although it remains to be proven whether this is the result of a pharmacologic effect. It is possible that antidepressant users have other characteristics that raise their odds of developing diabetes or are more likely to be diagnosed with diabetes or other medical conditions as a result of being in treatment for depression.

Cases of SSRI-associated hyponatremia and the syndrome of inappropriate antidiuretic hormone have been seen in patients, especially those who are older or treated with diuretics.

Endocrine and Allergic Reactions

The SSRIs can increase prolactin levels and cause mammoplasia and galactor-rhea in both men and women. Breast changes are reversible upon discontinuation of the drug, but this may take several months to occur.

Various types of rashes appear in about 4% of all patients; in a small subset of these patients, the allergic reaction may generalize and involve the pulmonary system, resulting rarely in fibrotic damage and dyspnea. Depending on severity, SSRI treatment may need to be discontinued in patients with drug-related rash.

Serotonin Syndrome

Concurrent administration of an SSRI with an MAOI, L-tryptophan, or lithium (Eskalith) can raise plasma serotonin concentrations to toxic levels, producing a constellation of symptoms called the *serotonin syndrome*. An outline of the progression of this serious and possibly fatal syndrome of serotonin overstimulation is provided in Table 33-3.

Treatment of serotonin syndrome consists of removing the offending agents and promptly instituting comprehensive supportive care with nitroglycerin, cyproheptadine, methysergide (Sansert), cooling blankets, chlorpromazine (Thorazine), dantrolene (Dantrium), benzodiazepines, anticonvulsants, mechanical ventilation, and paralyzing agents.

Sweating

Some patients experience sweating while being treated with SSRIs. The sweating is unrelated to ambient temperature. Nocturnal sweating may drench bed

TABLE 33-3: Symptoms of Serotonin Syndrome	
Stage 1	Diarrhea
Stage 2	Restlessness
Stage 3	Extreme agitation, hyperreflexia, and autonomic instability with possible rapid fluctuations in vital signs
Stage 4	Myoclonus, seizures, hyperthermia, uncontrollable shaking, and rigidity
Stage 5	Delirium, coma, status epilepticus, cardiovascular collapse, and death

sheets and require a change of night clothes. Terazosin, 1 or 2 mg per day, is often dramatically effective in counteracting sweating.

Overdose

The adverse reactions associated with overdose of SSRIs included serotonin syndrome, lethargy, restlessness, hallucinations, and disorientation.

SSRI Withdrawal

The abrupt discontinuance of SSRI use, especially one with a shorter half-life such as paroxetine or fluvoxamine, has been associated with a withdrawal syndrome that may include dizziness, weakness, nausea, headache, rebound depression, anxiety, insomnia, poor concentration, upper respiratory symptoms, paresthesia, and migraine-like symptoms. It usually does not appear until at least 6 weeks after treatment and usually resolves spontaneously in 3 weeks. Persons who experienced transient adverse effects in the first weeks of taking an SSRI are more likely to experience discontinuation symptoms.

Fluoxetine is the SSRI least likely to be associated with this syndrome because the half-life of its metabolite is more than 1 week, and it effectively tapers itself. Fluoxetine has therefore been used in some cases to treat the discontinuation syndrome caused by termination of other SSRIs. Nevertheless, a delayed and attenuated withdrawal syndrome occurs with fluoxetine as well.

Loss of Efficacy

Some patients report a diminished response or total loss of response to SSRIs with recurrence of depressive symptoms while remaining on a full dose of medication. The exact mechanism of this so-called "poop-out" is unknown, but the phenomenon is very real. Potential remedies for the attenuation of response to SSRIs include increasing or decreasing the dosage, tapering drug use, and then rechallenging with the same medication, switching to another SSRI or non-SSRI antidepressant, and augmenting with bupropion or another augmentation agent.

Pregnancy and Breastfeeding

SSRI Use During Pregnancy (Excluding Paroxetine)

With the exception of paroxetine, the SSRIs are safe to take during pregnancy when deemed necessary for treatment of the mother. There are no controlled human data regarding vilazodone use during pregnancy nor are there human data regarding drug concentrations in breast milk.

There is some evidence suggesting increased rates of special care nursery admissions after delivery for children of mothers taking SSRIs. There is also a potential for a discontinuation syndrome with paroxetine. Transient QTc prolongation has been noted in newborns whose mother was being treated with an SSRI during pregnancy. However, there is an absence of clinically significant neonatal complications associated with SSRI use.

Babies whose mothers are taking an SSRI in the latter part of pregnancy may be at a slight risk of developing pulmonary hypertension. Data about the risk of this side effect are inconclusive but is estimated to involve 1 to 2 babies out of 1,000 births.

Studies that have followed children into their early school years have failed to find any perinatal complications, congenital fetal anomalies, decreases in global intelligence quotient (IQ), language delays, or specific behavioral problems attributable to the use of fluoxetine during pregnancy.

Paroxetine Use During Pregnancy

The FDA has classified paroxetine as the most problematic of the SSRI medications. In 2005, the FDA issued an alert that paroxetine increases the risk of birth defects, particularly heart defects, when women take it during the first 3 months of pregnancy. Paroxetine should usually not be taken during pregnancy; but for some women who have already been taking paroxetine, the benefits of continuing paroxetine may be greater than the potential risk to the baby. Women taking paroxetine who are pregnant, think they may be pregnant, or plan to become pregnant should talk to their physicians about the potential risks of taking paroxetine during pregnancy.

The FDA alert was based on the findings of studies that showed that women who took paroxetine during the first 3 months of pregnancy were about one and a half to two times as likely to have a baby with a heart defect as women who received other antidepressants and women in the general population. Most of the heart defects in these studies were not life-threatening and happened mainly in the inside walls of the heart muscle where repairs can be done if needed (atrial and ventricular septal defects). Sometimes, these septal defects resolve without treatment. In one of the studies, the risk of heart defects in babies whose mothers had taken paroxetine early in pregnancy was 2%, compared to a 1% risk in the whole population. In the other study, the risk of heart defects in babies whose mothers had taken paroxetine in the first 3 months of pregnancy was 1.5% compared to 1% in babies whose mothers had taken other antidepressants in the first 3 months of pregnancy. This study also showed that women who took paroxetine in the first 3 months of pregnancy were about twice as likely to have a baby with any birth defect as women who took other antidepressants.

SSRI Use While Nursing

Very small amounts of SSRIs are found in breast milk and no harmful effects have been found in breastfed babies. Concentrations of sertraline and escitalopram are especially low in breast milk. However, in some cases, reported concentrations may be higher than average. No decision regarding the use of an SSRI is risk free and thus it is important to document that communication of potential risks to the patient has taken place.

Drug Interactions

The SSRIs do not interfere with most other drugs, though serotonin syndrome (see Table 33-3) can develop with concurrent administration of MAOIs, tryptophan, lithium, or other antidepressants that inhibit reuptake of serotonin. Fluoxetine, sertraline, and paroxetine can raise plasma concentrations of TCAs, which can cause clinical toxicity. A number of potential pharmacokinetic interactions have been described based on in vitro analyses of the CYP enzymes (see Table 33-2), but clinically relevant interactions are rare. SSRIs that inhibit CYP2D6 may interfere with the analgesic effects of hydrocodone and oxycodone. These drugs can also reduce the effectiveness of tamoxifen. Combined use of SSRIs and NSAIDs increases the risk of gastric bleeding.

The SSRIs, particularly fluvoxamine, should not be used with clozapine because it raises clozapine concentrations, increasing the risk of seizure. The SSRIs may increase the duration and severity of zolpidem (Ambien)-induced side effects, including hallucinations.

Fluoxetine

Fluoxetine can be administered with tricyclic drugs, but the clinician should use low dosages of the tricyclic drug. Since it is metabolized by the hepatic enzyme CYP2D6, fluoxetine may interfere with the metabolism of other drugs in the 7% of the population that has an inefficient isoform of this enzyme, the so-called poor metabolizers. Fluoxetine may slow down the metabolism of carbamazepine (Tegretol), antineoplastic agents, diazepam (Valium), and phenytoin (Dilantin). Drug interactions have been described for fluoxetine that may affect the plasma levels of benzodiazepines, antipsychotics, and lithium. Fluoxetine and other SSRIs may interact with warfarin (Coumadin) increasing the risk of bleeding and bruising.

Sertraline

Sertraline may displace warfarin from plasma proteins and may increase the prothrombin time. The drug interaction data on sertraline support a generally similar profile to that of fluoxetine, although sertraline does not interact as strongly with the CYP2D6 enzyme.

Paroxetine

Paroxetine has a higher risk for drug interactions than does either fluoxetine or sertraline because it is a more potent inhibitor of the CYP2D6 enzyme. Cimetidine (Tagamet) can increase the concentration of sertraline and paroxetine, and phenobarbital (Luminal) and phenytoin can decrease the concentration of paroxetine. Because of the potential for interference with the CYP2D6 enzyme, the coadministration of paroxetine with other antidepressants, phenothiazines, and antiarrhythmic drugs should be undertaken with caution. Paroxetine may increase the anticoagulant effect of warfarin. Coadministration of paroxetine and tramadol (Ultram) may precipitate a serotonin syndrome in elderly persons.

Fluvoxamine

Among the SSRIs, fluvoxamine appears to present the most risk for drug–drug interactions. Fluvoxamine is metabolized by the enzyme CYP3A4, which may be inhibited by ketoconazole (Nizoral). Fluvoxamine may increase the half-life of alprazolam (Xanax), triazolam (Halcion), and diazepam, and it should not be coadministered with these agents. Fluvoxamine may increase theophylline

(Slo-Bid, Theo-Dur) levels threefold and warfarin levels twofold, with important clinical consequences; thus, the serum levels of the latter drugs should be closely monitored, and doses adjusted accordingly. Fluvoxamine raises concentrations and may increase the activity of clozapine, carbamazepine, methadone (Dolophine, Methadose), propranolol (Inderal), and diltiazem (Cardizem). Fluvoxamine has no significant interactions with lorazepam (Ativan) or digoxin (Lanoxin).

Citalopram

Citalopram is not a potent inhibitor of any CYP enzymes. Concurrent administration of cimetidine increases concentrations of citalopram by about 40%. Citalopram does not significantly affect the metabolism of, nor is its metabolism significantly affected by, digoxin, lithium, warfarin, carbamazepine, or imipramine (Tofranil). Citalopram increases the plasma concentrations of metoprolol twofold, but this usually has no effect on blood pressure or heart rate. Data on coadministration of citalopram and potent inhibitors of CYP3A4 or CYP2D6 are not available.

Escitalopram

Escitalopram is a moderate inhibitor of CYP2D6 and has been shown to significantly raise desipramine and metoprolol concentrations.

Vilazodone

Vilazodone dose should be reduced to 20 mg when coadministered with CYP3A4 strong inhibitors. Concomitant use with inducers of CYP3A4 can result in inadequate drug concentrations and may diminish effectiveness. The effect of CYP3A4 inducers on systemic exposure of vilazodone has not been evaluated.

Laboratory Interferences

The SSRIs do not interfere with any laboratory tests.

Dosage and Clinical Guidelines

Fluoxetine

Fluoxetine is available in 10- and 20-mg capsules, in a scored 10-mg tablet, as a 90-mg enteric-coated capsule for once-weekly administration, and as an oral concentrate (20 mg/5 mL). Fluoxetine is also marketed as Sarafem for PMDD. For depression, the initial dosage is usually 10 or 20 mg orally each day, usually given in the morning, because insomnia is a potential adverse effect of the drug. Fluoxetine should be taken with food to minimize the possible nausea. The long half-lives of the drug and its metabolite contribute to a 4-week period to reach steady-state concentrations. 20 mg is often as effective as higher doses for treating depression. However, some patients may benefit from a dose increase after several weeks at the initial dose to a maintenance dosage of 20 mg taken twice a day, in the morning and at noon though this schedule may cause or worsen insomnia. If this dose is not well tolerated and symptoms do not improve, consider an alternative SSRI. The maximum dosage recommended by the manufacturer is 80 mg a day (see Table 33-11).

To minimize the early side effects of anxiety and restlessness, some clinicians initiate fluoxetine use at 5 to 10 mg a day, either with the scored 10-mg tablet or by using the liquid preparation. Alternatively, because of the long half-life of fluoxetine, its use can be initiated with an every-other-day administration schedule. The dosage of fluoxetine (and other SSRIs) that is effective in other indications may differ from the dosage generally used for depression (see Table 33-4).

In pediatric patients, doses should be initiated at 10 mg or 20 mg per day, taken once in the morning. After several weeks, consider an increase to 20 mg per day if symptom improvement is insufficient.

A combination treatment of fluoxetine and olanzapine (Symbax) is indicated for depressive episodes associated with bipolar I disorder and treatment-resistant depression. Symbax capsules are available in the following ratios:

1. 25 mg fluoxetine/3 mg olanzapine
2. 25 mg fluoxetine/6 mg olanzapine
3. 50 mg fluoxetine/6 mg olanzapine
4. 25 mg fluoxetine/12 mg olanzapine
5. 50 mg fluoxetine/12 mg olanzapine

For dosing guidelines, see Table 33-4.

TABLE 33-4: Dosing Guidelines for Fluoxetine

Indication	Adult Dosage		Pediatric Dosage	
	Initial	Maintenance	Initial	Maintenance
Major depressive disorder	20 mg/day in the morning	20–40 mg/day; 20 mg/day in the morning, or one 20-mg dose in the morning and one 20-mg dose at noon	10–20 mg/day in the morning	10–20 mg/day; 10 mg/day in the morning, or one 10-mg dose in the morning and one 10-mg dose at noon
Obsessive-compulsive disorder	20 mg/day in the morning	20–60 mg/day	10 mg/day in the morning	20–60 mg/day
Bulimia nervosa	60 mg/day in the morning	60 mg/day	N/A	N/A
Panic disorder	10 mg/day in the morning	10–60 mg/day	N/A	N/A
Depressive episodes associated with bipolar I disorder	20 mg/day in the morning with 5 mg oral olanzapine	20–50 mg/day with 5–12.5 mg oral olanzapine	20 mg/day in the morning with 2.5 mg oral olanzapine	20–50 mg/day with 2.5–12.5 mg oral olanzapine
Treatment-resistant depression	20 mg/day in the morning with 5 mg oral olanzapine	25–50 mg/day with 6–18 mg oral olanzapine	N/A	N/A

Note: Lower dosages should be used in geriatric populations, patients prescribed multiple medications, and patients with hepatic impairment.

TABLE 33-5: Dosing Guidelines for Sertraline

Indication	Adult Dosage		Pediatric Dosage	
	Initial	Maintenance	Initial	Maintenance
Major depressive disorder	50 mg/day	50–200 mg/day	N/A	N/A
Obsessive-compulsive disorder	50 mg/day	50–200 mg/day	25 mg/day (6–12 years old) 50 mg/day (13–17 years old)	50–200 mg/day
Panic disorder	25 mg/day	50–200 mg/day	N/A	N/A
Posttraumatic stress disorder	25 mg/day	50–200 mg/day	N/A	N/A
Social anxiety disorder	25 mg/day	50–200 mg/day	N/A	N/A
Premenstrual dysphoric disorder	50 mg/day	50–150 mg/day[a]	N/A	N/A

[a]When dosing continuously, patients may benefit from doses as high as 150 mg/day. When dosing intermittently and only during luteal phase of the menstrual cycle, the dosage should remain in the range of 50 to 100 mg/day.

Sertraline

Sertraline is available in scored 25-, 50-, and 100-mg tablets. An oral concentrate of 20 mg/mL (1 mL = 20 mg) is also available that has 12% alcohol content and must be diluted before use. Sertraline capsules containing dosages of 150 mg and 200 mg are also available for the treatment of MDD in adults and OCD in adults and pediatric patients 6 years of age and older.

For the initial treatment of depression, sertraline use should be initiated with a dosage of 50 mg once daily. To limit the GI effects, some clinicians begin at 25 mg a day and increase to 50 mg a day after 1 to 3 weeks. Patients who do not respond after 1 to 3 weeks may benefit from dosage increases of 50 mg every week, up to a maximum of 200 mg given once daily. Sertraline can be administered in the morning or the evening. Administration after eating may reduce the GI adverse effects. When used to treat panic disorder, sertraline should be initiated at 25 mg to reduce the risk of provoking a panic attack. For more guidance, see Table 33-5.

Paroxetine

Immediate-release paroxetine is available in scored 20-mg tablets; in unscored 10-, 30-, and 40-mg tablets; and as an orange-flavored 10-mg/5-mL oral suspension. Paroxetine use for the treatment of depression is usually initiated at a dosage of 10 or 20 mg a day. An increase in the dosage should be considered when an adequate response is not seen in 1 to 3 weeks. At that point, the clinician can initiate upward dose titration in 10-mg increments at weekly intervals to a maximum of 50 mg a day. Persons who experience GI upset may benefit by taking the drug with food. Paroxetine can be taken initially as a single daily dose in the evening; higher dosages may be divided into two doses per day. For more guidance, see Table 33-6.

A delayed-release formulation of paroxetine, paroxetine CR, is available in 12.5-, 25-, and 37.5-mg tablets. The starting dosages of paroxetine CR are 25 mg

TABLE 33-6: Dosing Guidelines for Paroxetine

Indication	Immediate-Release		Delayed-Release	
	Initial	Maintenance	Initial	Maintenance
Major depressive disorder	20 mg/day	20–50 mg/day	25 mg/day	25–62.5 mg/day
Obsessive-compulsive disorder	20 mg/day	20–60 mg/day	N/A	N/A
Panic disorder	10 mg/day	10–60 mg/day	12.5 mg/day	12.5–75 mg/day
Posttraumatic stress disorder	20 mg/day	20–50 mg/day	N/A	N/A
Social anxiety disorder	20 mg/day	20–60 mg/day	12.5 mg/day	12.5–37.5 mg/day
Generalized anxiety disorder	20 mg/day	20–60 mg/day	N/A	N/A
Premenstrual dysphoric disorder	N/A	N/A	12.5 mg/day	12.5–25 mg/day

Note: Paroxetine is not indicated for pediatric use.

per day for depression and 12.5 mg per day for panic disorder, social anxiety disorder, and PMDD.

Paroxetine is the SSRI most likely to produce a discontinuation syndrome because plasma concentrations decrease rapidly in the absence of continuous dosing. To limit the development of symptoms of abrupt discontinuation, paroxetine use should be tapered gradually, with dosage reductions every 2 to 3 weeks.

Fluvoxamine

Fluvoxamine is the only SSRI not approved by the FDA as an antidepressant. It is indicated for OCD, but often used off-label to treat social anxiety disorder. It is available in unscored 25-mg tablets and scored 50- and 100-mg tablets. The effective daily dosage range is 50 to 300 mg a day. A usual starting dosage is 50 mg once a day at bedtime for the first week, after which the dosage can be adjusted according to the adverse effects and clinical response. Dosages above 100 mg a day may be divided into twice-daily dosing.

A temporary dosage reduction or slower upward titration may be necessary if nausea develops over the first 2 weeks of therapy. In pediatric patients, the dosage should be 25 mg once a day at bedtime for the first week. Dosages can be increased in 25-mg increments very 4 to 7 days as tolerated. For patients 8 to 11 years old, the dosage should not exceed 200 mg a day. For patients 12 years of age and over, daily dosage should not exceed 300 mg (see Table 33-7). Although fluvoxamine

TABLE 33-7: Dosing Guidelines for Fluvoxamine

Indication	Adult Dosage		Pediatric Dosage	
	Initial	Maintenance	Initial	Maintenance
Obsessive-compulsive disorder	50 mg/day	50–300 mg/day	25 mg/day	25–200 mg day (8–11 years old) 25–300 mg/day (12–17 years old)

TABLE 33-8: Dosing Guidelines for Citalopram

Indication	Adult Dosage		Pediatric Dosage	
	Initial	Maintenance	Initial	Maintenance
Major depressive disorder	20 mg	20–40 mg/day	N/A	N/A

can also be administered as a single evening dose to minimize its adverse effects, its short half-life may lead to interdose withdrawal.

An extended-release formulation is available in 100- and 150-mg dose strengths. All fluvoxamine formulations should be swallowed with food without chewing the tablet. Abrupt discontinuation of fluvoxamine may cause a discontinuation syndrome owing to its short half-life.

Geriatric patients and patients with hepatic impairment may require dosage adjustments.

Citalopram

Citalopram is available in 10-, 20-, and 40-mg scored tablets and as a liquid (10 mg/5 mL). The usual starting dosage is 20 mg a day for the first week, after which it usually is increased to 40 mg a day. For elderly persons or persons with hepatic impairment, 20 mg a day is recommended, with an increase to 40 mg a day only if there is no response at 20 mg a day. Tablets should be taken once daily in either the morning or the evening with or without food (see Table 33-8).

Escitalopram

Escitalopram is available as 10- and 20-mg scored tablets, as well as an oral solution at a concentration of 5 mg/5 mL. The recommended dosage of escitalopram is 10 mg per day for both MDD and GAD (see Table 33-9), while the maximum daily dosage is 20 mg a day (see Table 33-11). Of note, in clinical trials, no additional benefit was noted when 20 mg per day was used though in clinical practice many patients benefit from a 20 mg per day dosage.

Vilazodone

Vilazodone is available as 10-, 20- and 40-mg tablets. The recommended therapeutic dose of vilazodone is 20 to 40 mg once daily with food for the treatment of MDD. Treatment should be titrated, starting with an initial dose of 10 mg once daily for 7 days, followed by 20 mg once daily for an additional 7 days, and then an increase to 40 mg once daily (see Table 33-10).

TABLE 33-9: Dosing Guidelines for Escitalopram

Indication	Adult Dosage		Pediatric Dosage	
	Initial	Maintenance	Initial	Maintenance
Major depressive disorder	10 mg/day	10 mg/day	10 mg/day	10 mg/day
Generalized anxiety disorder	10 mg/day	10 mg/day	N/A	N/A

TABLE 33-10: Dosing Guidelines for Vilazodone

Indication	Adult Dosage		Pediatric Dosage	
	Initial	Maintenance	Initial	Maintenance
Major depressive disorder	10 mg	20–40 mg/day	N/A	N/A

If vilazodone is taken without food, inadequate drug concentrations may result, and the drug's effectiveness may be diminished. Vilazodone is not approved for use in children. The safety and efficacy of vilazodone in pediatric patients have not been studied. No dose adjustment is recommended on the basis of age, in patients with mild or moderate hepatic impairment, or those with mild, moderate, or severe renal impairment. Vilazodone has not been studied in patients with severe hepatic impairment.

VORTIOXETINE

Vortioxetine (Trintellix, Brintellix) is an atypical SSRI that the FDA has designated as a serotonin modulator and stimulator. It is only approved for the treatment of MDD in adults. Vortioxetine was investigated as a treatment for GAD but was found to be no better than placebo.

Pharmacokinetics

Vortioxetine reaches maximal plasma concentration within 7 to 11 hours and has a bioavailability of 75%. It may be taken with or without food. Vortioxetine is extensively metabolized, mainly through the CYP450 isozymes 2D6, 3A4/5, 2C19, 2C9, 2A6, 2C8, and 2B6. After oxidation, it undergoes glucuronic acid conjugation. It is converted to a pharmacologically inactive metabolite through CYP2D6 oxidation. The pharmacologic activity of vortioxetine is entirely derived from the parent molecule and it has no active metabolites.

Poor metabolizers of CYP2D6 have nearly twice the plasma concentration of vortioxetine than do extensive metabolizers. No significant impact on plasma

TABLE 33-11: Maximum Dosages for SSRIs

Generic Name	Trade Name	Maximum Daily Adult Dosage
Fluoxetine	Prozac	80 mg
Sertraline	Zoloft	200 mg
Paroxetine	Paxil	60 mg
Paroxetine	Paxil CR	75 mg
Fluvoxamine	Luvox	300 mg
Citalopram	Celexa	40 mg
Escitalopram	Lexapro	20 mg
Vilazodone	Viibryd	40 mg
Vortioxetine	Trintellix, Brintellix	20 mg

protein binding or clearance has been demonstrated by hepatic or renal disease. Steady-state AUC and C_{max} of vortioxetine are increased when coadministered with bupropion, fluconazole, and ketoconazole. These are decreased when vortioxetine is used with rifampicin.

Vortioxetine has a mean terminal half-life of about 66 hours and steady-state plasma concentrations are usually achieved within 2 weeks.

Pharmacodynamics

Vortioxetine is classified as a "serotonin modulator and stimulator." It has been shown to possess a complex neuroreceptor profile with the following pharmacologic actions:

- Serotonin transporter blocker
- Norepinephrine transporter blocker
- 5-HT_{1A} receptor high-efficacy partial agonist/near-full agonist
- 5-HT_{1B} receptor partial agonist
- 5-HT_{1D} receptor antagonist
- 5-HT_{3A} receptor antagonist
- 5-HT_7 receptor antagonist
- β_1-Adrenergic receptor ligand

The clinical impact of these multiple receptor effects is not well understood.

Therapeutic Indications

Vortioxetine is approved for treatment of MDD in adults. There are no published data on the efficacy and safety of vortioxetine use in children and adolescents. It has been studied in elderly patients, with no evidence of unusual adverse events.

Precautions and Adverse Reactions

The most common side effects reported with vortioxetine are nausea, diarrhea, xerostomia, constipation, vomiting, flatulence, dizziness, and sexual dysfunction. Based on clinical trial data, the incidence of sexual dysfunction is reportedly higher in patients taking vortioxetine than in patients taking placebos but lower than in patients taking venlafaxine.

Warnings

As with other SSRIs, vortioxetine contains a black box warning about suicidal thoughts and behaviors (see above), serotonin syndrome (see above and Table 33-3), hematologic adverse effects (see above), and electrolyte and glucose disturbances (see above). Unlike other drugs described in this chapter, vortioxetine can be discontinued abruptly with minimal withdrawal effects.

Pregnancy and Nursing

Studies in animals have shown that use of vortioxetine during pregnancy may lead to an increased occurrence of fetal damage, the significance of which is considered uncertain in humans though its use is not recommended unless clearly needed. Use during breastfeeding is not recommended and a decision should be made to discontinue breastfeeding or discontinue the drug, depending on the

TABLE 33-12: Dosing Guidelines for Vortioxetine				
	Adult Dosage		Pediatric Dosage	
Indication	Initial	Maintenance	Initial	Maintenance
Major depressive disorder	10 mg	10–20 mg/day	N/A	N/A

risks and benefits of the drug to the mother. It is not known if it is excreted into human milk and effects on nursing infants are unknown.

Drug Interactions

Patients run a higher risk of developing serotonin syndrome (see Table 33-3) if vortioxetine is coadministered with MAOIs, tryptophan, lithium, or other antidepressants that inhibit reuptake of serotonin. MAOI use should be discontinued for at least 14 days before beginning treatment with vortioxetine. Drugs that interfere with hemostasis (e.g., NSAIDs, aspirin, warfarin) increase the risk of gastric bleeding when taken in conjunction with vortioxetine.

Vortioxetine dosages should be reduced by half if coadministered with a strong CYP2D6 inhibitor, while a strong inducer of CYP2D6 may require an increase in dosage.

Laboratory Interferences

Vortioxetine does not interfere with any laboratory tests.

Dosage and Clinical Guidelines

Vortioxetine is currently available in 5-, 10-, and 20-mg oral, immediate-release tablets under the trade name Trintellix and as immediate release tablets under the trade name Brintellix in 5-, 10-, 15-, and 20-mg oral, immediate-release tablets. Patients typically initiate drug therapy at 10 mg daily, which may be subsequently increased to 20 mg daily (as outlined in Table 33-12). If 10-mg dosing is poorly tolerated, the dose can be lowered to 5 mg per day. Clinical trial data do not indicate a clinically significant difference response and remission rates at doses above 20 mg per day.

34

Second-Generation or Atypical Antipsychotics (Serotonin–Dopamine Antagonists, Modulators, and Similarly Acting Drugs)

Generic Name	Trade Name	Adverse Effects	Drug Interactions	CYP Interactions
Aripiprazole	Abilify, Abilify Maintena, Aristada, Aristada Initio	Suicidality, sedation, agitation, GI symptoms, insomnia, headache	Carbamazepine, valproate, ketoconazole, fluoxetine, paroxetine, quinidine	2D6, 3A4, 3A5, 3A7
Asenapine	Saphris, Secudo	Suicidality, EPS, weight gain, sedation, dizziness, cardiac arrhythmia	Antihypertensives, QT	1A2, 2D6, 3A4
Brexpiprazole	Rexulti	Suicidality, EPS, weight gain, dizziness, agitation, sedation, headache	N/A	3A4, 2D6
Cariprazine	Vraylar	Suicidality, EPS, weight gain, insomnia, GI symptoms	N/A	3A4, 2D6, 3A5, 1A2, 2C9, 2C19, 2E1
Clozapine	Clozaril, FazaClo, Versacloz	Suicidality, sedation, anticholinergic effects, cardiac arrhythmia, weight gain, GI symptoms, fatigue, seizures	LITH, antiarrhythmics, antipsychotics, carbamazepine, phenytoin, propylthiouracil, sulfonamides, captopril, clomipramine, risperidone, fluoxetine, paroxetine, fluvoxamine, QT	1A2, 3A4, 2D6, 2C9, 2C19, 2A6, 2C8, 1A1
Iloperidone	Fanapt	Suicidality, cardiac arrhythmia, weight gain	Antihypertensives, QT	3A4, 2D6, 3A5, 3A7, 2E1
Lumateperone	Caplyta	Suicidality, sedation, dizziness, GI symptoms	Amisulpride, carbamazepine	3A4, 2C8, 1A2
Lurasidone	Latuda	Suicidality, EPS, sedation, agitation, GI symptoms	Bupropion	3A4
Olanzapine	Zyprexa, Zyprexa Zydis, Relprevv	Suicidality, weight gain, sedation, dizziness, GI symptoms, transaminase elevation, hypotension	CNS, fluoxetine, samidorphan, cimetidine, carbamazepine, phenytoin	1A2, 2D6, 2C19, 2C9, 3A4

Generic Name	Trade Name	Adverse Effects	Drug Interactions	CYP Interactions
Olanzapine and fluoxetine	Symbyax	Suicidality, weight gain, sedation, cardiac arrhythmia, insomnia, fatigue, increased prolactin levels, rash, dizziness, GI symptoms, transaminase elevation, hypotension, sexual dysfunction	CNS, MAOI, SERO, TRI, BENZ, antipsychotics, LITH, NSAID, warfarin, clozapine, zolpidem, samidorphan, cimetidine, carbamazepine, antineoplastic agents, phenytoin	2D6, 2B6, 3A4, 3A5, 1A2, 2C19, 2C9
Olanzapine and samidorphan	Lybalvi	Suicidality, weight gain, sedation, dizziness, GI symptoms, headache	CNS, opioids, fluoxetine, samidorphan, cimetidine, carbamazepine, phenytoin	1A2, 2D6, 2C19, 2C9, 3A4, 3A5, 2C8
Paliperidone	Invega, Invega Sustenna, Invega Trinza, Invega Hafyera	Suicidality, EPS, cardiac arrythmia, weight gain, hypotension	CNS, carbamazepine, QT	3A4, 3A5, 2D6
Pimavanserin	Nuplazid	Suicidality, confusion, GI symptoms	Antiarrhythmics, antipsychotics, QT	3A4, 3A5, 2J2, 2D6
Quetiapine	Seroquel, Seroquel XR	Suicidality, weight gain, sedation	Antiarrhythmics, antipsychotics, phenytoin, QT	2D6, 3A4, 3A5, 2C19, 3A7
Risperidone	Risperdal, Consta	Suicidality, EPS, weight gain, GI symptoms, sexual dysfunction, sedation	SSRI, DA	2D6, 3A4
Ziprasidone	Geodon	Suicidality, sedation, GI symptoms, headache	Antiarrhythmics, QT	3A4, 1A2

Introduction

The second-generation antipsychotics (SGAs) provide unique advantages in the treatment of schizophrenia and most of these drugs have also received approval from the Food and Drug Administration (FDA) as monotherapy or adjunctive therapy in the treatment of bipolar disorder. Also known as atypical antipsychotics, this class of pharmacologically diverse drugs are now considered as first-line agents for the treatment of psychotic and bipolar disorder. Besides being the most widely prescribed agents for schizophrenia and other illnesses associated with psychotic symptoms, some SGAs have also been approved as adjuncts to antidepressants in the treatment of major depressive disorder. Despite FDA warnings about their use in elderly patients with dementia-related psychoses, SGAs are prescribed for the treatment of agitation and behavioral disturbances in this patient population. Clinicians need to be aware of these risks and warnings and of higher rates of mortality associated with the use of atypical antipsychotics.

Initially, these agents were referred to as serotonin–dopamine antagonists (SDAs). The name came from the belief that they could be differentiated from the dopamine receptor antagonists (DRAs) by their high affinity for serotonin 2A (5-HT$_{2A}$) receptors, as well as dopamine (D$_2$) receptors. This simplistic conceptualization is now questioned, and the term SDA has been replaced by the terms SGAs and atypical antipsychotics. The term *atypical* is used because these drugs differ from the DRAs in their side-effect profiles and their low potential for extrapyramidal side effects (EPS), such as tardive dyskinesia. This makes them useful in the treatment of various neuropsychiatric conditions, while also showing better tolerability over conventional antipsychotics, especially in the treatment of young and older populations. Additionally, the FDA has classified some of these drugs as modulators, to reflect their ability to control and alter neurotransmission.

To date, more than a dozen SGAs have been approved by the FDA. These are listed in Table 34-1.

TABLE 34-1: Second-Generation Antipsychotics Approved by the Food and Drug Administration

Generic Name	Trade Name	Indication
Aripiprazole	Abilify	• Schizophrenia • Acute treatment of manic and mixed episodes associated with bipolar disorder I as monotherapy and adjunctive therapy • Major depressive disorder, as adjunctive treatment • Irritability associated with autism spectrum disorder • Tourette disorder • Agitation associated with bipolar mania or schizophrenia
Aripiprazole	Abilify Maintena	• Schizophrenia
Aripiprazole lauroxil	Aristada	• Schizophrenia
Aripiprazole lauroxil	Aristada Initio	• Coadminister Aristada Initio with oral aripiprazole when initiating treatment with Aristada
Asenapine	Saphris	• Schizophrenia in adults • Bipolar disorder I • As acute monotherapy for manic or mixed episodes in adults and pediatric patients 10–17 years old. • As adjunctive treatment with valproate and lithium in adults • As maintenance monotherapy treatment in adults
Asenapine (transdermal)	Secudo	• Schizophrenia in adults
Brexpiprazole	Rexulti	• Adjunctive therapy to antidepressants in the treatment of major depressive disorder in adults • Schizophrenia in adults and adolescent patients 13 years of age and older
Cariprazine	Vraylar	• Schizophrenia in adults • Acute treatment of manic or mixed episodes associated with bipolar I disorder in adults

TABLE 34-1: Second-Generation Antipsychotics Approved by the Food and Drug Administration (*continued*)

Generic Name	Trade Name	Indication
Clozapine	Clozaril	• Treatment-resistant schizophrenia in adults • The reduction of suicidal behavior in adult patients with schizophrenia or schizoaffective disorder
Clozapine	FazaClo	• Treatment-resistant schizophrenia in adults • The reduction of suicidal behavior in adult patients with schizophrenia or schizoaffective disorder
Clozapine	Versacloz	• Treatment-resistant schizophrenia in adults • The reduction of suicidal behavior in adult patients with schizophrenia or schizoaffective disorder
Iloperidone	Fanapt	• Schizophrenia in adults
Lumateperone	Caplyta	• Schizophrenia in adults • Depressive episodes associated with bipolar I or II disorder as monotherapy and as adjunctive therapy with lithium or valproate
Lurasidone	Latuda	• Schizophrenia in adults and pediatric patients aged 13–17 years old • Depressive episodes associated with bipolar I disorder in adults, as adjunctive therapy with valproate or lithium • Depressive episodes associated with bipolar I disorder in adults and adolescents aged 10–17 years old, as monotherapy
Olanzapine	Zyprexa, Zyprexa Zydis	• Schizophrenia in adults and pediatric patients aged 13–17 years old • Bipolar I disorder (manic or mixed episodes and maintenance treatment) in adults and pediatric patients aged 13–17 years old
Olanzapine IM	Zyprexa	• Agitation associated with schizophrenia and bipolar I disorder mania in adults
Olanzapine (IM long acting)	Relprevv	• Schizophrenia in adults
Olanzapine and fluoxetine	Symbyax	• Depressive episodes associated with bipolar I disorder in adults and adolescents 10–17 years of age • Treatment-resistant depression in adults
Olanzapine and samidorphan	Lybalvi	• Schizophrenia in adults • Bipolar I disorder in adults for acute treatment of manic or mixed episodes either as monotherapy or adjunct therapy with valproate or lithium; or for maintenance treatment as monotherapy
Paliperidone	Invega	• Acute and maintenance treatment of schizophrenia in adults • Acute treatment of schizoaffective disorder as monotherapy or as an adjunct to mood stabilizers or antidepressants in adults
Paliperidone (IM long acting [12/year])	Invega Sustenna	• Treatment of schizophrenia in adults • Acute treatment of schizoaffective disorder as monotherapy or as an adjunct to mood stabilizers or antidepressants in adults
Paliperidone (IM long acting [4/year])	Invega Trinza	• Treatment of schizophrenia in adults who have been adequately treated with Invega Sustenna

(*continued*)

TABLE 34-1: Second-Generation Antipsychotics Approved by the Food and Drug Administration (continued)

Generic Name	Trade Name	Indication
Paliperidone (IM long acting [2/year])	Invega Hafyera	• Treatment of schizophrenia in adults who have been adequately treated with Invega Sustenna or Invega Trinza
Pimavanserin	Nuplazid	• Treatment of hallucinations and delusions associated with Parkinson disease psychosis
Quetiapine	Seroquel	• Treatment of schizophrenia in adults and adolescents aged 13–17 years • Acute treatment of manic episodes associated with bipolar I disorder as monotherapy in adults and adolescents aged 10–17 years • Acute treatment of manic episodes associated with bipolar I disorder as adjunct to lithium or divalproex in adults • Acute treatment of depressive episodes associated with bipolar disorder and maintenance treatment of bipolar I disorder as monotherapy or as an adjunct to lithium or divalproex in adults
Quetiapine	Seroquel XR	• Treatment of schizophrenia in adults and adolescents aged 13–17 years • Acute treatment of manic episodes associated with bipolar I disorder as monotherapy in adults and adolescents aged 10–17 years • Acute treatment of manic episodes associated with bipolar I disorder as adjunct to lithium or divalproex in adults • Acute treatment of depressive episodes associated with bipolar disorder and maintenance treatment of bipolar I disorder as monotherapy or as an adjunct to lithium or divalproex in adults • Major depressive disorder in adults as an adjunctive treatment with antidepressants
Risperidone	Risperdal	• Acute and maintenance treatment of schizophrenia in adults and adolescents aged 13–17 years • Short-term treatment of acute manic or mixed episodes associated with bipolar I disorder in adults and adolescents aged 10–17 years, as monotherapy or in conjunction with lithium or valproate • Irritability associated with autistic spectrum disorder in children and adolescents aged 5–16 years
Risperidone (IM long acting)	Consta	• Schizophrenia in adults • Maintenance treatment in bipolar I disorder either as monotherapy or in conjunction with valproate or lithium
Ziprasidone	Geodon	• Schizophrenia in adults • Manic or mixed episodes associated with bipolar I disorder as monotherapy in adults • Maintenance treatment of bipolar I disorder as an adjunct to lithium or valproate in adults
Ziprasidone (IM)	Geodon	• Schizophrenia in adults • Manic or mixed episodes associated with bipolar I disorder as monotherapy in adults • Maintenance treatment of bipolar I disorder as an adjunct to lithium or valproate in adults

IM, Intramuscular.

General Overview of SGAs

Pharmacodynamics

The presumed antipsychotic effects of the SGAs are blockade of D_2 dopamine receptors. Where the SGAs differ from older antipsychotic drugs is their varied affinity for serotonin receptor subtypes, most notably the 5-HT_{2A} subtype, as well as with other neurotransmitter systems. It is hypothesized that these properties account for the distinct tolerability profiles associated with each of the SGAs. All SGAs have different chemical structures, receptor affinities, and side-effect profiles. *No SGA is identical in its combination of receptor affinities, and the relative contribution of each receptor interaction to the clinical effects is unknown.*

Warnings, Precautions, and Adverse Events

Black Box Warning—Dementia Patients. All drugs mentioned in this chapter contain a black box warning noting that elderly patients with dementia-related psychosis who are treated with antipsychotic drugs (both first and second generation) are at an increased risk of death.

Black Box Warning—Suicidal Ideation. Patients aged 24 and younger who are being treated for depression may be at an increased risk of suicidal thoughts and behaviors when taking aripiprazole, brexpiprazole, lurasidone, quetiapine, cariprazine and the combination treatment of olanzapine and fluoxetine (Symbax). Clinicians should monitor for worsening of clinical conditions and emergence of suicidal tendencies.

SGAs, Weight Gain, and Extrapyramidal Symptoms. Although SGAs represent an improvement over the DRAs with respect to a lowered, but not absent, risk of EPS, some still do cause EPS. However, the SGAs that typically have the lowest risk for EPS often produce substantial weight gain (see Table 34-2), which in turn increases the potential for development of obesity, metabolic syndrome, diabetes mellitus, and other diseases that are common comorbidities among extremely overweight individuals explored in greater detail in Chapter 40. Therefore, clinicians should consider existing risk factors in a patient-by-patient manner before administering a particular SGA and try to balance the risk of EPS with the risk of weight gain.

Olanzapine and clozapine appear to account for most cases of weight gain and drug-induced diabetes mellitus. The other agents pose less of a risk of these metabolic side effects, and that risk can vary (see Table 34-2); nevertheless, the FDA has requested that all SGAs carry a warning label that patients taking the drugs be monitored closely and has recommended the following factors be considered for all patients prescribed SGAs.

1. Personal and family history of obesity, diabetes, dyslipidemia, hypertension, and cardiovascular disease
2. Weight and height (so that body mass index can be calculated)
3. Waist circumference (at the level of the umbilicus)
4. Blood pressure
5. Fasting plasma glucose level
6. Fasting lipid profile

TABLE 34-2: Balancing the Risk of Extrapyramidal Symptoms and Weight Gain in Second-Generation Antipsychotics

Highest Risk of EPS	**Lowest Risk of Weight Gain**
Lurasidone	Aripiprazole
Paliperidone	Lumateperone
Risperidone	Lurasidone
	Pimavanserin
	Ziprasidone
Moderate Risk of EPS	**Moderate Risk of Weight Gain**
Asenapine	Asenapine
Brexpiprazole	Brexpiprazole
Cariprazine	Cariprazine
Quetiapine	Paliperidone
	Quetiapine
	Risperidone
Lowest Risk of EPS	**Highest Risk of Weight Gain**
Aripiprazole	Clozapine
Clozapine	Iloperidone
Iloperidome	Olanzapine
Lumateperone	
Olanzapine	
Pimavanserin	
Ziprasidone	

Patients with preexisting diabetes should have regular monitoring, including HgA1c and in some cases insulin levels. Among these drugs, clozapine sits apart. It is not considered a first-line agent because of side effects and need for weekly blood monitoring. Although highly effective in treating both mania and depression, clozapine does not have an FDA indication for these conditions. Tables 40-10, 40-11, and 40-12 outline potential monitoring schedules for patients on SGAs.

Neuroleptic Malignant Syndrome. A potentially fatal side effect of treatment with either first- or second-generation antipsychotics (FGAs or SGAs, respectively) is neuroleptic malignant syndrome, which can occur at any time during the course of the treatment. Symptoms include extreme hyperthermia, severe muscular rigidity and dystonia, akinesia, mutism, confusion, agitation, and increased pulse rate and blood pressure (BP). Laboratory findings include increased white blood cell (WBC) count, creatinine phosphokinase, liver enzymes, plasma myoglobin, and myoglobinuria, occasionally associated with renal failure. The symptoms usually evolve over 24 to 72 hours, and the untreated syndrome lasts 10 to 14 days. The diagnosis is often missed in the early stages, and the withdrawal or agitation may mistakenly be considered to reflect increased psychosis. Men are affected more frequently than are women, and young persons are affected more commonly than are elderly persons. The mortality rate can reach 20% to 30% or even higher when depot medications are involved. Rates are also increased when high doses of high-potency agents are used.

If neuroleptic malignant syndrome is suspected, causative agent should be stopped immediately and supportive care started without delay: Request medical support and patient may need care in an intensive care unit; use cooling blankets to lower fever; monitor vital signs, electrolytes, fluid balance, and renal output; and maintain cardiorespiratory stability. Antiparkinsonian medications may reduce muscle rigidity. Dantrolene (Dantrium), a skeletal muscle relaxant (0.8 to 2.5 mg/kg every 6 hours, up to a total dosage of 10 mg a day) may also be useful in the treatment of this disorder. When the person can take oral medications, dantrolene can be given in doses of 100 to 200 mg a day. Bromocriptine (20 to 30 mg a day in four divided doses) or amantadine can be added to the regimen. Treatment will typically need to be continued for 5 to 10 days. When drug treatment is restarted, the clinician should consider switching to a low-potency drug or an SGA, although these agents—including clozapine—may also cause neuroleptic malignant syndrome.

Tardive Dyskinesia.   As discussed in Chapter 42, medication-induced movement disorders can be one of the more concerning effects of long-term treatment with either FGAs or SGAs. Though far more common when using DRAs than SGAs, it is still important to monitor patients being treated with the latter.

Sexual Side Effects.   A wide range of sexual dysfunctions—including reduced libido, erectile dysfunction, and impairment in desire—can occur following the use of SGAs.

Hypotension, Syncope, and Falls.   Some patients may develop hypotension and syncope. This, in conjunction with drowsiness, may put some patients at risk of falls.

Use in Pregnancy and Lactation

A large review of the reproductive safety of SGAs found that the drugs did not raise the risk of major malformations significantly beyond those observed in the general population or those using other psychotropic medications. Despite their ostensible safety, SGAs have been classified as pregnancy category C drugs with the exception of clozapine, which is a pregnancy category B drug. SGA use by pregnant women has not been studied, but consideration should be given to the potential of risperidone to raise prolactin concentrations, sometimes up to three to four times the upper limit of the normal range. As these drugs can be excreted in breast milk, they should not be taken by nursing mothers.

Clinical Guidelines for SGAs

All SGAs, with the exception of pimavanserin and clozapine, are indicated for the management of an initial psychotic episode. Pimavanserin is used only for psychosis in Parkinson disease, generally a late-onset clinical manifestation. Clozapine is reserved for persons who are refractory to all other antipsychotic drugs.

If a person does not respond to the first SGA, a second SGA should be tried. The choice of drug should be based on the patient's clinical status and history of response to medication. It is an acceptable practice to augment an SGA with a high-potency DRA or benzodiazepine in the first few weeks of use. Lorazepam (Ativan) 1 to 2 mg orally or IM can be used as needed for acute agitation; and after the response is attained, their dosages can be lowered. In some treatment refractory patients, it may take up to 6 months of treatment with SGAs to attain clinical improvement, though some apparent benefits may be seen as early as

2 to 3 weeks. It should be noted that early response or failure may not be an indicator of subsequent response or failure.

Use of all SGAs must be initiated at low dosages and gradually titrated to therapeutic dosages. The gradual increase in dosage is necessary to offset the potential development of adverse effects. If a person stops taking an SGA for more than 36 hours, drug use should be resumed at the initial titration schedule. After the decision to terminate olanzapine or clozapine use, dosages should be tapered whenever possible to avoid cholinergic rebound symptoms such as diaphoresis, flushing, diarrhea, and hyperactivity.

After a clinician has determined that trial of an SGA is warranted for a particular person, the risks and benefits of SGA treatment must be explained to the person and the family. The patient's history should include information about blood disorders, epilepsy, cardiovascular disease, hepatic and renal diseases, and drug abuse. The presence of a hepatic or renal disease necessitates using low starting dosages of the drug. The physical examination should include supine and standing BP measurements to screen for orthostatic hypotension. The laboratory examination should include an EKG; several complete blood counts with WBC counts, which can then be averaged; as well as liver and renal function tests. Periodic monitoring of blood glucose, lipids, and body weight is recommended. In the case of clozapine, an informed consent procedure should be documented in the person's chart (see below).

Although the transition from a DRA to an SGA may be made abruptly, it is wiser to taper off the DRA slowly while titrating up the SGA. Clozapine and olanzapine both have anticholinergic effects, and the transition from one to the other can usually be accomplished with little risk of cholinergic rebound. The transition from risperidone to olanzapine is best accomplished by tapering the risperidone off over 3 weeks while simultaneously beginning olanzapine at 10 mg a day. Risperidone, quetiapine, and ziprasidone lack anticholinergic effects, and the abrupt transition from a DRA, olanzapine, or clozapine to one of these agents may cause cholinergic rebound, which consists of excessive salivation, nausea, vomiting, and diarrhea. The risk of cholinergic rebound can be mitigated by initially augmenting risperidone, quetiapine, or ziprasidone with an anticholinergic drug, which is then tapered off slowly. Any initiation and termination of SGA use should be accomplished gradually.

It is wise to overlap administration of the new drug with the old drug. Of interest, some people have a more robust clinical response while taking the two agents during the transition and then regressing on monotherapy with the newer drug. Little is known about the effectiveness and safety of a strategy of combining one SGA with another SGA or with a DRA.

Persons receiving regular injections of depot formulations of a DRA who are to switch to SGA use are given the first dose of the SGA on the day the next injection is due.

Persons who developed neutropenia while taking clozapine (see below) can safely switch to olanzapine use, although initiation of olanzapine use in the midst of clozapine-induced neutropenia can prolong the time of recovery from the usual 3 to 4 days up to 11 to 12 days. It is prudent to wait for resolution of neutropenia before initiating olanzapine use. Emergence or recurrence of neutropenia has not been reported with olanzapine, even in persons who developed it while taking clozapine.

The dosages for selected SGAs are given in Table 34-3.

TABLE 34-3: Dosages for Selected Second-Generation Antipsychotics

Antipsychotic	Typical Starting Dosage	Maintenance Therapy Dose Range	Titration	Maximum Recommended Dosage	TDM ng/mL	Alert Levels ng/mL
Aripiprazole (Abilify)	10–15-mg tablets once a day	10–30 mg/day	Dosage increases should not be made before 2 weeks	30 mg/day	150–500	1,000
Aripiprazole (Abilify Maintena)	400 mg/month	300–400 mg/month	Titration not necessary	400 mg/month	150–500	1,000
Aripiprazole lauroxil (Aristada)	441–882 mg/month	441–882 mg/month, or 882 mg every 6 weeks or 1,064 mg every 2 months	Titration not necessary	N/A	150–500	1,000
Aripiprazole lauroxil (Aristada Initio)	675 mg injection	N/A	N/A	N/A	N/A	N/A
Asenapine (Saphris)	5 mg twice a day	10 mg twice a day	Titration not necessary	20 mg/day	2–5	10
Asenapine (Secuado)	3.8 mg/day	3.8–7.6 mg/day	Can titrate to 5.7 mg/day or 7.6 mg/day on day 8	7.6 mg/day	2–5	10
Brexpiprazole (Rexulti)	1 mg/day through day 4	2–4 mg/day	Can titrate to 2 mg/day on day 5, and 4 mg/day on day 8	3 mg/day for MDD; 4 mg/day for schizophrenia	40–140	280
Cariprazine (Vraylar)	1.5 mg/day	3–6 mg once a day	Initial dose can be increased in 1.5-mg increments, depending on tolerability	6 mg/day	10–20	40
Clozapine (Clozaril, FazaClo, Versacloz)	12.5-mg tablets once or twice a day	150–300 mg/day in divided doses or 200 mg as a single dose in the evening	The dosage should be increased to 25–50 mg on the second day. Further increases may be made in daily increments of 25–50 mg to a target dosage of 300–450 mg/day. Subsequent dosage increases should be made no more than once or twice weekly in increments of no more than 100 mg	900 mg/day	350–600	1,000

(continued)

TABLE 34-3: Dosages for Selected Second-Generation Antipsychotics (*continued*)

Antipsychotic	Typical Starting Dosage	Maintenance Therapy Dose Range	Titration	Maximum Recommended Dosage	TDM ng/mL	Alert Levels ng/mL
Iloperidone (Fanapt)	1 mg twice a day	12–24 mg a day in divided dose	Start at 1 mg twice a day, then move to 2, 4, 6, 8 and 12 mg twice a day. Do this over the course of 7 days	24 mg/day	5–10	20
Lumateperone (Caplyta)	42 mg once daily	42 mg once daily	Titration not necessary	42 mg once daily	15–40	120
Lurasidone (Latuda)	40 mg/day	20–160 mg/day for adults; 20–80 mg/day for adolescents	Titration not necessary	160 mg/day	>70	120
Olanzapine (Zyprexa, Zyprexa Zydis)	5–10 mg/day tablets or orally disintegrating tablets	10–20 mg/day	Dosage increments of 5 mg once a day are recommended when required at intervals of not less than 1 week	20 mg/day	20–80	150
Olanzapine (Zyprexa IM)	5–10 mg	2.5–10 mg	N/A	30 mg/day	20–80	150
Olanzapine (Relprevv)	210–300 mg/fortnight or 405 mg/month	150–300 mg/fortnight or 300–405 mg/month	N/A	300 mg/fortnight	20–80	150
Olanzapine and fluoxetine (Symbyax)	6 mg olanzapine/25 mg fluoxetine once per day	6–12 mg olanzapine/25–50 mg fluoxetine once per day	N/A	12 mg olanzapine/50 mg fluoxetine once per day	N/A	N/A

Olanzapine and samidorphan (Lybalvi)	5, 10, or 15 mg olanzapine/10 mg samidorphan once per day	5–20 mg olanzapine/10 mg samidorphan once per day	Dosages should be increased in 5-mg increments (as measured by olanzapine content) at weekly intervals	20 mg olanzapine/20 mg samidorphan once per day	N/A	N/A
Paliperidone (Invega)	3–9-mg extended-release tablets once a day	3–6 mg/day	Plasma concentration rises to a peak approximately 24 hours after dosing	12 mg/day	20–60	120
Paliperidone (Invega Sustenna)	234-mg IM injection on day 1, then a 156-mg IM injection on day 8	39–234 mg/month	N/A	234 mg/month	20–60	120
Pimavanserin (Nuplazid)	17 or 34 mg once a day	34 mg once a day	No titration	34 mg/day	20–60	120
Quetiapine (Seroquel)	25-mg tablets twice a day	Lowest dose needed to maintain remission	Increase in increments of 25–50 mg two or three times a day on the second and the third day, as tolerated, to a target dosage of 500 mg daily by the fourth day (given in 2 or 3 doses/day). Further dosage adjustments, if required, should be of 25–50 mg twice a day and occur at intervals of not fewer than 2 days	800 mg/day	100–500	1,000
Quetiapine (Seroquel XR)	300 mg/day	400–800 mg/day	Increase in increments of 50–100 mg each day, as tolerated, to target dosage	800 mg/day	100–500	1,000
Risperidone (Risperdal)	1-mg tablet and oral solution once a day	2–6 mg once a day	Starting dose: 25 mg every 2 weeks	50 mg for 2 weeks (continued)	20–60	120

(continued)

TABLE 34-3: Dosages for Selected Second-Generation Antipsychotics (*continued*)

Antipsychotic	Typical Starting Dosage	Maintenance Therapy Dose Range	Titration	Maximum Recommended Dosage	TDM ng/mL	Alert Levels ng/mL
Risperidone IM long acting (Consta)	25–50-mg IM injection every 2 weeks	Start with oral risperidone for 3 weeks	Increase to 2 mg once a day on the second day and 4 mg once a day on the third day. In some patients, a slower titration may be appropriate. When dosage adjustments are necessary, further dosage increments of 1–2 mg/day at intervals of not less than 1 week are recommended	1–6 mg/day	20–60	120
Ziprasidone (Geodon)	20-mg capsules twice a day with food	20–80 mg twice a day	Dosage adjustments based on individual clinical status may be made at intervals of not fewer than 2 days	80 mg twice a day	50–200	400
Ziprasidone (IM)	For acute agitation: 10–20 mg, as required, up to a maximum of 40 mg/day	Not applicable	For acute agitation: doses of 10 mg may be administered every 2 hours, and doses of 20 mg may be administered every 4 hours up to a maximum of 40 mg/day	For acute agitation: 40 mg/day, for not more than three consecutive days	50–200	400

Note: Dosage adjustments may be required in special populations.
MDD, major depressive disorder; TDM, therapeutic drug monitoring.

ARIPIPRAZOLE

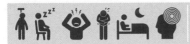 carbamazepine, valproate, ketoconazole, fluoxetine, paroxetine, quinidine

Pharmacokinetics

Aripiprazole is well absorbed, reaching peak plasma concentrations after 3 to 5 hours. Absorption is not affected by food. The mean elimination half-life of aripiprazole is about 75 hours. It has a weakly active metabolite, dehydro-aripiprazole, which has a half-life of 96 hours. These relatively long half-lives make aripiprazole suitable for once-daily dosing and clearance is reduced in elderly persons. Aripiprazole exhibits linear pharmacokinetics and is primarily metabolized by CYP3A4 and CYP2D6 enzymes and is 99% protein bound.

Pharmacodynamics

Mechanistically, aripiprazole acts as a modulator, rather than a blocker, and acts on both postsynaptic D_2 receptors and presynaptic autoreceptors. In theory, this mechanism of action addresses excessive limbic dopamine (hyperdopaminergic) activity, and decreased dopamine (hypodopaminergic) activity in frontal and prefrontal areas—abnormalities that are thought to be present in schizophrenia. The absence of complete D_2 blockade in the striatal areas would be expected to minimize EPS. Additionally, aripiprazole is an α_1-adrenergic receptor antagonist, which may cause some patients to experience orthostatic hypotension. Similar to several other atypical antipsychotic agents, aripiprazole is a 5-HT$_{2A}$ antagonist.

Therapeutic Indications

Aripiprazole is indicated for the treatment of schizophrenia (adults and adolescents aged 13 to 17 years). Short-term, 4- to 6-week studies comparing aripiprazole with haloperidol (Haldol) and risperidone in patients with schizophrenia and schizoaffective disorder have shown comparable efficacy. Dosages of 15, 20, and 30 mg a day were found to be effective. Long-term studies suggest that aripiprazole is effective as a maintenance treatment at a daily dose of 15 to 30 mg. In some cases, patients may benefit from the use of a monthly injection marketed under the name Abilify Maintena or another long-acting injection marketed under the name Aristada, which may be given once per month, once every six weeks, or once every 2 months.

Aripiprazole is also indicated for the acute and maintenance treatment of manic and mixed episodes associated with bipolar I disorder as monotherapy and as an adjunctive therapy to either lithium or valproate for the acute treatment of manic and mixed episodes associated with bipolar I disorder. This indication is for adults and pediatric patients aged 10 to 17 years.

It is also indicated for use as an adjunctive therapy to antidepressants for the treatment of MDD in adults, irritability associated with autistic spectrum disorder in patients aged 6 to 17 years old, and Tourette disorder in patients between the ages of 6 to 18 years.

Second-Generation or Atypical Antipsychotics

An injectable formulation of aripiprazole is indicated for the treatment of agitation associated with bipolar mania or schizophrenia.

Off-Label Uses

Some studies have found that aripiprazole may benefit individuals with anxiety disorders, dementia, and eating disorders like anorexia nervosa and bulimia nervosa.

A study of aggressive children and adolescents with oppositional-defiant disorder or conduct disorder found that there was a positive response in about 60% of the subjects. In this study, vomiting and somnolence led to a reduction in initial aripiprazole dosage.

Adverse Events

The most commonly reported side effects of aripiprazole are headache, somnolence, agitation, dyspepsia, anxiety, and nausea. Although it is not a frequent cause of EPS, aripiprazole does cause akathisia-like activation. Described as restlessness or agitation, it can be highly distressing and often leads to discontinuation of medication. Insomnia is another common complaint. Data so far do not indicate that weight gain or diabetes mellitus has an increased incidence with aripiprazole and prolactin elevation does not typically occur. In addition, aripiprazole does not cause significant QTc interval changes. There have been reports of seizures.

Drug Interactions

Whereas carbamazepine (Tegretol) and valproate reduce serum concentrations, ketoconazole, fluoxetine (Prozac), paroxetine (Paxil), and quinidine increase aripiprazole serum concentrations. Lithium and valproic acid, two drugs likely to be combined with aripiprazole when treating bipolar disorder, do not affect the steady-state concentrations of aripiprazole. Combined use with antihypertensives may cause hypotension. Drugs that inhibit CYP2D6 activity reduce aripiprazole elimination.

Dosage and Clinical Guidelines—Schizophrenia

Aripiprazole is available as 5-, 10-, 15-, 20-, and 30-mg tablets. The effective dosage range is 10 to 30 mg per day. Although the starting dosage is 10 to 15 mg per day for schizophrenia, problems with nausea, insomnia, and akathisia have led to use of lower than recommended starting dosages of aripiprazole. Many clinicians find that an initial dose of 5 mg increases tolerability. The FDA has approved aripiprazole as the first drug to have a digital ingestion tracking system. Abilify MyCite, the name of that formulation, has an ingestible sensor embedded in the pill that records that the medication was taken. It is available in 2-, 5-, 10-, 15-, 20-, and 30-mg tablets.

The initial dose for adolescent patients is 2 mg per day, titrated up to 5 mg after 2 days, and then titrated up again to a maintenance dose of 10 mg after another 2 days.

Additionally, schizophrenia patients may benefit from long-term injectables like Abilify Maintena or Aristada. Following the first 400-mg Abilify Maintena injection, patients continue taking 10 to 20 mg per day of oral aripiprazole.

TABLE 34-4: Aripiprazole Dosage Guidelines

	Initial Dose (mg/day)	Recommended Dose (mg/day)	Maximum Dose (mg/day)
Schizophrenia—adults	10–15	10–15	30
Schizophrenia—pediatric	2	10	30
Bipolar mania—adult monotherapy	15	15	30
Bipolar mania—adult adjunctive[a] therapy	10–15	15	30
Bipolar mania—pediatric monotherapy or as adjunctive[a] therapy	2	10	30
Major depressive disorder—as adjunct with antidepressants	2–5	5–10	15
Irritability associated with autism spectrum disorder—pediatric	2	5–10	15
Tourette disorder—<50 kg	2	5	10
Tourette disorder—≥50 kg	2	10	20

[a]Adjunct to lithium or valproate.

If well tolerated, continue administering doses of 400 mg no sooner than 26 days after the previous injection. If not well tolerated, consider reducing the monthly dosage to 300 mg. Aristada may be administered in 441-, 662, or 882-mg injections monthly, which corresponds to daily dosages of 10, 15, and 20 mg of aripiprazole, respectively. Aristada may also be administered every 6 weeks as an 882-mg dose or every 2 months as a 1064-mg dose. When starting or reinitiating treatment with Aristada, patients may be given a one-time, 675-mg injection of Aristada Initio in conjunction with an oral dose of aripiprazole.

An injectable formulation of aripiprazole is indicated for the treatment of agitation associated with bipolar mania or schizophrenia. The recommended dosage is 9.75 mg (range 5.25 to 15 mg). Cumulative doses up to 30 mg/day may be given.

For other indications, see Table 34-4.

ASENAPINE

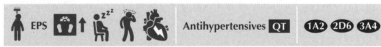
EPS   ↑   zᶻᶻ   Antihypertensives   QT   1A2 2D6 3A4

Pharmacokinetics

The bioavailability of asenapine is 35% via sublingual (preferred) route and achieves peak plasma concentration in 1 hour. Patients should avoid eating and drinking for at least 10 minutes after administration to ensure better absorption. Asenapine is metabolized through glucuronidation and oxidative metabolism by CYP1A2. Asenapine has a half-life of 24 hours and steady-state concentrations are reached after 3 days of dosing twice per day.

Pharmacodynamics

Asenapine has an affinity for several receptors, including serotonin (5-HT$_{2A}$ and 5-HT$_{2C}$), noradrenergic (α_2 and α_1), dopaminergic (D$_3$ and D$_4$ receptors is higher than its affinity for D$_2$ receptors), and histamine (H$_1$) receptors. It has negligible affinity for muscarinic-1 cholinergic receptors and hence less incidence of dry mouth, blurred vision, constipation, and urinary retention.

Therapeutic Indications

Asenapine is approved for the acute treatment of adults with schizophrenia and manic or mixed episodes associated with bipolar I disorder with or without psychotic features in adults. It has also been approved as maintenance monotherapy in adults and as an adjunctive therapy with lithium or valproate.

Off-Label Uses

Three open-label trials have evaluated asenapine for the treatment of borderline personality disorder with conflicting results. Other off-label uses include the treatment of PTSD, catatonia, delusional disorder, and cocaine-induced psychotic disorder.

Adverse Events

The most common side effects observed in schizophrenic and bipolar disorders are somnolence, dizziness, EPS other than akathisia, and increased weight. In clinical trials, the mean weight gain after 52 weeks is 0.9 kg and there were no clinically relevant differences in lipid profile and blood glucose after 52 weeks.

In clinical trials, asenapine was found to increase the QTc interval in a range of 2 to 5 ms compared to placebo. No patients treated with asenapine experienced QTc increases ≥60 ms from baseline measurements, nor did any experience a QTc of ≥500 ms. Nevertheless, asenapine should be avoided in combination with other drugs known to prolong QTc interval, in patients with congenital prolongation of QT interval or a history of cardiac arrhythmias, and in circumstances that may increase the occurrence of torsades de pointes. Asenapine can elevate prolactin levels, and the elevation can persist during chronic administration. Galactorrhea, amenorrhea, gynecomastia, and impotence may occur.

Asenapine is contraindicated in patients with severe hepatic impairment.

Drug Interactions

Since asenapine is metabolized by CYP1A2, coadministration with strong CYP1A2 inhibitors like fluvoxamine (Luvox) should be done cautiously. Dosage reductions may be necessary based on clinical responses. Asenapine may also enhance the effects of CYP2D6 substrates and inhibitors like paroxetine, so reductions in these drugs may be necessary. The effects of antihypertensive drugs may be enhanced due to the α_1-adrenergic antagonistic effects of asenapine. Monitor BP and adjust the dosage of the antihypertensive medication appropriately.

Dosage and Guidelines

Asenapine is available as 5- and 10-mg sublingual tablets and should be placed under the tongue. This is because the bioavailability of asenapine is less than 2% when swallowed, but is 35% when absorbed sublingually. Asenapine dissolves in saliva within seconds and is absorbed through the oral mucosa. Sublingual administration avoids first-pass hepatic metabolism.

The recommended starting and target dose for schizophrenia is 5 mg twice a day. In bipolar disorder, the patient may be started on 10 mg twice a day; and if necessary, the dosage may be lowered to 5 mg twice a day depending on the tolerability issues. In acute schizophrenia treatment, there is no evidence of added benefit with a 10-mg BID dose, but there is a clear increase in certain adverse reactions. In both bipolar I disorder and schizophrenia, the maximum dose should not exceed 10 mg BID. The safety of doses above 10 mg BID has not been evaluated in clinical studies.

In pediatric patients between 10 to 17 years of age, the initial dosage should be 2.5 mg twice per day but can be titrated up to 5 mg BID after 3 days, and then to 10 mg BID after another 3 days if well tolerated.

A transdermal system for the administration of asenapine is indicated for adults with schizophrenia. Marketed under the trade name Secuado, patches are available in strengths of 3.8, 5.7, and 7.6 mg that can be applied once per day. The recommended starting dosage is 3.8 mg per day. After 1 week, the dosage may be increased to 5.7 or 7.6 mg/day. No added benefit of the 7.6 mg/day formulation was observed during a short-term, placebo-controlled trial, but there was an increase in adverse reactions.

BREXPIPRAZOLE

Pharmacokinetics

Brexpiprazole has a bioavailability of 95% and reaches peak plasma levels within 4 hours of oral administration. Pharmacology of the drug is not affected by food. The drug is highly protein-bound (greater than 99%) and metabolism is primarily mediated by cytochrome P450 isoenzymes CYP3A4 and CYP2D6. The half-lives of brexpiprazole and its primary metabolite, DM-3411, are 91 and 86 hours, respectively.

Pharmacodynamics

Brexpiprazole is a D_2 dopamine partial agonist called serotonin–dopamine activity modulator (SDAM).

Therapeutic Indications

Brexpiprazole is indicated for use as an adjunctive therapy to antidepressants for the treatment of major depressive disorder and for the treatment of schizophrenia and pediatric patients aged 13 years and older.

Off-Label Uses

Brexpiprazole has been used off-label to treat mood lability in borderline personality disorder and symptoms associated with bipolar disorder. Some research has suggested that it could be used effectively to treat agitation in Alzheimer dementia, as well as an adjunctive treatment (with paroxetine or sertraline [Zoloft]) in the treatment of PTSD.

Some initial studies also suggested that brexpiprazole could help treat impulsivity in attention deficit hyperactivity disorder as an adjunctive treatment but was discontinued following phase 2 clinical trials for this indication.

Adverse Events

Common side effects of brexpiprazole reported in clinical trials include weight gain, agitation, distress, restlessness, constipation, fatigue, runny or stuffy nose, increased appetite, headache, drowsiness, tremor, dizziness, and anxiety.

Postmarketing case reports indicate that some patients may experience intense urges and impulsivity while taking brexpiprazole, and that they may manifest as pathologic gambling, unnecessary shopping episodes, binge eating, and increased sexual activity.

Drug Interactions

Brexpiprazole interacts with strong/moderate CYP2D6 or CYP3A4 inhibitors or strong CYP3A4 inducers.

Dosage and Guidelines

Brexpiprazole is available as 0.25-, 0.5-, 1-, 2-, 3-, and 4-mg tablets. The recommended starting dosage for brexpiprazole as adjunctive treatment for MDD is 0.5 or 1 mg once daily, taken orally. The recommended maintenance dose is 2 mg once daily and should not exceed 3 mg once daily. The recommended starting dosage for schizophrenia is 1 mg once daily for adults and 0.5 mg once daily for adolescents 13 to 17 years of age, while the recommended target brexpiprazole dosage to treat schizophrenia is 2 to 4 mg once daily for both adults and adolescents. The maximum recommended dose is 4 mg per day.

CARIPRAZINE

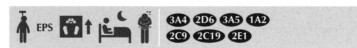

Pharmacokinetics

Peak plasma concentrations of cariprazine are reached within 3 to 6 hours or oral administration and absorption is not affected by food. Cariprazine and its metabolites are highly bound (91% to 97%) to plasma proteins and the parent compound is extensively metabolized by cytochrome P450 isoenzymes CYP3A4 and to a lesser extent CYP2D6. Cariprazine has a long half-life of 48 to 96 hours.

Pharmacodynamics

Cariprazine is a dopamine D_2 and D_3 receptor partial agonist, with higher affinity for D_3 receptors, as opposed to the D_2 antagonism.

Therapeutic Indications

Cariprazine is indicated in adults for the acute treatment of manic or mixed episodes associated with bipolar I disorder and the treatment of schizophrenia.

Off-Label Uses

There is limited evidence to suggest efficacy in the treatment of bipolar II depression and some symptoms associated with autism spectrum disorder.

Adverse Events

The most common side effects of cariprazine are EPS, especially akathisia. Also seen are insomnia, weight gain, sedation, nausea, dizziness, vomiting, and anxiety. Compared to other SGAs, cariprazine is less likely to impact metabolic variables or prolactin levels. It does not increase the QT interval. Some constipation may occur.

Use of cariprazine is not recommended in patients with severe liver disease.

Drug Interactions

Coadministration of cariprazine with either a strong CYP3A4 inhibitor or a CYP3A4 inducer may exacerbate adverse events. Reduce the dosage of cariprazine if concomitant use of a strong CYP3A4 inhibitor is necessary. Concomitant use of cariprazine and a CYP3A4 inducer is not recommended.

Dosage and Guidelines

Cariprazine is available as 1.5-, 3-, 4.5-, and 6-mg capsules. The dosage range is 1.5 to 6 mg a day in schizophrenia. The starting dose is 1.5 mg a day. The dose may be increased to 3 mg on day 2. Further dose adjustments can be made in 1.5- to 3-mg increments. The dosage range for bipolar disorder is 3 to 6 mg a day. The starting dose is 1.5 mg a day and should be increased to 3 mg on day 2. Further dose adjustments can be made in 1.5- to 3-mg increments.

When a strong CYP3A4 inhibitor is added when a patient is already on a stable dose of cariprazine, reduce the current cariprazine dose by 50%. For those patients taking a dosage of 4.5 mg/day, the dose should be reduced to 1.5 or 3 mg daily. For patients taking 1.5 mg daily, the dosing regimen should be adjusted to every other day. When a CYP3A4 inhibitor is discontinued, cariprazine dosage may need to be increased. When initiating cariprazine while already on a strong CYP3A4 inhibitor, use cariprazine 1.5 mg on days 1 and 3, with no dose on day 2. After day 4, the dose should be administered at 1.5 mg/day, then increased to a maximum of 3 mg/day. When a CYP3A4 inhibitor is discontinued, cariprazine dosage may need to be increased.

ILOPERIDONE

  Antihypertensives

Pharmacokinetics

Iloperidone has a peak concentration of 2 to 4 hours and a half-life that is dependent on hepatic isoenzyme metabolism. It is metabolized primarily through

CYP2D6 and CYP3A4, and the dosage should be reduced by half when administered concomitantly with strong inhibitors of these two isoenzymes. The half-life is 18 to 26 hours in CYP2D6 extensive metabolizers and is 31 to 37 hours in CYP2D6 poor metabolizers. Of note, approximately 7% to 10% of whites and 3% to 8% of African Americans lack the capacity to metabolize CYP2D6 substrates; hence, dosing should be done with this caveat in mind. Iloperidone should be used with caution in persons with severe hepatic impairment.

Pharmacodynamics

Iloperidone is not a derivative of another antipsychotic agent. It has complex multiple antagonist effects on several neurotransmitter systems. Iloperidone has a strong affinity for dopamine D_3 receptors, followed by decreasing affinities of α_{2C}-noradrenergic, 5-HT_{1A}, D_{2A}, and 5-HT_6 receptors. Iloperidone has a low affinity for histaminergic receptors. As with other antipsychotics, the clinical significance of this receptor binding affinity is unknown.

Therapeutic Indications

Iloperidone is indicated for the acute treatment of schizophrenia in adults. The safety and efficacy of iloperidone in children and adolescents has not been established.

Adverse Events

Iloperidone prolongs the QT interval by 9 ms at dosages of 12 mg twice daily and may be associated with arrhythmia and sudden death. Concurrent use with other agents that prolong the QTc interval may result in additive effects on the QTc interval. The concurrent use of iloperidone with agents that prolong the QTc interval may result in potentially life-threatening cardiac arrhythmias, including torsades de pointes. Concurrent administration of other drugs that are known to prolong the QTc interval should be avoided. Cardiovascular disease, hypokalemia, hypomagnesemia, bradycardia, congenital prolongation of the QT interval, and concurrent use of inhibitors of cytochrome P450 isoenzymes CYP3A4 or CYP2D6, which metabolize iloperidone, may increase the risk of QT prolongation.

The most common adverse effects reported are dizziness, dry mouth, fatigue, sedation, tachycardia, and orthostatic hypotension (depending on dosing and titration). Despite being a strong D_2 antagonist, the rate of EPS and akathisia are similar to those of placebo. The mean weight gain in short- and long-term trials is 2.1 kg. Weight-related studies suggest weight gain of approximately 3 lbs in the short term (up to 12 weeks) and modest weight gain of 7 lbs over 12 weeks. Some patients exhibit elevated prolactin levels.

At least three cases of priapism have been reported in the premarketing phase.

Drug Interactions

Inhibitors of CYP3A4 and CYP2D6 can inhibit iloperidone elimination and lead to increases in iloperidone exposure. Iloperidone may also enhance the effect of some hypertensive agents.

Dosage and Guidelines

Iloperidone must be titrated slowly to avoid orthostatic hypotension. It is available in a titration pack, and the effective dose (12 mg) should be reached in approximately 4 days based on a twice-a-day dosing schedule. It is usually started on day 1 at 1 mg twice a day and increased daily on a twice-a-day schedule to reach 12 mg by day 4. The maximum recommended dose is 12 mg twice a day (24 mg a day) and can be administered without regard to food.

LUMATEPERONE

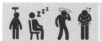 amisulpride, carbamazepine

Pharmacokinetics

Lumateperone has an absolute bioavailability of 4.4% and reaches peak concentrations (C_{max}) 1 to 2 hours after oral administration. It reaches steady-state concentrations with daily administration in approximately 5 days. Ingestion with food will reduce C_{max} by 33% and increase AUC by 9% and is, therefore, suggested. Protein binding is 97.4%. Lumateperone produces more than 20 metabolites while being metabolized and multiple enzymes are involved in the process, including 5′-diphospho-glucuronosyltransferases (UDP-glucuronosyltransferases, UGT) 1A1, 1A4, 1A4, and 2B15; aldo-keto reductase (AKR) 1C1, 1B10, and 1C4; and cytochrome P450 (CYP) 3A4, 2C8, and 1A2. It has a half-life of 18 hours.

Pharmacodynamics

Lumateperone's mechanism of action could be mediated through its antagonistic activity at 5-HT$_{2A}$ ($K_i = 0.54$ nM) receptors and postsynaptic antagonist activity at central D$_2$ receptors ($K_i = 32$ nM). It also has a moderate binding affinity for serotonin transports ($K_i = 33$ nM), D$_1$ ($K_i = 41$ nM), D$_4$ ($K_i \leq 100$ nM), α_{1A}-adrenergic ($K_i \leq 100$ nM), and α_{1B}-adrenergic ($K_i \leq 100$ nM) receptors. Lumateperone has low binding affinity for histaminic and muscarinic receptors.

Therapeutic Indications

Lumateperone is indicated in adults for the treatment of schizophrenia in adults. It has been approved for use in treating depressive episodes associated with bipolar I or II disorder as monotherapy and as adjunctive therapy with lithium or valproate.

Off-Label Uses

There is also some indication that it may be effective at treating behavioral disturbances in people with depression, dementia, and other neurologic conditions.

Adverse Events

The most common drug-related adverse effects are sedation, nausea, dry mouth, dizziness, increased creatine phosphokinase, fatigue, vomiting, increased hepatic transaminases, and decreased appetite. Some patients with a history of seizure disorders have reported increased seizures after taking lumateperone.

Drug Interactions

Coadministration of lumateperone with either a strong CYP3A4 inhibitor or a CYP3A4 inducer may exacerbate adverse events. UGT inhibitors may increase the exposure of lumateperone. Concomitant administration of lumateperone with either a strong CYP3A4 inhibitor, CYP3A4 inducer, or UGT inhibitor is not recommended.

Dosage and Guidelines

It is available as a 42-mg capsule and should be administered with food at a dosage of 42 mg per day. There is no need for titration.

Patients with moderate to severe hepatic impairment should avoid use of lumateperone.

LURASIDONE

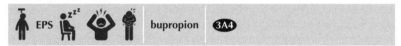

Pharmacokinetics

Peak concentrations of lurasidone are reached 1 to 3 hours after oral administration and with daily dosage, steady-state concentrations are reached within 7 days. Between 9% and 19% of an oral dose of lurasidone is absorbed and the drug is highly protein bound (approximately 99%). The AUC and peak concentrations are increased twofold and threefold, respectively, when consumed with a meal of at least 350 calories when compared to administration in a fasting state. It is metabolized primarily by cytochrome P450 isoenzyme CYP3A4 into two nonactive metabolites (ID-20219 and ID-20220) and two active metabolites (ID-14283 and ID-14326). The half-life of lurasidone is 18 hours.

Pharmacodynamics

Lurasidone is an antagonist at 5-HT$_{2A}$ (K$_i$ = 0.5 nM) and 5-HT$_7$ (K$_i$ = 0.5 nM) receptors, as well as at D$_2$ receptors (K$_i$ = 1 nM). Lurasidone has demonstrated partial agonistic activity at 5-HT$_{1A}$ receptors (K$_i$ = 6.4 nM) and moderate antagonistic activity at α_{2C}-adrenergic (K$_i$ = 11 nM) and α_{2A}-adrenergic (K$_i$ = 41 nM) receptors. It has low binding affinity for histaminic and muscarinic receptors.

Therapeutic Indications

Lurasidone is indicated for the treatment of adult and pediatric patients aged 13 to 17 years old with schizophrenia and for adult patients experiencing depressive episodes associated with bipolar I disorder as monotherapy and as adjunctive therapy with lithium or valproate. It is also approved for use as monotherapy for adolescent patients aged 10 to 17 years old with depressive episodes associated with bipolar I disorder.

Off-Label Uses

Lurasidone has shown some efficacy in the treatment of irritability and anger in autism spectrum disorder, as well as manic and hypomanic episodes in bipolar I disorder.

Adverse Events

The most commonly observed adverse reactions associated with the use of lurasidone are similar to those seen with other new-generation antipsychotics. These include, but are not limited to somnolence, akathisia, nausea, parkinsonism, and agitation. Based on clinical trial data, lurasidone appears to cause less weight gain and metabolic changes than the two other most recently approved SGAs, asenapine and iloperidone. Whether this is in fact the case awaits more extensive clinical experience with the drug.

Some patients with a history of seizure disorders have reported increased seizures after taking lurasidone.

Drug Interactions

If coadministrating with a moderate CYP3A4 inhibitor such as diltiazem (Cartia XT), the lurasidone dose should be halved and should not exceed 40 mg per day. It should not be used in combination with a strong CYP3A4 inhibitor (e.g., ketoconazole) or a strong CYP3A4 inducer (e.g., rifampin [Rifadin]).

Dosage and Guidelines

Lurasidone is available as 20-, 40-, 80-, and 120-mg tablets. Initial dose titration is not required. The recommended starting dose is 40 mg once daily for schizophrenia or 20 mg once daily for bipolar I disorder, and the medication should be taken with food. It has been shown to be effective in a dose range of 40 to 160 mg per day for adults with schizophrenia and 20 to 120 mg per day for adults being treated for depressive episodes associated with bipolar I disorder. In adolescents, the recommended range is 40 to 80 mg per day and 20 to 80 mg per day, respectively. There may be a dose-related increase in adverse reactions. Still, some patients may benefit from the maximum recommended dose of 160 mg per day.

Dose adjustment is recommended in patients with renal impairment. The dose in moderate to severe renal impairment should not exceed 80 mg per day. The dose in severe hepatic impairment patients should not exceed 40 mg per day.

OLANZAPINE

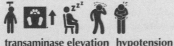

transaminase elevation   hypotension

CNS fluoxetine, samidorphan, cimetidine, carbamazepine, phenytoin

1A2 2D6 2C19 2C9 3A4

Pharmacokinetics

Approximately 85% of olanzapine is absorbed from the gastrointestinal (GI) tract, and about 40% of the dosage is inactivated by first-pass hepatic metabolism. It is extensively metabolized, but its two primary metabolites are inactive. The primary metabolic pathways for olanzapine are the flavin-containing monooxygenase system and cytochrome P450 isoenzymes CYP1A2 and CYP2D6. Peak concentrations are reached in 5 hours, and the half-life averages 31 hours (range: 21 to 54 hours). It is given in once-daily dosing and reaches steady-state concentrations in approximately 7 days with consistent dosing.

Pharmacodynamics

In addition to 5-HT_{2A} and D_2 antagonism, olanzapine is an antagonist of the D_1, D_4, α_1, 5-HT_{1A}, muscarinic $M_1\text{-}M_5$, and H_1 receptors.

Indications

Oral olanzapine is indicated for the treatment of schizophrenia in adults and adolescent patients. It is also indicated for use as monotherapy for the acute treatment of manic or mixed episodes associated with bipolar I disorder and maintenance treatment of bipolar I disorder. Oral olanzapine is also indicated for the treatment of manic or mixed episodes associated with bipolar I disorder as an adjunct to lithium or valproate.

A short-acting intramuscular (IM) injection of olanzapine has been approved for the treatment of agitation associated with schizophrenia and mania in bipolar I disorder in adults.

A long-acting IM injection marketed under the name Relprevv is indicated for adults with schizophrenia and can be administered either every 2 weeks or every 4 weeks.

Olanzapine can also be used in combination with fluoxetine (Symbyax) for the treatment of depressive episodes associated with bipolar I disorder in adults and adolescents 10 to 17 years of age. Symbyax is also indicated for treatment-resistant depression in adults.

Finally, olanzapine in combination with samidorphan (Lybalvi) is indicated for use in schizophrenia and bipolar I disorder in adults. For bipolar I disorder, it may be used either as acute treatment for manic or mixed episodes as monotherapy or in conjunction with valproate or lithium or as maintenance monotherapy treatment.

Adverse Events

Other than clozapine, olanzapine consistently causes a greater amount and more frequent weight gain than other SGAs. This effect is not dose-related and continues over time. Clinical trial data suggest that it peaks after 9 months, after which it may continue to increase more slowly. Somnolence, dry mouth, dizziness, constipation, dyspepsia, increased appetite, akathisia, and tremor are associated with olanzapine use. A small number of patients (2%) may need to discontinue use of the drug because of transaminase elevation. There is a dose-related risk of EPS. "Periodic" assessment of blood sugar and transaminases during treatment with olanzapine is recommended.

Olanzapine can elevate prolactin levels or lead to hypotension and syncope. Some patients with a history of seizure disorders have reported increased seizures, while others may develop motor or cognitive impairment.

When olanzapine is taken in conjunction with fluoxetine as Symbyax, patients may experience some of the adverse reactions discussed in Chapter 33. Common side effects for this formulation include somnolence, weight gain, increased appetite, increases in hepatic enzymes, tremor, increases in blood triglycerides, dry mouth, edema, fatigue, and restlessness.

When olanzapine is taken in conjunction with samidorphan as Lybalvi, patients may experience any of the adverse events described above. Common side effects for this formulation include weight gain, somnolence, dry mouth, headache, increases in blood insulin, sedation, dizziness, and decreases in neutrophil counts.

Drug Interactions

Fluvoxamine (Luvox) and cimetidine (Tagamet) increase while carbamazepine and phenytoin (Phenytek) decrease serum concentrations of olanzapine. Ethanol increases olanzapine absorption by more than 25%, leading to increased sedation and other central nervous system (CNS) depressants may produce similar effects. Olanzapine has little effect on the metabolism of most other drugs.

For drug interactions pertaining to fluoxetine (the other component in Symbyax), see Chapter 33.

In addition to the drug interactions noted above, Lybalvi is contraindicated in patients either using opioids or who are experiencing opioid withdrawal. Lybalvi's efficacy may be diminished if taken in conjunction with a strong CYP3A4 inhibitor or CYP1A2 inducer. Increases in Lybalvi adverse reactions may occur if coadministered with a strong CYP1A2 inhibitor. Meanwhile, Lybalvi may enhance the effects of some antihypertensive drugs and antagonize the effects of dopamine agonists and levodopa.

Dosages

Olanzapine is available as Zyprexa, which comes in 2.5-, 5-, 7.5-, 10-, 15-, and 20-mg oral tablets. An orally disintegrating tablet marketed under the name Zyprexa Zydis is available in 5-, 10-, 15-, and 20-mg tablets. The initial dosage for treatment of psychosis is usually 5 or 10 mg and for treatment of acute mania is usually 10 or 15 mg given once daily. The orally disintegrating tablets might be useful for patients who have difficulty swallowing pills or who "cheek" their medication.

When treating schizophrenia in adults, a starting daily dose of 5 to 10 mg is recommended. After 1 week, the dosage can be raised to 10 mg a day. Given the long half-life, 1 week must be allowed to achieve each new steady-state blood level. Dosages in clinical use ranges vary, with 5 to 20 mg a day being most commonly used but 30 to 40 mg a day being needed in treatment-resistant patients. A word of caution, however, is that the higher dosages are associated with increased EPS and other adverse events, and dosages above 20 mg a day were not studied in the pivotal trials that led to the approval of olanzapine. Some patients may benefit from the extended-release injectable suspension of olanzapine (Relprevv), which is a long-acting atypical IM injection indicated for the treatment of schizophrenia. It is injected deeply in the gluteal region and should not be administered intravenously or subcutaneously, nor is it approved for deltoid administration. Before administering the injection, the administrator should aspirate the syringe for several seconds to ensure no blood is visible. It carries a boxed warning for postinjection delirium sedation syndrome (PDSS). Patients are at risk for severe sedation (including coma) and must be observed for 3 hours after each injection in a registered facility. In controlled studies, all patients with PDSS recovered, and there were no deaths reported. It is postulated that PDSS is secondary to increased levels of olanzapine secondary to accidental rupture of a blood vessel. Patients should be managed as clinically appropriate and, if necessary, monitored in a facility capable of resuscitation. The injection can be given every 2 or 4 weeks depending on the dosing guidelines.

When treating manic or mixed states associated with bipolar I disorder in adults, the dosage should begin at 10 mg or 15 mg without regard for meals. Dose adjustments in increments of 5 mg are recommended and adjustments should be made in intervals of not less than 24 hours. Dosages in the range of 5 to 20 mg per day for the short-term (3 to 4 weeks) treatment of manic or mixed states or maintenance monotherapy are recommended. When coadministered with valproate or lithium, dosages of olanzapine should begin at 10 mg.

When treating schizophrenia in adolescents, the starting daily dosage should be 2.5 to 5 mg. After 1 week of treatment, the dose may be titrated. Dosage change increments of 2.5 mg or 5 mg are recommended. Efficacy of olanzapine has been demonstrated in adolescents with doses ranging from 2.5 to 20 mg/day, with a mean modal dose of 12.5 mg/day. Olanzapine has not been systematically evaluated as maintenance treatment for adolescent schizophrenia.

When treating manic or mixed states associated with bipolar I disorder in adults, the dosage should begin at 2.5 mg or 5 mg without regard for meals. Dose adjustments in increments of 2.5 mg or 5 mg are recommended and adjustments should be made in intervals of not less than 24 hours. Dosages in the range of 5 to 20 mg per day for the short-term (3 to 4 weeks) treatment of manic or mixed states were shown to be efficacious, with a mean modal dose of 10.7 mg/day.

The parenteral form of olanzapine is indicated for the treatment of acute agitation associated with schizophrenia and bipolar disorder, and the IM dosage is 10 mg. A lower dose of 2.5 mg or 5 mg may be warranted in some clinical conditions. If the first dosage does not reduce agitation, subsequent doses of 10 mg can be given, but the total daily dose should not exceed 30 mg; another 10-mg dose should not be administered after the first dose for at least 2 hours, and a tertiary, 10-mg dose should not be administered for at least 4 hours after the second dose. Coadministration with benzodiazepines is not approved.

Combined Formulations
Symbyax

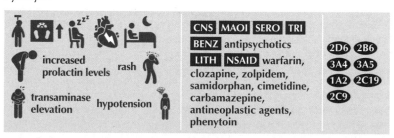

increased prolactin levels   rash

transaminase elevation   hypotension

CNS   MAOI   SERO   TRI
BENZ antipsychotics
LITH NSAID warfarin, clozapine, zolpidem, samidorphan, cimetidine, carbamazepine, antineoplastic agents, phenytoin

2D6 2B6
3A4 3A5
1A2 2C19
2C9

Symbyax is a fixed combination treatment of olanzapine and fluoxetine that is available in capsules containing 3 mg/25 mg, 6 mg/25 mg,

6 mg/50 mg, 12 mg/25 mg, and 12 mg/50 mg (mg olanzapine/mg equivalent fluoxetine).

When treating depressive episodes associated with bipolar I disorder, the adult starting dose for Symbyax is 6 mg/25 mg (mg olanzapine/mg equivalent fluoxetine) taken in the evening. Efficacy was demonstrated in dosages of 6 mg/25 mg (mg olanzapine/mg equivalent fluoxetine) to 12 mg/50 mg (mg olanzapine/mg equivalent fluoxetine). When treating adolescents for the same condition, the starting dose should be 3 mg/25 mg (mg olanzapine/mg equivalent fluoxetine).

When treating treatment-resistant depression in adults, the starting dose should be 6 mg/25 mg (mg olanzapine/mg equivalent fluoxetine) taken in the evening. Efficacy was demonstrated in dosages of 6 mg/25 mg (mg olanzapine/mg equivalent fluoxetine) to 12 mg/50 mg (mg olanzapine/mg equivalent fluoxetine).

Patients with a predisposition to hypotensive reactions, hepatic impairment, or any factors that may indicate slow metabolism of Symbyax should be started on a dose of 3 mg/25 mg (mg olanzapine/mg equivalent fluoxetine).

Lybalvi

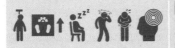
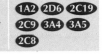

CNS opioids, fluoxetine, samidorphan, cimetidine, carbamazepine, phenytoin

1A2 2D6 2C19 2C9 3A4 3A5 2C8

Lybalvi is a fixed combination treatment of olanzapine and samidorphan, an opioid receptor antagonist, that is available in tablets containing 5 mg/10 mg, 10 mg/10 mg, 15 mg/10 mg, and 20 mg/10 mg olanzapine/samidorphan.

The recommended starting dosage in patients with schizophrenia is 5 mg/10 mg or 10 mg/10 mg administered once daily. The dosage may be maintained or, if deemed necessary and well tolerated, titrated up to 15 mg/10 mg or 20 mg/10 mg. Dosage adjustments should be made in 5-mg increments (based on olanzapine content) at weekly intervals. The maximum recommended daily dosage is 20 mg/10 mg.

In use as monotherapy for the treatment of mixed or manic episodes associated with bipolar I disorder, the recommended starting dosage is 10 mg/10 mg or 15 mg/10 mg once daily. After initiating treatment, the recommended daily dosage is 10 mg/10 mg, 15 mg/10 mg, or 20 mg/10 mg administered once daily. Maintenance monotherapy may be 5 mg/10 mg, 10 mg/10 mg, 15 mg/10 mg, or 20 mg/10 mg administered once daily. Dosage adjustments should be made in 5-mg increments (based on olanzapine content) in intervals of not less than 24 hours. In use as adjunctive therapy with lithium or valproate, the recommended starting dosage is 10 mg/10 mg once daily. After initiating treatment, the recommended daily dosage is 10 mg/10 mg, 15 mg/10 mg, or 20 mg/10 mg administered once daily. Maintenance monotherapy may be 5 mg/10 mg, 10 mg/10 mg, 15 mg/10 mg, or 20 mg/10 mg administered once daily. Dosage adjustments should be made in 5-mg increments (based on olanzapine content) in weekly intervals.

PALIPERIDONE

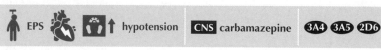

Pharmacokinetics

Paliperidone is the major active metabolite of risperidone. Peak plasma concentrations (C_{max}) are achieved approximately 24 hours after dosing, and steady-state concentrations of paliperidone are attained within 4 to 5 days. The hepatic isoenzymes CYP2D6 and CYP3A4 play a limited role in the metabolism and elimination of paliperidone, so no dose adjustment is required in patients with mild or moderate hepatic impairment. The terminal half-life of paliperidone is 23 hours.

Pharmacodynamics

Paliperidone is an antagonist at 5-HT$_{2A}$ (K_i = 0.8 to 1.2 nM) and at D$_2$ (K_i = 1.6 to 2.8 nM) receptors, through which it is believed to exert its therapeutic effects. It also acts an antagonist at α_1-adrenergic, α_2-adrenergic, and histamine (H$_1$) receptors.

Indications

Paliperidone is indicated for the acute and maintenance treatment of schizophrenia in adults and adolescents. It is also indicated for the acute treatment of schizoaffective disorder as monotherapy or as an adjunct to mood stabilizers, or antidepressants.

Adverse Events

The dose of paliperidone should be reduced in patients with renal impairment. It may cause more sensitivity to temperature extremes such as very hot or cold conditions. Paliperidone may cause an increase in QT (QTc) interval and should be avoided in combination with other drugs that cause prolongation of QT interval. It may cause orthostatic hypotension, tachycardia, somnolence, akathisia, dystonia, EPS, and parkinsonism.

Drug Interactions

Paliperidone should be used with caution with centrally acting drugs and alcohol, while an additive effect may be observed when paliperidone is administered in conjunction with drugs that can cause orthostatic hypotension.

Coadministration of paliperidone with carbamazepine caused a decrease of 37% of the mean steady-state C_{max} and AUC of paliperidone. If concomitant use is deemed necessary, the dosage of paliperidone should be increased. Coadministration with divalproex sodium resulted in an increase in the C_{max} and AUC of paliperidone by approximately 50%. If concomitant use is deemed necessary, the dosage of paliperidone may need to be decreased.

Dosage and Clinical Guidelines

When administered orally, paliperidone is available in 1.5-, 3-, 6-, and 9-mg tablets. The recommended dosage for adults is 6 mg once daily administered in the morning. It can be taken with or without food swallowed whole. It is also available as extended-release tablets, which are also available in 3-, 6-, and 9-mg tablets administered once daily. The recommended dosage is 3 to 12 mg/day, and it is recommended that no more than 12 mg should be administered per day. Dosage increases should occur at intervals of no more than 5 days.

In pediatric patients being treated for schizophrenia, the recommended starting dosage is 3 mg per day. For patients under 51 kg, the recommended daily dosage should range between 3 to 6 mg. For patients 51 kg and over, the recommended daily dosage is 3 to 12 mg.

Long-Acting Formulations

Invega Sustenna. A once monthly formulation of paliperidone marketed under the name Invega Sustenna is available as a white to off-white sterile aqueous extended-release suspension for IM injection in dose strengths of 39-, 78-, 117-, 156-, and 234-mg paliperidone palmitate. The drug product hydrolyzes to the active moiety, paliperidone, resulting in dose strengths of 25, 50, 75, 100, and 150 mg of paliperidone, respectively.

Invega Sustenna is provided in a prefilled syringe with a plunger stopper and tip cap. The kit also contains two safety needles (a 1.5-in, 22-gauge safety needle and a 1-in, 23-gauge safety needle). It has a half-life of 25 to 49 days. Monthly injections of 117 mg are recommended, although higher or lower dosages can be used depending on the clinical situation. The first two injections should be in the deltoid muscle because plasma concentrations are 28% higher with deltoid versus gluteal administration. Subsequent injections can alternate between gluteal and deltoid sites.

Invega Trinza. Adult patients with schizophrenia who have successfully been treated with Invega Sustenna for at least 4 months may transition to Invega Trinza, which is administered every 3 months.

- If their last dose of Invega Sustenna was 78 mg, then their dose of Invega Trinza should be 273 mg.
- If their last dose of Invega Sustenna was 117 mg, then their dose of Invega Trinza should be 410 mg.
- If their last dose of Invega Sustenna was 156 mg, then their dose of Invega Trinza should be 546 mg.
- If their last dose of Invega Sustenna was 234 mg, then their dose of Invega Trinza should be 819 mg.

Invega Hafyera. Adult patients with schizophrenia who have successfully been treated with Invega Sustenna for at least 4 months or Invega Trinza for at least 1 3-month cycle, may transition to Invega Hafyera, which is administered every 6 months.

If transitioning from Invega Sustenna:

- If their last dose of Invega Sustenna was 156 mg, then their dose of Invega Hafyera should be 1,092 mg.
- If their last dose of Invega Sustenna was 234 mg, then their dose of Invega Hafyera should be 1,560 mg.

If transitioning from Invega Trinza:

- If their last dose of Invega Trinza was 546 mg, then their dose of Invega Hafyera should be 1,092 mg.
- If their last dose of Invega Trinza was 819 mg, then their dose of Invega Hafyera should be 1,560 mg.

PIMAVANSERIN

 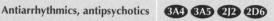
Antiarrhythmics, antipsychotics   3A4 3A5 2J2 2D6

Pharmacokinetics

Oral pimavanserin reaches peak concentrations in 6 hours (range: 4 to 24 hours) and is highly protein bound (approximately 95%) in human plasma. It is primarily metabolized by cytochrome P450 isoenzymes CYP3A4 and CYP3A5, with CYP3A4 being responsible for the formation of its active metabolite, AC-279. The half-lives of pimavanserin and AC-279 are 57 and 200 hours, respectively.

Pharmacodynamics

The mechanism of action of pimavanserin in treating hallucinations and delusions associated with Parkinson disease psychosis is not well understood. It is postulated that the effect of pimavanserin could be mediated through a combination of inverse agonist and antagonist activity at serotonin 5-HT$_{2A}$ receptors and to a lesser extent at serotonin 5-HT$_{2C}$ receptors.

Pimavanserin has high binding affinities at 5-HT$_{2A}$ and 5-HT$_{2C}$ receptors ($K_i = 0.087$ nM and $K_i = 0.44$ nM, respectively), and has low binding affinity to sigma 1 receptors ($K_i = 120$ nM). It has no appreciable binding affinity at 5-HT$_{2B}$, dopaminergic, muscarinic, histaminic, or adrenergic receptors, nor does it have significant affinity for calcium channels.

Indications

Pimavanserin is approved for the treatment of hallucinations and delusions associated with Parkinson disease psychosis. It is not indicated for treatment of schizophrenia or bipolar disorder.

Off-Label Uses

Despite recent attempts to obtain approval from the FDA for use in treating hallucinations and delusions in patients with Alzheimer disease, the FDA has not felt that there is sufficient evidence for this indication.

Adverse Events

Common side effects include nausea, constipation, swelling of the extremities, walking abnormally (gait disturbance), hallucinations, and confusion.

Drug Interactions

Coadministration of many drugs needs to be avoided or requires dosage adjustments. Strong CYP3A4 inhibitors, such as itraconazole (Sporanox), ketoconazole, clarithromycin, and indinavir (Crixivan), potentiate its effects. When using these drugs, its dose should be reduced by 50%. Strong CYP3A4 inducers, such as rifampin, carbamazepine, phenytoin, and St. John's wort, antagonize pimavanserin and concurrent use requires monitoring for reduced efficacy. Avoid concomitant use with other drugs known to prolong QT interval including Class 1A (e.g., quinidine, procainamide, disopyramide [Norpace]) or Class 3 antiarrhythmics (e.g., amiodarone [Pacerone], sotalol [Betapace]), certain antipsychotics (e.g., ziprasidone, chlorpromazine, thioridazine), and certain antibiotics (e.g., gatifloxacin [Zymaxid], moxifloxacin [Avelox]).

Dosage and Guidelines

The drug should be administered as 34 mg (taken as two 17-mg tablets) once daily. It is only available as 17-mg tablets. There is no need for titration.

QUETIAPINE

 antiarrhythmics, antipsychotics, phenytoin 2D6 3A4 3A5 2C19 3A7

Pharmacokinetics

Quetiapine is structurally related to clozapine, but it differs markedly from that agent in biochemical effects. It is rapidly absorbed from the GI tract, with peak plasma concentrations reached in 1 to 2 hours. Oral bioavailability is only 9% and is marginally impacted by administration with food, which causes C_{max} and AUC values to increase 25% and 15%, respectively. Quetiapine is extensively metabolized in the liver by the cytochrome P450 isoenzyme CYP3A4 into inactive metabolites. The steady-state half-life of quetiapine is about 7 hours with optimal dosing being two or three times per day, while the drug's mean terminal half-life is approximately 6 hours.

Following oral administration of quetiapine, clearance by patients 65 years of age and older was found to be 40% lower than younger patients, clearance by patients with severe renal impairment was found to be 25% lower than healthy adults, and clearance by patients with hepatic impairment was found to be 30% lower than healthy adults.

Pharmacodynamics

Quetiapine, in addition to being an antagonist of D_2 and 5-HT_{2A}, also blocks 5-HT_{1A}, 5-HT_6, D_1 and H_1, and α_1- and α_2-adrenergic receptors. It does not block muscarinic or benzodiazepine receptors. The receptor antagonism for quetiapine is generally lower than that for other antipsychotic drugs, and it is not associated with EPS. Quetiapine's mechanism of action is believed to be derived from its antagonistic activity at D_2 and 5-HT_{2A} receptors.

Indications

Quetiapine is indicated for the treatment of schizophrenia, as well as the acute treatment of manic episodes associated with bipolar I disorder, both as monotherapy and as an adjunct to lithium or divalproex. For adolescents, it is only indicated as a treatment for schizophrenia and as monotherapy for manic episodes associated with bipolar I disorder. The former indication applies to adolescents 13 to 17 years of age, while the latter indication applies to adolescents 10 to 17 years of age. For adults, quetiapine is also indicated as monotherapy for the acute treatment of depressive episodes associated with bipolar disorder and maintenance treatment of bipolar I disorder as an adjunct to lithium or divalproex.

An extended-release formulation marketed under the name Seroquel XR is indicated for each of these conditions, as well as a major depressive disorder as an adjunctive treatment with antidepressants in adults.

Off-Label Uses

Quetiapine has been used with some success to treat generalized anxiety disorder, psychosis in patients with Parkinson disease, PTSD, and insomnia as monotherapy. As adjunctive therapy with selective serotonin reuptake inhibitors (SSRIs), it has been used to treat OCD, borderline personality disorder, PTSD, insomnia, anxiety, major depressive disorder, and agitation.

Adverse Events

Somnolence, postural hypotension, and dizziness are the most common adverse events of quetiapine. These are usually transient and are best managed with initial gradual upward titration of the dosage. Quetiapine is the SGA least likely to cause EPS, regardless of dose. This makes it particularly useful in treating patients with Parkinson disease who develop dopamine-agonist–induced psychosis. Prolactin elevation is rare and both transient and mild when it occurs.

Quetiapine is associated with modest transient weight gain in some persons, but some patients occasionally gain a considerable amount of weight. The relationship between quetiapine and the development of diabetes is not as clearly established as are the cases involving the use of olanzapine, but clinicians should still monitor for signs of developing metabolic syndrome or other diseases associated with obesity (e.g., dyslipidemia, hypertension, hypercholesterolemia). Minor increases in heart rate, constipation, and a transient increase in liver transaminases may also occur. Initial concerns about cataract formation, based on animal studies, have not been borne out since the drug has been in clinical use. Nevertheless, it might be prudent to test for lens abnormalities early in treatment and periodically thereafter.

Increased BP has been observed in children and adolescents, particularly when initiating treatment, so clinicians should monitor for any anomalies.

Drug Interactions

The potential interactions between quetiapine and other drugs have been well studied. Phenytoin increases quetiapine clearance fivefold, but no major pharmacokinetic interactions have been noted. Coadministration of quetiapine with

CYP3A4 inhibitors can potentiate the drug's effects and should be reduced to one-sixth the original dosage if it is deemed necessary that both medications be continued. Conversely, coadministration of quetiapine with CYP3A4 inducers can diminish the effects of the drug, so the dose should be increased up to five-fold of the original dosage if coadministered with potent CYP3A4 inducers. If the CYP3A4 inducer is discontinued, the dosage of quetiapine should be reduced to original levels within 1 to 2 weeks.

Avoid use of quetiapine with drugs that increase the QT interval and in patients with risk factors for prolonged QT interval. The use of quetiapine should be avoided in combination with other drugs that are known to prolong QTc including Class 1A antiarrhythmics (e.g., quinidine, procainamide) or Class III antiarrhythmics (e.g., amiodarone, sotalol), antipsychotic medications (e.g., ziprasidone, chlorpromazine, thioridazine), antibiotics (e.g., gatifloxacin, moxifloxacin), or any other class of medications known to prolong the QTc interval (e.g., pentamidine, levomethadyl acetate [Orlaam], methadone). Quetiapine should also be avoided in circumstances that may increase the risk of occurrence of torsade de pointes and/or sudden death including (1) a history of cardiac arrhythmias such as bradycardia; (2) hypokalemia or hypomagnesemia; (3) concomitant use of other drugs that prolong the QTc interval; and (4) presence of congenital prolongation of the QT interval. Postmarketing cases also show increases in QT interval in patients who overdose on quetiapine.

Dosage and Guidelines

Quetiapine is available in 25-, 50-, 100-, 200-, 300-, and 400-mg tablets. When treating schizophrenia or bipolar mania in adolescents, quetiapine dosing should begin at 25 mg twice daily, with doses then raised by 25 to 50 mg per dose every 2 to 3 days up to the target dosage. In adults, the target dosage is 150 to 750 mg a day. In adolescents, the target dosage is 400 to 800 mg. When treating mania associated with bipolar I disorder either as monotherapy or adjunctive therapy in adults, the initial dosage should be 50 mg twice a day before titrating 25 to 50 mg per dose every 2 to 3 days until an effective and well tolerated dosage within the target range (400 to 800 mg/day) is reached. When used as monotherapy for the treatment of bipolar I disorder in adolescents, the initial dosage should be 25 mg twice daily and the target range is 400 to 600 mg/day.

When used as monotherapy for the acute treatment of depressive episodes associated with bipolar disorder in adults, the initial dosage should be 50 mg once daily at bedtime. In subsequent and consecutive days, the daily dosage may be titrated to 100 mg once at bedtime, 200 mg once at bedtime, and 300 mg once at bedtime on day 4. The target dose for this indication is 300 mg once at bedtime each night.

As a maintenance treatment of bipolar I disorder as an adjunct to lithium or divalproex, the dosage should be administered twice daily and total 400 to 800 mg/day.

Patients 65 years of age and older may benefit from a slower rate of dose titration in intervals of 50 mg/day and may respond better to an initial dosage of 50 mg/day.

Studies have shown efficacy in the range of 300 to 800 mg a day. In reality, more aggressive dosing is both tolerated and more effective. It has become evident that the target dose can be achieved more rapidly and that some patients benefit from dosages of as much as 1,200 to 1,600 mg a day. When used at higher doses, serial electrocardiograms (EKGs) should be performed. Despite its short elimination half-life, quetiapine can be given to many patients once a day. This is consistent with the observation that quetiapine receptor occupancy remains even when concentrations in the blood have markedly declined. Quetiapine in doses of 25 to 300 mg at night has been used for insomnia but may cause adverse effects in some patients.

The extended-release formulation of quetiapine, Seroquel XR, is available in 50-, 150-, 200-, 300-, and 400-mg tablets meant to be taken once daily. It has a comparable bioavailability to an equivalent dose of quetiapine administered 2 to 3 times daily. Seroquel XR is given once daily preferably in the evening 3 to 4 hours before bedtime without food or with a light meal to prevent an increase in C_{max}. When treating schizophrenia or manic episodes associated with bipolar I disorder in adults, the usual starting dose is 300 mg, and it may be increased to the target range of 400 to 800 mg the following day. When treating depressive episodes in bipolar I disorder, the initial dosage should be 50 mg, followed by dosages of 100, 200, and 300 mg in consecutive and subsequent days. When used as adjunctive treatment for adults with major depressive disorder, the dosage schedule should be 50 mg on the first day, 50 mg on the second day, and 150 mg on subsequent days.

When treating adolescents, the starting dosage should be 50 mg. Following the first day, the dosage may be titrated to 100, 200, 300, and 400 mg on subsequent and consecutive days.

RISPERIDONE

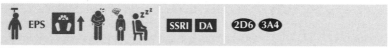

Pharmacokinetics

Risperidone has a bioavailability of 70% and undergoes extensive first-pass hepatic metabolism after oral administration primarily via the cytochrome P450 isoenzyme CYP2D6 to 9-hydroxyrisperidone, a metabolite with equivalent antipsychotic activity. Peak plasma levels of the parent compound occur within 1 and 3 hours for the metabolite. The combined half-life of risperidone and 9-hydroxyrisperidone averages 20 hours, so it is effective in once-daily dosing.

Pharmacodynamics

Risperidone is an antagonist of the serotonin 5-HT$_{2A}$, dopamine D$_2$, α_1- and α_2-adrenergic, and histamine H$_1$ receptors. It has a low affinity for α-adrenergic and muscarinic cholinergic receptors. Although it is as potent an antagonist of D$_2$ receptors, as is haloperidol (Haldol), risperidone is much less likely than haloperidol to cause EPS in humans when the dose of risperidone is below 6 mg per day.

Therapeutic Indications

Risperidone is indicated for the acute and maintenance treatment of schizophrenia in adults and for the treatment of schizophrenia in adolescents aged 13 to 17 years. Risperidone is also indicated for the short-term treatment of acute manic or mixed episodes associated with bipolar I disorder in adults and in children and adolescents aged 10 to 17 years either as monotherapy or with lithium or valproate. In addition, it is also indicated for the treatment of irritability associated with autistic spectrum disorder in children and adolescents aged 5 to 16 years, including symptoms of aggression toward others, deliberate self-injuriousness, temper tantrums, and quickly changing moods.

Off-Label Uses

Risperidone has frequently been used to treat psychotic symptoms, when present, in bipolar disorder, borderline personality disorder, conduct disorder, delusional disorder, delirium, depression, and PTSD. It has also been used to treat brain injury, developmental disorders, Lesch–Nyhan syndrome, movement disorders, pedophilia, Tourette syndrome, stuttering, and trichotillomania. It may also help treat aggression and agitation in some neurodegenerative diseases, as well as an add-on treatment in unipolar depression.

Adverse Events

The EPS of risperidone are largely dosage dependent, and there has been a trend of using lower doses than initially recommended. Weight gain, anxiety, nausea and vomiting, rhinitis, erectile dysfunction, priapism, orgasmic dysfunction, and increased pigmentation are associated with risperidone use. The most common drug-related reasons for discontinuation of risperidone use are EPS, dizziness, hyperkinesia, somnolence, and nausea. Marked elevation of prolactin may occur. Weight gain occurs more commonly with risperidone use in children than in adults.

Drug Interactions

Inhibition of CYP2D6 by drugs such as paroxetine and fluoxetine can block the formation of risperidone's active metabolite. Risperidone is a weak inhibitor of CYP2D6 and has little effect on other drugs. Combined use of risperidone and SSRIs may result in significant elevation of prolactin, with associated galactorrhea and breast enlargement.

Caution should be taken when risperidone is taken with alcohol or other centrally acting drugs. Coadministration of risperidone and drugs with hypotensive effects may enhance hypotensive effects, while coadministration with levodopa or dopamine agonists is not recommended, as risperidone may antagonize the effects of these medications.

Dosage and Clinical Guidelines

The recommended dose range and frequency of risperidone dosing have changed since the drug first came into clinical use. Risperidone is available in 0.25-, 0.5-, 1-, 2-, 3-, and 4-mg tablets and a 1-mg/mL oral solution.

For adults, the initial dosage is usually 1 to 3 mg at night, which can then be increased to 4 mg per day or more in increments of 1 mg at intervals of no less than 24 hours. The target dose for treating schizophrenia in adults is 4 to 8 mg per day (though in clinical practice 3 to 6 mg is the usual dose), but 1 to 6 mg per day when treating manic episodes associated with bipolar I disorder. In adolescents, the initial dose is 0.5 mg/day, titration should occur at 0.5 to 1 mg/day, and the target dosage is 3 mg per day for schizophrenia and 2.5 mg per day for mania associated with bipolar I disorder. When treating irritability associated with autism spectrum disorder, the initial dosage should be 0.25 mg per day for patients under 20 kg and 0.5 mg per day for patients who weigh 20 kg or more. After at least 4 days, the dose may be increased to the recommended dose of 0.5 mg per day for patients under 20 kg and 1 mg per day for patients who weigh 20 kg or more, and then maintained for at least 2 weeks. At this time, dose increases may be considered for patients who have not demonstrated sufficient clinical response in increments of 0.25 mg per day for patients under 20 kg and 0.5 mg per day for patients who weigh 20 kg or more.

Positron emission tomography (PET) studies have shown that dosages of 1 to 4 mg per day provide the required D_2 blockade needed for a therapeutic effect. At first it was believed that because of its short elimination half-life, risperidone should be given twice a day, but studies have shown equal efficacy with once-a-day dosing. Dosages above 6 mg a day are associated with a higher incidence of adverse events, particularly EPS. There is no correlation between plasma concentrations and therapeutic effect.

Risperidone is also available as an orally disintegrating tablet, though the brand name Risperdal M-Tab has been discontinued. These tablets are available in 0.5-, 1-, and 2-mg strengths, and have been indicated for the same uses detailed above.

Risperidone is also available in a depot formulation (Risperdal Consta), which is given as an IM injection formulation. The dose may be given as 25, 50, or 75 mg every 2 weeks. Oral risperidone should be coadministered with Risperdal Consta for the first 3 weeks before being discontinued. This formulation is currently only available for adults and for the treatment of schizophrenia or maintenance treatment in bipolar I disorder either as monotherapy or in conjunction with valproate or lithium.

ZIPRASIDONE

 antiarrhythmics

Pharmacokinetics

Following oral administration, peak plasma concentrations of ziprasidone are reached in 1 to 6 hours. Steady-state levels ranging from 5 to 10 hours are reached between the first and the third day of treatment. The mean terminal half-life at steady state ranges from 5 to 10 hours, which accounts for the recommendation that twice-daily dosing is necessary. Bioavailability doubles when ziprasidone is taken with food, and therefore should be taken with food.

Peak serum concentrations of IM ziprasidone occur after approximately 1 hour, with a half-life of 2 to 5 hours.

Ziprasidone is primarily metabolized by cytochrome P450 isoenzyme CYP3A4 and, to a lesser extent, CYP1A2.

Pharmacodynamics

Similar to other SGAs, ziprasidone blocks 5-HT_{2A} and D_2 receptors. It is also an antagonist of 5-HT_{1D}, 5-HT_{2C}, D_3, D_4, α_1, and H_1 receptors. It has very low affinity for D_1, M_1, and α_2 receptors. Ziprasidone also has agonist activity at the serotonin 5-HT_{1A} receptors and is a serotonin and norepinephrine reuptake inhibitor. This is consistent with clinical reports that ziprasidone has antidepressant-like effects in nonschizophrenic patients.

Indications

Ziprasidone is indicated for the treatment of schizophrenia. It is also indicated as monotherapy for the acute treatment of manic or mixed episodes associated with bipolar I disorder and as an adjunct to lithium or valproate for the maintenance treatment of bipolar I disorder.

Adverse Events

Somnolence, headache, dizziness, nausea, and light-headedness are the most common adverse events in patients taking ziprasidone. It has almost no significant effects outside the CNS, is associated with almost no weight gain, and does not cause sustained prolactin elevation. Concerns about prolongation of the QTc complex have deterred some clinicians from using ziprasidone as a first choice, since the QTc interval has been shown to increase in patients treated with 40 and 120 mg per day, respectively.

Ziprasidone should be avoided in patients with congenital long QT syndrome and in patients with a history of cardiac arrhythmias.

Drug Interactions

Ziprasidone is contraindicated in combination with other drugs known to prolong the QTc interval. These include, but are not limited to, dofetilide, sotalol, quinidine, other Class IA and III antiarrhythmics, mesoridazine, thioridazine, chlorpromazine, droperidol, pimozide, sparfloxacin, gatifloxacin, moxifloxacin, halofantrine, mefloquine, pentamidine, arsenic trioxide, levomethadyl acetate, dolasetron mesylate, probucol, and tacrolimus.

Inducers and inhibitors of CYP3A4 may alter the effects of ziprasidone. It should not be used in combination with a strong CYP3A4 inhibitor (e.g., ketoconazole) or a strong CYP3A4 inducer (e.g., rifampin [Rifadin]).

Dosage and Guidelines

Ziprasidone is available in 20-, 40-, 60-, and 80-mg capsules. Ziprasidone for IM use comes as a single-use 20-mg/mL vial. Oral ziprasidone dosing should be initiated at 40 mg a day divided into two daily doses. Studies have shown efficacy in the range of 80 to 160 mg a day, divided twice daily. In clinical practice, doses as high as 240 mg a day are being used. The recommended IM dosage is 10 to 20 mg every

2 hours for the 10-mg dose and every 4 hours for the 40-mg dose. The maximum total daily dose of IM ziprasidone is 40 mg.

Other than interactions with drugs that prolong the QTc complex, ziprasidone appears to have low potential for clinically significant drug interactions.

CLOZAPINE

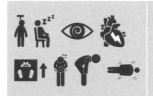

LITH antiarrhythmics, antipsychotics, carbamazepine, phenytoin, propylthiouracil, sulfonamides, captopril, clomipramine, risperidone, fluoxetine, paroxetine, fluvoxamine

1A2 3A4
2D6 2C9
2C19 2A6
2C8 1A1

Pharmacokinetics

Clozapine is rapidly absorbed and is 97% bound to serum proteins, with peak plasma levels reached in about 2 hours. Steady state is achieved in less than 1 week if twice-daily dosing is used. Clozapine is extensively metabolized in the liver by several cytochrome P450 isoenzymes, particularly CYP1A2, CYP2D6, and CYP3A4. It has two major metabolites, one of which, N-dimethyl clozapine, may have some pharmacologic activities and its elimination half-life is about 12 hours.

Pharmacodynamics

Clozapine is an antagonist of 5-HT$_{2A}$, D$_1$, D$_3$, D$_4$, and α-adrenergic (especially α$_1$) receptors. It has relatively low potency as a D$_2$ receptor antagonist. Data from PET scanning show whereas that 10 mg of haloperidol produces 80% occupancy of striatal D$_2$ receptors, clinically effective dosages of clozapine occupy only 40% to 50% of striatal D$_2$ receptors. This difference in D$_2$ receptor occupancy is probably why clozapine does not cause EPS. It has also been postulated that clozapine and other SGAs bind more loosely to the D$_2$ receptor, and as a result of this "fast dissociation," more normal dopamine neurotransmission is possible, though this may also lead to rebound psychoses much faster.

Therapeutic Indications

Clozapine is indicated for treatment-resistant schizophrenia in adults and for the reduction of suicidal behavior in adult patients with schizophrenia or schizoaffective disorder.

Off-Label Uses

In addition to being the most effective drug treatment for patients who have failed standard therapies, clozapine has been shown to benefit patients with severe tardive dyskinesia. Clozapine suppresses these dyskinesias, but the abnormal movements return when clozapine is discontinued. This is true even though clozapine, on rare occasions, may cause tardive dyskinesia.

Other clinical situations in which clozapine may be used include the treatment of psychotic patients who are intolerant of EPS caused by other agents, treatment-resistant mania, severe psychotic depression, idiopathic Parkinson disease, and Huntington disease. Other treatment-resistant disorders that have demonstrated response to clozapine include pervasive developmental disorder, autism spectrum disorder in childhood, and OCD (either as monotherapy or in combination with an SSRI).

Adverse Events

The most common drug-related adverse effects are sedation, dizziness, syncope, tachycardia, hypotension, EKG changes, nausea, and vomiting. Other common adverse effects include fatigue, weight gain, subjective muscle weakness, various GI symptoms (most commonly constipation), and anticholinergic effects. Clozapine has potent anticholinergic effects that may be particularly apparent in individuals with narrow-angle glaucoma and prostatic hypertrophy, as well as those who are taking concomitant anticholinergic medications. In some cases, the GI adverse reactions and constipation can lead to intestinal obstruction, fecal impaction, and paralytic ileus, which can prove fatal. If such side effects are reported, ensure that the patient is adequately hydrated and treat with bulk laxatives. In more serious cases, consult a gastroenterologist.

Patients exhibiting symptoms of chest pain, shortness of breath, fever, or tachypnea should be immediately evaluated for myocarditis or cardiomyopathy, an infrequent but serious adverse effect ending in death. Serial creatine phosphokinase with myocardial band fractions (CPK-MB), troponin levels, and EKG are recommended with immediate discontinuation of clozapine. Sialorrhea, or hypersalivation, is a side effect that begins early in treatment and is most evident at night. Patients report that their pillows are drenched with saliva. This side effect is most likely the result of impairment of swallowing. Although there are reports that clonidine or amitriptyline may help reduce hypersalivation, the most practical solution is to put a towel over the pillow. Other medications that are used for sialorrhea include glycopyrrolate, terazosin, diphenhydramine, chlorpheniramine, and benzamide derivatives. In addition, atropine 1% drops orally may be beneficial considering their low risk of inducing constipation.

The risk of seizures is about 4% in patients taking dosages above 600 mg a day and addition of an anticonvulsant may reduce this risk. Leukopenia, granulocytopenia, and fever occur in about 1% of patients. The new updated clozapine guidelines differentiate between the general population and those with benign ethnic neutropenia (BEN) and clinicians are advised to follow these recommendations for ANC monitoring.

During the first year of treatment, there is a 0.73% risk of clozapine-induced granulocytopenia but decreases to 0.07% during the second year. For neutropenia, the risk is 2.32% and 0.69% during the first and second years of treatment, respectively. The only contraindications to the use of clozapine are absolute neutrophile count (ANC) below 1,000 cells/µL in the general population and 500 cells/µL in patients with BEN; a history of myeloproliferative disorder or previous bone marrow disorder; a history of severe neutropenia during clozapine treatment; or the use of another drug that is known to suppress the bone marrow, such as carbamazepine. Clinicians are advised to monitor patients' absolute neutrophil count (ANC) to prevent severe neutropenia (see Risk Evaluation and Management Strategy for Clozapine and Tables 34-5 and 34-6 below).

Approximately 1% of patients taking clozapine have developed eosinophilia, which typically occurs within the first month of treatment. It may be associated with colitis, hepatitis, pancreatitis, nephritis, or myocarditis. If an eosinophil count above 700/μL is observed, evaluate promptly for systemic reactions. If clozapine-related systemic disease cannot be ruled out, discontinue clozapine immediately.

Used by itself, clozapine may very rarely induce obsessive–compulsive symptoms.

TABLE 34-5: Monitoring Absolute Neutrophil Count While Administering Clozapine in the General Population

ANC Level	Treatment Recommendation	ANC Monitoring

Normal Range ANC ≥ 1,500/μL	Initiate treatment
	If treatment is interrupted:
	  <30 days, continue monitoring as before
	  ≥30 days, monitor as if beginning anew
	  Discontinuation for reasons beside neutropenia
		Once per week for 6 months from initiation of treatment.
		Once every 2 weeks during months 6–12 of treatment
		Monthly after 12 months of treatment

Mild Neutropenia 1,000—1,499/μL[a]	Continue treatment	Three times per week until ANC ≥1,500/μL. Upon surpassing that threshold, return to patient's most recent "normal range" monitoring interval[b]
Moderate Neutropenia 500–999/μL[a]	Recommend hematology consultation Interrupt treatment for suspected clozapine-induced neutropenia Resume treatment once ANC ≥1,000/μL	Daily until ANC ≥1,000/μL, then three times per week until ANC ≥1,500/μL Upon surpassing that threshold and maintaining for 4 weeks, return to patient's most recent "normal range" monitoring interval[b]
Severe Neutropenia <500/μL[a]	Recommend hematology consultation Interrupt treatment for suspected clozapine-induced neutropenia DO NOT rechallenge unless prescriber determines that benefits outweigh risks	Daily until ANC ≥1,000/μL, then three times per week until ANC ≥1,500/μL. If patient is unchallenged, resume treatment as a new patient under "normal range" monitoring once ANC ≥1,500/μL
Discontinuation of therapy		
Moderate Neutropenia 500–999/μL[a]	Daily until ANC ≥1,000/μL, then three times per week until ANC ≥1,500/μL	
Severe Neutropenia <500/μL[a]	Daily until ANC ≥1,000/μL, then three times per week until ANC ≥1,500/μL	

[a]Confirm all initial reports of ANC less than 1,500/μL with a second ANC measurement within 24 hours.
[b]If clinically appropriate.

TABLE 34-6: Monitoring Absolute Neutrophil Count While Administering Clozapine in Patients with Benign Ethnic Neutropenia

ANC Level	Treatment Recommendation	ANC Monitoring
Normal BEN Range ANC ≥1,000/μL	Obtain at least two baseline ANC levels before initiating treatment If treatment is interrupted: <30 days, continue monitoring as before ≥30 days, monitor as if beginning anew Discontinuation for reasons beside neutropenia	Once per week for 6 months from initiation of treatment Once every 2 weeks during months 6–12 of treatment Monthly after 12 months of treatment
BEN Neutropenia 500–999/μL[a]	Recommend hematology consultation Continue treatment	Three times per week until ANC ≥1,000/μL or above patient's established baseline. Upon surpassing that threshold, check ANC weekly for 4 weeks, then return to patient's most recent "normal BEN range" monitoring interval[b]
BEN Severe Neutropenia <500/μL[a]	Recommend hematology consultation Interrupt treatment for suspected clozapine-induced neutropenia DO NOT rechallenge unless prescriber determines benefits outweigh risks	Daily until ANC ≥ 500/μL, then three times per week above patient's established baseline If patient is unchallenged, resume treatment as a new patient under "normal BEN range" monitoring once ANC ≥ 1,000/μL or at patient's established baseline
Discontinuation of therapy		
Severe Neutropenia <500/μL[a]	Daily until ANC ≥ 500/μL, then three times per week until ANC ≥ patient's established baseline	

[a]Confirm all initial reports of ANC less than 1,000/μL with a second ANC measurement within 24 hours.
[b]If clinically appropriate.

Drug Interactions

Clozapine should not be used with any other drug that is associated with the development of neutropenia or bone marrow suppression. Such drugs include carbamazepine, phenytoin, propylthiouracil, sulfonamides, and captopril (Capoten). Lithium combined with clozapine may increase the risk of seizures, confusion, and movement disorders and lithium should not be used by persons who have experienced an episode of neuroleptic malignant syndrome. However, lithium is combined with clozapine to boost neutrophil count though clinicians should be aware of the above-mentioned risks. Clomipramine (Anafranil) can increase the risk of seizure by lowering the seizure threshold and by increasing clozapine plasma concentrations. Similarly, risperidone, fluoxetine, paroxetine, and fluvoxamine may also increase serum concentrations of clozapine. Addition of paroxetine may precipitate clozapine-associated neutropenia.

The use of clozapine should be avoided in combination with other drugs that are known to prolong QTc including Class 1A antiarrhythmics (e.g., quinidine, procainamide) or Class III antiarrhythmics (e.g., amiodarone, sotalol), antipsychotic medications (e.g., ziprasidone, chlorpromazine, thioridazine), antibiotics (e.g., gatifloxacin, moxifloxacin), or any other class of medications known to prolong the QTc interval (e.g., pentamidine, levomethadyl acetate, methadone).

The dosage of clozapine should be reduced to one-third of the original dosage if coadministered with a strong CYP1A2 inhibitor, while use of weak CYP1A2 inhibitors, including oral contraceptives and caffeine, should be moderated. Use caution when coadministering clozapine with CYP3A4 and CYP2D6 inhibitors. Concomitant usage of clozapine with CYP1A2 and CYP3A4 inducers may warrant dosage adjustments, particularly with stronger inducers like phenytoin, rifampin, and St. John's wort.

Dosage and Guidelines

Clozapine is available in 25-, 50-, 100-, and 200-mg tablets; as orally disintegrating tablets marketed under the trade name FazaClo that are available in strengths of 12.5, 25, 100, 150, and 200 mg; as well as a 50-mg/mL oral suspension marketed under the trade name Versacloz. The initial dosage is usually 25 mg one or two times daily, although a conservative initial dosage is 12.5 mg twice daily. The dosage can then be raised gradually (25 mg a day every 1 to 3 days) to 300 mg a day in divided doses, usually two or three times daily though it is not unusual to dose all the medicine at bedtime. In such circumstances, patients should be advised and educated on risk of falls secondary to dizziness and postural hypotension when suddenly getting up from the bed. Dosages up to 900 mg a day can be used though risk of seizure increases beyond 600 mg and concomitant use of an anticonvulsant is warranted at times. Testing for blood concentrations of clozapine may be helpful in patients who fail to respond secondary to being a fast metabolizer or suspicion of cheeking. Studies have found that plasma concentrations greater than 350 mg/mL are associated with a better likelihood of response.

It may be necessary to reduce the dosage of clozapine in patients with moderate to severe hepatic or renal impairment.

Risk Evaluation and Management Strategy for Clozapine

- As of 2021, clozapine REMS was updated. To provide clozapine for outpatient use or to initiate treatment for inpatients, prescribers must:
- Certify in the clozapine REMS
- Enroll patients in clozapine REMS
- Provide baseline ANC when enrolling a new patient
- Comply with the clozapine prescribing information when ordering ANC testing for patients
- Verify and document each patient's ANC to the clozapine REMS each month and submit the patient status form

Outpatient pharmacies must:

- Certify in the clozapine REMS
- Obtain a REMS dispense authorization

Inpatient pharmacies must:

- Certify in the clozapine REMS
- Obtain a REMS dispense authorization

To obtain clozapine, patients must be enrolled in the clozapine REMS by a certified prescriber and comply with ANC testing requirements outlined below and in Tables 34-5 and 34-6.

During the first 6 months of treatment, weekly WBC counts are indicated to monitor the patient for the development of neutropenia. If the ANC remains normal, the frequency of testing can be decreased to every 2 weeks after 6 months and weekly after 12 months. Although monitoring is expensive, early indication of neutropenia can prevent a fatal outcome. As mentioned above, clozapine should be discontinued if ANC is below 1,000 cells/μL in the general population or 500 cells/μL in patients with BEN In addition, a hematologic consultation should be obtained, and obtaining bone marrow sample should be considered. Persons with severe neutropenia should not be reexposed to the drug. To avoid situations in which a physician or a patient fails to comply with the required blood tests, clozapine cannot be dispensed without proof of monitoring.

Second-Generation or Atypical Antipsychotics

35 Sympathomimetic Drugs and Atomoxetine

Generic Name	Trade Name	Adverse Effects	Drug Interactions	CYP Interactions
Amphetamine–dextroamphetamine	Adderall	Cardiac arrhythmia, GI symptoms, agitation, insomnia, dyskinesia	MAOI, TRI/TETR, warfarin, primidone, phenobarbital, phenytoin, phenylbutazone	2D6, 2A6
Atomoxetine	Strattera	Cardiac arrhythmia, GI symptoms, insomnia, skin rash	MAOI	2D6, 2C19
Dexmethylphenidate	Focalin, Focalin XR	Cardiac arrhythmia, GI symptoms, agitation, insomnia, dyskinesia	MAOI, TRI/TETR, warfarin, primidone, phenobarbital, phenytoin, phenylbutazone	N/A
Dextroamphetamine	Dexedrine, Dextrostat	Cardiac arrhythmia, GI symptoms, agitation, insomnia, dyskinesia	MAOI, TRI/TETR, warfarin, primidone, phenobarbital, phenytoin, phenylbutazone	2D6
Lisdexamfetamine	Vyvanse	Cardiac arrhythmia, GI symptoms, agitation, insomnia, dyskinesia	MAOI, TRI/TETR, warfarin, primidone, phenobarbital, phenytoin, phenylbutazone	N/A
Methamphetamine	Desoxyn	Cardiac arrhythmia, GI symptoms, agitation, insomnia, dyskinesia	MAOI, TRI/TETR, warfarin, primidone, phenobarbital, phenytoin, phenylbutazone	2D6
Methylphenidate	Ritalin, Methidate, Methylin, Attenade	Cardiac arrhythmia, GI symptoms, agitation, insomnia, dyskinesia	MAOI, TRI/TETR, warfarin, primidone, phenobarbital, phenytoin, phenylbutazone	N/A

Introduction

Sympathomimetic drugs, also known as stimulant drugs, are among the most widely used and abused drugs in the United States. Approximately 1.9% (over 5 million people) used cocaine and 6.4% (over 17 million people) were prescribed stimulants within the past year, while the prevalence rate of ADHD in the United States as of 2022 is 4.5%. Stimulants enhance motivation, attention, concentration, wakefulness, and stimulate the cardiovascular system. They also suppress appetite and interfere with sleep. These drugs achieve these effects by activating the sympathetic central nervous system (CNS) through effects on endogenous catecholamines. Several chemical classes are included in this group.

The first class of these drugs to be discovered were amphetamines, which were created in the late 19th century and were used by Bavarian soldiers in the mid-1880s to maintain wakefulness, alertness, energy, and confidence in combat.

They have been used in a similar fashion in most wars since then. They were not widely used clinically until the 1930s when they were marketed as Benzedrine inhalers for relief of nasal congestion. The inhalers were popular drugs of abuse until Benzedrine was made a prescription drug in 1959 that was used to treat sleepiness associated with narcolepsy.

Since the Controlled Substances Act of 1970, sympathomimetics have been classified as controlled drugs because of their rapid onset, immediate behavioral effects, and propensity to develop tolerance, which leads to the risk of abuse and dependence in vulnerable individuals. Their manufacture, distribution, and use are regulated by state and federal agencies.

Despite a relatively high potential for abuse, sympathomimetics have been found to be effective in treating certain cognitive disorders that result in secondary depression or profound apathy (e.g., acquired immunodeficiency syndrome [AIDS], multiple sclerosis, poststroke depression and dementia, closed head injury) as well as in the augmentation of antidepressant medications in specific treatment-resistant depressions. These drugs are most commonly used to treat symptoms of poor concentration and hyperactivity in children and adults with attention deficit hyperactivity disorder (ADHD). Paradoxically, many patients with ADHD find that these drugs can have a calming effect.

Even though it is not a psychostimulant, atomoxetine (Strattera) is included in this chapter because it is approved to treat ADHD. Modafinil (Provigil) and armodafinil (Nuvigil), which may be used off-label to treat ADHD, are discussed in Chapter 23.

Of note, all amphetamines have long been used to facilitate weight loss, but only one formulation, Evekeo, has been approved by the FDA as an adjunct in a regimen of weight reduction. For information about Evekeo, see Chapter 41.

Pharmacologic Actions

All sympathomimetics are well absorbed from the gastrointestinal tract. Amphetamine (Adderall) and dextroamphetamine (Dexedrine, Dextrostat) reach peak plasma concentrations in 2 to 3 hours and have a half-life of about 6 hours, thereby necessitating once- or twice-daily dosing. Methylphenidate is available in immediate-release (Ritalin), sustained-release (Ritalin SR), and extended-release (Concerta, Quillivant XR, Jornay, Adhansia XR, Aptensio XR) formulations. Immediate-release methylphenidate reaches peak plasma concentrations in 1 to 2 hours and has a short half-life of 2 to 3 hours, thereby necessitating multiple-daily dosing. The sustained release formulation reaches peak plasma concentrations in 4 to 5 hours and doubles the effective half-life of methylphenidate. The extended-release formulation reaches peak plasma concentrations in 6 to 8 hours and is designed to be effective for 12 hours in once-daily dosing. Dexmethylphenidate (Focalin) reaches peak plasma concentration in about 3 hours and is prescribed twice daily. The extended release of dexmethylphenidate (Focalin XR) produces two distinct peak plasma concentrations, one roughly 1.5 hours after administration (range 1 to 4 hours), the second 6.5 hours after administration (range 4.5 to 7 hours).

Lisdexamfetamine dimesylate, also known as L-lysine-D-amphetamine (Vyvanse), is an amphetamine prodrug. In this formulation, dextroamphetamine is coupled with the amino acid L-lysine. Lisdexamfetamine becomes active upon cleavage of the lysine portion of the molecule by enzymes in the red blood cells. This results in the gradual release of dextroamphetamine into the bloodstream. Apart from having an extended duration of action, this type of formulation reduces its abuse potential. It is the only prodrug of its kind. Lisdexamfetamine is indicated for the treatment of ADHD in children 6 to 12 years and in adults as an integral part of a total treatment program that may include other measures (i.e., psychological, educational, social). The safety and efficacy of lisdexamfetamine dimesylate in patients 3 to 5 years old has not been established. In contrast to Adderall, which contains approximately 75% dextroamphetamine and 25% levoamphetamine, lisdexamfetamine is a single, dextro-enantiomer amphetamine molecule. In most cases this makes the drug better tolerated, but there are some patients who experience greater benefit from the mixed isomer preparation.

Another amphetamine formulation is for all-day symptom control in Mydayis. It is indicated for patients 13 years of age or older. Mydayis consists of long-acting, triple-bead, mixed amphetamine salts—equal amounts (by weight) of four salts: dextroamphetamine sulfate and amphetamine sulfate, dextroamphetamine saccharate and amphetamine aspartate monohydrate. This results in a 3:1 mixture of dextro- to levoamphetamine base equivalent. In clinical studies, Mydayis was found to significantly improve ADHD symptoms in subjects when compared to a placebo, starting at 2 to 4 hours post dose and lasting up to 16 hours.

Methylphenidate, dextroamphetamine, and amphetamine are indirectly acting sympathomimetics, with the primary effect causing the release of catecholamines from presynaptic neurons. Their clinical effectiveness is associated with increased release of both dopamine and norepinephrine. Dextroamphetamine and methylphenidate are also weak inhibitors of catecholamine reuptake and inhibitors of monoamine oxidase.

Therapeutic Indications

Attention Deficit Hyperactivity Disorder

Sympathomimetics are the first-line drugs for treatment of ADHD in children and are effective about 75% of the time. Methylphenidate and dextroamphetamine are equally effective and work within 15 to 30 minutes. Sympathomimetic drugs decrease hyperactivity, increase attentiveness, and reduce impulsivity. They may also reduce comorbid oppositional behaviors associated with ADHD. Many persons take these drugs throughout their schooling and beyond. In responsive persons, use of a sympathomimetic may be a critical determinant of scholastic success.

Sympathomimetics improve the core ADHD symptoms of hyperactivity, impulsivity, and inattentiveness and permit improved social interactions with teachers, family, other adults, and peers. The success of long-term treatment of ADHD with sympathomimetics, which are efficacious for most of the various constellations of ADHD symptoms present from childhood to adulthood, supports a model in which ADHD results from a genetically determined neurochemical imbalance that requires lifelong pharmacologic management.

Methylphenidate is the most commonly used initial agent, at a dosage of 5 to 10 mg every 3 to 4 hours. Dosages may be increased to a maximum of 20 mg four times daily or 1 mg/kg a day. Use of the 20-mg sustained-release formulation to achieve 6 hours of benefit and eliminate the need for dosing at school is supported by many experts, although other authorities believe it is less effective than the immediate-release formulation. Dextroamphetamine is about twice as potent as methylphenidate on a per milligram basis and provides 6 to 8 hours of benefit.

Some 70% of nonresponders to one sympathomimetic may benefit from another. All the sympathomimetic drugs should be tried before switching to drugs of a different class. The previous dictum that sympathomimetics worsen tics and therefore should be avoided by persons with comorbid ADHD and tic disorders has been questioned. Small dosages of sympathomimetics do not appear to cause an increase in the frequency and severity of tics. Alternatives to sympathomimetics for ADHD include bupropion (Wellbutrin), venlafaxine (Effexor), guanfacine (Tenex), clonidine (Catapres), and tricyclic drugs.

Short-term use of the sympathomimetics induces a euphoric feeling. However, tolerance develops for both the euphoric feeling and the sympathomimetic activity.

Narcolepsy and Hypersomnolence

Narcolepsy consists of sudden sleep attacks (*narcolepsy*), sudden loss of postural tone (*cataplexy*), loss of voluntary motor control going into (hypnagogic) or coming out of (hypnopompic) sleep (*sleep paralysis*), and hypnagogic or hypnopompic *hallucinations*. Sympathomimetics reduce narcoleptic sleep attacks and improve wakefulness in other types of hypersomnolent states.

While several drugs have been developed to counteract narcolepsy and excessive daytime sleepiness, as covered in Chapter 23, sympathomimetics can also be used to maintain wakefulness and accuracy of motor performance, though only amphetamine–dextroamphetamine is specifically indicated for this purpose. Persons with narcolepsy, unlike persons with ADHD, may develop tolerance for the therapeutic effects of the sympathomimetics. In addition, they may also be prescribed to persons impacted by short-term sleep deprivation, such as those who have recently switched to new work schedules and are having a difficult time adjusting to the new work hours (shift work sleep disorder).

Binge Eating Disorder

Lisdexamfetamine is indicated for the treatment of moderate to severe binge eating disorder (BED). The underlying theory is that lisdexamfetamine increases dopamine and disrupts the dopaminergic pathways that reward binging behavior. Patients with BED who were given 30-, 50-, and 70-mg daily doses of lisdexamfetamine showed superior results compared to placebo.

Off-Label Uses

Depressive Disorders

Sympathomimetics may be used for treatment-resistant depressive disorders, usually as augmentation of standard antidepressant drug therapy. Possible indications for use of sympathomimetics as monotherapy include depression in elderly persons, who are at increased risk for adverse effects from standard antidepressant drugs; depression in medically ill persons, especially persons with

AIDS; obtundation caused by chronic use of opioids; and clinical situations in which a rapid response is important but for which electroconvulsive therapy is contraindicated. Depressed patients with abulia and anergia may also benefit.

Dextroamphetamine may be useful in differentiating pseudodementia of depression from dementia. A depressed person generally responds to a 5-mg dose with increased alertness and improved cognition. Sympathomimetics are thought to provide only short-term benefit (2 to 4 weeks) for depression because most persons rapidly develop tolerance for the antidepressant effects of the drugs. However, some clinicians report that long-term treatment with sympathomimetics can benefit some persons.

Encephalopathy Caused by Brain Injury

Sympathomimetics increase alertness, cognition, motivation, and motor performance in persons with neurologic deficits caused by strokes, trauma, tumors, or chronic infections. Treatment with sympathomimetics may permit earlier and more robust participation in rehabilitative programs. Poststroke lethargy and apathy may respond to long-term use of sympathomimetics.

Obesity

Sympathomimetics are used in the treatment of obesity because of their anorexia-inducing effects. Because tolerance develops for the anorectic effects and because of the drugs' high abuse potential, their use for this indication is limited. Of the sympathomimetic drugs, phentermine (Adipex-P, Fastin) is the most widely used for appetite suppression and is described in greater detail in Chapter 41. Additionally, phentermine was the other constituent of "fen-phen," an off-label combination of fenfluramine and phentermine, widely used to promote weight loss until fenfluramine and dexfenfluramine were withdrawn from commercial availability because of an association with cardiac valvular insufficiency, primary pulmonary hypertension, and irreversible loss of cerebral serotoninergic nerve fibers. The toxicity of fenfluramine is attributed to the fact that it stimulates release of massive amounts of serotonin from nerve endings, a mechanism of action not shared by phentermine. Use of phentermine alone has not been reported to cause the same adverse effects as those caused by fenfluramine or dexfenfluramine and is still indicated for use as a short-term adjunctive in a wider treatment regimen designed to promote weight reduction.

Careful limitation of caloric intake and judicious exercise are at the core of any successful weight loss program. Sympathomimetic drugs facilitate loss of, at most, an additional fraction of a pound per week. Sympathomimetic drugs are effective appetite suppressants only for the first few weeks of use; then the anorexigenic effects tend to decrease.

Fatigue

Between 70% and 90% of individuals with multiple sclerosis experience fatigue. Amphetamines, methylphenidate, and the dopamine receptor agonist amantadine (Symmctrcl) are sometimes effective in combating this symptom. Other causes of fatigue such as chronic fatigue syndrome or even cancer may respond to stimulants in many cases.

Apathy in Alzheimer Disease

One of the primary behavioral problems with Alzheimer disease (AD) is apathy. In conjunction with loneliness, apathy can accelerate functional impairment and lead to higher caregiver burden, higher service utilization, and higher mortality rates for patients. A prospective, double-blind, randomized, placebo-controlled trial held over 12 weeks found methylphenidate improved apathy in a group of 60 male veterans with mild AD. It also improved functional status, cognition, caregiver burden, depression, and Clinical Global Impressions Scale scores.

Precautions and Adverse Reactions

The most common adverse effects associated with amphetamine-like drugs are stomach pain, anxiety, irritability, insomnia, tachycardia, cardiac arrhythmias, and dysphoria. Sympathomimetics cause a decrease in appetite, although tolerance usually develops for this effect. The treatment of common adverse effects in children with ADHD is usually straightforward (see Table 35-1). The drugs can also cause increases in heart rate and blood pressure (BP) and may cause palpitations.

TABLE 35-1: Management of Common Stimulant-Induced Adverse Effects in Attention Deficit Hyperactivity Disorder

Adverse Effect	Management
Anorexia, nausea, weight loss	• Administer stimulant with meals. • Use caloric-enhanced supplements. Discourage forcing meals.
Insomnia, nightmares	• Administer stimulants earlier in the day. • Change to short-acting preparations. • Discontinue afternoon or evening dosing. • Consider adjunctive treatment (e.g., antihistamines, clonidine, antidepressants).
Dizziness	• Monitor BP. • Encourage fluid intake. • Change to long-acting form.
Rebound phenomena	• Overlap stimulant dosing. • Change to long-acting preparation or combine long- and short-acting preparations. • Consider adjunctive or alternative treatment (e.g., clonidine, antidepressants).
Irritability	• Assess timing of phenomena (during peak or withdrawal phase). • Evaluate comorbid symptoms. • Reduce dose. • Consider adjunctive or alternative treatment (e.g., lithium, antidepressants, anticonvulsants).
Dysphoria, moodiness, agitation	• Consider comorbid diagnosis (e.g., mood disorder). • Reduce dosage or change to long-acting preparation. • Consider adjunctive or alternative treatment (e.g., lithium, anticonvulsants, antidepressants).

BP, blood pressure.
Reprinted from *Prim Care Companion CNS Disord*, Vol. 15, Wilens TE, Biederman J. The Stimulants, pp. 191–222, Copyright 1992, with permission from Elsevier.

Less common adverse effects include the possible induction of movement disorders, such as tics, Tourette disorder–like symptoms, and dyskinesias, all of which are often self-limited over 7 to 10 days. If a person taking a sympathomimetic develops one of these movement disorders, a correlation between the dose of the medication and the severity of the disorder must be firmly established before adjustments are made in the medication dosage. In severe cases, augmentation with risperidone (Risperdal), clonidine (Catapres), or guanfacine (Tenex) may be necessary. Methylphenidate may worsen tics in one-third of persons; these persons fall into two groups: Those whose methylphenidate-induced tics resolve immediately upon metabolism of the dosage and a smaller group in whom methylphenidate appears to trigger tics that persist for several months but eventually resolve spontaneously.

Longitudinal studies do not indicate that sympathomimetics cause growth suppression. Sympathomimetics may exacerbate glaucoma, hypertension, cardiovascular disorders, hyperthyroidism, anxiety disorders, psychotic disorders, and seizure disorders.

High dosages of sympathomimetics can cause dry mouth, pupillary dilation, bruxism, formication, excessive ebullience, restlessness, emotional lability, and occasionally seizures. Long-term use of high dosages can cause a delusional disorder that resembles paranoid schizophrenia. Overdosages of sympathomimetics result in hypertension, tachycardia, hyperthermia, toxic psychosis, delirium, hyperpyrexia, convulsions, coma, chest pain, arrhythmia, heart block, hyper- or hypotension, shock, and nausea. Toxic effects of amphetamines can be seen at 30 mg, but idiosyncratic toxicity can occur at doses as low as 2 mg. Conversely, survival has been reported up to 500 mg. Seizures can be treated with benzodiazepines, cardiac effects with ß-adrenergic receptor antagonists, fever with cooling blankets, and delirium with dopamine receptor antagonists (DRAs).

The most limiting adverse effect of sympathomimetics is their association with psychological and physical dependence. At the doses used for treatment of ADHD, development of psychological dependence virtually never occurs. A larger concern is the presence of adolescent or adult cohabitants who might confiscate the supply of sympathomimetics for abuse or sale.

Use in Pregnancy and Lactation

When weighing the potential risks and benefits of different treatment strategies for ADHD in young women of reproductive age and in pregnant women, it is important to consider that there might be a small increase in the risk of cardiac malformations associated with intrauterine exposure to methylphenidate. No association has been observed between amphetamines and any congenital or cardiac malformations.

Both dextroamphetamine and methylphenidate pass into the breast milk.

Drug Interactions

The coadministration of sympathomimetics and tricyclic or tetracyclic antidepressants, warfarin (Coumadin), primidone (Mysoline), phenobarbital (Luminal), phenytoin (Dilantin), or phenylbutazone (Butazolidin) decreases the metabolism of these compounds, resulting in increased plasma levels. Sympathomimetics decrease the therapeutic efficacy of many antihypertensive drugs, especially guanethidine (Esimil, Ismelin).

The sympathomimetics should be used with extreme caution with monoamine oxidase inhibitors (MAOIs).

Laboratory Interferences

Dextroamphetamine may elevate plasma corticosteroid levels and interfere with some assay methods for urinary corticosteroids.

Dosage and Administration

Sympathomimetics have been controversial for decades, despite their wide usage. Many pundits and social commentators are worried that they are being over-prescribed. Conversely, many psychiatrists believe that amphetamine use has been overly regulated by governmental authorities. Amphetamines are listed as schedule II drugs by the Drug Enforcement Agency (DEA). Some states keep a registry of patients who receive amphetamines. Such mandates worry both patients and physicians about breaches in confidentiality, and physicians are concerned that their prescribing practices may be misinterpreted by official agencies. Consequently, some physicians may withhold prescription of sympathomimetics, even from persons who may benefit from the medications.

Dextroamphetamine, methylphenidate, amphetamine, and methamphetamine are schedule II drugs, requiring strict prescribing rules governed by each individual state. Several sympathomimetic amines that are closely related to the drugs covered in this chapter but are only indicated in the management of obesity are also considered controlled substances. This includes benzphetamine (Didrex), which is a Schedule II drug; phendimetrazine (Adipost, Bontril), which is a Schedule III drug; and phentermine and diethylpropion (Tenuate), which are both Schedule IV drugs. All four will be covered in Chapter 41. Modafinil (Provigil) and armodafinil (Nuvigil) are also Schedule IV drugs that were covered in Chapter 23.

Pretreatment evaluation should include an evaluation of the person's cardiac function, with particular attention to the presence of hypertension or tachyarrhythmias. The clinician should also examine the person for the presence of movement disorders, such as tics and dyskinesia, because these conditions can be exacerbated by the administration of sympathomimetics. If tics are present, many experts will not prescribe sympathomimetics but will instead choose clonidine or antidepressants. However, recent data indicate that sympathomimetics may cause only a mild increase in motor tics and may actually suppress vocal tics. Liver function and renal function should be assessed, and dosages of sympathomimetics should be reduced for persons with impaired metabolism.

The dosage ranges and the available preparations for sympathomimetics are presented in Table 35-2. Persons with ADHD can take immediate-release methylphenidate at 8 AM, 12 noon, and 4 PM. The starting dose of methylphenidate ranges from 2.5 mg of regular to 20 mg for some sustained-release formulations (Jornay) and 25 mg for others (Adhansia XR). If this is inadequate, dosages may be increased to a maximum dose as noted in Table 35-3. For individuals 6 years of age and above, extended-release capsules of methylphenidate hydrochloride

TABLE 35-2: Sympathomimetics Commonly Used in Psychiatry

Generic Name	Trade Name	Preparations	Initial Daily Dose	Usual Daily Dose for ADHD[a]	Usual Daily Dose for Disorders Associated with Excessive Daytime Somnolence	Maximum Daily Dose
Amphetamine–dextroamphetamine	Adderall	5-, 7.5-, 10-, 12.5-, 15-, 20-, and 30-mg tablets; 5-, 10-, 12.5-, 15-, 20-, 25-, 30-, 37.5-, and 50-mg ER capsules	5–10 mg	20–30 mg	5–60 mg	Children: 40 mg; adults: 60 mg
Atomoxetine	Strattera	10-, 18-, 25-, 40-, 60-, 80-, and 100-mg tablets	20 mg	40–80 mg	Not used	Children: 80 mg; adults: 100 mg
Dexmethylphenidate	Focalin	2.5-, 5-, and 10-mg oral tablets	5 mg	5–20 mg	Not used	20 mg
Dexmethylphenidate	Focalin XR	5-, 10-, 15-, 20-, 25-, 30-, 35-, and 40-mg XR oral capsules	Children: 5 mg; adults: 10 mg	Children: 5–30 mg; adults: 10–40 mg	Not used	Children: 30 mg; adults: 40 mg
Dextroamphetamine	Dexedrine, Dextrostat	5-, 10-, and 15-mg SR capsules; 5- and 10-mg tablets	5–10 mg	20–30 mg	5–60 mg	Children: 40 mg; adults: 60 mg
Lisdexamfetamine	Vyvanse	10-, 20-, 30-, 40-, 50-, 60-, and 70-mg capsules; 10-, 20-, 30-, 40-, 50-, and 60-mg chewable tablets	20–30 mg	Children: 30–70 mg; adults: 50–70 mg	Not used	70 mg
Equal amounts (by weight) of: dextroamphetamine sulfate and amphetamine sulfate, dextroamphetamine saccharate and amphetamine aspartate monohydrate. This results in a 3:1 mixture of dextro- to levoamphetamine base equivalent.	Mydayis	Each pill contains equal portions of the following: amphetamine aspartate, amphetamine sulfate, dextroamphetamine saccharate, and dextroamphetamine capsules: 12.5 mg 25 mg 37.5 mg 50 mg	12.5 mg once daily in the morning upon awakening.	12.5–50 mg/day	Not used	Adults: 50 mg/day; pediatrics: 25 mg/day

Methamphetamine	Desoxyn	5-mg tablets; 5-, 10-, and 15-mg XR tablets	5–10 mg	20–25 mg	Not generally used	45 mg
Methylphenidate	Ritalin, Methidate, Methylin, Attenace	5-, 10-, and 20-mg tablets; 10- and 20-mg SR tablets	5–10 mg	5–60 mg	20–30 mg	Children: 80 mg; adults: 90 mg
Methylphenidate	Concerta	18- and 36-mg ER tablets	18 mg	18–54 mg	Not used	54 mg
Methylphenidate	Jornay	20-, 40-, 60-, 80-, and 100-mg XR oral capsules	20 mg	20–100 mg	Not used	100 mg
Methylphenidate	Adhansia XR	25-, 35-, 45-, 55-, 70-, and 85-mg XR oral capsules	25 mg	Children: 25–70 mg; adults: 25–85 mg	Not used	Children: 70 mg; adults: 85 mg
Methylphenidate hydrochloride	Quillivant XR	25-mg/5-mL oral solution	20 mg	20–60 mg	Not used	60 mg
Methylphenidate hydrochloride	Aptensio XR	10-, 15-, 20-, 30-, 40-, 50-, and 60-mg ER capsules	10 mg	10–60 mg	Not used	60 mg

ᵃFor children 6 years of age and older.
ER, extended release; SR, sustained release.

TABLE 35-3: Lisdexamfetamine (Vyvanse) Dosage Equivalency Conversions

Vyvanse and Adderall XR

Vyvanse (mg)	Adderall XR (mg)
20	5
30	10
40	15
50	20
60	25
70	30

Vyvanse, Adderall IR, and Dexedrine

Vyvanse (mg)	Adderall IR (mg)	Dexedrine (mg)
70	30	22.5
50	20	15
30	10	7.5

IR, immediate release; XR, extended release.

(Aptensio XR) can be initiated once daily with or without food in the morning at a dosage of 10 mg per day. Dosages may be increased weekly at intervals of 10 mg per day and should not exceed 60 mg/day.

Immediate-release Adderall and dextroamphetamine (Dexedrine) can be taken once or twice daily to start at dosages of 5 mg for children over 6 and at dosages of 2.5 mg for children aged 3 to 5 years. Dosages can then be increased in increments of 5 mg per week (2.5 mg per week for children aged 3 to 5 years) until the optimal dose is achieved. If needed, doses can be given on awakening, and then at intervals of 4 or 6 hours. Adderall extended-release capsules should be administered in the morning. For children (ages 6 to 12 years old), dosages should be initiated at 10 mg. Dosages can then be adjusted in increments of 5 mg or 10 mg at weekly intervals. The maximum recommended dosage is 30 mg. For adolescents and adults, the initial dosage should be 10 mg/day. The dose may be increased to 20 mg/day after 1 week.

Dexmethylphenidate should be administered twice daily, 4 hours apart with or without food. The dosage for patients who are new to dexmethylphenidate is 2.5 mg taken twice daily. Dosages may be titrated in weekly intervals by 2.5 to 5 mg intervals to a maximum dosage of 20 mg/day (10 mg twice daily). When administering extended-release capsules, pediatric patients should begin treatment with a dose of 5 mg/day and adults should begin treatment with a dose of 10 mg/day. Doses can be titrated by 5 mg for pediatric patients and 10 mg for adults in weekly intervals and should not exceed 30 mg for children and 40 mg for adults.

Quillivant XR (methylphenidate hydrochloride) is a once-daily, extended-release liquid formulation of methylphenidate HCL. Quillivant XR is supplied as a liquid solution designed for oral administration. Quillivant XR is taken once a day. The recommended dose for patients 6 years and above is 20 mg orally once daily in the morning with or without food. The dose may be titrated weekly in increments of 10 to 20 mg. Daily doses above 60 mg have not been studied and are not recommended. Before administering the dose, vigorously shake the bottle of Quillivant XR for at least 10 seconds, to ensure that the proper dose is administered. The clinical effects of the drug are evident from 45 minutes to 12 hours after dosing.

Lisdexamfetamine (Vyvanse) dosing requires special consideration, since many patients are switched to this formulation after being treated with other stimulants. A conversion table is shown in Table 35-3. It is available in 20-, 30-, 40-, 50-, 60-, and 70-mg capsules, as well as 10-, 20-, 30-, 40-, 50-, and 60-mg chewable tablets. Dosage should be individualized according to the therapeutic needs and response of the patient and should be administered at the lowest effective dosage. In patients who are either starting treatment for the first time or switching from another medication, 30 mg once daily in the morning is the recommended dose. Dosages may be increased or decreased in 10- or 20-mg increments in intervals of approximately 1 week. Afternoon doses should be avoided because of the potential for insomnia. The drug may be taken with or without food.

ATOMOXETINE

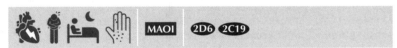

Atomoxetine is the first nonstimulant drug to be approved by the FDA as a treatment of ADHD in children, adolescents, and adults. It is included in this chapter because it shares this indication with the stimulants described above.

Pharmacologic Actions

Atomoxetine is well absorbed after oral administration and is minimally affected by food. High-fat meals may decrease the rate but not the extent of absorption. Maximum plasma concentrations are reached after approximately 1 to 2 hours. At therapeutic concentrations, 98% of atomoxetine in plasma is bound to protein, mainly albumin. Atomoxetine has a half-life of approximately 5 hours and is metabolized principally by the CYP2D6 pathway. Poor metabolizers of this compound reach a fivefold higher area under the curve and fivefold higher peak plasma concentration than normal or extensive metabolizers. This is important to consider in patients receiving medications that inhibit the CYP2D6 enzyme. For example, the antidepressant-like pharmacology of atomoxetine has led to its use as an add-on to selective serotonin reuptake inhibitors (SSRIs) or other antidepressants. Drugs such as fluoxetine (Prozac), paroxetine (Paxil), and bupropion (Wellbutrin) are CYP2D6 inhibitors and may raise atomoxetine levels.

Atomoxetine is believed to produce a therapeutic effect through selective inhibition of the presynaptic norepinephrine transporter.

Therapeutic Indications

Atomoxetine is used for the treatment of ADHD. It should be considered for use in patients who find stimulants too activating or who experience other intolerable side effects. Because atomoxetine has no abuse potential, it is a reasonable choice in the treatment of patients with both ADHD and substance abuse, patients who complain of ADHD symptoms but are suspected of seeking stimulant drugs, and patients who are in recovery.

Atomoxetine may enhance cognition when used to treat patients with schizophrenia. It may also be used as an alternative or add-on to antidepressants in patients who fail to respond to standard therapies.

Precautions and Adverse Reactions

Common side effects of atomoxetine include abdominal discomfort, decreased appetite with resulting weight loss, sexual dysfunction, dizziness, vertigo, irritability, and mood swings. Minor increases in BP and heart rate have also been observed. There have been cases of severe liver injury in a small number of patients taking atomoxetine. The drug should be discontinued in patients with jaundice (yellowing of the skin or whites of the eyes, itching) or laboratory evidence of liver injury. Atomoxetine should not be taken at the same time, or within 2 weeks of taking, as an MAOI or by patients with narrow-angle glaucoma.

The effects of overdose greater than twice the maximum recommended daily dose in humans is unknown. No specific information is available on the treatment of overdose with atomoxetine.

Dosage and Clinical Guidelines

Atomoxetine is available as 10-, 18-, 25-, 40-, and 60-mg capsules. In children and adolescents who weigh up to 70 kg in body weight, atomoxetine should be initiated at a total daily dose of approximately 0.5 mg/kg, and increased after a minimum of 3 days to a target total daily dose of approximately 1.2 mg/kg administered either as a single daily dose in the morning or as evenly divided doses in the morning and late afternoon or early evening. The total daily dose in smaller children and adolescents should not exceed 1.4 mg/kg or 100 mg, whichever is less. Dosing of children and adolescents, who weigh more than 70 kg, and adults should start at a total daily dose of 40 mg and then be increased after a minimum of 3 days to a target total daily dose of approximately 80 mg. The doses can be administered either as a single daily dose in the morning or as evenly divided doses in the morning and late afternoon or early evening. After 2 to 4 additional weeks, the dose may be increased to a maximum of 100 mg in patients who have not achieved an optimal response. The maximum recommended total daily dose in children and adolescents over 70 kg and adults is 100 mg.

Thyroid Hormones

36

Generic Name	Trade Name	Adverse Effects	Drug Interactions	CYP Interactions
Liothyronine	Cytomel	GI symptoms, tachycardia, insomnia, hypertension, headache	SSRI, TRI/TETR, LITH, anticoagulants, insulin, stimulants, ketamine, maprotiline, carbamazepine	
Levothyroxine	Synthroid, Levothroid, Levoxine	GI symptoms, tachycardia, insomnia, hypertension, headache	SSRI, TRI/TETR, LITH, anticoagulants, insulin, stimulants, ketamine, maprotiline, carbamazepine	2C8

Introduction

The thyroid plays a significant role in mental health and use of synthetic thyroid hormones that mimic triiodothyronine (T_3) or tetraiodothyronine (T_4) have been used in psychiatry either alone or as augmentation to treat persons with depression or rapid-cycling bipolar I disorder. The synthetic thyroid hormone liothyronine (Cytomel) mimics triiodothyronine, while levothyroxine (Synthroid, Levothroid, Levoxine) mimics tetraiodothyronine. Use of synthetic thyroid hormones can convert an antidepressant-nonresponsive person into an antidepressant-responsive person. They are also used as replacement therapy for persons treated with lithium (Eskalith) who have developed a hypothyroid state.

Successful use of thyroid hormone as an intervention for treatment-resistant patients was first reported in the early 1970s. Study results since then have been mixed, but most show that patients taking liothyronine are twice as likely to respond to antidepressant treatment versus placebo. These studies have also found that augmentation with liothyronine is effective with tricyclic antidepressants and selective serotonin reuptake inhibitors (SSRIs). Despite these findings, many endocrinologists object to the use of thyroid hormones as antidepressant augmentation agents, citing such risks as osteoporosis and cardiac arrhythmias.

Pharmacologic Actions

Thyroid hormones are administered orally, and their absorption from the gastrointestinal tract is variable. Absorption is increased if the drug is administered on an empty stomach. In the brain, T_4 (or the synthetic levothyroxine) crosses the blood–brain barrier and diffuses into neurons, where it is converted into T_3, which is the physiologically active form. The half-life of T_4 is 6 to 7 days, and that of T_3 is 1 to 2 days.

The mechanism of action for thyroid hormone effects on antidepressant efficacy is unknown. Thyroid hormone binds to intracellular receptors that regulate the transcription of a wide range of genes, including several receptors for neurotransmitters.

Therapeutic Indications

The major indication for thyroid hormones in psychiatry is as an adjuvant to antidepressants. There is no clear correlation between the laboratory measures of thyroid function and the response to thyroid hormone supplementation of antidepressants. If a patient has not responded to a 6-week course of antidepressants at appropriate dosages, adjuvant therapy with either lithium or a thyroid hormone is an alternative. Most clinicians use adjuvant lithium before trying a thyroid hormone. Several controlled trials have indicated that liothyronine use converts about 50% of antidepressant nonresponders to responders.

The dosage of liothyronine is 25 or 50 μg a day added to the patient's antidepressant regimen. Liothyronine has been used primarily as an adjuvant for tricyclic drugs, but evidence suggests that liothyronine augments the effects of all of the antidepressant drugs.

Thyroid hormones have not been shown to cause significant problems in pediatric or geriatric patients. Despite their relative safety, the hormones should be used with caution in elderly persons, who may have occult heart disease.

Precautions and Adverse Reactions

At the dosages usually used for augmentation—25 to 50 μg a day—adverse effects occur infrequently. The most common adverse effects associated with thyroid hormones are transient headache, weight loss, palpitations, nervousness, diarrhea, abdominal cramps, sweating, tachycardia, increased blood pressure, tremors, and insomnia. Osteoporosis may also occur with long-term treatment, but this has not been found in studies involving liothyronine augmentation. Overdoses of thyroid hormones can lead to cardiac failure and death.

Thyroid hormones should not be taken by persons with cardiac disease, angina, or hypertension. The hormones are contraindicated in thyrotoxicosis and uncorrected adrenal insufficiency and in persons with acute myocardial infarctions.

Use in Pregnancy and Lactation

Thyroid hormones can be administered safely to pregnant women, provided that laboratory thyroid indexes are monitored. Thyroid hormones are minimally excreted in breast milk and have not been shown to cause problems in nursing babies. Both liothyronine and levothyroxine are classified as pregnancy category A drugs.

Drug Interactions

Thyroid hormones can potentiate the effects of warfarin (Coumadin) and other anticoagulants by increasing the catabolism of clotting factors. They may increase the insulin requirement for diabetic persons and the digitalis requirement for persons with cardiac disease. Thyroid hormones should not be coadministered with sympathomimetics, ketamine (Ketalar, Esketamine), or maprotiline (Ludiomil) because of the risk of cardiac decompensation. Administration of SSRIs, tricyclic and tetracyclic drugs, lithium, or carbamazepine (Tegretol) can mildly lower serum T_4 and raise serum thyrotropin concentrations in euthyroid persons or persons taking thyroid replacements. This interaction warrants close serum monitoring and may require an increase in the dosage or initiation of thyroid hormone supplementation.

Laboratory Interferences

Levothyroxine has not been reported to interfere with any laboratory test other than thyroid function indexes. Liothyronine, however, suppresses the release of endogenous T_4, thereby lowering the result of any thyroid function test that depends on the measure of T_4.

Thyroid Function Tests

Several thyroid function tests are available, including tests for T_4 by competitive protein binding (T_4 [D]) and by radioimmunoassay (T_4 RIA) involving a specific antigen–antibody reaction. Over 90% of T_4 is bound to serum protein and is responsible for thyroid-stimulating hormone (TSH) secretion and cellular metabolism. Other thyroid measures include the free T_4 index (FT_4I), T_3 uptake, and total serum T_3 measured by radioimmunoassay (T_3 RIA). Those tests are used to rule out hypothyroidism, which can be associated with symptoms of depression. In some studies, up to 10% of patients complaining of depression and associated fatigue had incipient hypothyroid disease. Lithium can cause hypothyroidism and, more rarely, hyperthyroidism. Neonatal hypothyroidism results in intellectual disability and is preventable if the diagnosis is made at birth.

Thyrotropin-Releasing Hormone Stimulation Test

The thyrotropin-releasing hormone (TRH) stimulation test is indicated for patients who have marginally abnormal thyroid test results with suspected subclinical hypothyroidism, which may account for clinical depression. It is also used in patients with possible lithium-induced hypothyroidism. The procedure entails an intravenous injection of 500 mg of protirelin (TRH), which produces a sharp increase in serum TSH levels measured at 15, 30, 60, and 90 minutes. An increase in serum TSH of 5 to 25 mIU/mL above the baseline is normal. An increase of less than 7 mIU/mL is considered a blunted response, which may correlate with a diagnosis of depression. Eight percent of all patients with depression have some thyroid illness.

Dosage and Clinical Guidelines

Liothyronine is available in 5-, 25-, and 50-µg tablets. Levothyroxine is available in 12.5-, 25-, 50-, 75-, 88-, 100-, 112-, 125-, 150-, 175-, 200-, and 300-µg tablets. It is also available in a 200- and 500-µg parenteral form.

For psychiatric purposes, the dosage of liothyronine is 25 or 50 µg a day added to the person's antidepressant regimen. Liothyronine has been used as an adjuvant for all the available antidepressant drugs. An adequate trial of liothyronine supplementation should last 2 to 3 weeks. If liothyronine supplementation is successful, it should be continued for 2 months and then tapered off at the rate of 12.5 µg a day every 3 to 7 days.

37 Tricyclics and Tetracyclics

Generic Name	Trade Name	Adverse Effects	Drug Interactions	CYP Interactions
Imipramine	Tofranil	Suicidality, anticholinergic effects, cardiac arrhythmia, hypotension, sedation, tremors, sexual dysfunction	CNS, MAOI, DRA, LITH, QT, stimulants, antihypertensives, antiarrhythmic, oral contraceptives, barbiturates, ascorbic acid, ammonium chloride, carbamazepine, chloral hydrate, primidone, acetazolamide, sodium bicarbonate, acetylsalicylic acid, cimetidine, thiazide diuretics, fluoxetine, paroxetine, fluvoxamine	1A2, 3A4, 2C19, 2D6, 3A7, 2B6, 2C18, 2E1
Desipramine	Norpramin, Pertofrane	Suicidality, anticholinergic effects, cardiac arrhythmia, hypotension, sedation, tremors, sexual dysfunction	CNS, MAOI, DRA, LITH, QT, stimulants, antihypertensives, antiarrhythmic, oral contraceptives, barbiturates, ascorbic acid, ammonium chloride, carbamazepine, chloral hydrate, primidone, acetazolamide, sodium bicarbonate, acetylsalicylic acid, cimetidine, thiazide diuretics, fluoxetine, paroxetine, fluvoxamine	1A2, 3A4, 2D6, 2B6, 2E1
Trimipramine	Surmontil	Suicidality, anticholinergic effects, cardiac arrhythmia, hypotension, sedation, tremors, sexual dysfunction	CNS, MAOI, DRA, LITH, QT, stimulants, antihypertensives, antiarrhythmic, oral contraceptives, barbiturates, ascorbic acid, ammonium chloride, carbamazepine, chloral hydrate, primidone, acetazolamide, sodium bicarbonate, acetylsalicylic acid, cimetidine, thiazide diuretics, fluoxetine, paroxetine, fluvoxamine	2D6, 2C9, 2C19
Amitriptyline	Elavil, Endep	Suicidality, anticholinergic effects, cardiac arrhythmia, hypotension, sedation, tremors, sexual dysfunction	CNS, MAOI, DRA, LITH, QT, stimulants, antihypertensives, antiarrhythmic, oral contraceptives, barbiturates, ascorbic acid, ammonium chloride, carbamazepine, chloral hydrate, primidone, acetazolamide, sodium bicarbonate, acetylsalicylic acid, cimetidine, thiazide diuretics, fluoxetine, paroxetine, fluvoxamine	2D6, 3A4, 3A5, 2B6, 2C8, 1A2, 2C9, 2C19

Generic Name	Trade Name	Adverse Effects	Drug Interactions	CYP Interactions
Nortriptyline	Pamelor, Aventyl	Suicidality, anticholinergic effects, cardiac arrhythmia, hypotension, sedation, tremors, sexual dysfunction	CNS, MAOI, DRA, LITH, QT, stimulants, antihypertensives, antiarrhythmic, oral contraceptives, barbiturates, ascorbic acid, ammonium chloride, carbamazepine, chloral hydrate, primidone, acetazolamide, sodium bicarbonate, acetylsalicylic acid, cimetidine, thiazide diuretics, fluoxetine, paroxetine, fluvoxamine	2D6, 3A4, 3A5, 2E1, 1A2, 2C19
Protriptyline	Vivactil	Suicidality, anticholinergic effects, cardiac arrhythmia, hypotension, sedation, tremors, sexual dysfunction	CNS, MAOI, DRA, LITH, QT, stimulants, antihypertensives, antiarrhythmic, oral contraceptives, barbiturates, ascorbic acid, ammonium chloride, carbamazepine, chloral hydrate, primidone, acetazolamide, sodium bicarbonate, acetylsalicylic acid, cimetidine, thiazide diuretics, fluoxetine, paroxetine, fluvoxamine	N/A
Amoxapine	Asendin	Suicidality, anticholinergic effects, cardiac arrhythmia, hypotension, sedation, tremors, sexual dysfunction	CNS, MAOI, DRA, LITH, QT, stimulants, antihypertensives, antiarrhythmic, oral contraceptives, barbiturates, ascorbic acid, ammonium chloride, carbamazepine, chloral hydrate, primidone, acetazolamide, sodium bicarbonate, acetylsalicylic acid, cimetidine, thiazide diuretics, fluoxetine, paroxetine, fluvoxamine	2D6
Doxepin	Adapin, Sinequan	Suicidality, anticholinergic effects, cardiac arrhythmia, hypotension, sedation, tremors, sexual dysfunction	CNS, MAOI, DRA, LITH, QT, stimulants, antihypertensives, antiarrhythmic, oral contraceptives, barbiturates, ascorbic acid, ammonium chloride, carbamazepine, chloral hydrate, primidone, acetazolamide, sodium bicarbonate, acetylsalicylic acid, cimetidine, thiazide diuretics, fluoxetine, paroxetine, fluvoxamine	3A4, 2D6, 2C19, 2C9, 1A2
Maprotiline	Ludiomil	Suicidality, anticholinergic effects, cardiac arrhythmia, hypotension, sedation, tremors, sexual dysfunction	CNS, MAOI, DRA, LITH, QT, stimulants, antihypertensives, antiarrhythmic, oral contraceptives, barbiturates, ascorbic acid, ammonium chloride, carbamazepine, chloral hydrate, primidone, acetazolamide, sodium bicarbonate, acetylsalicylic acid, cimetidine, thiazide diuretics, fluoxetine, paroxetine, fluvoxamine	2D6, 1A2

Generic Name	Trade Name	Adverse Effects	Drug Interactions	CYP Interactions
Clomipramine	Anafranil	Suicidality, anticholinergic effects, cardiac arrhythmia, hypotension, sedation, tremors, sexual dysfunction	CNS, MAOI, DRA, LITH, QT, stimulants, antihypertensives, antiarrhythmic, oral contraceptives, barbiturates, ascorbic acid, ammonium chloride, carbamazepine, chloral hydrate, primidone, acetazolamide, sodium bicarbonate, acetylsalicylic acid, cimetidine, thiazide diuretics, fluoxetine, paroxetine, fluvoxamine	2D6, 2C19, 1A2, 3A4

Introduction

Imipramine was first synthesized in the early 1950s. In 1955, the Swiss psychiatrist Roland Kuhn examined the effects of imipramine (Tofranil) on a small group of schizophrenic patients in a remote Swiss village of Münsterlingen. Kuhn initially hoped the drug would possess antipsychotic effects similar to the recently discovered chlorpromazine. While imipramine did not affect the psychotic symptoms of his patients, many with comorbid depression reported some relief from their depressive symptoms. This discovery led to the development of a new class of antidepressant compounds, the tricyclics (TRIs) and an increased understanding in the role that norepinephrine and other catecholamines play in depression.

After the introduction of imipramine, several other antidepressant compounds were developed that shared a basic tricyclic structure and had relatively similar effects. Later, other heterocyclic compounds were also marketed that were somewhat similar in structure and that had relatively comparable secondary properties. At one time, amitriptyline (Elavil, Endep) and imipramine were the two most commonly prescribed antidepressants in the United States, but because of their anticholinergic and antihistaminic side effects, their use declined, and nortriptyline (Pamelor) and desipramine (Norpramin, Pertofrane) became more popular. Nortriptyline has the least effect on orthostatic hypotension, and desipramine is the least anticholinergic.

Although introduced as antidepressants, the therapeutic indications for these agents have grown to include panic disorder, generalized anxiety disorder, posttraumatic stress disorder (PTSD), obsessive-compulsive disorder (OCD), and pain syndromes. The introduction of newer antidepressant agents with more selective actions on neurotransmitters or with unique mechanisms of action has sharply reduced the prescribing of TRIs and tetracyclics (TETs). The improved safety profiles of the newer drugs, especially when taken in overdose, also contributed to the decline in use of the older drugs. Nevertheless, the TCAs and TETs (TCAs to denote both) remain unsurpassed in terms of their antidepressant efficacy. Table 37-1 lists the TCAs and their available preparations.

Pharmacologic Actions

The absorption of most TCAs is complete after oral administration, and there is significant metabolism from the first-pass effect. Peak plasma concentrations

TABLE 37-1: Tricyclic and Tetracyclic Drug Preparations

Drug	Tablets (mg)	Capsules (mg)	Parenteral (mg/mL)	Solution
Imipramine (Tofranil)	10, 25, and 50	75, 100, 125, and 150	12.5	—
Desipramine (Norpramin, Pertofrane)	10, 25, 50, 75, 100, and 150	—	—	—
Trimipramine (Surmontil)	—	25, 50, and 100	—	—
Amitriptyline (Elavil)	10, 25, 50, 75, 100, and 150	—	10	—
Nortriptyline (Aventyl, Pamelor)	—	10, 25, 50, and 75	—	10 mg/5 mL
Protriptyline (Vivactil)	5 and 10	—	—	—
Amoxapine (Asendin)	25, 50, 100, and 150	—	—	—
Doxepin (Sinequan)	—	10, 25, 50, 75, 100, and 150	—	10 mg/mL
Maprotiline (Ludiomil)	25, 50, and 75	—	—	—
Clomipramine (Anafranil)	—	25, 50, and 75	—	—

occur within 2 to 8 hours, and the half-lives of the TCAs vary from 10 to 70 hours; nortriptyline, maprotiline (Ludiomil), and particularly protriptyline (Vivactil) have longer half-lives. The long half-lives allow all the compounds to be given once daily. Steady-state plasma concentrations are typically reached in 5 to 7 days. Imipramine pamoate (Tofranil) is a depot form of the drug for intramuscular (IM) administration; indications for the use of this preparation are limited. The oral formulation should supplant the IM formulation as soon as possible.

The TCAs undergo hepatic metabolism by the CYP450 enzyme system (see Drug Interactions below).

The TCAs block the transporter site for norepinephrine and serotonin, thus increasing synaptic concentrations of these neurotransmitters. Each drug differs in its affinity for each of these transporters, with clomipramine (Anafranil) being the most serotonin selective and desipramine the most norepinephrine selective of the TCAs. Secondary effects of the TCAs include antagonism at the muscarinic acetylcholine, histamine H_1, and a_1- and a_2-adrenergic receptors. The potency of these effects on other receptors largely determines the side-effect profile of each drug. Amoxapine, nortriptyline, desipramine, and maprotiline have the least anticholinergic activity; doxepin has the most antihistaminergic activity. Although they are more likely to cause constipation, sedation, dry mouth, or light-headedness than the selective serotonin reuptake inhibitors (SSRIs), the TCAs are less prone to cause sexual dysfunction, significant long-term weight gain, and sleep disturbances than the SSRIs. The half-life and plasma clearance for most TCAs are very similar.

Therapeutic Indications

Each of the following indications is also an indication for the SSRIs, which have widely replaced the TCAs in clinical practice. However, the TCAs represent a reasonable alternative for persons who cannot tolerate the adverse effects of the SSRIs.

Major Depressive Disorder

The treatment of a major depressive episode and the prophylactic treatment of major depressive disorder are the principal indications for using TCAs. Although the TCAs are effective in the treatment of depression in persons with bipolar I disorder, they are more likely to induce mania, hypomania, or cycling than the newer antidepressants, most notably the SSRIs and bupropion. It is thus not advised that TCAs be routinely used to treat depression associated with bipolar I or bipolar II disorder.

Melancholic features, prior major depressive episodes, and a family history of depressive disorders increase the likelihood of a therapeutic response. All of the available TCAs are equally effective in the treatment of depressive disorders. In the case of an individual person, however, one TCA may be effective, and another one may be ineffective. The treatment of a major depressive episode with psychotic features almost always requires the coadministration of an antipsychotic drug and an antidepressant.

Generalized Anxiety Disorder

The use of doxepin for the treatment of anxiety disorders is approved by the Food and Drug Administration (FDA). Some research data show that imipramine may also be useful. Although rarely used anymore, a chlordiazepoxide–amitriptyline combination (Limbitrol) is available for mixed anxiety and depressive disorders.

Obsessive-Compulsive Disorder

Although it is used worldwide as an antidepressant, clomipramine is only approved in the United States for the treatment of OCD. OCD appears to respond specifically to clomipramine, as well as the SSRIs. Some improvement is usually seen in 2 to 4 weeks, but a further reduction in symptoms may continue for the first 4 to 5 months of treatment. None of the other TCAs appear to be nearly as effective as clomipramine for treatment of this disorder. Clomipramine may also be a drug of choice for depressed persons with marked obsessive features.

Childhood Enuresis

Though imipramine is typically considered solely an antidepressant, it is also indicated for childhood enuresis.

Off-Label Uses

Panic Disorder with Agoraphobia

Imipramine is the TCA most studied for panic disorder with agoraphobia, but other TCAs are also effective when taken at the usual antidepressant dosages. Because of the potential initial anxiogenic effects of the TCAs, starting dosages should be small, and the dosage should be titrated upward slowly. Small doses of benzodiazepines may be used initially to deal with this side effect.

Pain

The TCAs are widely used to treat chronic neuropathic pain and in prophylaxis of migraine headache. Amitriptyline is the TCA most often used in this role. During treatment of pain, doses are generally lower than those used in depression; for example, 75 mg of amitriptyline may be effective. These effects also appear more rapidly.

Additionally, TCAs have shown efficacy in treating postherpetic neuralgia, diabetic neuropathy, myofascial pain, and orofacial pain.

Other Disorders

Peptic ulcer disease can be treated with doxepin, which has marked antihistaminergic effects. Desipramine has been used to treat irritable bowel syndrome and overactive bladder, while amitriptyline has demonstrated some efficacy in treating interstitial cystitis and fibromyalgia. Amoxapine may reduce amyloid-ß formulation through actions at $5HT_6$.

Other indications for the TCAs are narcolepsy, insomnia, nightmare disorder, and PTSD. The drugs are sometimes used for treatment of children and adolescents with attention deficit hyperactivity disorder (ADHD), sleepwalking disorder, separation anxiety disorder, and sleep terror disorder. Clomipramine has also been used to treat premature ejaculation, movement disorders, and compulsive behavior in children with autistic disorders; however, because the TCAs have caused sudden death in several children and adolescents, they should not be used in children.

Precautions and Adverse Reactions

The TCAs are associated with a wide range of problematic side effects and can be lethal when taken in overdose. The drugs should be used with caution in persons with hepatic and renal diseases. The TCAs should not be administered during a course of electroconvulsive therapy, primarily because of the risk of serious cardiac adverse effects.

Psychiatric Effects

The TCAs can induce a switch to mania or hypomania in susceptible individuals. The TCAs may also exacerbate psychotic disorders in susceptible persons. At high plasma concentrations (levels above 300 ng/mL), the anticholinergic effects of the TCAs can cause confusion or delirium. Patients with dementia are particularly vulnerable to this development.

Anticholinergic Effects

Anticholinergic effects often limit the tolerable dosage to relatively low ranges, though some patients may develop a tolerance for the anticholinergic effects with continued treatment. Anticholinergic effects include dry mouth, constipation, blurred vision, delirium, and urinary retention. Sugarless gum, candy, or fluoride lozenges can alleviate dry mouth. Bethanechol (Urecholine), 25 to 50 mg three or four times a day, may reduce urinary hesitancy and may be helpful in erectile dysfunction when the drug is taken 30 minutes before sexual intercourse. Narrow-angle glaucoma can also be aggravated by anticholinergic drugs, and the precipitation of glaucoma requires emergency treatment with a miotic agent. The TCAs should be avoided in persons with narrow-angle glaucoma, and an SSRI should be substituted. Severe anticholinergic effects can lead to a central nervous system (CNS) anticholinergic syndrome with confusion and delirium, especially if the TCAs are administered with dopamine receptor antagonists (DRAs) or anticholinergic drugs. IM or intravenous physostigmine (Antilirium, Eserine) is used to diagnose and treat anticholinergic delirium.

Cardiac Effects

When administered in their usual therapeutic dosages, the TCAs may cause tachycardia, flattened T waves, prolonged QT intervals, and depressed ST segments in the electrocardiographic (EKG) recording. Imipramine has a quinidine-like effect at therapeutic plasma concentrations and may reduce the number of premature ventricular contractions. Because the drugs prolong conduction time, their use in persons with preexisting conduction defects is contraindicated. In persons with a history of any type of heart disease, the TCAs should be used only after SSRIs or other newer antidepressants have been found ineffective. If used, they should be introduced at low dosages, with gradual increases in dosage and monitoring of cardiac functions. All the TCAs can cause tachycardia, which may persist for months and is one of the most common reasons for drug discontinuation, especially in younger persons. At high plasma concentrations, as seen in overdoses, the drugs become arrhythmogenic.

Other Autonomic Effects

Orthostatic hypotension is the most common cardiovascular autonomic adverse effect and the most common reason TCAs are discontinued. It can result in falls and injuries in affected persons. Nortriptyline may be the drug least likely to cause this problem. Orthostatic hypotension is treated with avoidance of caffeine, intake of at least 2 L of fluid per day, and addition of salt to the diet unless the person is being treated for hypertension. In persons taking antihypertensive agents, reduction of the dosage may reduce the risk of orthostatic hypotension. Other possible autonomic effects are profuse sweating, palpitations, and increased blood pressure (BP). Although some persons respond to fludrocortisone (Florinef), 0.02 to 0.05 mg twice a day, substitution of an SSRI is preferable to addition of a potentially toxic mineralocorticoid such as fludrocortisone. The TCAs' use should be discontinued several days before elective surgery because of the occurrence of hypertensive episodes during surgery in persons receiving TCAs.

Sedation

Sedation is a common effect of the TCAs and may be welcomed if sleeplessness has been a problem. The sedative effect of the TCAs is a result of anticholinergic and antihistaminergic activities. Amitriptyline, trimipramine, and doxepin are the most sedating agents; imipramine, amoxapine, nortriptyline, and maprotiline are less sedating; and desipramine and protriptyline are the least sedating agents.

Neurologic Effects

A fine, rapid tremor may occur with use of TCAs. Myoclonic twitches and tremors of the tongue and the upper extremities are common. Rare effects include speech blockage, paresthesia, peroneal palsies, and ataxia.

Amoxapine is unique in causing parkinsonian symptoms, akathisia, and even dyskinesia because of the dopaminergic blocking activity of one of its metabolites. Amoxapine may also cause neuroleptic malignant syndrome in rare cases. Maprotiline may cause seizures when the dosage is increased too quickly or is kept at high levels for too long. Clomipramine and amoxapine may lower the seizure threshold more than other drugs in the class. As a class, however, the TCAs have a relatively low risk for inducing seizures, except in persons who are at risk for seizures (e.g., persons with epilepsy and those with brain lesions). Although the TCAs can still be used by such persons, the initial dosages should be lower than usual, and subsequent dosage increases should be gradual.

Allergic and Hematologic Effects

Exanthematous rashes are seen in 4% to 5% of all persons treated with maprotiline. Jaundice is rare. Agranulocytosis, leukocytosis, leukopenia, and eosinophilia are rare complications of TCA treatment. However, a person who has a sore throat or a fever during the first few months of TCA treatment should have a complete blood count (CBC) done immediately.

Hepatic Effects

Mild and self-limited increases in serum transaminase concentrations may occur and should be monitored. The TCAs can also produce a fulminant acute hepatitis in 0.1% to 1% of persons. This can be life threatening, and the antidepressant should be discontinued.

Other Adverse Effects

Modest weight gain is common with use of TCAs. Amoxapine exerts a DRA effect and may cause hyperprolactinemia, impotence, galactorrhea, anorgasmia, and ejaculatory disturbances. Other TCAs have also been associated with gynecomastia and amenorrhea. The syndrome of inappropriate secretion of antidiuretic hormone (SIADH) has also been reported with TCAs. Other effects include nausea, vomiting, and hepatitis.

Use in Pregnancy and Lactation

A definitive link between the TCAs and teratogenic effects has not been established, but isolated reports of morphogenesis have been reported. TCAs cross the placenta, meaning neonatal drug withdrawal can occur. This syndrome includes tachypnea, cyanosis, irritability, and poor sucking reflex. If possible, these medications should be discontinued 1 week before delivery. Norepinephrine and serotonin transporters have been identified in the placenta and appear to play an important role in the clearance of these amines in the fetus. The understanding of the effects of reuptake inhibitors on these transporters during pregnancy is limited, but one study compared intelligence and language development in 80 children exposed to

TCAs during pregnancy with 84 children exposed to other nonteratogenic agents and found no deleterious effects of the TCAs.

The TCAs are excreted in breast milk at concentrations similar to plasma. The actual quantity delivered, however, is small, so drug levels in the infant are usually undetectable or very low.

Because the risk of relapse is a serious concern in patients with recurrent depression and these risks may be increased during pregnancy or the postpartum period, the risks and benefits of continuing or withdrawing treatment need to be discussed with the patient and weighed carefully.

Drug Interactions

Clinically relevant drug interactions may result from competition for enzyme CYP2D6 among TCAs and quinidine, cimetidine (Tagamet), fluoxetine (Prozac), sertraline (Zoloft), paroxetine (Paxil), phenothiazines, carbamazepine (Tegretol), and the type IC antiarrhythmics propafenone (Rythmol) and flecainide (Tambocor). Concomitant administration of TCAs and these inhibitors may slow down the metabolism and raise the plasma concentrations of TCAs. Additionally, genetic variations in the activity of CYP2D6 may account for up to a 40-fold difference in plasma TCA concentrations in different persons. The dosage of the TCA may need to be adjusted to correct changes in the rate of hepatic TCA metabolism.

Monoamine Oxidase Inhibitors

The TCAs should not be taken within 14 days of administration of a monoamine oxidase inhibitor.

Antihypertensives

The TCAs block the therapeutic effects of antihypertensive medication. The antihypertensive effects of the β-adrenergic receptor antagonists (e.g., propranolol [Inderal] and clonidine [Catapres]) may be blocked by the TCAs. The coadministration of a TCA and methyldopa (Aldomet) may cause behavioral agitation.

Antiarrhythmic Drugs

The antiarrhythmic properties of TCAs can be additive to those of quinidine, an effect that is further exacerbated by the inhibition of TCA metabolism by quinidine.

Dopamine Receptor Antagonists

Concurrent administration of TCAs and DRAs increases the plasma concentrations of both drugs. Desipramine plasma concentrations may increase twofold during concurrent administration with perphenazine (Trilafon). The DRAs also add to the anticholinergic and sedative effects of the TCAs. Concomitant use of serotonin–dopamine antagonists also increases those effects.

Central Nervous System Depressants

Opioids, alcohol, anxiolytics, hypnotics, and over-the-counter cold medications have additive effects by causing CNS depression when coadministered with

TCAs. Persons should be advised to avoid driving or using dangerous equipment if sedated by TCAs.

Sympathomimetics

TCA use with sympathomimetic drugs may cause serious cardiovascular effects.

Oral Contraceptives

Birth control pills may decrease TCA plasma concentrations through the induction of hepatic enzymes.

Other Drug Interactions

Nicotine may reduce TCA concentrations. Plasma concentrations may also be lowered by ascorbic acid, ammonium chloride, barbiturates, carbamazepine, chloral hydrate, lithium (Eskalith), and primidone (Mysoline). TCA plasma concentrations may be increased by concurrent use of acetazolamide (Diamox), sodium bicarbonate, acetylsalicylic acid, cimetidine, thiazide diuretics, fluoxetine, paroxetine, and fluvoxamine (Luvox). Plasma concentrations of the TCAs may rise three- to fourfold when administered concurrently with fluoxetine, fluvoxamine, and paroxetine.

Laboratory Interferences

TCAs are present at low concentrations and are not likely to interfere with other laboratory assays. It is possible that they may interfere with the determination of conventional neuroleptic blood concentrations because of their structural similarity and the low concentrations of some neuroleptics.

Dosage and Clinical Guidelines

Persons who intend to take TCAs should undergo routine physical and laboratory examinations, including a CBC, a white blood cell count with differential, and serum electrolytes with liver function tests. An EKG should be obtained for all persons, especially women older than 40 years of age and men older than 30 years of age. The TCAs are contraindicated in persons with a QT_c greater than 450 ms. The initial dose should be small and should be raised gradually. Because of the availability of highly effective alternatives to TCAs, a newer agent should be used if there is any medical condition that may interact adversely with the TCAs.

Elderly persons and children are more sensitive to TCA adverse effects than are young adults. In children, the EKG should be regularly monitored during use of a TCA.

The available preparations of TCAs are presented in Table 37-1. The dosages and therapeutic blood levels for the TCAs vary among the drugs (as shown in Table 37-2). With the exception of protriptyline, all of the TCAs should be started at 25 mg a day and increased as tolerated. Divided doses at first reduce the severity of the adverse effects, although most of the dosage should be given at night to help induce sleep if a sedating drug such as amitriptyline is used. Eventually, the entire daily dose can be given at bedtime. A common clinical mistake is to stop increasing the dosage when the person is tolerating the drug

TABLE 37-2: General Information for the Tricyclic and Tetracyclic Antidepressants

Generic Name	Trade Name	Usual Adult Dosage Range (mg/day)	Therapeutic Plasma Concentrations (mg/mL)
Imipramine	Tofranil	150–300	150–300[a]
Desipramine	Norpramin, Pertofrane	150–300	150–300[a]
Trimipramine	Surmontil	150–300	?
Amitriptyline	Elavil, Endep	150–300	100–250[b]
Nortriptyline	Pamelor, Aventyl	50–150	50–150[a] (maximum)
Protriptyline	Vivactil	15–60	75–250
Amoxapine	Asendin	150–400	?
Doxepin	Adapin, Sinequan	150–300	100–250[a]
Maprotiline	Ludiomil	150–230	150–300[a]
Clomipramine	Anafranil	130–250	?

Where "?" denotes unknown therapeutic plasma levels.
[a]Exact range may vary among laboratories.
[b]Includes parent compound and desmethyl metabolite.

but taking less than the maximum therapeutic dose and does not show clinical improvement. The clinician should routinely assess the person's pulse and orthostatic changes in BP while the dosage is being increased.

Nortriptyline use should be started at 25 mg a day. Most patients need only 75 mg a day to achieve a blood level of 100 mg/nL. However, the dosage may be raised to 150 mg a day if needed. Amoxapine use should be started at 150 mg a day and raised to 400 mg a day. Protriptyline use should be started at 15 mg a day and raised to 60 mg a day. Maprotiline has been associated with an increased incidence of seizures if the dosage is raised too quickly or is maintained at too high a level. Maprotiline use should be started at 25 mg a day and increased over 4 weeks to 225 mg a day. It should be kept at that level for only 6 weeks and then be reduced to 175 to 200 mg a day.

Persons with chronic pain may be particularly sensitive to adverse effects when TCA use is started. Therefore, treatment should begin with low dosages that are raised in small increments. However, persons with chronic pain may experience relief on long-term, low-dosage therapy, such as amitriptyline or nortriptyline at 10 to 75 mg a day.

The TCAs should be avoided in children, except as a last resort. Dosing guidelines in children for imipramine include initiation at 1.5 mg/kg a day. The dosage can be titrated to no more than 5 mg/kg a day. In enuresis, the dosage is usually 50 to 100 mg a day taken at bedtime. Clomipramine use can be initiated at 50 mg a day and increased to no more than 3 mg/kg or 200 mg a day.

When TCA treatment is discontinued, the dosage should first be decreased to three-fourths the maximal dosage for a month. At that time, if no symptoms are present, drug use can be tapered by 25 mg (5 mg for protriptyline) every 4 to 7 days. Slow tapering avoids a cholinergic rebound syndrome consisting of nausea, upset stomach, sweating, headache, neck pain, and vomiting. This syndrome can be treated by reinstituting a small dosage of the drug and tapering more slowly than before. Several case reports note the appearance of rebound mania or hypomania after the abrupt discontinuation of TCA use.

Plasma Concentrations and Therapeutic Drug Monitoring

Clinical determinations of plasma concentrations should be conducted after 5 to 7 days on the same dosage of medication and 8 to 12 hours after the last dose. Because of variations in absorption and metabolism, there may be a 30- to 50-fold difference in the plasma concentrations in persons given the same dosage of a TCA. Nortriptyline is unique in its association with a therapeutic window—that is, plasma concentrations below 50 ng/mL or above 150 ng/mL may reduce its efficacy.

Plasma concentrations may be useful in confirming compliance, assessing reasons for drug failures, and documenting effective plasma concentrations for future treatment. Clinicians should always treat the person and not the plasma concentration. Some persons have adequate clinical responses with seemingly subtherapeutic plasma concentrations, and other persons only respond at supratherapeutic plasma concentrations without experiencing adverse effects. The latter situation, however, should alert the clinician to monitor the person's condition with, for example, serial EKG recordings.

Overdose Attempts

Overdose attempts with TCAs are serious and can often be fatal. Prescriptions for these drugs should be nonrefillable and for no longer than a week at a time for patients at risk for suicide. Amoxapine may be more likely than the other TCAs to result in death when taken in overdose. The newer antidepressants are safer in overdose.

Symptoms of overdose include agitation, delirium, convulsions, hyperactive deep tendon reflexes, bowel and bladder paralysis, dysregulation of BP and temperature, and mydriasis. The patient then progresses to coma and perhaps respiratory depression. Cardiac arrhythmias may not respond to treatment. Because of the long half-lives of TCAs, the patients are at risk of cardiac arrhythmias for 3 to 4 days after the overdose, so they should be monitored in an intensive care medical setting.

38 Valproate

Introduction

Also known as valproic acid, valproate (Depakene, Depakote) was originally used as an anticonvulsant, but is also approved for the treatment of manic episodes associated with bipolar I disorder. It is one of the most widely prescribed mood stabilizers in psychiatry since it has a rapid onset of action and is well tolerated. Additionally, numerous studies have found that it reduces the frequency and intensity of recurrent manic episodes over extended periods of time. Even though lithium is still considered as the first-line treatment for bipolar disorder, many patients who cannot tolerate lithium or develop renal complications find valproate to be a preferable alternative treatment.

Valproate is a branched short-chain carboxylic acid. It is called valproic acid because it is rapidly converted to the acid form in the stomach. Multiple formulations of valproic acid are marketed. These include valproic acid (Depakene); divalproex sodium (Depakote), an enteric-coated delayed-release 1:1 mixture of valproic acid and sodium valproate available in tablet and sprinkle formulation (can be opened and spread on food); and sodium valproate injection (Depacon). An extended-release preparation is also available. Each of these is therapeutically equivalent because at physiologic pH, valproic acid dissociates into valproate ion.

Pharmacologic Actions

Regardless of how it is formulated, valproate is rapidly and completely absorbed within 1 to 2 hours of oral ingestion, with peak concentrations occurring 4 to 5 hours following administration. The plasma half-life of valproate is 10 to 16 hours and is highly protein bound. Protein binding becomes saturated at higher dosages, and concentrations of therapeutically effective free valproate increase at serum concentrations above 50 to 100 mg/mL. The unbound portion of valproate is considered to be pharmacologically active and can cross the blood–brain barrier. The extended-release preparation produces lower peak concentrations with higher minimum concentrations and can be given once a day. Valproate is metabolized primarily by the cytochrome P450 isoenzymes CYP2A6, CYP2B6, CYP2C9, and CYP3A5, as well as the UDP-glucuronosyltransferase enzymes UGT1A3, UGT1A4, UGT1A6, UGT1A8, UGT1A9, UGT1A10, UGT2B7, and UGT2B15. Valproate is also metabolized by mitochondrial β-oxidation. Less than 3% of the parent compound is excreted unchanged in urine.

The biochemical basis of valproate's therapeutic effects remains poorly understood. Evidence suggests that it inhibits the degradation of γ-aminobutyric acid (GABA) and thereby increases GABA concentration; reducing the high-frequency firing of neurons by voltage-gated potassium, calcium, and sodium; by stimulating the Wnt/β-catenin signaling pathway; and by inhibiting histone deacetylase.

Therapeutic Indications

Valproate is currently approved as monotherapy or adjunctive therapy of complex partial seizures, monotherapy and adjunctive therapy of simple and complex absence seizures, and adjunctive therapy for patients with multiple seizures that include absence seizures.

Divalproex sodium has additional indications for prophylaxis of migraine and as a treatment of manic episodes in bipolar disorder.

Bipolar I Disorder

Acute Mania. About two-thirds of persons with acute mania respond to valproate. The majority of patients with mania usually respond within 1 to 4 days after achieving valproate serum concentrations above 50 mg/mL. Antimanic response is generally associated with levels greater than 50 mg/mL, in a range of 50 to 100 mg/mL though in some cases levels up to 150 mg/mL have been used. Using gradual dosing strategies, this serum concentration may be achieved within 1 week of initiation of dosing, but rapid oral loading strategies achieve therapeutic serum concentrations in 1 day and can control manic symptoms within 5 days. The short-term antimanic effects of valproate can be augmented with addition of lithium, carbamazepine (Tegretol), serotonin–dopamine antagonists (SDAs), or dopamine receptor antagonists (DRAs). Numerous studies have suggested that the irritable manic subtype respond significantly better to divalproex sodium than lithium or placebo. Because of its more favorable profile of cognitive, dermatologic, thyroid, and renal adverse effects, valproate is preferred to lithium for treatment of acute mania in children and elderly persons.

Off-Label Uses

Bipolar I Disorder

Acute Bipolar Depression. Valproate possesses some activity as a short-term treatment of depressive episodes in bipolar I disorder, but this effect is far less pronounced than for treatment of manic episodes. Among depressive symptoms, valproate is more effective for treatment of agitation than dysphoria. In clinical practice, valproate is most often used as add-on therapy to an antidepressant to prevent the development of mania or rapid cycling.

Prophylaxis. Studies suggest that valproate is effective in the prophylactic treatment of bipolar I disorder, resulting in fewer and less severe and shorter manic episodes. In direct comparison, valproate is at least as effective as lithium. It is also better tolerated than lithium. It may be particularly effective in persons with rapid-cycling and ultrarapid-cycling bipolar disorders, dysphoric or mixed mania, and mania caused by a general medical condition, as well as in persons who have comorbid substance abuse or panic attacks and in persons who have not had complete favorable responses to lithium treatment.

Schizophrenia and Schizoaffective Disorder

Valproate may accelerate response to antipsychotic therapy in patients with schizophrenia or schizoaffective disorder. Valproate alone is generally less effective in schizoaffective disorder than in bipolar I disorder. Valproate alone is ineffective for treatment of psychotic symptoms and is typically used in combination with other drugs in patients with these symptoms.

Other Mental Disorders

Valproate has been studied for possible efficacy in a broad range of psychiatric disorders. These include alcohol withdrawal and relapse prevention, panic disorder, posttraumatic stress disorder, impulse control disorder, and borderline personality disorder. Evidence supporting use in these cases is weak, and any observed therapeutic effects may be related to treatment of comorbid bipolar disorder.

Some evidence suggests that valproate's inhibition of histone deacetylase could slow the progression of neurodegenerative disorders.

Other Medical Conditions

Some evidence suggests that valproate may be an effective adjuvant therapy in cancer and HIV/AIDS. However, far more research is needed.

Precautions and Adverse Reactions

Although valproate treatment is generally well tolerated and safe, it carries quite a few black box and other warnings (Table 38-1). The two most serious adverse effects of valproate treatment affect the pancreas and liver. Clinicians should carefully assess before administering the drug to persons with hepatic diseases.

Risk factors for potentially fatal hepatotoxicity include young age (younger than 3 years); concurrent use of phenobarbital; and the presence of neurologic disorders, especially inborn errors of metabolism. The rate of fatal hepatotoxicity in persons who have been treated with only valproate is 0.85 per 100,000 persons; no persons older than the age of 10 years have been reported to have died from hepatotoxicity. Therefore, the risk of this adverse reaction in adult psychiatric patients is low. Nevertheless, if symptoms of lethargy, malaise, anorexia, nausea and vomiting, edema, and abdominal pain occur in a person treated with valproate, the clinician must consider the possibility of severe hepatotoxicity. A modest increase in liver function test results does not correlate with the development of serious hepatotoxicity.

Rare cases of pancreatitis have been reported; they occur most often in the first 6 months of treatment, and the condition occasionally results in death. Pancreatic function can be assessed and followed with serum amylase concentrations. Other potentially serious consequences of treatment include hyperammonemia-induced encephalopathy and thrombocytopenia. Thrombocytopenia and platelet dysfunction occur most commonly at high dosages and result in the prolongation of bleeding times.

TABLE 38-1: Black Box Warnings and Other Warnings for Valproate

More Serious Side Effect	Management Considerations
Hepatotoxicity	Rare, idiosyncratic event
	Estimated risk: 1:118,000 (adults)
	Greatest risk profile (polypharmacy, younger than 2 years of age, mental retardation): 1:800
Pancreatitis	Rare, similar pattern to hepatotoxicity
	Incidence in clinical trial data is 2 in 2,416 (0.0008%)
	Postmarketing surveillance shows no increased incidence
	Relapse with rechallenge
	Asymptomatic amylase not predictive
Hyperammonemia	Rare; more common in combination with carbamazepine (Tegretol)
	Associated with coarse tremor and may respond to L-carnitine administration
Associated with urea cycle disorders	Discontinue valproate and protein intake and assess underlying urea cycle disorder
	Divalproex sodium is contraindicated in patients with urea cycle disorders
Teratogenicity	Neural tube defect: 1–4% with valproate
	Preconceptual education and folate–vitamin B complex supplementation for all young women of childbearing potential
Somnolence in elderly persons	Slower titration than conventional doses. Regular monitoring of fluid and nutritional intake
Thrombocytopenia	Decrease dose if clinically symptomatic (i.e., bruising, bleeding gums)
	Thrombocytopenia more likely with valproate levels ≥110 mg/mL (women) and ≥135 mg/mL (men)

The common adverse effects associated with valproate (Table 38-2) are those affecting the gastrointestinal (GI) system, such as nausea, vomiting, dyspepsia, and diarrhea. The GI effects are generally most common in the first month of treatment, particularly if the dosage is increased rapidly. Unbuffered valproic acid (Depakene) is more likely to cause GI symptoms than the enteric-coated "sprinkle" or the delayed-release divalproex sodium formulations. Other common adverse effects involve the nervous system, such as sedation, ataxia, dysarthria, and tremor. Valproate-induced tremor may respond well to treatment with β-adrenergic receptor antagonists or gabapentin. Treatment of the other neurologic adverse effects usually requires lowering the valproate dosage.

Weight gain is a common adverse effect, especially in long-term treatment, and can best be treated by strict limitation of caloric intake. Hair loss may occur in 5% to 10%, and rare cases of complete loss of body hair have been reported. Some clinicians have recommended treatment of valproate-associated hair loss with vitamin supplements that contain zinc and selenium.

Five to 40% of persons experience a persistent but clinically insignificant elevation in liver transaminases up to three times the upper limit of normal,

TABLE 38-2: Adverse Effects of Valproate
Common
GI irritation
Nausea
Sedation
Tremor
Weight gain
Hair loss
Uncommon
Vomiting
Diarrhea
Ataxia
Dysarthria
Persistent elevation of hepatic transaminases
Rare
Fatal hepatotoxicity (primarily in pediatric patients)
Reversible thrombocytopenia
Platelet dysfunction
Coagulation disturbances
Edema
Hemorrhagic pancreatitis
Agranulocytosis
Encephalopathy and coma
Respiratory muscle weakness and respiratory failure
GI, gastrointestinal.

which is usually asymptomatic and resolves after discontinuation of the drug. High dosages of valproate (above 1,000 mg a day) may rarely produce mild to moderate hyponatremia, most likely secondary to syndrome of secretion of inappropriate antidiuretic hormone (SIADH), which is reversible upon lowering the dosage.

Overdoses of valproate can lead to coma and death.

Use in Pregnancy and Lactation

Valproate has been classified as a pregnancy category D drug.

There are multiple concerns regarding the use of valproate during pregnancy. Women who require valproate therapy should therefore inform their physicians if they intend to become pregnant. First trimester use of valproate has been associated with a 3% to 5% risk of neural tube defects, as well as an increased risk of other malformations affecting the heart and other organ systems. Multiple reports have also indicated that in utero exposure to valproate may also negatively affect cognitive development in children of mothers who take valproate during pregnancy. They have lower IQ scores at age 6 compared to those exposed to other antiepileptic drugs. Fetal valproate exposure has dose-dependent associations with reduced cognitive abilities across a range of domains at 6 years of age. Prenatal valproate exposure may also increase the risk of a child developing autistic spectrum disorder.

Valproate is also associated with teratogenicity, most notably neural tube defects (e.g., spina bifida). The risk is about 1% to 4% of all women who take valproate during the first trimester of the pregnancy. The risk of valproate-induced neural tube defects can be reduced with daily folic acid supplements (1 to 4 mg a day). *All women with childbearing potential who take the drug should be given folic acid supplements.* Infants breastfed by mothers taking valproate develop serum valproate concentrations that are 1% to 10% of maternal serum concentrations, but no data suggest that this poses a risk to the infant. Valproate is not contraindicated in nursing mothers.

Valproate may be especially problematic for adolescents and young women. Cases of polycystic ovarian disease have been reported in women using valproate. Even when the full syndromal criteria for this syndrome are not met, many of these women develop menstrual irregularities, hair loss, and hirsutism. These effects are thought to result from a metabolic syndrome that is driven by insulin resistance and hyperinsulinemia.

Drug Interactions

Valproate is commonly prescribed as part of a regimen involving other psychotropic agents. The only consistent drug interaction with lithium, if both drugs are maintained in their respective therapeutic ranges, is the exacerbation of drug-induced tremors, which can usually be treated with β-receptor antagonists. The combination of valproate and DRAs may result in increased sedation, as can be seen when valproate is added to any central nervous system (CNS) depressant (e.g., alcohol), and an increased severity of extrapyramidal symptoms, which usually responds to treatment with antiparkinsonian drugs. Valproate can usually be safely combined with carbamazepine or SDAs.

Perhaps the most worrisome interaction of valproate and a psychotropic drug involves lamotrigine. Since the approval of lamotrigine for the treatment of bipolar disorder, the likelihood that patients will be treated with both agents has increased. Valproate more than doubles lamotrigine concentrations, increasing the risk of a serious rash, including Stevens–Johnson syndrome and toxic epidermal necrolysis. Appropriate dose reduction is recommended.

The plasma concentrations of carbamazepine, diazepam (Valium), amitriptyline (Elavil), nortriptyline (Pamelor), and phenobarbital (Luminal) may also be increased when these drugs are coadministered with valproate, and the plasma concentrations of phenytoin (Dilantin) and desipramine (Norpramin) may be decreased when they are combined with valproate. The plasma concentrations of valproate may be decreased when the drug is coadministered with carbamazepine and may be increased when coadministered with guanfacine (Tenex), amitriptyline, or fluoxetine (Prozac). Valproate can be displaced from plasma proteins by carbamazepine, diazepam, and aspirin. Persons who are treated with anticoagulants (e.g., aspirin and warfarin [Coumadin]) should also be monitored when valproate use is initiated to assess the development of any undesired augmentation of the anticoagulation effects. Interactions of valproate with other drugs are listed in Table 38-3.

TABLE 38-3: Interactions of Valproate with Other Drugs

Drug	Interactions Reported with Valproate
Lithium	Increased tremor
Antipsychotics	Increased sedation; increased extrapyramidal effects; delirium and stupor (single report)
Clozapine	Increased sedation; confusional syndrome (single report)
Carbamazepine	Acute psychosis (single report); ataxia, nausea, lethargy (single report); may decrease valproate serum concentrations
Antidepressants	Amitriptyline and fluoxetine may increase valproate serum concentrations
Diazepam	Serum concentration increased by valproate
Clonazepam	Absence status (rare; reported only in patients with preexisting epilepsy)
Phenytoin	Serum concentration decreased by valproate
Phenobarbital	Serum concentration increased by valproate; increased sedation
Other CNS depressants	Increased sedation
Anticoagulants	Possible potentiation of effect

CNS, central nervous system.

Laboratory Interferences

Valproate may cause laboratory increase of serum-free fatty acids. Valproate metabolites may produce a false-positive test result for urinary ketones as well as falsely abnormal thyroid function test results.

Dosage and Clinical Guidelines

When starting valproate therapy, a baseline hepatic panel, complete blood cell and platelet counts, and pregnancy testing should be ordered. Additional testing should include amylase and coagulation studies if baseline pancreatic disease or coagulopathy is suspected. In addition to baseline laboratory tests, hepatic transaminase concentrations should be obtained 1 month after initiation of therapy and every 6 to 12 months thereafter. However, because even frequent monitoring may not predict serious organ toxicity, it is more prudent to reinforce the need for prompt evaluation of any illnesses when reviewing the instructions with patients. Asymptomatic elevation of transaminase concentrations up to three times the upper limit of normal are common and do not require any change in dosage. Table 38-4 lists the recommended laboratory tests for valproate treatment.

Valproate is available in a number of formulations (Table 38-5). For treatment of acute mania, an oral loading strategy of initiation with 20 to 30 mg/kg a day can be used to accelerate control of symptoms. This is usually well tolerated but can cause excessive sedation and tremor in elderly persons. Agitated behavior can be rapidly stabilized with intravenous infusion of valproate. If acute mania is absent, it is best to initiate drug treatment gradually to minimize the common adverse effects of nausea, vomiting, and sedation.

The dose on the first day should be 250 mg administered with a meal. The dosage can be raised up to 250 mg orally three times daily over the course of 3 to

TABLE 38-4: Recommended Laboratory Tests During Valproate Therapy

Before treatment
    Standard chemistry screen with special attention to liver function tests
    CBC, including WBC and platelet count

During treatment
    Liver function tests at 1 month; then every 6–12 months if no abnormalities are found
    Complete blood work with platelet count at 1 month; then every 6–12 months if findings are normal

Liver function test results become abnormal
    Mild transaminase elevation (less than three times normal): monitoring every 1–2 weeks; if stable
    and patient is responding to valproate, results are monitored monthly to every 3 months
    Pronounced transaminase elevation (more than three times normal): dosage reduction or
    discontinuation of valproate; increase dose or rechallenge if transaminases normalize and if the
    patient is a valproate responder

CBC, complete blood count; WBC, white blood cell.

6 days. The plasma concentrations can be assessed in the morning before the first daily dose is administered. Therapeutic plasma concentrations for the control of seizures range between 50 to 150 mg/mL, but concentrations up to 200 mg/mL are usually well tolerated.

It is reasonable to use the same range for the treatment of mental disorders; most of the controlled studies have used 50 to 125 mg/mL. Most persons attain therapeutic plasma concentrations on a dosage between 1,200 to 1,500 mg a day in divided doses. After a person's symptoms are well controlled, the full daily dose can be taken all at once before sleep.

TABLE 38-5: Valproate Preparations Available in the United States		
Generic Name	**Trade Name, Form (Doses)**	**Time to Peak**
Valproate sodium injection	Depacon injection (100 mg valproic acid/mL)	1 hour
Valproic acid	Depakene, syrup (250 mg/5 mL)	1–2 hours
	Depakene, capsules (250 mg)	1–2 hours
Divalproex sodium	Depakote, delayed-released tablets (125, 250, 500 mg)	3–8 hours
Divalproex sodium–coated particles in capsules	Depakote, sprinkle capsules (125 mg)	Compared with tablets, divalproex sodium sprinkle has earlier onset and slower absorption, with slightly lower peak plasma concentration

39 Nutritional Supplements and Medical Foods

Introduction

The herbal and dietary supplement industry has seen tremendous growth in recent years. While there is no doubt that a healthy diet and proper nutrition play an enormous role in one's physical and mental health, many of the supplements that are being marketed today are purported to have psychoactive properties and are being used less for their nutritional value and more so for their medicinal value. This should not come as a surprise, since cultures throughout the world have long used plant-based medicines to treat a wide range of disorders. Controlled studies have even shown that a number of these compounds could be used to treat certain psychiatric symptoms. The cannabinoid cannabidiol (see Chapter14) is just one example.

While certain compounds may be beneficial, in many cases, the quantity and quality of data have been insufficient to make definitive conclusions. Nevertheless, some patients prefer to use these substances in place of, or in conjunction with, conventional pharmaceutical treatments. While many clinicians many disagree with this course of action, it is important that they listen to their patients' reasoning and respectfully discuss any potential benefits and risks of using herbal or dietary supplements. Clinicians should also note that the use of herbal drugs or nutritional supplements comes at the expense of proven interventions and that adverse effects are possible.

In addition, herbal and nonherbal supplements may augment or antagonize the actions of prescription and nonprescription drugs. Thus, it is important for clinicians to remain informed on the latest research involving these substances. Because of the paucity of clinical trials, the clinician must be extraordinarily alert to the possibility of adverse effects as a result of drug–drug interactions, especially if psychotropic agents are prescribed, because many phytomedicinals have ingredients that produce physiologic changes in the body.

Nutritional Supplements

In the United States, the term nutritional supplement is used interchangeably with the term dietary supplement. The Dietary Supplement Health and Education Act (DSHEA) of 1994 defined nutritional supplements as items taken by mouth that contain a "dietary ingredient" meant to supplement the diet. These ingredients may include vitamins, minerals, herbs, botanicals, amino acids, and substances such as enzymes, tissues, glandulars, and metabolites. By law, such products must be labeled as supplements and may not be marketed as conventional food.

DSHEA places dietary supplements in a special category governed by far less stringent regulations than those for prescription and over-the-counter drugs.

Unlike pharmaceutical drugs, nutritional supplements are not required to seek the approval of the Food and Drug Administration (FDA), and the FDA does not evaluate their effectiveness. Because dietary supplements are not regulated by the FDA, the contents and quality on store shelves vary dramatically. Contamination, mislabeling, and misidentification of herbs and supplements are important problems. Patients must play the part of educated consumers and recognize that there are many companies that are not interested in providing quality products. As there is no governmental oversight to hold these companies accountable, reliance on third-party certifiers is oftentimes necessary.

See Table 39-1 for a list of dietary supplements used in psychiatry.

Medical Foods

In recent years, the FDA has introduced a new category of nutritional supplement called "medical foods." According to the FDA, the term medical food, as defined in the Orphan Drug Act, is "a food which is formulated to be consumed or administered enterally under the supervision of a physician and which is intended for the specific dietary management of a disease or condition for which distinctive nutritional requirements, based on recognized scientific principles, are established by medical evaluation."

A clear distinction can be made between the regulatory classifications of medical foods and dietary supplements. Medical foods must be shown, by medical evaluation, to meet the distinctive nutritional needs of a specific population of patients with a specific disease being targeted. Dietary supplements, on the other hand, are intended for normal, healthy adults and may not require proof of efficacy of the finished product. Medical foods are distinguished from the broader category of foods for special dietary use and from foods that make health claims by the requirement that medical foods are to be used under medical supervision.

Medical foods do not have to undergo premarket approval by FDA. However, medical food firms must comply with other requirements, such as good manufacturing practices and registration of food facilities. Medical foods do have some additional regulations that dietary supplements do not because medical foods are intended to treat illnesses. For example, a compliance program requires annual inspections of all medical food manufacturers.

In summary, to be considered a medical food, a product must, at a minimum, meet the following criteria:

1. The product must be a food for oral or tube feeding
2. The product must be labeled for the dietary management of a specific medical disorder, disease, or condition for which there are distinctive nutritional requirements
3. The product must be intended to be used under medical supervision

The most common medical foods with psychoactive claims are listed in Table 39-2.

TABLE 39-1: Dietary Supplements Used in Psychiatry

Name	Ingredients/What Is It?	Uses	Adverse Effects	Interactions	Dosage	Comments
Docosahexaenoic acid (DHA)	Omega-3 polyunsaturated fatty acid	ADD, dyslexia, cognitive impairment, dementia	Anticoagulant properties, mild GI distress	Warfarin	Varies with indication	Stop using prior to surgery
Choline	Derived from soy lecithin	Fetal brain development, manic conditions, cognitive disorders, tardive dyskinesia, cancers	Restrict in patients with primary genetic trimethylaminuria, sweating, hypotension, depression	Methotrexate, works with B_6, B_{12}, and folic acid in metabolism of homocysteine	300–1,200 mg BID doses >3 g associated with fishy body odor	Needed for structure and function of all cells
l-alpha-glyceryl-phosphorylcholine (a-GPC)	Derived from soy lecithin	To increase growth hormone secretion, cognitive disorders	None known	None known	500 mg–1 g daily	Remains poorly understood
Phosphatidylcholine	Phospholipid that is part of cell membranes	Manic conditions, Alzheimer disease, and cognitive disorders, tardive dyskinesia	Diarrhea, steatorrhea in those with malabsorption, avoid with antiphospholipid antibody syndrome	None known	3–9 g/day in divided doses	Soybeans, sunflower, and rapeseed are major sources
Phosphatidylserine	Phospholipid isolated from soya and egg yolks	Cognitive impairment including Alzheimer disease, may reverse memory problems	Avoid with antiphospholipid antibody syndrome, GI side effects	None known	For soya-derived variety, 100 mg TID	Type derived from bovine brain carries hypothetical risk of bovine spongiform encephalopathy
Zinc	Metallic element	Immune impairment, wound healing, cognitive disorders, prevention of neural tube defects	GI distress, high doses can cause copper deficiency, immunosuppression	Bisphosphonates, quinolones, tetracycline, penicillamine, copper, cysteine-containing foods, caffeine, iron	Typical dose 15 mg/day, adverse effects >30 mg	Claims that zinc can prevent and treat the common cold are supported in some studies but not in others; more research needed

Acetyl-l-carnitine	Acetyl ester of l-carnitine	Neuroprotection, Alzheimer disease, Down syndrome, strokes, antiaging, depression in geriatric patients	Mild GI distress, seizures, increased agitation in some with Alzheimer disease	Nucleoside analogs, valproic acid, and pivalic acid–containing antibiotics	500 mg–2 g daily in divided doses	Found in small amounts in milk and meat
Huperzine A	Plant alkaloid derived from Chinese club moss	Alzheimer disease, age-related memory loss, inflammatory disorders	Seizures, arrhythmias, asthma, irritable bowel disease	Acetylcholinesterase inhibitors and cholinergic drugs	60–200 mg/day	Huperzia serrata has been used in Chinese folk medicine for the treatment of fevers and inflammation
Nicotinamide adenine dinucleotide (NADH)	Dinucleotide located in mitochondria and cytosol of cells	Parkinson disease, Alzheimer disease, chronic fatigue, CV disease	GI distress	None known	5 mg/day or 5 mg BID	Precursor of NADH is nicotinic acid
S-Adenosyl-l-methionine (SAMe)	Metabolite of essential amino acid l-methionine	Mood elevation, osteoarthritis	Hypomania, hyperactive muscle movement, caution in patients with cancer	None known	200–1,600 mg daily in divided doses	Several trials demonstrate some efficacy in the treatment of depression
5-Hydroxytryptophan (5-HTP)	Immediate precursor of serotonin	Depression, obesity, insomnia, fibromyalgia, headaches	Possible risk of serotonin syndrome in those with carcinoid tumors or taking MAOIs	SSRIs, MAOIs, methyldopa, St. John's wort, phenoxybenzamine, 5-HT antagonists, 5-HT receptor agonists	100 mg–2 g daily, safer with carbidopa	5-HTP along with carbidopa is used in Europe for the treatment of depression
Folinic acid (Leucovorin)		Depression; Prevention of side effects of methotrexate				

(continued)

TABLE 39-1: Dietary Supplements Used in Psychiatry (*continued*)

Name	Ingredients/What Is It?	Uses	Adverse Effects	Interactions	Dosage	Comments
Phenylalanine	Essential amino acid	Depression, analgesia, vitiligo	Contraindicated in patients with PKU, may exacerbate tardive dyskinesia or hypertension	MAOIs and neuroleptic drugs	Comes in two forms: 500 mg–1.5 g daily for DL-phenylalanine, 375 mg–2.25 g for DL-phenylalanine	Found in vegetables, juices, yogurt, and miso
Myoinositol	Major nutritionally active form of inositol	Depression, panic attacks, OCD	Caution in patients with bipolar disorder, GI distress	Possible additive effects with SSRIs and 5-HT receptor agonists (sumatriptan)	12 g in divided doses for depression and panic attacks	Studies have *not* shown effectiveness in treating Alzheimer disease, autism, or schizophrenia
Vinpocetine	Semisynthetic derivative of vincamine (plant derivative)	Cerebral ischemic stroke, dementia	GI distress, dizziness, insomnia, dry mouth, tachycardia, hypotension, flushing	Warfarin	5–10 mg daily with food, no more than 20 mg/day	Used in Europe, Mexico, and Japan as pharmaceutical agent for treatment of cerebrovascular and cognitive disorders
Vitamin E family	Essential fat-soluble vitamin, family made of tocopherols and tocotrienols	Immune-enhancing, antioxidant, some cancers, protection in CV disease, neurologic disorders, diabetes, premenstrual syndrome	May increase bleeding in those with propensity to bleed, possible increased risk of hemorrhagic stroke, thrombophlebitis	Warfarin, antiplatelet drugs, neomycin, may be additive with statins.	Depends on form: tocotrienols, 200–300 mg daily with food; tocopherols, 200 mg/day	Stop members of vitamin E family 1 month prior to surgical procedures

Glycine	Amino acid	Schizophrenia, alleviating spasticity, and seizures	Avoid in those who are anuric or have hepatic failure	Additive with antispasmodics	1 g/day in divided doses for supplement; 40–90 g/day for schizophrenia	
Melatonin	Hormone of pineal gland	Insomnia, sleep disturbances, jet lag, cancer	May inhibit ovulation in 1 g doses, seizures, grogginess, depression, headache, amnesia	Aspirin, NSAIDs, b-blockers, INH, sedating drugs, corticosteroids, valerian, kava kava, 5-HTP, alcohol	0.3–3 mg for short periods of time	Melatonin sets the timing of circadian rhythms and regulates seasonal responses
Fish oil	Lipids found in fish	Bipolar disorder, lowering triglycerides, hypertension, decrease blood clotting	Caution in hemophiliacs, mild GI upset, "fishy"-smelling excretions	Coumadin, aspirin, NSAIDs, garlic, ginkgo	Varies depending on form and indication—usually about 3–5 g daily	Stop prior to any surgical procedure

ADD, attention deficit disorder; CV, cardiovascular; 5-HTP, 5-hydroxytryptophan; GI, gastrointestinal; INH, isoniazid; MAOIs, monoamine oxidase inhibitors; NSAIDs, nonsteroidal anti-inflammatory drugs; OCD, obsessive-compulsive disorder; PKU, phenylketonuria; SSRIs, selective serotonin reuptake inhibitors.
Table by Mercedes Blackstone, MD.

TABLE 39-2: Some Common Medical Foods

Medical Food	Indication	Mechanism of Action
Caprylic-triglyceride (Axona)	Alzheimer disease	Increases plasma concentration of ketones as an alternative energy source in the brain; metabolized in the liver.
L-methylfolate (Deplin)	Depression	Regulates synthesis of serotonin, norepinephrine, and dopamine; adjunctive to SSRIs; 15 mg/day.
S-adenosyl-L-methionine (SAMe)	Depression	Naturally occurring molecule involved in synthesis of hormones and neurotransmitters including serotonin and norepinephrine.
L-Tryptophan	Sleep disturbance Depression	Essential amino acid; precursor of serotonin; reduces sleep latency; usual dose 4–5 g/day.
Omega-3 fatty acid	Depression Cognition	Eicosapentaenoic (EPA) and docosahexaenoic (DHA) acids; direct effect on lipid metabolism; used for augmentation of antidepressant drugs.
Theramine (Sentra)	Sleep disturbances Cognitive enhancer	Cholinergic modulator; increases acetylcholine and glutamate.
N-Acetylcysteine	Depression Obsessive-compulsive disorder	Amino acid that attenuates glutamatergic neurotransmission; used to augment SSRIs.
L-Tyrosine	Depression	Amino acid precursor to biogenic amines epinephrine and norepinephrine.
Glycine	Depression	Amino acid that activates N-methyl-D-aspartate (NMDA) receptors; may facilitate excitatory transmission in the brain.
Citicoline	Alzheimer disease Ischemic brain injury	Choline donor involved in synthesis of brain phospholipids and acetylcholine; 300–1,000 mg/day; may improve memory.
Acetyl-L-carnitine (Alcar)	Alzheimer disease Memory loss	Antioxidant that may prevent oxidative damage in the brain.

SSRIs, selective serotonin reuptake inhibitors.

Phytomedicinals

The term phytomedicinals (from the Greek *phyto,* meaning plant) refers to herb and plant preparations that are used or have been used for centuries for the treatment of a variety of medical conditions. Phytomedicinals are categorized as dietary supplements and not drug products. Therefore, they are exempt from the regulations that govern prescriptions and over-the-counter medications.

Manufacturers of phytomedicinals are not required to provide the FDA with safety information before marketing a product or give the FDA postmarketing safety reports. Thousands of herbal drugs are being marketed today; the most common with psychoactive properties are listed in Table 39-3. Many of the identified ingredients as well as their indications, adverse events, dosages, and comments are also listed. The latter category is particularly important considering the interactions with commonly prescribed drugs used in psychiatry. For example, St. John's wort (*wort* is an old English word meaning root or herb), which is used

Name	Ingredients	Use	Adverse Effects[a]	Interactions	Dosage[a]	Comments
Arctic weed, golden root	MAOI and b-endorphin	Anxiolytic, mood enhancer, antidepressant	No side effect yet documented in trials		100 mg BID–200 mg TID	Use caution with drugs that mimic MAOIs
Areca, areca nut, betel nut, L. *Areca catechu*	Arecoline, guvacoline	For alteration of consciousness to reduce pain and elevate mood	Parasympathomimetic overload: increased salivation, tremors, bradycardia, spasms, GI disturbances, ulcers of the mouth	Avoid with parasympathomimetic drugs; atropine-like compounds reduce effect	Undetermined; 8–10 g is toxic dose for humans	Used by chewing the nut; used in the past as a chewing balm for gum disease and as a vermifuge; long-term use may result in malignant tumors of the oral cavity
Ashwagandha	Also called Indian winter cherry or Indian ginseng, native to India. Flavonoids	Antioxidant, may decrease anxiety levels. Improved libido in men and women May lower levels of the stress hormone, cortisol	Drowsiness and sleepiness	None	Dosage is 1 tablet twice daily before meals with a gradual increase to 4 tablets per day	None
Belladonna, L. *Atropa belladonna*, deadly nightshade	Atropine, scopolamine, flavonoids[b]	Anxiolytic	Tachycardia, arrhythmias, xerostomia, mydriasis, difficulties with micturition and constipation	Synergistic with anticholinergic drugs; avoid with TCAs, amantadine, and quinidine	0.05–0.10 mg a day; maximum single dose is 0.20 mg BID	Has a strong smell, tastes sharp and bitter, and is poisonous
Biota, *Platycladus orientalis*	Plant derivative	Used as a sedative. Other uses are to treat heart palpitations, panic, night sweats, and constipation. May be useful in attention deficit hyperactivity disorder (ADHD)	No known adverse effects	None	No clearly established doses exist	None

TABLE 39-3: Phytomedicinals with Psychoactive Effects

Nutritional Supplements and Medical Foods

TABLE 39-3: Phytomedicinals with Psychoactive Effects (continued)						
Name	Ingredients	Use	Adverse Effects[a]	Interactions	Dosage[a]	Comments
Bitter orange flower, *Citrus aurantium*	Flavonoids, limonene	Sedative, anxiolytic, hypnotic	Photosensitization	Undetermined	Tincture, 2–3 g/day; drug, 4–6 g/day; extract, 1–2 g/day	Contradictory evidence; some refer to it as a gastric stimulant
Black cohosh, *L. Cimicifuga racemosa*	Triterpenes, isoferulic acid	For PMS, menopausal symptoms, dysmenorrhea	Weight gain, GI disturbances	Possible adverse interaction with male or female hormones	1–2 g/day; over 5 g can cause vomiting, headache, dizziness, cardiovascular collapse	Estrogen-like effects, questionable because root may act as an estrogen receptor blocker
Black haw, cramp bark, *L. Viburnum prunifolium*	Scopoletin, flavonoids, caffeic acids, triterpenes	Sedative, antispasmodic action on uterus; for dysmenorrhea	Undetermined	Anticoagulant-enhanced effects	1–3 g/day	Insufficient data
California poppy, *L. Eschscholtzia californica*	Isoquinoline alkaloids, cyanogenic glycosides	Sedative, hypnotic, anxiolytic; for depression	Lethargy	Combination of California poppy, valerian, St. John's wort, and passion flowers can result in agitation.	2 g/day	Clinical or experimental documentation of effects is unavailable
Casein	Casein peptides	Antistress agent. May improve sleep	Usually consumed through milk products. May interact with antihypertensive medicine and lower the blood pressure. May cause drowsiness and should be avoided when taking alcohol or benzodiazepines	None	1–2 tablets once or twice daily	

Catnip, L. Nepeta cataria	Valeric acid	Sedative, antispasmodic; for migraine	Headache, malaise, nausea, hallucinogenic effects	Undetermined	Undetermined	Delirium produced in children
Chamomile, L. Matricaria chamomilla	Flavonoids	Sedative, anxiolytic	Allergic reaction	Undetermined	2–4 g/day	Maybe GABAergic
Coastal water hyssop		Anxiolytic, sedative, epilepsy, asthma	Mild GI discomfort	May stimulate	300–450 mg QID	Insufficient data
Cordyceps sinensis	A genus of fungi that includes about 400 described species, found primarily in the high altitude of the Tibetan plateau in China. Antioxidant	Has been used for weakness, fatigue, to improve sexual drive in the elderly	GI discomfort, dry mouth, and nausea	None	Dosage in ranges of 3–6 g daily	None
Corydalis, L. Corydalis cava	Isoquinoline alkaloids	Sedative, antidepressant; for mild depression	Hallucination, lethargy	Undetermined	Undetermined	Clonic spasms and muscular tremor with overdose
Cyclamen, L. Cyclamen europaeum	Triterpene	Anxiolytic; for menstrual complaints	Small doses (e.g., 300 mg) can lead to nausea, vomiting, and diarrhea.	Undetermined	Undetermined	High doses can lead to respiratory collapse
Echinacea, L. Echinacea purpurea	Flavonoids, polysaccharides, caffeic acid derivatives, alkamides	Stimulates immune system; for lethargy, malaise, respiratory infections, and lower UTIs	Allergic reaction, fever, nausea, vomiting	Undetermined	1–3 g/day	Use in HIV and AIDS patients is controversial; may not be effective in coryza

(continued)

TABLE 39-3: Phytomedicinals with Psychoactive Effects (*continued*)

Name	Ingredients	Use	Adverse Effects[a]	Interactions	Dosage[a]	Comments
Ephedra, ma-huang *L. Ephedra sinica*	Ephedrine, pseudoephedrine	Stimulant; for lethargy, malaise, diseases of respiratory tract	Sympathomimetic overload: arrhythmias, increased BP, headache, irritability, nausea, vomiting	Synergistic with sympathomimetics, serotonergic agents; avoid with MAOIs	1–2 g/day	Tachyphylaxis and dependence can occur (taken off market)
Ginkgo, *L. Ginkgo biloba*	Flavonoids, ginkgolide A, B	Symptomatic relief of delirium, dementia; improves concentration and memory deficits; possible antidote to SSRI-induced sexual dysfunction	Allergic skin reactions, GI upset, muscle spasms, headache	Anticoagulant: use with caution because of its inhibitory effect on PAF; increased bleeding possible	120–240 mg/day	Studies indicate improved cognition in persons with Alzheimer disease after 4–5 weeks of use, possibly because of increased blood flow
Ginseng, *L. Panax ginseng*	Triterpenes, ginsenosides	Stimulant; for fatigue, elevation of mood, immune system	Insomnia, hypertonia, and edema (called Ginseng abuse syndrome)	Not to be used with sedatives, hypnotic agents, MAOIs, antidiabetic agents, or steroids	1–2 g/day	Several varieties exist; Korean (most highly valued), Chinese, Japanese, American (*Panax quinquefolius*)
Heather, *L. Calluna vulgaris*	Flavonoids, triterpenes	Anxiolytic, hypnotic	Undetermined	Undetermined	Undetermined	Efficacy for claimed uses is not documented
Holy Basil formula, *Ocimum tenuiflorum*	*Ocimum tenuiflorum*, an aromatic plant native to the tropics, part of the Lamiaceae family. Flavonoids	Used to combat stress, also used for common colds, headaches, stomach disorders, inflammation, heart disease	No data exists regarding the long-term effects. May prolong clotting time, increase the risk of bleeding during surgery and lower blood sugar	None	Dosage depends on the formulation type; recommended dose is 2 softgel capsules taken with 8-oz water daily	None

Name	Constituents	Uses/Action	Adverse Effects	Interactions	Dose	Comments
Hops, L. *Humulus lupulus*	Humulone, lupulone, flavonoids	Sedative, anxiolytic, hypnotic; for mood disturbances, restlessness	Contraindicated in patients with estrogen-dependent tumors (breast, uterine, cervical)	Hyperthermia effects with phenothiazine antipsychotics and with CNS depressants	0.5 g/day	May decrease plasma levels of drugs metabolized by CYP450 system
Horehound, L. *Ballota nigra*	Diterpenes, tannins	Sedative	Arrhythmias, diarrhea, hypoglycemia, possible spontaneous abortions	May enhance serotonergic drug effects, may augment hypoglycemic effects of drugs	1–4 g/day	May cause abortion
Jambolan, L. *Syzygium cumini*	Oleic acid, myristic acid, palmitic and linoleic acids, tannins	Anxiolytic, antidepressant	Undetermined	Undetermined	1–2 g/day	In folk medicine, a single dose is 30 seeds (1.9 g) of powder
Kanna, *Sceletium tortuosum*	Alkaloid, mesembrine	Anxiolytic, mood enhancer, empathogen, COPD treatment	Sedation, vivid dreams, headache	Potentiates cannabis, PDE inhibitor	50–100 mg QID	Insufficient data
Kava kava, L. *Piperis methysticum*	Kava lactones, kava pyrone	Sedative, hypnotic antispasmodic	Lethargy, impaired cognition, dermatitis with long-term usage, liver toxicity	Synergistic with anxiolytics, alcohol; avoid with levodopa and dopaminergic agents	600–800 mg/day	Maybe GABAergic; contraindicated in patients with endogenous depression; may increase the danger of suicide
Kratom, *Mitragyna speciosa*	Alkaloid	Stimulant and depressant	Priapism, testicular enlargement, withdrawal, depression, fatigue, insomnia	Structurally similar to yohimbine	Undetermined	Chewed, extracted into water, tar formulations
Lavender, L. *Lavandula angustifolia*	Hydroxycoumarin, tannins, caffeic acid	Sedative, hypnotic	Headache, nausea, confusion	Synergistic with other sedatives	3–5 g/day	May cause death in overdose

(continued)

TABLE 39-3: Phytomedicinals with Psychoactive Effects (*continued*)

Name	Ingredients	Use	Adverse Effects[a]	Interactions	Dosage[a]	Comments
Lemon balm, sweet Mary, *L. Melissa officinalis*	Flavonoids, caffeic acid, triterpenes	Hypnotic, anxiolytic, sedative	Undetermined	Potentiates CNS depressant; adverse reaction with thyroid hormone	8–10 g/day	Insufficient data
L-methylfolate	Folate is a B-vitamin found in some foods, needed to form healthy cells, especially red blood cells. L-methylfolate and levomefolate are names for the active form of folic acid.	Adjunctive L-methylfolate is used for major depression, not an antidepressant when used alone. Folate and L-methylfolate are also used to treat folic acid deficiency in pregnancy, to prevent spinal cord birth defects	GI side effects reported	None	15-mg, once a day by mouth with or without food	Considered a "medical food" by the FDA and only available by prescription. Safe to take during pregnancy when used as directed
Mistletoe, *L. Viscum album*	Flavonoids, triterpenes, lectins, polypeptides	Anxiolytic; for mental and physical exhaustion	Berries said to have emetic and laxative effects	Contraindicated in patients with chronic infections (e.g., TB)	10 mg per day	Berries have caused death in children
Mugwort, *L. Artemisia vulgaris*	Sesquiterpene lactones, flavonoids	Sedative, antidepressant, anxiolytic	Anaphylaxis, contact dermatitis, may cause hallucinations	Potentiates anticoagulants	5–15 g/day	May stimulate uterine contractions, can induce abortion
N-acetylcysteine (NAC)	Amino acid	Used as an antidote for acetaminophen overdose, augmentation of SSRIs in the treatment of trichotillomania	Rash, cramps, and angioedema may occur	Activated charcoal, ampicillin, carbamazepine, cloxacillin, oxacillin, nitroglycerin, and penicillin G	1,200–2,400 mg/day	Acts as an antioxidant and a glutamate-modulating agent. When used as an antidote for acetaminophen overdose, the doses 20–40 times higher than those used in OCD trials. It has not been shown to be effective in treating schizophrenia

Nux vomica, L. Strychnos nux vomica, poison nut	Indole alkaloids: strychnine and brucine, polysaccharides	Antidepressant; for migraine, menopausal symptoms	Convulsions, liver damage, death; severely toxic because of strychnine	Undetermined	0.02–0.05 g/day	Symptoms of poisoning can occur after ingestion of one bean; lethal dose is 1–2 g
Oats, L. Avena sativa	Flavonoids, oligo and polysaccharides	Anxiolytic, hypnotic; for stress, insomnia, opium, and tobacco withdrawal	Bowel obstruction or other bowel dysmotility syndromes, flatulence	Undetermined	3 g/day	Oats have sometimes been contaminated with aflatoxin, a fungal toxin linked with some cancers
Omega-3 fatty acid	Comes in three forms, eicosapentaenoic acid (EPA), docosahexaenoic acid (DHA), and alpha-linolenic acid (LNA)	Used as a supplement in the treatment of heart disease, high cholesterol, high blood pressure. May also be helpful in treatment of depression, b polar disorder, schizophrenia, and ADHD. May reduce the risk of ulcers when used in conjunction with NSAID pain relievers	Can cause gas, bloating, belching, and diarrhea	May increase effectiveness of blood thinners, may increase fasting blood sugar levels when used with diabetes medications, such as insulin and metformin.	Doses vary from 1–4 g/day	Can be contaminated with mercury and PCBs
Passion flower, L. Passiflora incarnata	Flavonoids, cyanogenic glycosides	Anxiolytic, sedative, hypnotic	Cognitive impairment	Undetermined	4–8 g/day	Overdose causes depression
Phosphatidylserine and Phosphatidylcholine	Phospholipids	Used for Alzheimer disease, age-related decline in mental function, improving thinking skills in young people, ADHD, depression, preventing exercise-induced stress, and improving athletic performance	Insomnia and stomach upset	None	100 mg three times daily	None

(continued)

TABLE 39-3: Phytomedicinals with Psychoactive Effects *(continued)*

Name	Ingredients	Use	Adverse Effects[a]	Interactions	Dosage[a]	Comments
Polygala	Polygala is a genus of about 500 species of *flowering plants* belonging to the family Polygalaceae, commonly known as milkwort or snakeroot.	Used for insomnia, forgetfulness, mental confusion, palpitation, seizures, anxiety, and listlessness	Contraindicated in patients who have ulcers or gastritis, should not be used long term	None	Dosage of polygala is 1.5–3 g of dried root, 1.5–3 g of a fluid extract or 2.5–7.5 g of a tincture. A polygala tea can also be made, with a maximum of three cups per day.	None
Rehmannia	Iridoid glycosides	Stimulates the release of cortisol. Used in lupus, rheumatoid arthritis (RA), fibromyalgia, and multiple sclerosis. May improve asthma and urticaria. Used to treat menopause, hair loss, and impotence	Loose bowel movements, bloating, nausea, and abdominal cramps	None	Exact dosage unknown	None
Rhodiola rosea	Potentiator, monoterpene alcohols, flavonoids					
S-adenosyl methionine (SAMe)	S-adenosyl methionine (SAMe)	Used for arthritis and fibromyalgia, may be effective as an augmentation strategy for SSRI in depression	GI symptoms, anxiety, nightmares, insomnia, and worsening of Parkinson symptoms	Use with SSRIs or SNRIs may result in serotonin syndrome. Interacts with levodopa, meperidine, pentazocine, and tramadol	400–1,600 mg/day	A naturally occurring molecule made from the amino acid methionine and ATP, serves as a methyl donor in human cellular metabolism

Scarlet Pimpernel, L. Anagallis arvensis	Flavonoids, triterpenes, cucurbitacins, caffeic acids	Antidepressant	Overdose or long-term doses may lead to gastroenteritis and nephritis	Undetermined	1.8 g of powder four times a day	Flowers are poisonous
Skullcap, L. Scutellaria lateriflora	Flavonoid, monoterpenes	Anxiolytic, sedative, hypnotic	Cognitive impairment, hepatotoxicity	Disulfiram-like reaction may occur if used with alcohol	1–2 g/day	Little information exists to support the use of this herb in humans
St. John's wort, L. Hypericum perforatum	Hypericin, flavonoids, xanthones	Antidepressant, sedative, anxiolytic	Headaches, photosensitivity (may be severe), constipation	Report of manic reaction when used with sertraline (Zoloft); do not combine with SSRIs or MAOIs; possible serotonin syndrome; do not use with alcohol, opioids	100–950 mg/day	Under investigation by the NIH; may act as MAOI or SSRI; 4- to 6-week trial for mild depressive moods; if no apparent improvement, another therapy should be tried
Strawberry leaf, L. Fragaria vesca	Flavonoids, tannins	Anxiolytic	Contraindicated with strawberry allergy	Undetermined	1 g/day	Little information exists to support the use of this herb in humans.
Tarragon, L. Artemisia dracunculus	Flavonoids, hydroxycoumarins	Hypnotic, appetite stimulant	Undetermined	Undetermined	Undetermined	Little information exists to support the use of this herb in humans
Valerian, L. Valeriana officinalis	Valepotriates, valerenic acid, caffeic acid	Sedative, muscle relaxant, hypnotic	Cognitive and motor impairment, GI upset, hepatotoxicity; long-term use: contact allergy, headache, restlessness, insomnia, mydriasis, cardiac dysfunction	Avoid concomitant use with alcohol or CNS depressants	1–2 g/day	Maybe chemically unstable

(continued)

TABLE 39-3: Phytomedicinals with Psychoactive Effects (*continued*)

Name	Ingredients	Use	Adverse Effects[a]	Interactions	Dosage[a]	Comments
Wild lettuce, *Lactuca, Virosa*	Flavonoids, coumarins, lactones	Sedative, anesthetic, galactagogue	Tachycardia, tachypnea, visual disturbance, diaphoresis		Undetermined	Bitter taste, added to salad or drinks, active compound closely resembles opium
Winter cherry, *Withania, somnifera*	Alkaloids, steroidal lactones	Sedative, treatment for arthritis, possible anticarcinogenic	Thyrotoxicosis, unfavorable effects on heart and adrenal gland		Undetermined	Smoke inhaled

[a]There are no reliable, consistent, or valid data exist on dosages or adverse effects of most phytomedicinals.

[b]Flavonoids are common to many herbs. They are plant byproducts that act as antioxidants (i.e., agents that prevent the deterioration of material such as DNA via oxidation).

ATP, adenosine triphosphate; BID, twice a day; BP, blood pressure; CNS, central nervous system; COPD, chronic obstructive pulmonary disease; GABA, gamma-aminobutyric acid; GI, gastrointestinal; MAOI, monoamine oxidase inhibitor; NIH, National Institutes of Health; NSAID, nonsteroidal anti-inflammatory drug; OCD, obsessive-compulsive disorder; PAF, platelet-activating factor; PDE, phosphodiesterase; PMS, premenstrual syndrome; QID, four times a day; SSRI, selective serotonin reuptake inhibitor; TB, tuberculosis; TCA, tricyclic antidepressant; TID, three times a day; UTI, urinary tract infection.

to treat depression, decreases the effectiveness of certain psychotropic drugs such as amitriptyline, alprazolam, paroxetine, and sertraline, among others. Kava kava, which is used to treat anxiety, has been associated with liver toxicity.

Adverse Effects

Adverse effects are possible, and toxic interactions with other drugs may occur with all phytomedicinals, dietary supplements, and medicinal foods. There are few or no consistent standard preparations available for most herbs. Medical foods are not tested by the FDA, even if strict voluntary compliance is required. Moreover, safety profiles and knowledge of adverse effects of most of these substances have not been studied rigorously. Adulteration is also possible, especially with phytomedicinals.

Because of the lack of standardization and paucity of clinical trials, all these agents should be avoided during pregnancy. Because most of these substances or their metabolites are secreted in breast milk, they are contraindicated during lactation.

Clinicians should always attempt to obtain a history of herbal use or the use of medical foods or nutritional supplements during the psychiatric evaluation, and it is important to be nonjudgmental in dealing with patients who use these substances. Many do so for various reasons: (1) As part of their cultural tradition, (2) because they mistrust physicians or are dissatisfied with conventional medicine, or (3) because they experience relief of symptoms with the particular substance. It is more likely for patients to be cooperative with traditional psychiatric treatments if they are allowed to continue using their preparations, psychiatrists should try to keep an open mind and not attribute all effects to suggestion. If psychotropic agents are prescribed, the clinician must be extraordinarily alert to the possibility of adverse effects as a result of drug–drug interactions because many of these compounds have ingredients that produce actual physiologic changes in the body. Patients should be educated about these concerns and potential adverse effects.

40 Assessment and Treatment of Obesity and Metabolic Syndrome

Introduction

Patients with psychiatric illnesses are at an increased risk of being overweight with higher rates of cardiovascular and metabolic disorders such as type 2 diabetes and hyperlipidemia. Obesity and metabolic syndrome are associated phenomena that can impact patient quality of life and adversely affect overall health, particularly in patients with schizophrenia, who already have a 20% shorter lifespan compared to the general population. As a result, assessment of physical health is imperative in this population.

Genetics, lifestyle, and medications, all contribute to these conditions and clinicians should be vigilant in assessing for these risk factors. It is important to obtain baseline tests, coordinate with medical experts, and intervene at the earliest point in time.

Patients with obesity are also at a greater risk of developing conditions like hypertension, sleep apnea, gallstones, osteoarthritis, stroke, and certain types of cancer (e.g., gall bladder, breast, colon, endometrial). Obesity is also associated with decreased sexual function, impaired fertility, menstrual abnormalities, and increased pregnancy risks. In addition to physiologic effects, obesity can lead to sociologic and psychological challenges, as people who are obese may face prejudices in multiple domains. For those who find solace in food or cope with difficult emotional situations by overeating, this may perpetuate a cycle that both worsens their mental health and leads to further weight gain.

Obese patients—particularly patients with excessive abdominal fat—are also at a greater risk of developing metabolic syndrome, which is more commonly precipitated by unhealthy behaviors, particularly a sedentary lifestyle and/or lack of exercise; insufficient sleep; chronic stress; and unhealthy diet. Without corrective action, patients may go on to develop type 2 diabetes, as well as a host of chronic inflammatory disorders.

From a clinical standpoint, the dangers of obesity and metabolic syndrome are relevant to psychiatry because some medications can lead to weight gain and increased risk of metabolic syndrome, which is twofold higher in patients with schizophrenia. There also appears to be a bidirectional relationship between type 2 diabetes and psychiatric illnesses, particularly schizophrenia, bipolar disorder, and depression. People with type 2 diabetes are two to four times more likely to have these disorders than people without diabetes. Moreover, depression is a significant predictor of rapid weight gain, with a fivefold increase a year later compared to baseline. Depression is also associated with inflammation, abdominal fat, and insulin resistance. In addition, certain features of psychiatric illnesses appear to exacerbate the underlying causes of metabolic syndrome and diabetes mellitus, most notably sleep disturbances, autonomic hyperactivation, increased psychological stress, and excessive drug and alcohol use. It is also

TABLE 40-1: Percentage Body Fat Ranges

	Women	Men
Essential fat	10–13%	2–5%
Athlete	13–20%	5–13%
Fit	20–25%	13–18%
Acceptable	25–30%	18–25%
Obese	30–40%	25–35%
Morbidly obese	>40%	>35%

relevant because the challenges of being obese and/or struggling with metabolic syndrome can affect patients' mental health.

Definitions

Obesity

Obesity is defined as abnormal or excessive fat accumulation (see Table 40-1). In healthy men, body fat may account for between 5% and 25% of total weight. Obesity is defined as having a body weight that is composed of above 26% body fat. In healthy women, body fat may account for between 10% and 31% of total weight. Obesity is defined as having a body weight that is composed of above 32% body fat.

Body Mass Index

A healthy body mass index (BMI) for an adult can range from 18.5 to 25 kg/m^2, while a BMI out of this range signifies that a person is either underweight or overweight (see Table 40-2). BMI is a poor tool in assessing obesity since it does not take body composition (muscle, fat, and water content) into account, meaning an obese person with a high percentage of body fat and a professional bodybuilder with high muscle mass can have the same BMI.

Metabolic Syndrome

Metabolic syndrome is a constellation of metabolic abnormalities strongly associated with obesity, poor glucose tolerance, and insulin resistance. While not a disease in itself, metabolic syndrome is diagnosed when a patient presents with three or more of the following:

- Abdominal obesity (BMI >30 kg/m^2) and/or a waistline of 40 inches or more for men or 35 inches for women

TABLE 40-2: Body Mass Index Ranges (kg/m^2)

Underweight	<18.5
Healthy weight	18.5–25
Overweight	25–30
Obesity	>30

- High triglyceride levels (≥150 mg/dL or ≥1.7 mmol/L)
- Low high-density lipoprotein (HDL) cholesterol levels (≤40 mg/dL for men; ≤50 mg/dL for women)
- Hypertension (≥130/85 mm Hg)
- Elevated fasting blood glucose levels/impaired glucose tolerance (≥100 mg/dL)

Approximately 30% of adults in the United States are believed to meet criteria for metabolic syndrome. Clinicians should be aware that patients who are prescribed certain psychiatric drugs, especially some atypical antipsychotics (noted below), may experience weight gain, which may put them at increased risk of developing metabolic syndrome and some of the myriad conditions with which it is associated, including cardiovascular diseases, coagulopathy, abnormalities of uric acid metabolism, nonalcoholic fatty liver disease, cognitive decline, and cancer. Rapid weight gain is also associated with increased abdominal circumference, high fasting glucose, hypertriglyceridemia, and high diastolic blood pressure. Many of these conditions can significantly impact quality of life or prove fatal.

Epidemiology

As of 2018, it is estimated that 73.1% of adults over 20 years of age in the United States have a BMI above the healthy range, while 42.4% are obese. As Tables 40-3, 40-4, and 40-5 reveal, these figures have been steadily rising since at least the late 1990s for men and women.

Etiology

There is no one cause for obesity or metabolic disorders. Typically, weight gain occurs following increased caloric intake, decreased energy expenditure, or a

TABLE 40-3: Percentage of Overweight, Obese, and Severely Obese Adults Over 20 Years of Age in the United States, 1999–2018

Survey Period	Above Healthy Weight	Overweight	Obese	Severely Obese
1999–2000	64.5	34.0 (1.0)	30.5 (1.5)	4.7 (0.6)
2001–2002	65.6	35.1 (1.1)	30.5 (1.5)	5.1 (0.5)
2003–2004	66.3	34.1 (1.1)	32.2 (1.2)	4.8 (0.6)
2005–2006	66.9	32.6 (0.8)	34.3 (1.4)	5.9 (0.5)
2007–2008	68.0	34.3 (0.8)	33.7 (1.1)	5.7 (0.4)
2009–2010	68.7	33.0 (1.0)	35.7 (0.9)	6.3 (0.2)
2011–2012	68.5	33.6 (1.3)	34.9 (1.4)	6.4 (0.6)
2013–2014	70.2	32.5 (0.8)	37.7 (0.9)	7.7 (0.7)
2015–2016	71.2	31.6 (0.8)	39.6 (1.6)	7.7 (0.6)
2017–2018	73.1	30.7 (1.1)	42.4 (1.8)	9.2 (0.9)

Severely obese individuals included as both "obese" and within a separate subset of "severely obese."
Data from Fryar CD, Carroll MD, Afful J. Prevalence of overweight, obesity, and severe obesity among adults aged 20 and over: United States, 1960–1962 through 2017–2018. NCHS Health E-Stats. 2020.

TABLE 40-4: Percentage of Overweight, Obese, and Severely Obese Men Over 20 Years of Age in the United States, 1999–2018

Survey Period	Above Healthy Weight	Overweight	Obese	Severely Obese
1999–2000	67.2	39.7 (1.4)	27.5 (1.5)	3.1 (0.7)
2001–2002	69.9	42.2 (1.3)	27.7 (1.0)	3.6 (0.6)
2003–2004	70.8	39.7 (1.5)	31.1 (1.3)	2.8 (0.4)
2005–2006	73.2	39.9 (1.3)	33.3 (2.0)	4.2 (0.5)
2007–2008	72.3	40.1 (1.4)	32.2 (1.4)	4.2 (0.5)
2009–2010	73.9	38.4 (1.1)	35.5 (1.7)	4.4 (0.3)
2011–2012	71.3	37.8 (1.5)	33.5 (1.4)	4.4 (0.9)
2013–2014	73.7	38.7 (1.2)	35.0 (1.1)	5.5 (0.6)
2015–2016	74.4	36.5 (1.6)	37.9 (2.7)	5.6 (0.7)
2017–2018	77.1	34.1 (1.8)	43.0 (2.7)	6.9 (1.0)

Severely obese individuals included as both "obese" and within a separate subset of "severely obese."
Data from Fryar CD, Carroll MD, Afful J. Prevalence of overweight, obesity, and severe obesity among adults aged 20 and over: United States, 1960–1962 through 2017–2018. NCHS Health E-Stats. 2020.

combination of the two. In addition, patients with psychiatric disorders are more likely to eat unhealthily and remain inactive, which may be a function of the underlying disorder, as well as a side effect of the medications. Consequently, several psychiatric disorders may drive individuals to behave in ways that are likely to lead to obesity (see Table 40-6).

In addition, dysfunction in the signaling of certain neurotransmitters may lead to abnormalities in feeding behavior. In particular, serotonin, dopamine, and norepinephrine have been implicated in the control of satiety.

TABLE 40-5: Percentage of Overweight, Obese, and Severely Obese Women Over 20 Years of Age in the United States, 1999–2018

Survey Period	Above Healthy Weight	Overweight	Obese	Severely Obese
1999–2000	62.0	28.6 (1.6)	33.4 (1.7)	6.2 (0.7)
2001–2002	61.4	28.2 (1.7)	33.2 (1.5)	6.5 (0.6)
2003–2004	61.8	28.6 (1.2)	33.2 (1.7)	6.9 (0.9)
2005–2006	60.8	25.5 (1.2)	35.3 (1.4)	7.4 (0.7)
2007–2008	64.0	28.6 (1.2)	35.4 (1.1)	7.3 (0.6)
2009–2010	63.7	27.9 (1.4)	35.8 (0.9)	8.1 (0.5)
2011–2012	67.8	29.7 (1.8)	36.1 (1.7)	8.3 (0.7)
2013–2014	66.9	26.5 (0.8)	40.4 (1.3)	9.9 (0.9)
2015–2016	68.0	26.9 (1.0)	41.1 (1.6)	9.7 (0.7)
2017–2018	69.4	27.5 (1.0)	41.9 (2.0)	11.5 (1.3)

Severely obese individuals included as both "obese" and within a separate subset of "severely obese."
Data from Fryar CD, Carroll MD, Afful J. Prevalence of overweight, obesity, and severe obesity among adults aged 20 and over: United States, 1960–1962 through 2017–2018. NCHS Health E-Stats. 2020.

TABLE 40-6: Disorders Capable of Causing Obesity
Agoraphobia
Cushing syndrome
Depressive disorders
Fröhlich syndrome
Growth hormone deficiency
Hypogonadism
Hypothalamic syndrome
Hypothyroidism
Insulinoma and hyperinsulinism
Myxedema
Neuroendocrine obesities
Polycystic ovarian syndrome (Stein–Leventhal syndrome)
Prader–Willi syndrome
Pseudohypoparathyroidism

Stress is also associated with weight gain. On the one hand, it can modify dietary preferences (leading to what is colloquially known as "stress eating"), encourage alcohol consumption, and affect sleep patterns. On the other, psychological stress is associated with hormonal dysfunction, cytokine release, and other physiologic mechanisms that can contribute to weight gain and the redistribution of fat to the abdominal region.

Tobacco Cessation

Given the numerous risks associated with tobacco and the synergy of risks for those who use tobacco and are obese, clinicians should always advise patients to give up tobacco use. However, tobacco cessation is associated with weight gain if other lifestyle adjustments are not made.

Medications

Iatrogenic obesity can arise following the use of several medications for psychiatric conditions, particularly major depression, psychotic disturbances, and bipolar disorder (see Table 40-7). Long-term use of steroid medications and many oral hypoglycemics may also lead to weight gain. Other iatrogenic cardiometabolic risks associated with psychiatric medications are noted in Table 40-8. Therefore, patients should be screened for certain risk factors (see Table 40-9) before being prescribed psychiatric medications. Clinicians should obtain baseline measurements of:

- Weight
- Waist circumference
- Pulse
- Blood pressure
- Fasting blood glucose
- Hemoglobin A1c
- Blood lipid profile

TABLE 40-7: Medications with Potential to Increase Weight Gain and Increased Appetite

	Greatest	Intermediate	Least	Weight Loss Possible
Antidepressant drugs	Amitriptyline (Elavil)	Doxepin (Adapin, Sinequan) Imipramine (Tofranil) Mirtazapine (Remeron) Nortriptyline (Pamelor) Phenelzine (Nardil) Trimipramine (Surmontil)	Amoxapine (Asendin) Bupropion (Wellbutrin) Desipramine (Norpramin) Fluoxetine (Prozac) Sertraline (Zoloft) Tranylcypromine (Parnate) Trazodone (Desyrel) Venlafaxine (Effexor)	Bupropion (Wellbutrin) Fluoxetine (Prozac) Sertraline (Zoloft) Venlafaxine (Effexor)
Mood stabilizers	Lithium (Eskalith) Valproic acid (Depakene)	Carbamazepine (Tegretol)	Topiramate (Topamax)	
Antipsychotic drugs	Chlorpromazine (Thorazine) Clozapine (Clozaril) Mesoridanazine (Serentil) Olanzapine (Zyprexa) Quetiapine (Seroquel) Risperidone (Risperdal) Thioridazine (Mellaril)	Fluphenazine (Permitil, Prolixin) Haloperidol (Haldol) Perphenazine (Trilafon) Trifluoperazine (Stelazine) Thiothixene (Navane)	Aripiprazole (Abilify) Asenapine (Saphris) Molindone (Moban) Ziprasidone (Geodon)	Molindone (Moban)

If prescribing risperidone or paliperidone, prolactin levels should also be measured. Clinicians should also inquire about any movement disorders, diet, and level of physical activity at baseline and potentially make recommendations based on this information.

TABLE 40-8: Medications Associated Cardiometabolic Risks

	Dyslipidemia	Diabetes Mellitus/Insulin Resistance	Hypertension
Antidepressant drugs	Mirtazapine (Remeron) SSRIs	Tricyclic antidepressants	SNRIs Tricyclic antidepressants
Mood stabilizers	Valproic acid (Depakene)	Valproic acid (Depakene)	Valproic acid (Depakene)
Antipsychotic drugs	Clozapine (Clozaril) Olanzapine (Zyprexa)	Some first-generation antipsychoticsSecond-generation antipsychotics, particularly: • Clozapine (Clozaril) • Olanzapine (Zyprexa)	Aripiprazole (Abilify) Clozapine (Clozaril) Olanzapine (Zyprexa) Ziprasidone (Geodon)

SNRIs, Serotonin-norepinephrine reuptake inhibitors; SSRIs, Selective serotonin reuptake inhibitors

TABLE 40-9: Conditions to Screen for Prior to Prescribing Antipsychotics
Cardiovascular disease
Diabetes mellitus
Dyslipidemia
Hypertension
Family history of obesity
Personal history of obesity

Before prescribing psychotropic medication, and particularly atypical antipsychotics, clinicians should obtain the baseline measurements described in Tables 40-10 and 40-11, and then at subsequent appointments. Clinicians need not strictly adhere to any one guideline when monitoring a patient's progress. Rather, they should create a framework tailored to suit the individual patient.

Effects on Health—Metabolic Syndrome and Beyond

Being sensitive to, fighting against, and working to prevent discrimination against people with obesity is both admirable and necessary. The primary goal of any weight management intervention should always be to promote wellness, and to prevent, reverse, or stay the progression of metabolic syndrome, as well as the several types of conditions and diseases that obesity can exacerbate (see Table 40-12). These strategies can both prolong patients' lives and improve the quality of their lives.

TABLE 40-10: American Psychiatric Association's Recommended Monitoring for Patients Prescribed Atypical Antipsychotics							
Measure	Baseline	Initial 4 Weeks	Initial 8 Weeks	Initial 12 Weeks	Initial 16 Weeks	Quarterly	Annually
Body mass index, weight, height	X	X	X	X	X	X	X
Waist circumference							
Blood pressure[a]	X						
Fasting plasma glucose	X				X		X
Fasting lipid panel[b]	X						
Personal/family history	X						

[a]As clinically indicated, particularly as prescription doses are titrated.
[b]At least every 5 years.
Data from American Psychiatric Association's Recommended Monitoring for Patients Prescribed Atypical Antipsychotics, Third Edition.

TABLE 40-11: Mt. Sinai Recommended Monitoring for Patients Prescribed Atypical Antipsychotics

Measure	Baseline	Initial 4 Weeks	Initial 8 Weeks	Initial 12 Weeks	Initial 16 Weeks	Quarterly	Annually
Body mass index, weight, height	X	X	X	X	X	X	X
Waist circumference	X	X	X	X	X	X	X
Blood pressure							
Fasting plasma glucose[a]	X				X		X
Fasting lipid panel[b]	X						
Personal/family history	X						

[a]For patients at risk of developing diabetes mellitus, 4 months after starting, then annually.
[b]At least every 2 years when LDL-C is within normal range or every 6 months when LDL-C is >130 mg/dL (3.37 mmol/L).
Data from Lehman AF, Lieberman JA, Dixon LB, et al. Practice guideline for the treatment of patients with schizophrenia, second edition. *Am J Psychiatry*. 2004;161(2 Suppl):1–56.

TABLE 40-12: Selected List of Health Disorders Exacerbated by Obesity

Heart	Angina pectoris Congestive heart failure Left ventricular hypertrophy Premature coronary heart disease Right ventricular hypertrophy Ventricular arrhythmia
Vascular system	Arteriovenous fistula Carotid artery stenosis Carotid-cavernous fistula Hypertension Transient ischemic attack and stroke Venous stasis
Respiratory system	Obstructive sleep apnea Pickwickian syndrome (alveolar hypoventilation) Secondary polycythemia
Hepatobiliary system	Cholecystitis Cholelithiasis Hepatic steatosis
Hormonal and metabolic functions	Diabetes mellitus Gout Hyperlipidemia Hypertriglyceridemia

TABLE 40-12: Selected List of Health Disorders Exacerbated by Obesity *(continued)*	
Kidney	Proteinuria
	Renal vein thrombosis
Joints, muscles, and connective tissue	Bone spurs
	Chronic pain
	Osteoarthritis
	Osteoarthrosis
Cancers	Biliary passages
	Breast
	Cervix
	Colon
	Endometrium
	Gallbladder
	Ovary
	Prostate
	Rectum

Assessment and Interventions When Prescribing Psychotropic Medications

Clinicians should intervene early to prevent subsequent complications including weight gain, obesity, high blood sugar, and hyperlipidemia, which may occur as a result of psychotropic medication. Clinicians should explain these risks to the patient, as well as the need for regular monitoring. Various clinical guidelines have been established for monitoring patients, specifically those on atypical antipsychotics. Regardless of the medication class, patients with hereditary risk factors or those prescribed medicines with weight gain potential should be monitored for the length of the treatment. It is important to plan a strategy prior to initiation of the treatment to prevent subsequent weight gain and metabolic disorders.

Mental health professionals should coordinate with the patient's primary care provider to communicate any relevant abnormal tests and discuss treatment changes and necessary interventions. Strategies that help patients maintain a healthy weight should include reducing caloric intake, eliminating processed foods, increasing the consumption of nutrient-dense foods, lifestyle changes, getting regular exercise, and incorporating stress management as core components. An appropriate initial goal may be to lose 5% to 10% of one's baseline weight over the course of 3 to 6 months or a loss of 0.5% to 1% of one's baseline weight each week. More aggressive interventions may be warranted if these first-line therapies are not successful and include pharmacotherapy and surgery.

Patients with chronic mental disorders have difficulty ascribing to strict guidelines regarding diet and exercise and consequently may require other strategies, including medication adjustment or weight loss medicines in addition to psychotropics. The following strategies can be utilized to assist patients who are struggling with weight gain and related medical complications:

- Ask for support from friends and family
- Get a full night of sleep

- Drink plenty of water (3.7 L for men; 2.7 L for women)
- Limit sugar intake
- Keep a food journal and monitor diet
- Change diet to incorporate more fruits and nonstarchy vegetables
- Do at least 30 minutes of cardiovascular exercise five times per week
- Add strength-training exercises to fitness routine

Diet

Specific strategies for diet should be tailored to the patient. In some cases, a low-calorie diet, where caloric intake is limited to between 1,200 and 1,500 calories per day, may be beneficial in reducing weight, but may not be manageable if it is too restrictive. Many elimination diets, particularly those that are very low in sugars and complex carbohydrates, can produce very swift reductions in weight. However, they are very difficult to maintain regardless of whether one decides to follow a ketogenic, paleo, raw food, or carnivore diet. As maintenance is key to any weight management program, these diets should not be regularly encouraged. Moreover, the data on the benefits and risks of these types of diets remain limited. The strongest available evidence suggests that severely limiting heavily processed foods that contain added preservatives, sugars, fats, and salts is always good, and that patients should strive to eat a wide variety of whole grains, legumes, vegetables, fruits, nuts, seeds, fish, lean meats, and fermented foods.

Lifestyle Changes

Lifestyle changes are also encouraged. These include major changes, such as quitting the use of tobacco products and limiting alcohol consumption, as well as minor ones that address behaviors during meals and eating cues. For a partial list of such modifications, see Table 40-13.

TABLE 40-13: Behavioral Modifications	
Modify eating behavior during a meal	Eat slowly, savoring each mouthful
	Chew each bite 30 times before swallowing
	Put the fork down between bites
	Intermittently delay eating for 2–3 minutes and converse
	Serve food on a smaller plate
	Divide portions in half so that another portion may be permitted
Modify behavior before/after a meal	Stock home with healthier food choices
	Grocery shop following a full meal
	Plan meals ahead of time
	Keep a food diary to link eating with hunger and nonhunger episodes
	Postpone a snack for 10 minutes
Eliminate eating cues	Eat only at one designated location
	Leave the table immediately after the meal
	Do not combine other activities with eating
	Substitute other activities for snacking
	Do not leave unhealthy food in the open

Exercise

Increased physical activity and exercise is vital for caloric expenditure and any weight management regimen. While it is difficult to overcome the inertia resulting from a sedentary lifestyle, or drug-induced fatigue and sedation, those who do begin exercising and making dietary changes will likely experience weight loss. This often encourages them to overcome the inertia and to maintain an increasingly rigorous exercise regimen. For many, simply walking and taking 8,000 to 10,000 steps a day would suffice in terms of physical activity.

Stress Management

Stress management can help encourage patients to maintain an exercise regimen, a healthier diet, and certain lifestyle changes. Stress management may also promote more restful sleep. Examples of stress management include mindfulness meditation, yoga, breathing exercises, and light exercise.

Psychotherapy

In some cases, psychotherapy may help patients stay motivated and address the sources of pathologic associations with food. Behavior modification is the most common therapeutic approach and has demonstrated some success. Patients are advised to monitor their eating behavior to uncover external cues, emotional states, or circumstances that trigger compulsive feeding behaviors. This practice can help patients develop new eating patterns. Group therapy may also help some patients feel encouraged as they work to make lifestyle changes. Any form of psychotherapy without concurrent treatment modalities rarely alters patient behavior and, therefore, is not recommended.

Pharmacotherapy

Several pharmaceuticals have been developed for the treatment of obesity, as noted in Table 40-14. Many drugs may also be used off-label to produce similar

TABLE 40-14: FDA-Approved Medications for the Treatment of Obesity

Generic Name	Trade Name(s)
Benzphetamine	Didrex
Diethylpropion	Tenuate
Liraglutide	Saxenda
Naltrexone HCl/Bupropion HCl	Contrave
Orlistat	Xenical, Alli
Phendimetrazine	Bontril PDM, Adipost, Phendiet, Statobex
Phentermine	Adipex-P
Phentermine resin	Ionamin
Phentermine-topiramate	Qsymia
Semaglutide	Wegovy, Ozempic

TABLE 40-15: Non–FDA-Approved Medications for the Treatment of Obesity	
Name	Trade Name(s)
Amphetamine and dextroamphetamine	Adderall
Metformin	Glucophage
Topiramate	Topamax
Zonisamide	Zonegran
Naltrexone	Vivitrol, Reviva
Amantadine	Gocovri

effects (see Table 40-15). Virtually all drugs mentioned in the two tables suppress appetite with the notable exception of orlistat (Xenical), which is a selective gastric and pancreatic lipase inhibitor that prevents the full absorption of dietary fat.

While efficacy may vary from patient to patient, it should be stressed that pharmaceuticals should be used in conjunction with interventions already noted. Patients can quickly gain a tolerance to many of these drugs within just a few weeks, thereby nullifying their benefits in reducing caloric intake. An initial trial period of 4 weeks with any specific drug is recommended. If effective, its use can be continued for a longer time until the desired weight is achieved or until tolerance is developed.

Numerous medications are used for weight loss strategy and include both Food and Drug Administration (FDA) approved as well as some for off-label use. Clinicians need to assess each patient's needs and individualize treatment considering risk factors, current medications, and long-term effects. When using off-label medicines, clinicians should discuss the off-label use, explain risks and benefits, and document this appropriately. Clinicians can familiarize themselves with these medicines in more detail by reviewing the chapter entitled Weight Loss Drugs.

Surgery

In some cases, patients may benefit from bariatric surgeries that reduce the size of the stomach (gastric bypass) or slow the passage of food into the stomach (gastroplasty). Side effects of these procedures include vomiting, electrolyte imbalance, and discomfort. Procedures like lipectomy and liposuction, where adipose tissue is removed, may have a temporary effect on weight, but do not address the underlying cause of the obesity. Surgery of any kind is often seen as a last resort when safer, more conventional options have been exhausted.

Conclusion

Obesity and metabolic syndrome have long been known to exacerbate risks to patients' cardiovascular health. However, these conditions can also affect patients' mental health in a variety of ways. Patients who can lose weight are more likely to adhere to psychotropic medication. Consequently, clinicians should encourage interventions and lifestyle modifications for better weight management not as a means of making cosmetic changes, but to promote optimal health.

41 Weight Loss Drugs

Generic Name	Trade Name	Adverse Effects	Drug Interactions	CYP Interactions
FDA Approved				
Phentermine	Adipex-P	Dizziness, GI symptoms	MAOI, insulin, guanethidine	3A4
Phentermine-topiramate	Qsymia	Cardiac arrhythmia, dizziness, GI symptoms, memory impairment, sedation, cognitive problems	MAOI, insulin, guanethidine, anticonvulsants, carbonic anhydrase inhibitors	3A4, 2C19
Phentermine resin	Ionamin	Dizziness, GI symptoms, sedation	MAOI, insulin, guanethidine	3A4
Phendimetrazine	Bontril PDM, Adipost, Phendiet, Statobex	Dizziness, GI symptoms, sexual dysfunction, confusion, cardiac arrhythmia	MAOI, alcohol, insulin, guanethidine, oral hypoglycemic agents	N/A
Diethylpropion	Tenuate	Dizziness, sedation, tremors, GI symptoms, tachycardia, skin rash, swelling	MAOI	N/A
Orlistat	Xenical, Alli	GI symptoms, liver injury	Cyclosporine, amiodarone	3A4
Benzphetamine	Didrex	Dizziness, GI symptoms	MAOI	3A4, 2B6
Liraglutide	Saxenda	GI symptoms, headache, acute pancreatitis	GLP-1 agonists,	N/A
Naltrexone HCl/ Bupropion HCl	Contrave	GI symptoms, insomnia, dizziness, headache, fatigue, skin rash	Opioids, DRA, disulfiram	2B6
Semaglutide	Wegovy, Ozempic	Suicidality, GI symptoms	N/A	N/A
Amphetamine	Evekeo	Cardiac arrhythmia, GI symptoms, agitation, insomnia, dyskinesia	MAOI, TRI/TETR, warfarin, primidone, phenobarbital, phenytoin, phenylbutazone	2D6, 2A6
Non-FDA Approved				
Topiramate	Topamax	Cardiac arrhythmia, dizziness, memory impairment, sedation, cognitive problems	Anticonvulsants, carbonic anhydrase inhibitors	3A4, 2C19
Zonisamide	Zonegran	GI symptoms, dizziness, sedation, mood swings, memory impairment, skin rash	Carbonic anhydrase inhibitors	3A

Generic Name	Trade Name	Adverse Effects	Drug Interactions	CYP Interactions
Metformin	Glucophage	GI symptoms, headache, lactic acidosis	N/A	N/A
Amphetamine and dextroam-phetamine	Adderall	Cardiac arrhythmia, GI symptoms, agitation, insomnia, dyskinesia	MAOI, TRI/TETR, warfarin, primidone, phenobarbital, phenytoin, phenylbutazone	2D6, 2A6
Naltrexone	Vivitrol, Reviva	GI symptoms, insomnia, dizziness, fatigue, headache, rash	Opioids, DRA, disulfiram	N/A
Amantadine	Gocovri	Dizziness, insomnia, agitation, seizures, GI symptoms, skin rash	Anticholinergics, stimulants, MAOI	N/A
Tirzepatide	Mounjaro	GI symptoms	None	N/A

Introduction

Patients with psychiatric disorders are more likely to struggle with weight gain and obesity. This is either due to poor self-care or as a side effect of psychotropic drug treatment and may lead to noncompliance resulting in relapse and hospitalization. Apart from negatively affecting self-esteem, it can also induce or exacerbate medical conditions such as hypertension, diabetes mellitus, and hyperlipidemia. Effects on body weight, glucose, and lipid regulation need to be taken into consideration when selecting medications. Unfortunately, with few exceptions, most psychotropic drugs used to manage mood disorders, anxiety disorders, and psychosis significantly increase the risk of weight gain, and are a common cause of treatment refusal or discontinuation. Consequently, it is important for clinicians to be well informed about treatment strategies for mitigating drug-induced weight gain, and obesity in general.

Early assessment and intervention are the key to preventing weight gain and other complications. The standard recommendation for weight loss requires consistent dietary modifications and regular physical activity. This may be difficult for psychiatric patients since their ability to be disciplined in this effort can be compromised by their mental disorder. Also, the physiologic effects of some psychotropic drugs on body metabolism and the regulation of satiety are difficult, if not impossible, to overcome through diet and exercise alone. For these reasons, it may be necessary to use prescription medications to facilitate weight loss.

In this section, drugs used to manage obesity can be categorized in two ways: (1) drugs approved by the Food and Drug Administration (FDA) as "diet pills"; and (2) drugs with primary indications other than weight loss, but that produce weight loss as a side effect.

Drugs with FDA Approval for Weight Loss

All the drugs approved by the FDA as weight loss agents are specifically indicated as an adjunct to a reduced calorie diet and increased physical activity for chronic weight management in adult patients with an initial body mass index

(BMI) of 30 kg/m² or greater (obese), or 27 kg/m² or greater (overweight) in the presence of at least one weight-related comorbidity, such as hypertension, type 2 diabetes mellitus, or dyslipidemia.

PHENTERMINE

 MAOI insulin, guanethidine   3A4

Phentermine hydrochloride is a sympathomimetic amine with pharmacologic activity similar to the amphetamines. It is indicated as a short-term adjunct in a regimen of weight reduction, but in fact, many patients use the drug for extended periods. As with all sympathomimetics, contraindications include advanced arteriosclerosis, cardiovascular disease, moderate to severe hypertension, hyperthyroidism, known hypersensitivity or idiosyncrasy to the sympathomimetic amines, agitated states, and glaucoma.

The drug should be prescribed with caution to patients with a history of drug abuse. Phentermine is a Schedule IV drug, meaning there is some potential for abuse.

Hypertensive crises may result if phentermine is used during or within 14 days following the administration of monoamine oxidase inhibitors (MAOIs). Insulin requirements in diabetes mellitus may be altered in association with the use of phentermine hydrochloride and the concomitant dietary regimen. Phentermine hydrochloride may decrease the hypotensive effect of guanethidine. Phentermine is contraindicated during pregnancy. Studies have not been performed with phentermine hydrochloride to determine the potential for carcinogenesis, mutagenesis, or impairment of fertility.

Phenterime may be administered orally as an immediate-release tablet (8 mg) or in controlled-release tablets (15 to 37.5 mg). Immediate-release tablets should be taken 30 minutes before meals. Extended-release tablets should be taken once per day before breakfast or between 1 and 2 hours after breakfast. Tablets may be broken or cut in half but should not be crushed. To avoid disrupting normal sleep patterns, it should be dosed early in the day. If taking more than one dose a day, the last dose should be taken approximately 4 to 6 hours prior to going to bed. An oral resin formulation is available in 15- and 30-mg capsules, which should be taken once per day before breakfast.

PHENTERMINE/TOPIRAMATE EXTENDED RELEASE (QSYMIA)

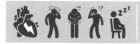 **MAOI** insulin, guanethidine, anticonvulsants, carbonic anhydrase inhibitors   3A4 2C19

A combination of phentermine, a sympathomimetic amine, and topiramate (Topamax), an anticonvulsant, can be effective at decreasing appetite and can serve as part of a larger weight loss strategy that includes dieting and exercise.

It is approved for use in both adults and pediatric patients aged 12 and over with a BMI in the 95th percentile or greater for their age and sex.

Use of this drug is associated with a fivefold increased risk of infants with cleft palate and is contraindicated in pregnancy. As a result, it can only be prescribed through certified pharmacies by clinicians who have been certified in the use of this drug. Clinicians should monitor for the emergence of kidney stones, metabolic acidosis, and secondary angle closure glaucoma. More common side effects can be found in Table 41-1. As phentermine is a Schedule IV drug, there is some potential for abuse.

TABLE 41-1: FDA-Approved Medications for the Treatment of Obesity

Name	Standard Dosage Range (mg/day)	Schedule	Common Side Effects
Phentermine (Adipex-P)	18.75–37.5	IV	Dizziness, dry mouth, troubled sleep, irritability, nausea, vomiting, diarrhea, and constipation
Phentermine-topiramate (Qsymia)	3.75–23 phentermine 15–92 topiramate	IV	Dizziness, drowsiness, dry mouth, unpleasant taste, difficulty sleeping, tingling sensation in extremities, constipation, and tiredness
Phentermine resin (Ionamin)	15–30	IV	Dizziness, dry mouth, unpleasant taste, restlessness, troubled sleep, hyperactivity, irritability, nausea, and vomiting
Phendimetrazine (Bontril PDM, Adipost, Phendiet, Statobex)	105	III	Dizziness, dry mouth, blurred vision, restlessness, troubled sleep, hyperactivity, headache, psychosis, altered libido, and tremors
Diethylpropion (Tenuate)	75	IV	Dizziness, drowsiness, dry mouth, unpleasant taste, restlessness, troubled sleep, irritability, anxiety, depression, tremors, nausea, vomiting, diarrhea, frequent urination, and constipation
Orlistat (Xenical, Alli)	360	—	Oily stool, flatulence, increased defecation, fecal incontinence, and diarrhea
Benzphetamine (Didrex)	75–150	III	Dizziness, dry mouth, troubled sleep, irritability, nausea, vomiting, diarrhea, and constipation
Liraglutide (Saxenda)	0.6–1.8	—	Nausea, headache, constipation, heartburn, running nose, cough, sneezing, tiredness, difficulty urinating or pain during urination, and redness or rash at site of injection
Naltrexone HCl/ Bupropion HCl (Contrave)	32/360	—	Nausea, vomiting, diarrhea, constipation, stomach pain, headaches, dizziness, dry mouth, troubled sleep, flushing, increased sweating, and strange taste
Semaglutide (Wegovy, Ozempic)	.25–2.4	—	Nausea, vomiting diarrhea, abdominal pain, constipation, heartburn, and burping
Amphetamine (Evekeo)	15–30	II	Tachycardia, hypertension, palpitations, restlessness, dizziness, insomnia, dysphoria, tremor, headache, dry mouth, constipation, urticaria, impotence, changes in libido, and rhabdomyolysis

Weight Loss Drugs

Phentermine-topiramate is administered as an extended-release capsule that is taken whole orally once per day with or without food. The medication should be taken early in the day, as it can cause sleep difficulties (insomnia) if taken in the late afternoon or evening. The initial dosage should be 3.75 mg/23 mg phentermine/topiramate. The dosage may be increased after 14 days to 7.5 mg/46 mg phentermine/topiramate. If weight loss is less than 3% of baseline weight in adults or the pediatric patient has not lost at least 3% of baseline BMI, the medication can be discontinued or the dosage can be increased to 11.25 mg/69 mg phentermine/topiramate for 2 weeks, and then increased to the maximum recommended daily dose of 15 mg/92 mg phentermine/topiramate. Evaluate weight loss following dose escalation to 15 mg/92 mg after an additional 12 weeks of treatment. If at least 5% of baseline body weight in adults or 5% of baseline BMI for pediatric patients has not been lost on 15 mg/92 mg, discontinue the medication gradually.

PHENTERMINE RESIN (IONAMIN)

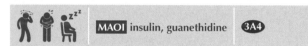

MAOI insulin, guanethidine 3A4

Phentermine resin is a sympathomimetic amine and an appetite suppressant that is indicated for short-term monotherapy only and should be used as part of a larger weight loss strategy that includes lifestyle changes. Phentermine resin may be administered orally in 15- or 30-mg capsules. The initial dosage should be one 15-mg capsule daily taken before breakfast. The dosage can be increased to 30 mg once daily in less responsive patients.

Phentermine resin is a Schedule IV drug, meaning there is some potential for abuse. For a list of potential side effects, see Table 41-1.

PHENDIMETRAZINE (BONTRIL PDM, ADIPOST, PHENDIET, STATOBEX)

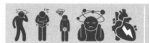

MAOI alcohol, insulin, guanethidine, oral hypoglycemic agents

Phendimetrazine is a sympathomimetic amine that is closely related to the amphetamines. It is classified by the Drug Enforcement Administration (DEA) as a Schedule III substance and is related chemically and pharmacologically to the amphetamines. Amphetamines and related stimulant drugs have been extensively abused, and the possibility of abuse of phendimetrazine should be kept in mind when evaluating the desirability of including a drug as part of a weight reduction program.

Overall, prescribing of this agent is limited. Phendimetrazine may be administered orally as an immediate-release tablet (35 mg) or in controlled-release tablets (105 mg). Immediate-release tablets should be taken 1 hour before meals, two or three times per day. Extended-release tablets should be taken 30 to 60 minutes before the first meal of the day. Use of the 105-mg extended-release capsule is more common and approximates the action of three 35-mg immediate-release doses taken at 4-hour intervals. The average half-life of elimination, when studied under controlled conditions, is about 3.7 hours for both the extended-release and immediate-release forms. The absorption half-life of the drug from the immediate-release 35-mg phendimetrazine tablets is appreciably more rapid than the absorption rate of the drug from the extended-release formulation. The major route of elimination is via the kidneys where most of the drug and metabolites are excreted.

Phendimetrazine contraindications are similar to those of phentermine. They include history of cardiovascular disease (e.g., coronary artery disease, stroke, arrhythmias, congestive heart failure, uncontrolled hypertension, pulmonary hypertension); use during or within 14 days following the administration of MAOIs; hyperthyroidism; glaucoma; agitated states; history of drug abuse; pregnancy; nursing; use in combination with other anorectic agents or central nervous system (CNS) stimulants; and known hypersensitivity or idiosyncratic reactions to sympathomimetics. Given the lack of systematic research, phendimetrazine should not be used in combination with over-the-counter preparations and herbal products that claim to promote weight loss.

Phendimetrazine tartrate is contraindicated during pregnancy because weight loss offers no potential benefit to a pregnant woman and may result in fetal harm. Studies with phendimetrazine tartrate sustained release have not been performed to evaluate carcinogenic potential, mutagenic potential, or effects on fertility.

Interactions may occur with MAOIs, alcohol, insulin, and oral hypoglycemic agents. Phendimetrazine may decrease the hypotensive effect of adrenergic neuron-blocking drugs. The effectiveness and the safety of phendimetrazine in pediatric patients have not been established. It is not recommended in patients less than 17 years of age.

For a list of adverse reactions, see Table 41-1.

Acute overdose with phendimetrazine may manifest itself by restlessness, confusion, belligerence, hallucinations, and panic states. Fatigue and depression usually follow the central stimulation. Cardiovascular effects include tachycardia, arrhythmias, hypertension or hypotension, and circulatory collapse. Gastrointestinal symptoms include nausea, vomiting, diarrhea, and abdominal cramps. Poisoning may result in convulsions, coma, and death. The management of acute overdose is largely symptomatic. It includes lavage and sedation with a barbiturate. If hypertension is marked, the use of a nitrate or rapid acting a receptor-blocking agent should be considered.

DIETHYLPROPION (TENUATE)

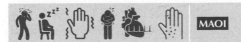

MAOI

Diethylpropion is a sympathomimetic amine and an appetite suppressant that is indicated for short-term monotherapy only and should be used as part of a larger weight loss strategy that includes lifestyle changes. It preceded its analog, the antidepressant drug bupropion (Wellbutrin). Diethylpropion comes in two formulations: a 25-mg tablet and a 75-mg extended-release tablet (Tenuate Dospan).

Immediate-release tablets should be taken 1 hour before meals, three times per day. An additional midevening dose may be useful in preventing night hunger but should only be prescribed if night eating is a problem. Controlled-release tablets should be swallowed whole in midmorning and should never be chewed, crushed, or cut. The maximum daily dose is 75 mg.

Diethylpropion is pregnancy category B and has a low-abuse potential, though it is listed as a Schedule IV drug by the DEA. For a list of common side effects, see Table 41-1. Side effects that warrant medical attention include tachycardia, palpitations, blurred vision, skin rash, itching, difficulty breathing, chest pain, fainting, swelling of the ankles or feet, fever, sore throat, chills, and painful urination.

ORLISTAT (XENICAL, ALLI)

 cyclosporine, amiodarone **3A4**

Orlistat interferes with the absorption of dietary fats, causing reduced caloric intake. It works by inhibiting gastric and pancreatic lipases, the enzymes that break down triglycerides in the intestine. When lipase activity is blocked, triglycerides from the diet are not hydrolyzed into absorbable free fatty acids and are excreted undigested instead. Absorption of fat-soluble vitamins and other fat-soluble nutrients is inhibited by the use of orlistat. Multivitamin supplements that contain vitamins A, D, E, and K, as well as β-carotene should be taken once a day, preferably at bedtime.

Only trace amounts of orlistat are absorbed systemically; it is almost entirely eliminated through the feces, and many patients experience steatorrhea, flatulence, fecal incontinence, and frequent or urgent bowel movements. These side effects may be minimized by avoiding high-fat foods. Contrarily, orlistat can be used in conjunction with a high-fat diet to treat medication-induced constipation. As the drug does not act systemically, orlistat may be a suitable candidate for obese patients who are already taking several other medications.

The effectiveness of orlistat in promoting weight loss is definite, though modest. When used as part of weight loss program, between 30% and 50% of patients can expect a 5% or greater decrease in body mass. About 20% achieve at least a 10% decrease in body mass. Patients may also see a decrease in blood pressure and a reduced risk of developing type 2 diabetes. After orlistat is stopped, up to a third of people gain the weight they lose.

In 2010, new safety information about rare cases of severe liver injury was added to the product label of orlistat. The rate of acute kidney injury is more common among orlistat users than nonusers. It should be used with caution in patients with impaired liver function and renal function, as well as those with an obstructed bile duct and pancreatic disease. Orlistat is contraindicated in malabsorption syndromes, hypersensitivity to orlistat, reduced gallbladder function, and in pregnancy and breastfeeding. Orlistat should not be used during pregnancy. For a list of common side effects, see Table 41-1.

Orlistat can reduce plasma levels of the immunosuppressant cyclosporine (Sandimmune), so the two drugs should therefore not be administered concomitantly. Orlistat can also impair absorption of the antiarrhythmic amiodarone (Nexterone).

The recommended starting dose is 120 mg given three times per day with meals. Orlistat is also available in a reduced-strength formula without a prescription. Decreases in total triglycerides, total cholesterol, and low-density lipoprotein (LDL) cholesterol have been observed with administration of orlistat. An increase in high-density lipoprotein (HDL) cholesterol has also been observed.

An over-the-counter formulation of orlistat (Alli) is available as 60-mg capsules—half the dosage of prescription orlistat.

BENZPHETAMINE (DIDREX)

Benzphetamine is a sympathomimetic amine and an appetite suppressant that is indicated for short-term monotherapy only and should be used as part of a larger weight loss strategy that includes lifestyle changes. Benzphetamine is administered orally as a tablet. The initial dose should be 25 to 50 mg once per day in the morning or midafternoon. Dosage may be increased to 25 to 50 mg one to three times per day. The dose and frequency of the medication should be individualized based on patient response and needs, but a maintenance dose should not exceed a total of 150 mg per day.

Benzphetamine should not be used in conjunction with MAOIs. Pulmonary hypertension has been reported when used with other diet medications, so concomitant use of even over-the-counter medications is strongly discouraged. Benzphetamine is contraindicated during pregnancy and for people with coronary artery disease, arrhythmia, severe hypertension, thyroid conditions, and glaucoma. As benzphetamine is a Schedule III drug and does have a low to moderate potential for abuse, clinicians should be cautious when prescribing it to patients with a history of drug or alcohol use disorders. For a list of potential side effects, see Table 41-1.

LIRAGLUTIDE INJECTION (SAXENDA)

 GLP-1 agonists

Liraglutide is a glucagon-like peptide-1 (GLP-1) receptor agonist or incretin mimetics and works by increasing insulin release from the pancreas and decreasing glucagon release. Liraglutide has been approved as a treatment for type 2

diabetes and can also treat chronic obesity. It should be used as part of a larger weight loss strategy that includes dieting and exercise. Liraglutide is administered once daily by subcutaneous injection at patient's convenience. The initial dose should be 0.6 mg. After 1 week of use, the dosage may be increased to 1.2 mg. The maximum recommended daily dose is 1.8 mg.

Saxenda and Victoza both contain the same active ingredient, liraglutide, and therefore should not be used together. Victoza is only indicated for type 2 diabetes and not for weight loss. Saxenda should not be used in combination with any other GLP-1 receptor agonist. Saxenda has not been studied in patients taking insulin. Saxenda and insulin should not be used together.

The drug may promote thyroid C-cell tumors. If serum calcitonin is measured and found to be elevated, the patient should be further evaluated. Patients with thyroid nodules noted on physical examination or neck imaging should also be further evaluated. Based on spontaneous postmarketing reports, acute pancreatitis, including fatal and nonfatal hemorrhagic or necrotizing pancreatitis, has been observed in patients treated with liraglutide. After initiation of Saxenda, patients should be monitored for signs and symptoms of pancreatitis (including persistent severe abdominal pain, sometimes radiating to the back and which may or may not be accompanied by vomiting). If pancreatitis is suspected, Saxenda should promptly be discontinued, and appropriate management should be initiated. If pancreatitis is confirmed, Saxenda should not be restarted. The incidence of acute gallbladder disease is increased in patients treated with Saxenda. Saxenda is contraindicated in pregnancy.

Common side effects can be found in Table 41-1.

NALTREXONE/BUPROPION (CONTRAVE)

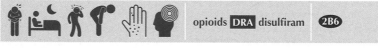

opioids DRA disulfiram 2B6

The combination of naltrexone, an opiate antagonist, and bupropion, an antidepressant medication used to treat major depressive disorder and seasonal affective disorder, has shown promise in treating obesity possibly by acting on food reward networks in the brain. Dosage should begin with a sustained-release tablet of 8 mg of naltrexone and 90 mg of bupropion. As risk of seizure and increased blood pressure are associated with rapid increases in bupropion, dosages should be gradually increased over the course of 1 month to 2 tablets twice per day for a total dosage of 32 mg of naltrexone and 360 mg of bupropion. The pill should be swallowed whole and not used with high-fat meals. When administered in conjunction with lifestyle interventions and a calorie-restrictive diet, the combination of naltrexone and bupropion has been shown to be more effective than with monotherapy and can produce sustained results over the course of 6 months or even 1 year. If after 12 weeks a ≥5% weight loss is not achieved, the drug should be discontinued.

With concomitant CYP2B6 inhibitors (e.g., ticlopidine, clopidogrel) and moderate or severe renal impairment, the maximum dose should be two tablets daily (one tablet each in the morning and evening). With hepatic impairment, one tablet in the morning is the maximum dose.

Contrave is not recommended for use during pregnancy, as it may harm a fetus. This drug passes into breast milk and is not recommended for use while breastfeeding. Withdrawal symptoms may occur if you suddenly stop taking this medication. For a list of potential side effects, see Table 41-1.

SEMAGLUTIDE (WEGOVY, OZEMPIC)

Semaglutide is a GLP-1 receptor agonist that increases insulin secretion and is indicated for chronic weight management in patients with obesity who have at least one weight-related ailment or in patients with a BMI greater than 30 kg/m². Semaglutide should be used as part of a larger weight loss strategy that includes dieting and exercise. It is administered by once-weekly subcutaneous injection at patient's convenience. The initial dose of 0.25 mg per week should last for 4 weeks, and thereafter can be increased to 0.5 mg per week for weeks 5 to 8, 1 mg per week for weeks 9 to 12, 1.7 mg per week for weeks 13 to 16, and then reach a maintenance dose of 2.4 mg per week.

Semaglutide is contraindicated in patients with multiple endocrine neoplasia type 2, medullary thyroid cancer, or a family history of medullary thyroid carcinoma. Patients with low blood pressure, diabetic retinopathy, gallbladder disease, kidney disease, and pancreatitis should not use semaglutide. If pancreatitis is suspected, it should be discontinued immediately. Semaglutide is a category D pregnancy drug and women who plan to become pregnant should discontinue use at least 2 months before planned pregnancy.

For a list of side effects, see Table 41-1.

AMPHETAMINE (EVEKEO)

  dyskinesia 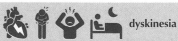 MAOI TRI/TETR warfarin, primidone, phenobarbital, phenytoin, phenylbutazone 2D6 2A6

Evekeo is an amphetamine, consisting of racemic amphetamine sulfate (i.e., 50% levoamphetamine sulfate and 50% dextroamphetamine sulfate). Amphetamines have long been known to promote weight loss. Interestingly, this is the only formulation to have been approved by the FDA for use as a weight loss treatment but only in the short term. Evekeo is available in 5- and 10-mg tablets. Tablets are scored, so they can be split in half. Dosages should be taken 30 to 60 minutes before meals. Daily dosage should not exceed 30 mg. Please refer to the chapter on psychostimulants for more information on the clinical effects and use of amphetamines. Evekeo is a category C pregnancy drug. It is a Schedule II drug, which means it has a high potential for abuse. For a partial list of side effects, side Table 41-1.

Weight Loss Drugs

Drugs without FDA Approval for Weight Loss

TOPIRAMATE (TOPAMAX)

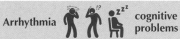 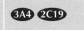

| Arrhythmia | | | cognitive problems | anticonvulsants, carbonic anhydrase inhibitors | 3A4 2C19 |

Topiramate and the next drug zonisamide are discussed in Chapter 5 but are mentioned here because both agents can have a substantial effect on weight loss.

Topiramate is approved as an antiepileptic drug and is used for prevention of migraine headaches in adults. The degree of weight loss associated with topiramate may be comparable to the weight loss that other FDA-approved antiobesity drugs induce. Small studies and extensive anecdotal reports indicate that topiramate can help to offset weight gain associated with selective serotonin reuptake inhibitors (SSRIs) and second-generation antipsychotic drugs. A review of 10 studies found that patients treated with topiramate lost an average of 5.34 kg over a span of 6 to 7 months.

Its impact on body weight may be due to its effects on both appetite suppression and satiety enhancement. These may be the result of a combination of pharmacologic effects including augmenting γ-aminobutyric acid activity, modulation of voltage-gated ion channels, inhibition of excitatory glutamate receptors, or inhibition of carbonic anhydrase.

The duration and dosage of treatment affect the weight loss benefits of topiramate. Weight loss is higher when the drug is prescribed at doses of 100 to 200 mg per day for more than a month compared with less than a month. In a large study, it was shown that compared to those who took placebo, topiramate-treated patients were seven times more likely to lose more than 10% of their body weight. In clinical practice, many patients experience weight loss at a starting dose of 25 mg per day. Topiramate is available as 25-, 50- 100-, and 200-mg tablets and as 15-, 25-, and 50-mg capsules.

There are no established dosage guidelines for weight loss, but clinicians are recommended to titrate slowly, considering its cognitive effects. Dosage should begin at 25 mg at night and increase by no more than 25 mg every week to an average dosage of 100 mg. In rare instances, the dosage can be increased to 150 to 200 mg, provided there are no adverse effects. Metformin can be added to topiramate in individuals on psychotropic medication. *Topiramate may cause serious side effects including kidney stones and clinicians need to be aware of these potential risks.* Discontinuation should be gradual considering its antiepileptic effects.

The most common side effects of topiramate are paresthesias—typically around the mouth, impaired taste (taste perversion) and psychomotor disturbances, including slowed cognition and reduced physical movements. Impaired concentration and memory impairment, characterized by word-finding and name-recall problems, are often reported. Some patients may experience emotional lability and mood changes. Medical side effects include increased risk of kidney stones and acute-angle closure glaucoma. Patients should report

TABLE 41-2: Non–FDA-Approved Medications for the Treatment of Obesity

Name	Standard Dosage Range (mg/day)	Schedule	Common Side Effects
Topiramate (Topamax)	25–400	—	Tiredness, dry mouth, unpleasant taste, dizziness, drowsiness, loss of coordination, tingling sensation in extremities, nervousness, and diarrhea
Zonisamide (Zonegran)	100–600	—	Nausea, vomiting, weight loss, altered taste, diarrhea, constipation, heartburn, and dry mouth
Metformin (Glucophage)	500–2550	—	Headache, muscle pain, weakness, nausea, vomiting, diarrhea, stomach pain, gas, and feeling cold
Amphetamine and dextroamphetamine (Adderall)	5–20	II	Dry mouth, troubled sleep, nausea, dizziness, headache, diarrhea, and nervousness
Naltrexone (Vivitrol, Reviva)	50	—	Nausea, vomiting, diarrhea, constipation, stomach pain, headaches, dizziness, anxiety, troubled sleep, joint or muscle pain, and unusual tiredness
Amantadine (Gocovri)	100–300	—	Dizziness, falls, dry mouth, swelling in appendages, nausea, constipation, and insomnia
Tirzepatide (Mounjaro)	5–15	—	Nausea, diarrhea, reduced appetite, vomiting, dyspepsia, constipation, and abdominal pain

Weight Loss Drugs

any change in visual acuity. Those with a history of kidney stones should be instructed to drink adequate amounts of fluid. For a listing of other common side effects, see Table 41-2.

ZONISAMIDE (ZONEGRAN)

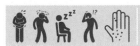 carbonic anhydrase inhibitors

Zonisamide (Zonegran) is a sulfonamide-related drug and antiseizure medication, similar to topiramate. Its exact mechanism of action is not known. Studies have found that the drug is tolerated well, with few adverse effects. One small study found that the zonisamide group experienced a mean weight loss of 9.2 kg at week 32 compared to 1.5 kg in the placebo group.

Considering its off-label use, there are no dosage guidelines. The starting dose is 100 mg a day and can be increased every 2 weeks to an average dose of 400 mg per day with a further increase to a maximum dose of 600 mg a day (can be in divided doses) in those patients losing less the 5% of body weight after 12 weeks. Discontinuation should be gradual, considering its antiepileptic effects.

Like topiramate, it can cause cognitive problems, but the incidence is lower compared to topiramate. The most common side effects include drowsiness, loss of appetite, dizziness, headache, nausea, and agitation/irritability (see Table 41-2). Zonisamide has also been associated with hypohidrosis. There is a 2% to 4% risk of developing kidney stones. Other drugs known to increase risk of renal stones, such as topiramate or acetazolamide, should not be combined with zonisamide. Serious, but rare, adverse drug reactions include Stevens–Johnson syndrome, toxic epidermal necrolysis, and metabolic acidosis.

Zonisamide has been assigned to pregnancy category C. Animal studies have revealed evidence of teratogenicity. Fetal abnormalities or embryo–fetal deaths have been reported in animal tests at maternal plasma levels similar to, or lower than, human therapeutic levels. Therefore, use of this drug in human pregnancy may expose the fetus to significant risks.

METFORMIN (GLUCOPHAGE)

Metformin belongs to a class of drugs known as biguanides and is used to control high blood sugar in treating type 2 diabetes and may help patients lose weight when used in conjunction with diet and exercise. It has also been found to help with weight loss even in patients without type 2 diabetes, especially if the patient is taking psychotropic medicines, though the effect only lasts as long as the patient takes the medicine. Its actions include reduction of hepatic glucose production, reduced intestinal glucose absorption, increased insulin sensitivity, and improved peripheral glucose uptake and regulation. It does not increase insulin secretion.

When used as an adjunct to second-generation antipsychotics, it has consistently been shown to reduce body weight and waist circumference. Metformin probably has the best evidence of therapeutic benefit for the treatment of antipsychotic drug–induced metabolic syndrome. In several studies, metformin has been shown to attenuate or reverse some of the weight gain induced by antipsychotics. The degree of effect on body weight compares favorably with the effect of other treatment options that are approved for weight reduction. The weight loss effect of adjunctive metformin appears to be stronger in drug-naive patients treated with second-generation antipsychotic medications. This effect is most evident for those being treated with clozapine and olanzapine. Based on the existing evidence, if weight gain occurs after second-generation antipsychotic initiation, despite lifestyle intervention, metformin should be considered.

Metformin is available in 500-, 850-, and 1,000-mg tablets, all now generic. Metformin SR (slow release) or XR (extended release) is available in 500- and 750-mg strengths. These formulations are intended to reduce gastrointestinal side effects, and to increase patient compliance by reducing pill burden. Though the dose varies based on various factors, the usual starting dosage is 500 mg once a day and can be increased to a maximum dosage of 2,500 mg given once as an extended-release tablet or in divided dosages for regular formulation.

Common side effects include nausea, vomiting, abdominal pain, and loss of appetite (see Table 41-2). Gastrointestinal side effects can be mitigated by dividing the dose, taking the drug after meals, or using delayed-release formulations.

One serious treatment risk is that of lactic acidosis. This side effect is more common in those with reduced renal function. Though quite rare (9/100,000 persons/year), it has a 50% mortality rate. Alcohol use along with metformin can increase the risk of acidosis. Renal function monitoring and alcohol avoidance are important.

The weight loss effects of metformin are also evident in chronically ill patients with schizophrenia. Long-term use of metformin appears to be safe and effective.

AMPHETAMINE AND DEXTROAMPHETAMINE (ADDERALL)

 MAOI TRI/TETR warfarin, primidone, phenobarbital, phenytoin, phenylbutazone 2D6 2A6

The combination of amphetamine and dextroamphetamine is approved for the use in treating attention deficit hyperactive disorder (ADHD) but may be effective at decreasing appetite. Immediate-release tablets (administered orally one to three times per day) and extended-release capsules that are taken once per day are both available in a variety of dosages. There are no dosing guidelines for weight loss. Clinicians can follow the same dosage as for ADHD with initial recommended dose in adults of 5-mg tablets taken once or twice per day. Dosage can be increased by 5 mg at weekly intervals. Only in rare cases should a dosage exceed 40 mg per day.

Amphetamine and dextroamphetamine are both Schedule II stimulants and may be abused. Clinicians should carefully screen for underlying mood, anxiety, and psychotic disorders before prescribing these medicines. For a list of potential side effects, see Table 41-2.

NALTREXONE (VIVITROL, REVIVA)

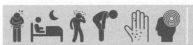 opioids DRA disulfiram

The opioid antagonist naltrexone was covered in Chapter 29 but is also considered an off-label medicine when used alone for the treatment of weight loss. It has been indicated for weight loss when used in conjunction with bupropion.

Naltrexone has been shown to decrease food cravings and therefore induce weight loss. Starting and maintenance dose is 50 mg per day. Patients should be educated about its antagonistic effects on opioid drugs, especially in patients requiring analgesics for various pain syndromes. Liver function monitoring is recommended for those requiring long-term treatment. For a list of potential side effects, see Table 41-2. For more information, consult Chapter 29.

AMANTADINE (GOCOVRI)

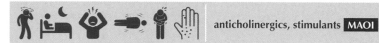
anticholinergics, stimulants **MAOI**

Amantadine was initially developed as an antiviral and has been used to treat Parkinson disease. It has been shown to induce weight loss, particularly in patients on atypical antipsychotics. Clinicians should closely monitor psychiatric symptoms as there are rare but severe psychological side effects, including agitation, hallucinations, anxiety, insomnia, and depression. Amantadine is available as an oral immediate-release capsule, extended-release capsule, immediate-release tablet, extended-release tablet, and syrup. The usual starting dose for immediate-release formulation is 100 to 200 mg per day in a divided dosage. It can be increased to 300 mg per day. For a list of potential side effects, see Table 41-2. For more information, consult Chapter 18.

TIRZEPATIDE (MOUNJARO)

Tirzepatide was granted FDA approval to control blood sugar levels in adults with type 2 diabetes in May 2022, and recent studies have shown that it may also help nondiabetic adults lose weight. Tirzepatide is a combination of two incretins, GLP-1 and glucose-dependent insulinotropic polypeptide (GIP). It is administered as a once-a-week injection and is designed to mimic the effects of incretins, which are responsible for lowering blood sugar. In addition, tirzepatide decreases food intake, slows gastric emptying, reduces glucagon levels, increases insulin sensitivity, and enhances first- and second-phase insulin secretion.

A clinical trial over 72 weeks showed weight loss of 22.5% on 15 mg of tirzepatide compared to 2.4% on placebo. Another 72-week study whose participants were obese adults without diabetes reported similar results. Individuals who took a 5-mg dose reported an average loss of 16 kg, those who took a 10-mg dose lost an average of 22 kg, and those who received a 15-mg dose lost an average of 23.6 kg. The most common side effects observed included nausea, diarrhea, and reduced appetite, and only a small percentage of participants found these effects severe enough to exit the study. Tirzepatide was associated with an increased risk of thyroid C-cell tumors in animal models. This includes medullary thyroid carcinoma (MTC). Consequently, tirzepatide is contraindicated in patients with a personal or family history of MTC or multiple endocrine neoplasia syndrome type 2 (MEN 2).

42 Medication-Induced Movement Disorders

Generic Name	Trade Name	Adverse Effects	Drug Interactions	CYP Interactions
Valbenazine	Ingrezza	Cardiac arrhythmia, sedation	CNS, MAOI, QT, reserpine, valbenazine	3A4, 3A5, 2D6
Deutetrabenazine	Austedo	Cardiac arrhythmia, sedation, nasopharyngitis	CNS, MAOI, QT, reserpine, valbenazine	2D6, 1A2, 3A4, 3A5

Introduction

Patients taking psychotropic drugs may experience medication-induced movement disorders. Drugs that block dopamine type 2 (D_2) receptors, such as dopamine receptor antagonists (DRAs), or inhibit serotonin reuptake are associated with movement disorders, though abnormal motor activity may occur with other types of medications as well. Sometimes, it can be difficult to determine if abnormal motor movements are an adverse event or a symptom of an underlying disorder. For example, anxiety can resemble akathisia and alcohol or benzodiazepine withdrawal can cause tremor.

The most common medication-induced movement disorders are parkinsonism, acute dystonia, and acute akathisia. Neuroleptic malignant syndrome is a life-threatening and often misdiagnosed condition. Neuroleptic-induced tardive dyskinesia is a late-appearing adverse effect of neuroleptic drugs and can be irreversible; recent data, however, indicate that the syndrome, although still serious and potentially disabling, is less pernicious than was previously thought in patients taking DRAs. Dopaminergic blockade is less complete with serotonin-dopamine antagonists (SDAs) and are presumed to be less likely to produce such movement disorders. Nevertheless, the risk of movement disorders remains, and caution and vigilance is still required when prescribing SDAs. Consequently, the term "antipsychotic" will be used to discuss the impact of these medicines rather than make distinction between DRAs and SDAs.

Note: While the term *neuroleptic* may seem dated, the American Psychiatric Association has decided to retain the term when discussing side effects associated with drugs used to treat psychosis—including the DRAs and second-generation antipsychotics (SGAs). The rationale for continued use of the term is that it was originally used to describe the tendency of these drugs to cause abnormal movements. The term *neuroleptic* will be used in this chapter to reflect this principle. Based on the specific agent and type of movement disturbance, various strategies are employed to counter these adverse effects.

Table 42-1 lists the selected medications associated with movement disorders and their impact on relevant neuroreceptors.

TABLE 42-1: Selected Medications Associated with Movement Disorders: Impact on Relevant Neuroreceptors

Type (Subtype)	Name (Brand)	D_2 Blockade	5-HT$_2$ Blockade	mACh Blockade
Antipsychotics				
Phenothiazine (aliphatic)	Chlorpromazine (Thorazine)	Low	High	High
Phenothiazine (piperidines)	Thioridazine (Mellaril)	Low	Med	High
	Mesoridazine (Serentil)	Low	Med	High
Phenothiazine (piperazines)	Trifluoperazine (Stelazine)	Med	Med	Med
	Fluphenazine (Prolixin)	High	Low	Low
	Perphenazine (Trilafon)	High	Med	Low
Thioxanthenes	Thiothixene (Navane)	High	Med	Low
	Chlorprothixene (Taractan)	Med	High	Med
Dibenzoxazepine	Loxapine (Loxitane)	Med	High	Low
Butyrophenones	Haloperidol (Haldol)	High	Low	Low
	Droperidol (Inapsine)	High	Med	—
Diphenyl-butylpiperidine	Pimozide (Orap)	High	Med	Low
Dihydroindolone	Molindone (Moban)	Med	Low	Low
Dibenzodiazepine	Clozapine (Clozaril)	Low	High	High
Benzisoxazole	Risperidone (Risperdal)	High	High	Low
Thienobenzodiazepine	Olanzapine (Zyprexa)	Low	High	High
Dibenzothiazepine	Quetiapine (Seroquel)	Low/med	Low/med	Low
Benzisothiazolinone	Ziprasidone (Geodon)	Med	High	Low
Quinolone	Aripiprazole (Abilify)	High (as partial agonist)	High	Low
Nonantipsychotic psychotropic	Lithium (Eskalith)	N/A	N/A	N/A
Anticonvulsants		Low	Low	Low
Antidepressants		Low (except amoxapine)	(Varies)	(Varies)
Nonpsychotropics	Prochlorperazine (Compazine)	High	Med	Low
	Metoclopramide (Reglan)	High	High	—

D_2, dopamine type 2; 5-HT$_2$, 5-hydroxytryptamine type 2; mACh, muscarinic acetylcholine; N/A, not applicable.
Adapted from Janicak PG, Davis JM, Preskorn SH, et al. *Principles and Practice of Psychopharmacotherapy.* 3rd ed. Lippincott Williams & Wilkins; 2001.

Neuroleptic-Induced Parkinsonism and Other Medication-Induced Parkinsonism

Diagnosis, Signs, and Symptoms

Symptoms of neuroleptic-induced parkinsonism and other medication-induced parkinsonism include muscle stiffness (lead pipe rigidity), cogwheel rigidity, shuffling gait, stooped posture, and drooling. The pill-rolling tremor of idiopathic parkinsonism is rare, but a regular, coarse tremor similar to essential tremor may be present. The so-called *rabbit syndrome*, a tremor affecting the lips and perioral muscles, is another parkinsonian effect seen with antipsychotics, although perioral tremor is more likely than other tremors to occur late in the course of treatment.

Epidemiology

Parkinsonian adverse effects typically occur within 5 to 90 days of the initiation of treatment. Patients who are elderly and female are at the highest risk for neuroleptic-induced parkinsonism, although the disorder can occur at all ages.

Etiology

Neuroleptic-induced parkinsonism is caused by the blockade of D_2 receptors in the caudate nucleus at the termination of the nigrostriatal dopamine neurons. All antipsychotics can cause these symptoms, especially high-potency drugs with low levels of anticholinergic activity, most notably haloperidol (Haldol).

Differential Diagnosis

Included in the differential diagnosis are idiopathic parkinsonism, other organic causes of parkinsonism, and depression, which can also be associated with parkinsonian symptoms. Decreased psychomotor activity and blunted facial expression are symptoms of depression and idiopathic parkinsonism.

Treatment

Parkinsonism can be treated with anticholinergic agents, benztropine (Cogentin), amantadine (Symmetrel), or diphenhydramine (Benadryl) (Table 42-2). Anticholinergics should be withdrawn after 4 to 6 weeks to assess whether tolerance to the parkinsonian effects has developed. About half of the patients with neuroleptic-induced parkinsonism require continued treatment. Even after the antipsychotics are withdrawn, parkinsonian symptoms can last up to 2 weeks and even up to 3 months in some elderly patients. In such patients, the clinician may continue the anticholinergic drug after the antipsychotic has been stopped until the parkinsonian symptoms resolve completely.

Neuroleptic Malignant Syndrome

Diagnosis, Signs, and Symptoms

Neuroleptic malignant syndrome is a life-threatening complication that can occur anytime during the course of antipsychotic treatment. The motor and behavioral symptoms include muscular rigidity and dystonia, akinesia, mutism, obtundation, and agitation. The autonomic symptoms include hyperthermia, diaphoresis, and increased pulse and blood pressure. Laboratory findings include an increased white blood cell (WBC) count and increased levels of creatinine phosphokinase, liver enzymes, plasma myoglobin, and myoglobinuria, occasionally associated with renal failure.

Epidemiology

About 0.01% to 0.02% of patients treated with antipsychotics develop neuroleptic malignant syndrome. Men are affected more frequently than women, and

TABLE 42-2: Drug Treatments of Extrapyramidal Disorders

Generic Name	Trade Name	Usual Daily Dosage	Indications
Anticholinergics			
Benztropine	Cogentin	PO 0.5–2 mg TID; IM or IV 1–2 mg	Acute dystonia, parkinsonism, akinesia, akathisia
Biperiden	Akineton	PO 2–6 mg TID; IM or IV 2 mg	
Procyclidine	Kemadrin	PO 2.5–5 mg BID-QID	
Trihexyphenidyl	Artane, Tremin	PO 2–5 mg TID	
Orphenadrine	Norflex, Disipal	PO 50–100 mg BID-QID; IV 60 mg	Rabbit syndrome
Antihistamine			
Diphenhydramine	Benadryl	PO 25 mg QID; IM or IV 25 mg	Acute dystonia, parkinsonism, akinesia, rabbit syndrome
Amantadine	Symmetrel	PO 100–200 mg BID	Parkinsonism, akinesia, rabbit syndrome
b-Adrenergic antagonist			
Propranolol	Inderal	PO 20–40 mg TID	Akathisia, tremor
a-Adrenergic antagonist			
Clonidine	Catapres	PO 0.1 mg TID	Akathisia
Benzodiazepines			
Clonazepam	Klonopin	PO 1 mg BID	Akathisia, acute dystonia
Lorazepam	Ativan	PO 1 mg TID	
Buspirone	BuSpar	PO 20–40 mg QID	Tardive dyskinesia
Vitamin E	—	PO 1,200–1,600 IU/day	Tardive dyskinesia

PO, orally; IM, intramuscularly; IV, intravenously; BID, twice a day; TID, three times a day; QID, four times a day.

young patients are affected more commonly than elderly patients. The mortality rate can reach 10% to 20% or even higher when depot antipsychotic medications are involved.

Course and Prognosis

The symptoms usually evolve over 24 to 72 hours, and the untreated syndrome lasts 10 to 14 days. The diagnosis is often missed in the early stages, and the withdrawal or agitation may mistakenly be considered to reflect an exacerbation of the psychosis.

Treatment

In addition to supportive medical treatment, the most commonly used medications for the condition are dantrolene (Dantrium) and bromocriptine (Parlodel), although amantadine is sometimes used. Bromocriptine and amantadine pose direct DRA effects and may serve to overcome the antipsychotic-induced

TABLE 42-3: Treatment of Neuroleptic Malignant Syndrome

Intervention	Dosing	Effectiveness
Amantadine	200–400 mg PO/day in divided doses	Beneficial as monotherapy or in combination; decrease in death rate
Bromocriptine	2.5 mg PO BID or TID, may increase to a total of 45 mg/day	Mortality reduced as a single or combined agent
Levodopa/ carbidopa	Levodopa 50–100 mg/day IV as continuous infusion	Case reports of dramatic improvement
Electroconvulsive therapy	Reports of good outcome with both unilateral and bilateral treatments; response may occur in as few as three treatments	Effective when medications have failed; may also treat underlying psychiatric disorder
Dantrolene	1 mg/kg/day for 8 days, then continue as PO for 7 additional days	Benefits may occur in minutes or hours as a single agent or in combination
Benzodiazepines	1–2 mg IM as test dose; if effective, switch to PO; consider use if underlying disorder has catatonic symptoms	Has been reported effective when other agents have failed
Supportive measures	IV hydration, cooling blankets, ice packs, ice water enema, oxygenation, antipyretics	Often effective as initial approach early in the episode

PO, orally; BID, twice a day; TID, three times a day; IV, intravenously; IM, intramuscularly.
Adapted with permission of SLACK Incorporated, from Davis JM, Caroff SN, Mann SC. Treatment of neuroleptic malignant syndrome. *Psychiatr Ann.* 2000;30:325–331; permission conveyed through Copyright Clearance Center, Inc.

dopamine receptor blockade. The lowest effective dosage of the antipsychotic drug should be used to reduce the chance of neuroleptic malignant syndrome. High-potency drugs, such as haloperidol, pose the greatest risk. Antipsychotic drugs with anticholinergic effects seem less likely to cause neuroleptic malignant syndrome. Electroconvulsive therapy has been used to treat alterations in temperature, level of consciousness, catatonia, and diaphoresis.

Table 42-3 summarizes treatments for neuroleptic malignant syndrome.

Medication-Induced Acute Dystonia

Diagnosis, Signs, and Symptoms

Dystonias are brief or prolonged contractions of muscles that result in visibly abnormal movements or postures, including oculogyric crises, tongue protrusion, trismus, torticollis, laryngeal–pharyngeal dystonia, and dystonic postures of the limbs and trunk. Other dystonias include blepharospasm and glossopharyngeal dystonia; the latter results in dysarthria, dysphagia, and even difficulty in breathing, which can cause cyanosis. Children are particularly likely to evidence opisthotonos, scoliosis, lordosis, and writhing movements. Dystonia can be painful and frightening and often results in noncompliance with future drug treatment regimens.

Epidemiology

The development of acute dystonic symptoms is characterized by their early onset during the course of treatment with neuroleptics. There is a higher incidence of acute dystonia in men, in patients younger than age 30 years, and in patients given high dosages of high-potency medications.

Etiology

Although it is most common with intramuscular (IM) doses of high-potency antipsychotics, dystonia can occur with any antipsychotic. The mechanism of action is thought to be dopaminergic hyperactivity in the basal ganglia that occurs when central nervous system (CNS) levels of the antipsychotic drug begin to fall between doses.

Differential Diagnosis

The differential diagnosis includes seizures and tardive dyskinesia.

Course and Prognosis

Dystonia can fluctuate spontaneously and respond to reassurance, so the clinician gets the false impression that the movement is hysterical or completely under conscious control.

Treatment

Prophylaxis with anticholinergics or related drugs usually prevents dystonia, although the risks of prophylactic treatment weigh against that benefit. Treatment with IM anticholinergics or intravenous or IM diphenhydramine (Benadryl, 50 mg) almost always relieves the symptoms. Diazepam (Valium, 10 mg intravenously), amobarbital (Amytal) though rarely used, and caffeine sodium benzoate have also been reported to be effective. Although tolerance for the adverse effects usually develops, it is prudent to change the antipsychotic if the patient is particularly concerned that the reaction may recur.

Medication-Induced Acute Akathisia

Diagnosis, Signs, and Symptoms

Akathisia is defined by subjective feelings of restlessness, objective signs of restlessness, or both. *It is derived from the Greek word "akathemi" which means never to sit down.* Examples include a sense of anxiety, inability to relax, jitteriness, pacing, rocking motions while sitting, and rapid alternation of sitting and standing. Akathisia has been associated with the use of a wide range of psychiatric drugs, including antipsychotics, antidepressants, and sympathomimetics. Once akathisia is recognized and diagnosed, the antipsychotic dose should be reduced to the minimal effective level. Akathisia may be associated with a poor treatment outcome.

Epidemiology

Middle-aged women are at increased risk of akathisia, and the time course is similar to that for neuroleptic-induced parkinsonism.

Treatment

Three basic steps in the treatment of akathisia are reducing medication dosage, attempting treatment with appropriate drugs, and considering changing medications. The most efficacious drugs are β-adrenergic receptor antagonists, although anticholinergic drugs, benzodiazepines, and cyproheptadine (Periactin) may benefit some patients. In some cases of akathisia, no treatment seems to be effective.

Tardive Dyskinesia

Diagnosis, Signs, and Symptoms

Tardive dyskinesia is a delayed effect of antipsychotics; it rarely occurs until after 6 months of treatment. The disorder consists of abnormal, involuntary, and irregular choreoathetoid movements of the muscles of the head, limbs, and trunk. Movement severity ranges from minimal—often missed by patients and their families—to grossly incapacitating. Perioral movements are the most common and include darting, twisting, and protruding movements of the tongue; chewing and lateral jaw movements; lip puckering; and facial grimacing. Finger movements and hand clenching are also common. Torticollis, retrocollis, trunk twisting, and pelvic thrusting occur in severe cases. In the most serious cases, patients may have breathing and swallowing irregularities that result in aerophagia, belching, and grunting. Respiratory dyskinesia has also been reported. Dyskinesia is exacerbated by stress and disappears during sleep.

Epidemiology

Tardive dyskinesia develops in about 10% to 20% of patients who are treated for more than a year. About 20% to 40% of patients who require long-term hospitalization have tardive dyskinesia. Women are more likely to be affected than men. Children, patients who are more than 50 years of age, and patients with brain damage or mood disorders are also at high risk.

Course and Prognosis

Between 5% and 40% of all cases of tardive dyskinesia eventually remit, and between 50% and 90% of all mild cases remit. Tardive dyskinesia is less likely to remit in elderly patients than in young patients, however.

Treatment

The three basic approaches to tardive dyskinesia are prevention, diagnosis, and management. Prevention is best achieved by using antipsychotic medications only when clearly indicated and in the lowest effective doses. The atypical antipsychotics are associated with less tardive dyskinesia than the older antipsychotics. Clozapine (Clozaril) is the only antipsychotic to have minimal risk of tardive dyskinesia and can even help improve pre-existing symptoms of tardive dyskinesia. This has been attributed to its low affinity for D_2 receptors and high affinity for 5-hydroxytryptamine (5-HT) receptor antagonism. Patients who are receiving antipsychotics should be examined regularly for the appearance of abnormal movements, preferably with the use of a standardized rating scale. Patients frequently experience an exacerbation of their symptoms when the DRA is withheld or its dose is lowered, whereas substitution of an SDA may limit the abnormal movements without worsening the progression of the dyskinesia.

Once tardive dyskinesia is recognized, the clinician should consider reducing the dose of the antipsychotic or even stopping the medication altogether. Alternatively, the clinician may switch the patient to clozapine or to an SDA. In patients who cannot continue taking any antipsychotic medication, lithium (Eskalith), carbamazepine (Tegretol), or benzodiazepines may effectively reduce the symptoms of both the movement disorder and the psychosis.

Valbenazine and Deutetrabenazine. In 2017, valbenazine (Ingrezz) became the first FDA-approved drug to treat adults with tardive dyskinesia. Also in 2017, a second drug, deutetrabenazine (Austedo), was approved by the FDA for the treatment of chorea associated with Huntington disease and tardive dyskinesia. Both drugs inhibit the vesicular monoamine transporter 2 (VMAT2), which results in reversible reduction of dopamine release. Since tardive dyskinesia is believed to be associated with dopamine hypersensitivity, the reduction in levels of available dopamine in the synaptic cleft alleviates symptoms of the disorder.

Valbenazine is available as a 40-mg capsule. The initial dose is 40 mg once daily. After 1 week, the dose can be increased to the recommended dose of 80 mg once daily. It can be taken with or without food. The recommended dose for patients with moderate or severe hepatic impairment is 40 mg once daily.

Deutetrabenazine is available in 6-, 9-, and 12-mg tablets. The initial dose is 12 mg per day and can be titrated at weekly intervals by 6 mg daily. Total daily doses of 12 mg or above should be divided into two doses and should be administered with food. Deutetrabenazine is contraindicated in patients with hepatic impairment or who are concurrently taking valbenazine, monoamine oxidase inhibitors (MAOIs), or reserpine. Patients who have discontinued MAOI treatment should wait 14 days after final dose before initiating treatment with deutetrabenazine. Patients should wait 20 days after their final dose of reserpine before beginning treatment with deutetrabenazine.

For both drugs, consider dose reduction based on tolerability in known CYP2D6 poor metabolizers. Its use should also be avoided in patients with congenital or drug-induced long QT syndrome or with abnormal heartbeats associated with a prolonged QT interval. Serious side effects include sleepiness and QT prolongation, as well as nasopharyngitis particularly with deutetrabenazine. Patients taking either drug should not drive or operate heavy machinery or do other dangerous activities until it is known how the drug affects them. Alcohol and sedating drugs may have additive effects.

Valbenazine may interact with MAOIs, itraconazole, ketoconazole, clarithromycin, paroxetine, fluoxetine, quinidine, rifampin, carbamazepine, phenytoin, St. John's wort, and digoxin.

Tardive Dystonia and Tardive Akathisia

On occasion, dystonia and akathisia emerge late in the course of treatment. These symptoms may persist for months or years despite drug discontinuation or dose reduction.

Medication-Induced Postural Tremor

Diagnosis, Signs, and Symptoms

Tremor is a rhythmic alteration in movement that is usually faster than 1 beat/second. Fine tremor (8 to 12 Hz) is most common.

Epidemiology

Typically, tremors decrease during periods of relaxation and sleep and increase with stress or anxiety.

Etiology

Whereas all the above diagnoses specifically include an association with a neuroleptic, a range of psychiatric medications can produce tremor—most notably, lithium, stimulants, antidepressants, caffeine, and valproic acid (Depakene).

Treatment

The treatment involves four principles:

1. The lowest possible dose of the psychiatric drug should be taken.
2. Patients should minimize caffeine consumption.
3. The psychiatric drug should be taken at bedtime to minimize the amount of daytime tremor.
4. β-Adrenergic receptor antagonists (e.g., propranolol [Inderal]) can be given to treat drug-induced tremors.

Other Medication-Induced Movement Disorders

Periodic Limb Movement Disorder

Periodic Limb Movement Disorder (PLMD), formerly called nocturnal myoclonus, consists of highly stereotyped, abrupt contractions of certain leg, and occasionally of upper extremity muscles during sleep. Patients lack any subjective awareness of the leg jerks. The condition may be present in about 40% of persons over 65 years of age. The cause is unknown, but it is a rare side effect of SSRIs.

The repetitive movements occur every 20 to 60 seconds, most commonly with extensions of the large toe and flexion of the ankle, the knee, and the hips. Frequent awakenings, unrefreshing sleep, and daytime sleepiness are major symptoms. No treatment for nocturnal myoclonus is universally effective. Treatments that may be useful include dopamine agonists, anticonvulsants, benzodiazepines, levodopa, quinine, and, in rare cases, opioids. Gabapentinoids and dopamine agonists are considered appropriate first-line therapies.

Restless Legs Syndrome

In *restless legs syndrome*, persons feel deep sensations of creeping inside the calves whenever sitting or lying down. The dysesthesias are rarely painful but are agonizingly relentless and cause an almost irresistible urge to move the legs; thus, this syndrome interferes with sleep and with falling asleep. It peaks in

TABLE 42-4: Drug-Induced Central Hyperthermic Syndromes[a]

Condition (and Mechanism)	Common Drug Causes	Frequent Symptoms	Possible Treatment[b]	Clinical Course
Hyperthermia (↓ heat dissipation) (↑ heat production)	Atropine, lidocaine, meperidine, NSAID toxicity, pheochromocytoma, thyrotoxicosis	Hyperthermia, diaphoresis, malaise	Acetaminophen per rectum (325 mg every 4 hours), diazepam oral or per rectum (5 mg every 8 hours) for febrile seizures	Benign, febrile seizures in children
Malignant hyperthermia (↑ heat production)	NMJ blockers (succinylcholine), halothane	Hyperthermia muscle rigidity, arrhythmias, ischemia, hypotension,[c] rhabdomyolysis; disseminated intravascular coagulation	Dantrolene sodium (1–2 mg/kg/minute IV infusion)[d]	Familial, 10% mortality if untreated
Tricyclic overdose (↑ heat production)	Tricyclic antidepressants, cocaine	Hyperthermia, confusion, visual hallucinations, agitation, hyperreflexia, muscle relaxation, anticholinergic effects (dry skin, pupil dilation), arrhythmias	Sodium bicarbonate (1 mEq/kg IV bolus) if arrhythmia is present, physostigmine (1–3 mg IV) with cardiac monitoring	Fatalities have occurred if untreated
Autonomic hyperreflexia (↑ heat production)	CNS stimulants (amphetamines)	Hyperthermia, excitement, hyperreflexia	Trimethaphan (0.3–7 mg/minute IV infusion)	Reversible
Lethal catatonia (↓ heat dissipation)	Lead poisoning	Hyperthermia, intense anxiety, destructive behavior, psychosis	Lorazepam (1–2 mg IV every 4 hours), antipsychotics may be contraindicated	High mortality if untreated
Neuroleptic malignant syndrome (mixed; hypothalamic, ↓ heat dissipation, ↑ heat production)	Antipsychotics (neuroleptics), methyldopa, reserpine	Hyperthermia, muscle rigidity, diaphoresis (60%), leukocytosis, delirium, rhabdomyolysis, elevated CPK, autonomic deregulation, extrapyramidal symptoms	Bromocriptine (2–10 mg every 8 hours orally or nasogastric tube), lisuride (0.02–0.1 mg/hour IV infusion), carbidopa–levodopa (Sinemet) (25/100 PO every 8 hours), dantrolene sodium (0.3–1 mg/kg IV every 6 hours)	Rapid onset, 20% mortality if untreated

[a]Boldface indicates features that may be used to distinguish one syndrome from another.
[b]Gastric lavage and supportive measures, including cooling, are required in most cases.
[c]Oxygen consumption increases by 7% for every 1°F increase in body temperature.
[d]Has been associated with idiosyncratic hepatocellular injury, as well as severe hypotension in one case.
NSAID, nonsteroidal anti-inflammatory drug; NMJ, neuromuscular junction; CNS, central nervous system; CPK, creatine phosphokinase; PO, orally; IV, intravenously.
From Theoharides TC, Harris RS, Weckstein D. Neuroleptic malignant-like syndrome due to cyclobenzaprine? *J Clin Psychopharmacol.* 1995;15:79–81, with permission.

middle age and occurs in 5% of the population. The cause is unknown, but it is a rare side effect of SSRIs.

Symptoms are relieved by movement and by leg massage. The dopamine receptor agonists, ropinirole (Requip) and pramipexole (Mirapex), are effective in treating this syndrome. Other treatments include the benzodiazepines, levodopa, quinine, opioids, propranolol, valproate, and carbamazepine.

Hyperthermic Syndromes

All the medication-induced movement disorders may be associated with hyperthermia. Table 42-4 summarizes the drugs associated with hyperthermia, possible mechanisms as well their symptoms, treatments, and their clinical course.

Pharmacogenomic Testing $\quad$ 43

Introduction

Medical genetics is an emerging field, particularly in the field of psychiatry. It helps us understand the role of genes and their use for medical applications. In addition, it helps us identify risks for developing disease as well as personalize treatment through a very targeted approach using specific drugs based on genetic profile. Pharmacogenomics is the study of how genetics affects individual patients' metabolism and response to therapeutic drugs. Its name is a combination of the words "pharmacology" and "genomics," which is the study of the function and structure of genomes (for a refresher on the terminology of genetics, see Table 43-1).

Pharmacogenomics is already playing a crucial role in personalized and precision medicine and will continue to become more integral to patient care as the technology improves and the costs of testing come down. However, it needs to be emphasized that pharmacogenomics as a field of research, particularly in psychiatry, is still in its infancy. Despite the limitations, it helps provide clarity on the link between genomic variations in the cytochrome P450 (CYP) enzyme system and the variability in the rate of drug metabolism. The CYP enzyme system is responsible for the metabolism of drugs and this variation in an individual can range from being a poor to ultrarapid metabolizer. While pharmacogenomic testing can help clinicians assess these genomic variations to predict the metabolism of various medicines, thereby allowing them to modify dosages and predict drug interactions, the technology still needs time to be developed for more accurate and personalized approach. Clinicians should continue to monitor patients for

TABLE 43-1: Commonly Used Terminology in Genetics	
Term	Definition
Allele	The variant of a given gene. Each person inherits two alleles, one from each parent, that occur at a specific site on a chromosome.
Chromosome	A deoxyribonucleic acid (DNA) molecule containing all or part of an organism's genetic material.
DNA bases	The bases serve as the building blocks of DNA nucleotides and provide structure to the human genome. There are four: adenine, thymine, cytosine, and guanine.
Genome	The DNA of a cell, including mitochondrial DNA and nuclear chromosomes.
Nucleotide	Organic molecules consisting of a nucleoside and a phosphate. Nucleotides are the basic units of DNA and ribonucleic acid (RNA).
Polymorphisms	DNA variants occurring within a single population at a frequency of greater than 1%.
Single nucleotide polymorphisms (SNPs)	A polymorphism involving the substitution of one nucleotide for another nucleotide.

adverse events and view pharmacogenomics as a tool to enhance rather than substitute good judgment.

Humans share approximately 99.9% of their DNA with other people. Despite this seemingly minor variance, 0.1% difference provides an enormous amount of variability and accounts for the vast diversity among the billions of people on Earth. These genetic differences account for our differences in appearance and aptitudes, as well as our chances of developing certain diseases and how we respond to individual treatments. Even minor shifts and substitutions contained in a single gene can have a major clinical impact.

Research into the field of pharmacogenomics is ongoing and has accelerated rapidly following the completion of the Human Genome Project in 2003, which mapped and sequenced the base pairs of nucleotides that comprise human DNA. Since that time, numerous key single-nucleotide polymorphisms (SNPs) have been identified that can influence gene expression and the activity of enzymes responsible for drug metabolism, particularly those found in the CYP system. By testing for these SNPs, clinicians should be able to better predict potentially abnormal responses to specific medications and adjust treatment accordingly, at least theoretically.

Just as certain traits are more common among groups with a similar lineage and genetic profile, certain SNPs are more common among certain ethnic groups. For example, SNPs affecting vitamin K epoxide reductase complex subunit 1 (VKORC1) and CYP2C9 liver enzymes are more common in individuals of East Asian ancestry than individuals of Western European ancestry. These SNPs have been shown to slow clearance rates of drugs like warfarin. Unsurprisingly, individuals of East Asian ancestry frequently experience adverse effects when on the drug warfarin and oftentimes require lower initiation and maintenance doses than people who can trace their lineage back to Western Europe.

Effect of SNPs on Drug Metabolism

Several clinical variables can affect how a patient responds to drug treatment. Age, organ function, sex, diet, and drug regimen can all influence an individual drug's effect. Genetics is just one more piece of the puzzle, and researchers have found that several dozen individual genes are responsible for encoding the cells that produce individual CYP enzymes. An SNP at one such loci can affect one or more of the CYP enzymes responsible for metabolizing a drug, thereby altering the rate with which it is metabolized.

If a patient metabolizes a drug at a fast rate, a larger dose may be necessary to obtain the desired effect. Conversely, a patient who metabolizes a drug slower than others may experience a prolonged or enhanced effect of the drug that may potentially lead to adverse events. Consequently, a lower dose may be necessary for patients with these SNPs.

CYP genotyping can be used to screen patients for SNPs that can affect the metabolism of drugs, and there are four metabolizer categories: Poor metabolizers, intermediate metabolizers, extensive metabolizers, and ultrarapid metabolizers. Metabolism can also be altered by SNPs that affect transport proteins such as P-glycoprotein. For a list of common variations, see Table 43-2.

TABLE 43-2: Pharmacokinetic Genetic Variations and Their Clinical Significance

Gene Result	Allele	Effect on Metabolism	Clinical Significance
ACBC1 (rs2032583)	A/A	N/A	Associated with normal activity
ABCB1 (rs1045642)	A/A	N/A	Reduced activity of P-glycoprotein, which affects intestinal absorption and blood–brain barrier penetration. May lead to increased absorption of some medications, including opioids and second-generation antipsychotics.
CYP1A2	*1F/*1F	Extensive in presence of inducers	Use of inducers like coffee, cannabis, and tobacco associated with decreased serum levels and possible increased risk of drug interactions with active metabolites
CYP2B6	*1/*5	Extensive	Associated with normal activity
CYP2C9	*1/*3	Intermediate	Increased risk of drug interactions and elevated serum levels
CYP2C19	*1/*2	Intermediate	Increased risk of drug interactions and elevated serum levels
CYP2D6	*1/*4	Intermediate	Increased risk of drug interactions and elevated serum levels
CYP3A4	*1/*1	Extensive	Associated with normal activity
CYP3A5	*3/*3	Extensive	Associated with normal activity
UGT1A4	*1a/*1a	Extensive	Associated with normal activity
UGT2B15	*2/*2	Intermediate	Increased risk of drug interactions and elevated serum levels

The Indiana University School of Medicine has produced a far more exhaustive CYP drug interaction table that includes commonly prescribed drugs that interact with CYP substrates (https://drug-interactions.medicine.iu.edu/MainTable.aspx).

Effect of SNPs on Pharmacodynamics

In addition to affecting how the body absorbs, distributes, metabolizes, or excretes a drug, SNPs can impact the protein expression or the structural integrity of individual proteins. Consequently, this can have an impact on the efficacy of drugs that are meant to target these protein receptors. To use an analogy, if these receptors are locks and the drugs are keys, SNPs may slightly alter the shape of the lock, thereby changing how well the key slides into the lock. Some common pharmacodynamic genetic variations can be found in Table 43-3.

It should be noted that pharmacogenomic testing has advanced at a far quicker pace with pharmacokinetics than pharmacodynamics. Consequently, clinicians should not purely depend on these tests regarding the choice of medicine. Rather, the treatment decision regarding medication should be based on clinical response and potential risks. The tests are ancillary to good clinical judgment. It is important to note that genetic testing for medical conditions like cancer,

TABLE 43-3: Pharmacodynamic Genetic Variations and Their Clinical Significance

Gene	Allele	Affected Protein	Protein Type	Clinical Significance
5HTR2A	A/A	Serotonin receptor 2A (5HT$_{2A}$)	Serotonin receptor	Improved chances of response to citalopram; Decreased changes of response to non-SSRI antidepressants
5HT2C	T/T	Serotonin receptor 2C (5HT$_{2C}$)	Serotonin receptor	Decreased risk of weight gain with use of second-generation antipsychotics.
ADRA2A	C/G	Alpha-2A adrenergic receptor	Adrenoceptor and target for many catecholamines, particularly norepinephrine	Increased response to stimulants in treating symptoms associated with ADHD
ANK3	C/T	Ankyrin-3	Protein associated with sodium channel function	Aberrant sodium channel function may affect mood regulation. Several therapeutic agents may modulate sodium channel signaling and necessitate mood stabilizers
BDNF	Val/Val	Brain-derived neurotrophic factor	Protein integral to neural plasticity and neuronal development	Normal activity
CACNA1C	G/G	Calcium channel	Subunit of L-type voltage-gated calcium channels	Normal activity
COMT	Val/Met	Catechol-O-Methyl-transferase	Catabolic enzyme involved in the breakdown of dopamine in the frontal cortex	Normal activity
DRD2	C/C	Dopamine receptor D2	Dopamine receptor	Normal activity
GRIK1	C/C	Glutamate receptor kainite-1	Neurotransmitter receptor	Increased chance of response to topiramate for treatment of alcohol use disorder
HLA-A *31:01	Negative	Major histocompatibility complex, class I, A	Part of a group of genes known as the human leukocyte antigen complex	Some variants increase the risk of drug-induced skin reactions, particularly with use of carbamazepine
HLA-B *15:02	Negative	Major histocompatibility complex, class I, B	Part of a group of genes known as the human leukocyte antigen complex	Some variants increase the risk of drug-induced skin reactions, particularly with use of carbamazepine, oxcarbazepine, phenytoin, and fosphenytoin

MC4R	A/A	Melacortin 4 receptor	Receptor integral to feeding behavior, metabolism, and sexual function	increased risk of weight gain with use of second-generation antipsychotics. • Highest risk: clozapine, olanzapine • Medium risk: aripiprazole, brexpiprazole, iloperidone, paliperidone, quetiapine, risperidone Lower risk: asenapine, cariprazine, lurasidone, ziprasidone
MTHFR	C667T: C/C	Methylene-tetrahydrofolate	Catabolic enzyme responsible for the breakdown of conversion of folic acid to methylfoate	Normal activity
MTHFR	A1298C: A/A	Methylene-tetrahydrofolate	Catabolic enzyme involved in the conversion of folic acid to methylfolate	Normal activity
OPRM1	A/A	μ-Opioid receptor	Opioid receptor	Normal activity
SLC6A4	L(G)	Serotonin transporter and solute carrier family 6 member 4	Transporter involved in serotonin reuptake	Increased risk of side effects, especially those affecting the GI tract, with SSRIs.
SLC6A4	S	Serotonin transporter and solute carrier family 6 member 4	Transporter involved in serotonin reuptake	Increased risk of side effects, especially those affecting the GI tract, with SSRIs.

ADHD, Attention-deficit/hyperactivity disorder; GI, Gastrointestinal; SSRI, Selective serotonin reuptake inhibitor specifically breast cancer, tests for biomarkers and provides specific data and information. Consequently, the treatment based on such data can be lifesaving. Unfortunately, the same is not true for psychiatric disorders and clinicians should not expect the same degree of accuracy with pharmacogenomic testing while treating mental health conditions. More research is needed to predict specific medications purely based on pharmacogenomic testing for psychiatric disorders.

Conclusion

In the coming years, pharmacogenomics will offer a wealth of opportunities for clinicians to better treat patients. By having a clearer understanding of a patient's DNA, clinicians will be able to create a more personalized treatment algorithm. For clinicians and patients alike, this will translate into a more efficient use of resources, with fewer adverse events, hospitalizations, and overdoses. As of now, there are no treatment guidelines on the use of pharmacogenomic testing in psychiatric disorders and clinicians should continue to recommend treatments that incorporate various modalities to help patients regain functional status.

Brain Stimulation or Neuromodulation Procedures

44

Introduction

The first recorded use of brain stimulation occurred in ancient Greece more than 2,000 years ago. Writing in the first century CE, Scribonius Largus, a physician familiar with the practice, claimed that electric eels (*torpedo nigra*) could be used to treat patients with headaches, chronic pain, gout, seizures, and depression.

Modern brain stimulation techniques were pioneered in the 1930s, following the work of Hungarian psychiatrist Laszlo Meduna, who first studied how the administration of convulsion-inducing drugs could reduce psychiatric symptoms. In 1938, Ugo Cerletti and his assistant, Lucio Bini, first administered electroconvulsive therapy (ECT) to a human patient after years of using animal models to study the effects of electric current on epilepsy. After 11 treatments, their patient's symptoms remitted. Subsequently, ECT was used for the first time in the United States in 1939.

Though ECT became increasingly common throughout the 1940s, by today's standards, the procedure was significantly unpleasant for patients, and many experienced bone fractures on account of the intensity of the convulsions, as well as anticipatory anxiety prior to treatments. Advances in anesthetics and the development of muscle relaxants in the 1950s eliminated these problems, but the 1950s also saw the rise of more sophisticated psychiatric medications that made ECT look antiquated. In addition, negative depictions of ECT in films such as *The Snakepit* (1948) and *One Flew Over the Cuckoo's Nest* (1975) took a toll on patients' perception of the treatment, which seemed at best old-fashioned and at worst barbaric. These perceptions persist to this day, and many patients may be shocked to find that ECT is still widely considered to be an effective and safe treatment modality.

Despite the enduring public stigma against it, ECT has been used safely for decades, and several additional brain stimulation procedures have been developed within the past three decades to treat a host of psychiatric disorders. These treatments include minimally invasive and transcranial techniques such as transcranial magnetic stimulation (TMS), cranial electrotherapy stimulation (CES), and transcranial direct current stimulation (tDCS—also called direct current polarization). More invasive and surgical techniques include vagus nerve stimulation (VNS) and deep brain stimulation (DBS). Experimental procedures that will be briefly mentioned in this chapter include magnetic seizure therapy (MST) and low field magnetic stimulation (LFMS).

All the devices mentioned here are classified by the FDA into one of three classes; I, II, or III based on their risk, safety, and effectiveness. In terms of their risks, class I devices carry the lowest risk while class III devices pose the highest risk.

Pretreatment Evaluation

For patients who have not responded to more conventional treatments or cannot tolerate pharmaceutical interventions due to severe side effects, neuromodulation interventions can offer hope, but clinicians should strive to provide them with a full understanding of the benefits, risks, adverse events, and side effects involved with these treatments. Patients should also recognize that some procedures are more invasive than others.

Before initiating any of these procedures, clinicians should conduct a pretreatment evaluation to:

- Confirm that the treatment is indicated
- Establish baseline psychiatric and cognitive status
- Perform a standard physical, neurologic, and preanesthesia examinations and obtain a complete medical history with laboratory evaluations that include blood and urine chemistries, a chest x-ray, and an electrocardiogram (ECG)
- Identify, and then treat, any medical conditions that could increase the risks associated with the procedure
- Complete the informed consent process

Mechanism of Action

All brain activity is a combination of electrical and chemical communication. Pharmacology concerns itself with modulating the chemical communication system, which in turn can affect electrical signaling in the central nervous system (CNS). Conversely, brain stimulation focuses on modulating the electrical signaling in the CNS, which then produces localized neurochemical changes.

Pregnancy

Pregnant patients may benefit from these treatments and the procedures may be safely performed without serious risk. Particularly in cases where patients are suffering from life-threatening depression, brain stimulation therapies are considered safe and effective treatment options.

Electroconvulsive Therapy

ECT uses electric current to induce a generalized cerebral seizure. Since the 1950s, the procedure has been performed while patients are under general anesthesia. There is a dose–response relationship with right unilateral ECT and that bilateral ECT is likely to be ineffective with ultrabrief pulse widths. The induction of a bilateral generalized seizure is necessary for both the beneficial and the adverse effects since it affects the cellular mechanisms of memory and mood regulation as well as raises the seizure threshold. The latter effect may be blocked by the opiate antagonist naloxone (Narcan).

Therapeutic Indications and Uses

ECT is indicated as a Class II device by the Food and Drug Administration (FDA) for catatonia and severe major depressive episodes associated with major depressive disorder or bipolar disorder in patients who are both treatment resistant and 13 years of age or older. ECT devices are also in premarket approval (Class III) for the following indications: schizophrenia, schizoaffective disorder, schizophreniform disorder, and episodes of mania associated with bipolar disorder. There is limited evidence that ECT can help treat suicidality, severe psychosis, and depression-related food refusal.

Procedure

Though there are no standard number of ECT treatments and no way to predict patient response, most patients show improvement after 6 to 12 treatments, though some may require only 3 while others may need as many as 20. Standard practice in the United States is to conduct three ECT treatments per week. Maintenance ECT treatments may be given in intervals of every 1 to 8 weeks during the first 6 months of remission.

Warnings

The seizures induced by ECT can cause transient increases in blood pressure, myocardial oxygen consumption, heart rate, and intracranial pressure. Extreme caution should be used when treating patients with compromised cardiovascular, pulmonary, or central nervous systems.

Contraindications. Absolute contraindications for ECT include pheochromocytoma and elevated intracranial pressure with mass effect. Relative contraindications include elevated intracranial pressure without mass effect, cardiovascular conduction defects, aortic and cerebral aneurysms, and high-risk pregnancies.

Drug Interactions. Clinicians should review patients' current medications prior to the procedure. Antidepressants (including tricyclics, selective serotonin reuptake inhibitors [SSRIs], serotonin–norepinephrine reuptake inhibitors [SNRIs], and monoamine oxidase inhibitors [MAOIs]) are generally safe to use with ECT and have little effect on tolerability. Antipsychotic medications, particularly second-generation antipsychotics (SGAs), may provide some synergistic antipsychotic effects.

Concomitant lithium use with ECT is safe. However, it may increase delirium following treatment, prolong the effects of succinylcholine (which is administered during the procedure), and lower seizure threshold, thereby leading to prolonged seizures.

Mortality. The mortality rate with ECT is about 0.002% per treatment and 0.01% for each patient.

Adverse Events

Headache, confusion, and delirium are possible shortly after the seizure and marked confusion may occur in up to 10% of patients. However, acute confusion tends to clear within 10 to 30 minutes of the procedure. Conversely, delirium characteristically clears within several days or a few weeks at the longest. Temporary jaw or neck discomfort are also common side effects and typically fade within a few days. On occasion, patients may experience dental and tongue injuries if the oral bite block is not properly in place during the procedure and loose teeth are at an increased risk of dislodgement.

Anterograde amnesia (the inability or decreased ability to create new memories) is frequently reported during the course of ECT and tends to resolve within 2 weeks. Consequently, it is advised that patients not drive or make important decisions within 2 to 3 weeks of completing the treatment. Retrograde amnesia may affect memories from weeks or months prior to the treatment and in some cases, the amnesia may affect memories that are more than a year old. Oftentimes these memories return, but rarely may lead to permanent loss. Memory deficits tend to be most persistent in impersonal knowledge (world events or news) and are far less pronounced in more intimate knowledge about the self.

Approximately 75% of all patients who undergo ECT say that the memory impairment is the worst adverse effect, but almost all patients are back to their cognitive baseline after 6 months.

Transcranial Magnetic Stimulation

TMS or repetitive transcranial magnetic stimulation (rTMS) is a noninvasive procedure that induces electrical fields in the brain with alternating magnetic fields measured in units known as tesla (T). It is the international system unit of field intensity for magnetic fields used in magnetic resonance imaging (MRI) and is named after the Serbian American inventor and engineer who discovered the rotating magnetic field, Nikolai Tesla.

The strength of the magnetic field used in TMS is typically 1.5 tesla (T) and produced by an insulated coil that is applied directly to the scalp. TMS allows clinicians to target focal regions of the brain without the need for anesthesia. TMS frequencies equal to or below 1 Hz (slow TMS) are believed to affect inhibitory neuronal networks by activating γ-aminobutyric acid-ergic (GABAergic) interneurons within the cortex. Frequencies above 1 Hz (fast TMS) have more glutamatergic or excitatory effects.

Therapeutic Indications and Uses

rTMS is indicated for the treatment of major depressive disorder in patients who have not responded to at least one antidepressant drug treatment and are currently not undergoing antidepressant therapy.

Beyond treatment-resistant depression, studies have shown some therapeutic potential for rTMS in the treatment of obsessive-compulsive disorder (OCD), posttraumatic stress disorder (PTSD), generalized anxiety disorder (GAD), Tourette disorder, bipolar disorder, movement disorders, and chronic pain.

Procedure

rTMS sessions are usually carried out five times per week. In addition, since there is no need for sedation, patients are alert for the procedure. The number of treatments ranges from 20 to 30 for an acute treatment course.

Warnings

The most concerning risk of TMS is seizure during the procedure, which has an incidence rate of approximately 1 per 10,000 TMS sessions.

Contraindications. TMS should not be administered to patients with pacemakers or implantable medical devices; ferrous implants, shrapnel, or bullet fragments near or in their neck and head; or facial tattoos that contain metallic or magnetic-sensitive ink. Risk of seizure is higher in patients with a history of seizure or epilepsy.

Adverse Events

Site application pain and headaches are common adverse events, with upward of 20% of patients reporting the latter. In most cases, headaches are mild and dissipate after the first week of treatment. TMS device emits a loud clicking sound, and therefore, patients are advised to wear earplugs.

Cranial Electrotherapy Stimulation

CES involves the use of a weak electrical current (1 to 4 mA) to stimulate or modulate central and/or peripheral nervous system activity. First marketed in the 1970s, CES treatment involves attaching electrodes to bilateral anatomical positions located on the head (e.g., earlobes, mastoids, temples). The treatment has been shown to be effective in treating anxiety, insomnia, and depression.

Therapeutic Indications and Uses

The FDA has approved the use of CES devices for the treatment of anxiety and insomnia and classified them as Class II devices. CES devices used to treat depression are classified as Class III devices.

Procedure

The device is small, portable, and battery operated and therefore, patients can use it from the comfort of their own homes.

Contraindications

There are no known contraindications for CES devices.

Adverse Events

It is believed that the CES stimulation is not harmful, primarily due to its low-voltage power supply (9-V battery) and lack of any reported adverse event by the FDA. Mild discomfort due to local skin effects and a general feeling of dizziness following use have been reported.

Transcranial Direct Current Stimulation

Although tDCS has not been approved by the FDA for any use at this time, the treatment is noninvasive and appears to cause limited side effects or discomfort in patients. The treatment involves passing a weak (oftentimes ≤1 mA) direct DC current between two electrodes applied directly to the scalp. The current enters from the anode, travels through patient tissue, and then passes into the cathode.

tDCS is believed to act via the alteration of neuronal membrane polarization, but little is known about the actual mechanism of action.

Therapeutic Indications and Uses

Unfortunately, currently there is paucity of strong evidence to support the use of tDCS, but small studies suggest promising results in the treatment of major depressive disorder. There is notably weaker evidence about its use in treating Parkinson disease, Alzheimer disease, chronic pain, and schizophrenia.

Procedure

The device is small, portable, and battery operated and specialized electrodes are not necessary. Instead, researchers have even been known to use damp sponges as the electrodes. Typical sessions last about 20 to 30 minutes and can be repeated daily for several weeks. In time, patients may be able to use the device without clinician supervision.

Contraindications

Patients with implantable medical devices or metallic implants should not use tDCS, as the implants may alter current flow. Patients with a history of migraines or scalp conditions may be at a greater risk of discomfort following tDCS administration.

Adverse Events

There are no known serious adverse effects of this treatment. The most common side effects in the literature consist of mostly minimal tingling at the site of stimulation, skin irritation, nausea, headache, and dizziness.

Vagus Nerve Stimulation

VNS is a treatment involving an implanted device that stimulates the left vagus nerve with weak electrical pulses. Though originally approved by the FDA in 1997 as adjunctive therapy in reducing the frequency of seizures in children over 12 years of age and adults, the treatment has since been approved for use in children as young as 4 years of age with partial-onset seizures who have not responded to more conventional medications. Anecdotal reports of improved mood among epilepsy patients and subsequent studies into the treatment's efficacy in treating depression led to its approval by the FDA for this use in 2005.

Several studies have also suggested that VNS could treat a wide range of inflammatory conditions, including rheumatoid arthritis, diabetes, and lung injury.

Psychiatric Indications

VNS is currently approved by the FDA as an adjunctive treatment for adults with treatment-resistant and severe unipolar or bipolar depression. As the treatment often takes upward of 10 to 12 months to produce the full and desired effect, it is not considered a rapid treatment for depression.

Procedure

Surgery is required to implant electrodes that stimulate the left vagus nerve with weak electrical pulses. A bipolar lead is also wrapped around the left nerve in the neck and connected to a generator that is implanted in the chest wall, typically just below the left clavicle. The stimulating current is unidirectional to minimize efferent side effects.

The device is only turned on several weeks after the operation.

Adverse Events

With VNS, adverse events can be divided into those related to the surgery and those related to the operation of the device and side effects of stimulation.

Surgical Complications.   Surgical complications may include infection, left vocal cord paresis, and temporary asystole. No known deaths have occurred due to asystole and normal cardiac rhythm has always been restored. Moreover, no cardiac events have been reported following the activation of the device.

Side Effects Associated with Stimulation.   Once the device has been turned on, patients may experience voice alteration, cough, pain, and dyspnea in the initial days following device activation. Voice alteration and dyspnea may persist far longer, while other side effects typically abate.

More importantly, patients with bipolar disorder may be at risk of episodes of hypomania or frank mania.

Deep Brain Stimulation

Initially developed to treat patients with Parkinson disease, DBS is a more invasive procedure that requires the use of MRI and electrophysiologically guided stereotaxic placement of electrodes in specific regions with the brain. These electrodes can be placed in subdural or extradural neural tissue, and then stimulated electronically. Extradural stimulation is oftentimes referred to as cortical stimulation.

Therapeutic Indications and Uses

DBS is currently indicated for use in treating Parkinson disease, but is also effective in treating dystonia, essential tremor, epilepsy, and severe medically intractable Tourette syndrome. In addition, it has received licensing approval in the United States for treatment of refractory OCD. Existing evidence does not support the use of DBS for the treatment of depression, though clinical studies for this indication are ongoing.

Extradural cortical stimulation has been used to mitigate certain types of pain with promising results, but its efficacy in the field of psychiatry remains an open question.

Procedure

Implanting the electrodes in neural tissue requires patients to undergo surgery where burr holes are drilled into the skull bone. The leads are then guided by multimodal imaging and precise stereotactic landmarking. Thereafter, a "pacemaker" (also known as an implantable neurostimulator or pulse generator) is implanted under the skin, typically in the upper chest wall. The two are then connected via extension wires tunneled under the skin.

The device is turned on after several weeks.

Contraindications

This therapy is contraindicated for patients who are incapable of operating the neurostimulator, as well as patients with dementia, active psychiatric disorders, and structural CNS abnormalities.

Adverse Events

The vast majority of adverse effects are related to the initial surgery rather than the operation of the neurostimulator. Complications may include bleeding in the brain, stroke, infection, seizure, breathing problems, or heart problems. Following the surgery, patients may experience confusion, headache, difficulty concentrating, stroke, nausea, or temporary pain or swelling at the site of the implant.

Once the device has been turned on, patients may experience numbness or tingling sensations, lightheadedness, double vision, muscle tightness, difficulties with balance, speech problems, and mood lability.

Experimental Treatments

Magnetic Seizure Therapy

MST is a novel form of convulsive treatment that uses rTMS at higher rates to induce therapeutic seizures under general anesthesia. MST is a convulsive treatment in many ways similar to ECT, and it requires approximately the same preparation and infrastructure as ECT. Though researchers have been studying the use of MST since the 1990s, it has yet to receive FDA approval for use in treating any condition.

Low Field Magnetic Stimulation

LFMS uses low-strength, high-frequency electromagnetic fields to treat unipolar depression, bipolar depression, and anxiety. Though the device is not FDA approved for any indication at this time, the noninvasive treatment has been shown to reduce depressive symptom severity in patients with treatment-resistant depression in as little as three 20-minute sessions and to improve symptoms in bipolar disorder in as little as one 20-minute session. Larger studies need to be conducted to better determine the permanence of these effects.

Conclusion

The many techniques of neuromodulation explored in this chapter are by and large safe and effective. While they may be used in conjunction with pharmaceutical treatments, these techniques also offer hope to patients who have not responded to conventional interventions or for patients who cannot tolerate many medications due to severe adverse events. Moreover, many are noninvasive and offer patients the convenience of using the devices in their own homes.

Unfortunately, many of the brain stimulation techniques explored in this chapter are still relatively new technologies with limited evidence due to a lack of large, well-designed studies. As these devices become more popular, this will likely change, though there are several obstacles facing those responsible for developing the studies. For one, pharmaceutical treatments allow for the use of placebo to compare effects between active and inactive agents. However, it is far more difficult to "blind" patients when using devices that are designed to produce stimulation during treatment. Second, questions persist about best practices when using different devices. It remains to be seen if there is a specific location on the head where individual devices should be placed for maximum effect and if this location is universal or something that needs to be determined on a patient-by-patient basis. Questions also persist about the frequency and duration of sessions. Without standardization, it can make it very difficult to compare research.

Finally, while there is mounting evidence to support the use of these techniques, particularly rTMS and ECT, there are still questions about the mechanism of action of brain stimulation. While research suggests that these techniques enhance neuronal plasticity, the intercellular changes that are responsible for the therapeutic effects of these interventions need to be better·elucidated. In time, these findings may help explain not only why neuromodulation is effective, but also provide clinicians with reasoning for choosing one neuromodulation technique over another.

Index

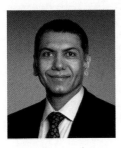

Samoon Ahmad, M.D. is a Clinical Professor of Psychiatry at NYU Grossman School of Medicine and recently completed 30 years of service at Bellevue Hospital Center serving as Unit Chief of Inpatient Psychiatry. A graduate of Allama Iqbal Medical College in Lahore, Pakistan, where he trained in Internal Medicine, General Surgery, and Cardiology, Dr. Ahmad completed his psychiatric training at Bellevue Hospital/NYU Medical Center, serving as chief resident in his final year. Upon completion, he became an Attending at Bellevue and joined the faculty of the NYU School of Medicine. Dr. Ahmad supervises and mentors trainees, and lectures globally on various topics, including antipsychotics, obesity, metabolic disorders, and medical marijuana. He is a Diplomate of the American Board of Psychiatry and Neurology, a Distinguished Life Fellow of the American Psychiatric Association, and an International Associate member of the Royal College of Psychiatrists.

During his tenure, Dr. Ahmad has served as Director of the Division of Continuing Medical Education (CME), on the board of Governors of Bellevue Psychiatric Society, and on various committees including Grand Rounds, CME Advisory, CME Task Force, Educational Steering, Bellevue Collaboration Council, and Bellevue Psychiatry's Oversight Committee. He developed Bellevue Hospital Psychiatry Department's Integrated Systems Conference, based on the morbidity and mortality conference in medicine, to better coordinate services and treatment in the department. He was recognized for 25 years of distinguished service at Bellevue and was named Bellevue's Physician of the Year in Psychiatry (2014) for his continued pursuit of clinical excellence, leadership, and dedication at the institution.

Dr. Ahmad's research has focused primarily on the prevalence of metabolic abnormalities in the chronically mentally ill, specifically the association of psychiatric medications, diet, physical activity, and obesity. He has conducted other research on the role of faith, religion, and resilience in disasters. His documentary "The Wrath of God: A Faith Based Survival Paradigm" about the aftermath of the earthquake in Pakistan was awarded "The Frank Ochberg Award for Media and Trauma" by the International Society for Traumatic Stress Studies.

Dr. Ahmad specializes in the psychopharmacological treatment of psychotic, mood, anxiety, and substance use disorders. He is the founder of Integrative Center for Wellness in New York City. He is an author, contributor and consulting editor for several medical textbooks. His most recent book is *Coping with COVID-19, The Medical, Mental and Social Consequences of the Pandemic.* He also coauthored *Medical Marijuana: A Clinical Handbook* and *Pocket Handbook of Clinical Psychiatry.* He lives in New York City with his wife and son, and enjoys photography, travel, classic cars, and vinyl in his spare time.